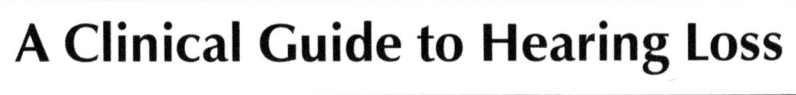

A Clinical Guide to Hearing Loss

A Clinical Guide to Hearing Loss

Editor: Peter Barry

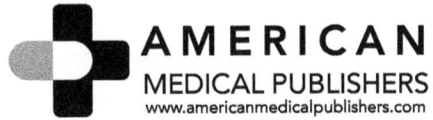
www.americanmedicalpublishers.com

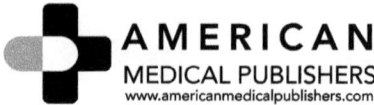

Cataloging-in-Publication Data

A clinical guide to hearing loss / edited by Peter Barry.
   p. cm.
Includes bibliographical references and index.
ISBN 979-8-88740-171-3
  1. Deafness. 2. Hearing disorders--Therapy. 3. Deafness--Treatment. 4. Deafness--Diagnosis. I. Barry, Peter.
RF290 .C55 2023
617.8--dc23

© American Medical Publishers, 2023

American Medical Publishers,
41 Flatbush Avenue,
1st Floor, New York,
NY 11217, USA

ISBN 979-8-88740-171-3 (Hardback)

This book contains information obtained from authentic and highly regarded sources. Copyright for all individual chapters remain with the respective authors as indicated. All chapters are published with permission under the Creative Commons Attribution License or equivalent. A wide variety of references are listed. Permission and sources are indicated; for detailed attributions, please refer to the permissions page and list of contributors. Reasonable efforts have been made to publish reliable data and information, but the authors, editors and publisher cannot assume any responsibility for the validity of all materials or the consequences of their use.

Trademark Notice: Registered trademark of products or corporate names are used only for explanation and identification without intent to infringe.

Contents

Preface VII

Chapter 1 **Caffeine Induces Autophagy and Apoptosis in Auditory Hair Cells via the SGK1/HIF-1α Pathway** 1
Xiaomin Tang, Yuxuan Sun, Chenyu Xu, Xiaotao Guo, Jiaqiang Sun, Chunchen Pan and Jingwu Sun

Chapter 2 **Gpr125 Marks Distinct Cochlear Cell Types and is Dispensable for Cochlear Development and Hearing** 16
Haiying Sun, Tian Wang, Patrick J. Atkinson, Sara E. Billings, Wuxing Dong and Alan G. Cheng

Chapter 3 **Generation of a Spiral Ganglion Neuron Degeneration Mouse Model** 29
Zhengqing Hu, Fnu Komal, Aditi Singh and Meng Deng

Chapter 4 **Cochlear Sox2+ Glial Cells are Potent Progenitors for Spiral Ganglion Neuron Reprogramming Induced by Small Molecules** 38
Zhen Chen, Yuhang Huang, Chaorong Yu, Qing Liu, Cui Qiu and Guoqiang Wan

Chapter 5 **Sirtuin-3 Protects Cochlear Hair Cells Against Noise-Induced Damage via the Superoxide Dismutase 2/Reactive Oxygen Species Signaling Pathway** 55
Wenqi Liang, Chunli Zhao, Zhongrui Chen, Zijing Yang, Ke Liu and Shusheng Gong

Chapter 6 **A Model of Waardenburg Syndrome Using Patient-Derived iPSCs with a *SOX10* Mutation Displays Compromised Maturation and Function of the Neural Crest that Involves Inner Ear Development** 67
Jie Wen, Jian Song, Yijiang Bai, Yalan Liu, Xinzhang Cai, Lingyun Mei, Lu Ma, Chufeng He and Yong Feng

Chapter 7 **Tlr2/4 Double Knockout Attenuates the Degeneration of Primary Auditory Neurons: Potential Mechanisms from Transcriptomic Perspectives** 87
Quan Wang, Yilin Shen, Yi Pan, Kaili Chen, Rui Ding, Tianyuan Zou, Andi Zhang, Dongye Guo, Peilin Ji, Cui Fan, Ling Mei, Haixia Hu, Bin Ye and Mingliang Xiang

Chapter 8 **Hearing Loss in Neurological Disorders** 101
Siyu Li, Cheng Cheng, Ling Lu, Xiaofeng Ma, Xiaoli Zhang, Ao Li, Jie Chen, Xiaoyun Qian and Xia Gao

Chapter 9 **Promising Applications of Nanoparticles in the Treatment of Hearing Loss** 117
Zilin Huang, Qiang Xie, Shuang Li, Yuhao Zhou, Zuhong He, Kun Lin, Minlan Yang, Peng Song and Xiong Chen

Chapter 10	**Single-Cell RNA Sequencing Analysis Reveals Greater Epithelial Ridge Cells Degeneration During Postnatal Development of Cochlea in Rats** 125
	Jianyong Chen, Dekun Gao, Junmin Chen, Shule Hou, Baihui He, Yue Li, Shuna Li, Fan Zhang, Xiayu Sun, Fabio Mammano, Lianhua Sun, Jun Yang and Guiliang Zheng
Chapter 11	**Use of a Network-Based Method to Identify Latent Genes Associated with Hearing Loss in Children** 142
	Feng Liang, Xin Fu, ShiJian Ding and Lin Li
Chapter 12	**Stem Cell-Based Therapies in Hearing Loss** 152
	Zuhong He, Yanyan Ding, Yurong Mu, Xiaoxiang Xu, Weijia Kong, Renjie Chai and Xiong Chen
Chapter 13	**Endolymphatic Hydrops is a Marker of Synaptopathy Following Traumatic Noise Exposure** 161
	Ido Badash, Patricia M. Quiñones, Kevin J. Oghalai, Juemei Wang, Christopher G. Lui, Frank Macias-Escriva, Brian E. Applegate and John S. Oghalai
Chapter 14	**Treatment with Calcineurin Inhibitor FK506 Attenuates Noise-Induced Hearing Loss** 174
	Zu-Hong He, Song Pan, Hong-Wei Zheng, Qiao-Jun Fang, Kayla Hill and Su-Hua Sha
Chapter 15	**Syndromic Deafness Gene *ATP6V1B2* Controls Degeneration of Spiral Ganglion Neurons Through Modulating Proton Flux** 187
	Shiwei Qiu, Weihao Zhao, Xue Gao, Dapeng Li, Weiqian Wang, Bo Gao, Weiju Han, Shiming Yang, Pu Dai, Peng Cao and Yongyi Yuan
Chapter 16	**N-Acetylcysteine Combined with Dexamethasone Treatment Improves Sudden Sensorineural Hearing Loss and Attenuates Hair Cell Death Caused by ROS Stress** 201
	Xue Bai, Sen Chen, Kai Xu, Yuan Jin, Xun Niu, Le Xie, Yue Qiu, Xiao-Zhou Liu and Yu Sun
Chapter 17	**CCDC154 Mutant Caused Abnormal Remodeling of the Otic Capsule and Hearing Loss in Mice** 210
	Kai Xu, Xue Bai, Sen Chen, Le Xie, Yue Qiu, He Li and Yu Sun
Chapter 18	**Local Drug Delivery for Prevention of Hearing Loss** 219
	Leonard P. Rybak, Asmita Dhukhwa, Debashree Mukherjea and Vickram Ramkumar

Permissions

List of Contributors

Index

Preface

Over the recent decade, advancements and applications have progressed exponentially. This has led to the increased interest in this field and projects are being conducted to enhance knowledge. The main objective of this book is to present some of the critical challenges and provide insights into possible solutions. This book will answer the varied questions that arise in the field and also provide an increased scope for furthering studies.

Hearing loss is defined as the inability to apprehend sound. There are mainly three forms of hearing loss, namely, sensorineural hearing loss, conductive hearing loss and mixed hearing loss. A number of factors like genetics, ageing, exposure to noise, infections, birth complications, trauma to the ear, and certain medications or toxins can lead to hearing loss. Its primary symptoms of hearing loss involve difficulty in understanding speech, and pain or pressure in the ears. Hyperacusis, tinnitus, vertigo and tympanophonia are some secondary symptoms associated with hearing loss. Diagnostic methods include otoscopy, tympanometry and differential testing. MRI and CT scans are also used to determine the pathology of causes related to hearing loss. The management of this medical issue includes cochlear implants, hearing aids, middle ear implants and assistive technology. The various advancements in the study of hearing loss are glanced at and the management strategies are looked at in detail within this book. Clinicians in search of information to further their knowledge will be greatly assisted by it.

I hope that this book, with its visionary approach, will be a valuable addition and will promote interest among readers. Each of the authors has provided their extraordinary competence in their specific fields by providing different perspectives as they come from diverse nations and regions. I thank them for their contributions.

Editor

Caffeine Induces Autophagy and Apoptosis in Auditory Hair Cells via the SGK1/HIF-1α Pathway

Xiaomin Tang, Yuxuan Sun, Chenyu Xu, Xiaotao Guo, Jiaqiang Sun, Chunchen Pan* and Jingwu Sun*

Departments of Otolaryngology-Head and Neck Surgery, The First Affiliated Hospital of University of Science and Technique of China, Hefei, China

***Correspondence:**
Chunchen Pan
panchunchen@hotmail.com
Jingwu Sun
entsun@ustc.edu.cn

Caffeine is being increasingly used in daily life, such as in drinks, cosmetics, and medicine. Caffeine is known as a mild stimulant of the central nervous system, which is also closely related to neurologic disease. However, it is unknown whether caffeine causes hearing loss, and there is great interest in determining the effect of caffeine in cochlear hair cells. First, we explored the difference in auditory brainstem response (ABR), organ of Corti, stria vascularis, and spiral ganglion neurons between the control and caffeine-treated groups of C57BL/6 mice. RNA sequencing was conducted to profile mRNA expression differences in the cochlea of control and caffeine-treated mice. A CCK-8 assay was used to evaluate the approximate concentration of caffeine. Flow cytometry, TUNEL assay, immunocytochemistry, qRT-PCR, and Western blotting were performed to detect the effects of SGK1 in HEI-OC1 cells and basilar membranes. *In vivo* research showed that 120 mg/kg caffeine injection caused hearing loss by damaging the organ of Corti, stria vascularis, and spiral ganglion neurons. RNA-seq results suggested that SGK1 might play a vital role in ototoxicity. To confirm our observations *in vitro*, we used the HEI-OC1 cell line, a cochlear hair cell-like cell line, to investigate the role of caffeine in hearing loss. The results of flow cytometry, TUNEL assay, immunocytochemistry, qRT-PCR, and Western blotting showed that caffeine caused autophagy and apoptosis *via* SGK1 pathway. We verified the interaction between SGK1 and HIF-1α by co-IP. To confirm the role of SGK1 and HIF-1α, GSK650394 was used as an inhibitor of SGK1 and $CoCl_2$ was used as an inducer of HIF-1α. Western blot analysis suggested that GSK650394 and $CoCl_2$ relieved the caffeine-induced apoptosis and autophagy. Together, these results indicated that caffeine induces autophagy and apoptosis in auditory hair cells *via* the SGK1/HIF-1α pathway, suggesting that caffeine may cause hearing loss. Additionally, our findings provided new insights into ototoxic drugs, demonstrating that SGK1 and its downstream pathways may be potential therapeutic targets for hearing research at the molecular level.

Keywords: apoptosis, caffeine, autophagy, SGK1, auditory hair cells

INTRODUCTION

According to the WHO's report on hearing, more than 1.5 billion people now suffer from hearing loss worldwide, and nearly 2.5 billion people will be living with different degrees of hearing loss by 2050. Societal changes have made hearing loss more common owing to excessive exposure to loud noise and ototoxic drugs being more common (Brown et al., 2018). Hearing loss is closely associated with decreased quality of life, especially by impacting speech and language development in children and causing social problems for adults (Lasak et al., 2014). The clinical treatment of hearing loss depends on the cause and type of hearing loss. Medical therapy, surgery, amplification, or hearing implants have been used to improve the threshold (Lee and Bance, 2019). However, the effect of these clinical treatments is limited. There are still a substantial number of people suffering from cureless hearing loss. Thus, it is urgent to identify an effective method to prevent or improve hearing loss.

For all the reasons leading to hearing loss, ototoxic drugs are regarded as the major preventable factors (Liu W. et al., 2019; Gao S. et al., 2019; Guo et al., 2019; Zhang et al., 2019; Zhong et al., 2020; Fu et al., 2021b). Some general therapeutic drugs, such as antineoplastic drugs and aminoglycosides, directly kill inner ear cells, ultimately leading to serious hearing loss (He et al., 2015; Liu et al., 2016; Zhang et al., 2017; Li et al., 2018). Different drugs may damage different parts of the cochlea. Previous studies have confirmed that cisplatin damages hair cells, spiral neurons, supporting cells, and vascular veins (Gao D. et al., 2019). Additionally, aminoglycoside antibiotics can cause vestibulotoxicity, characterized by vertigo and dizziness, and cochleotoxicity. Thus, preventative treatment and mechanisms of ototoxic drugs have become one of the hot topics in hearing research.

Caffeine, as one of the most widely used drugs worldwide, is well known as a major component of common drinks, and it has an incitant effect on the nervous system, stimulating the cerebral cortex and relieving fatigue (Carolyn Brice, 2001; Mielgo-Ayuso et al., 2019). Paul et al. (2019) had found that caffeine intake protects against Parkinson's disease. Moreover, some studies have shown that long-term coffee consumption is linked to a lower risk of type 2 diabetes (Salazar-Martinez et al., 2004; van Dam et al., 2020). In contrast, a large dose of caffeine causes a negative impact on the human body. Excessive caffeine intake can cause obvious arrhythmias, palpitations, and other cardiovascular diseases (Hartley et al., 2004; Zulli et al., 2016). Caffeine has also been demonstrated to stimulate hypersecretion of stomach glands and increase in stomach acid, leading to the formation of gastric ulcers (Kwiecien and Konturek, 2003; Liszt et al., 2017). A previous study has indicated that caffeine may have a detrimental effect on hearing recovery after a single event of acoustic trauma (Mujica-Mota et al., 2014). In contrast, some researchers have found that coffee consumption is associated with a lower risk of disabling hearing impairment in men (Machado-Fragua et al., 2021). Hearing loss is one of the major symptoms in Ménière's disease. Restriction of salt, caffeine, and alcohol intake is recommended to patients with Ménière's disease as a first-line treatment (Hussain et al., 2018). Caffeine may result in a reduction in the blood supply to the inner ear, which may worsen the symptoms of patients. Overall, it is not clear whether caffeine has a direct effect on hearing cells; thus, exploring the regulatory mechanism of caffeine may provide new insights into the protection of hearing loss.

Autophagy, a dynamic mechanism of cellular defense and self-protection, is an effective mechanism that promotes cell survival by removing impaired proteins and nonfunctional organelles (Mizushima et al., 2001). Autophagy have been reported in many previous studies to protect the cochlear hair cells (He et al., 2017; He et al., 2020; Zhou et al., 2020; He et al., 2021) and spiral ganglion neurons (Liu et al., 2021). Apoptosis is the most well-known form of programmed cell death in the inner ear cochlea (Sun et al., 2014; Yan et al., 2018; He et al., 2019; Ding et al., 2020; Fu et al., 2021a; Cheng et al., 2021) and is responsible for removing aging, damaged, or mutated cells. Apoptosis and autophagy are functionally interrelated. Caffeine has been revealed to induce apoptosis and mitochondrial dysfunction in the neonatal rat brain (Kasala et al., 2020). Moreover, caffeine is regarded as a potent stimulator of hepatic autophagic flux in mice (Sinha et al., 2014). Endoplasmic reticulum stress has been found to mediate autophagy, which enhances caffeine-induced apoptosis in hepatic stellate cells (Li et al., 2017). However, it remains unknown whether caffeine regulates autophagy and apoptosis in hair cells.

In the present study, we explored the effect of caffeine on HEI-OC1 cells and cochlear hair cells as well as the underlying mechanism to better understand caffeine ototoxicity in hearing.

MATERIALS AND METHODS
Animals
Twenty-seven C57BL/6 mice (weight 20 g each, 2 months, male) were purchased from the Model Animal Research Center of Nanjing University, China. The animal research was completed with the approval of the Ethics Board of the first affiliated hospital of USTC (2021-N(A)-019). These mice were kept in a specific pathogen-free environment, where humidity was maintained in the range of 50%–60% and temperature was at 25°C. These mice were randomly decided into four groups: group I received daily normal saline injection of 0.2 ml as control ($n = 8$); group II received daily caffeine (Sigma-Aldrich, St. Louis, MO, USA) injection of 120 mg/kg for 7 days ($n = 8$); group III received daily caffeine injection of 120 mg/kg for 14 days ($n = 8$); group IV received daily caffeine injection of 20 mg/kg for 14 days ($n = 3$). These were sacrificed by overdose of ketamine after Auditory Brainstem Response (ABR) tests.

Twenty-four Sprague-Dawley (SD) rats [postnatal day 3 (P3)] were purchased from the Model Animal Research Center of Nanjing University, China. These SD rats were sacrificed by overdose of ketamine. Cochlear basilar membranes were cultured in Neurobasal medium (Gibco, Grand Island, NY, USA) after being gently isolated from SD rats. The 24 SD rats were equally allocated to two experiments. In one, 12 neonatal SD rats were divided into four groups: no caffeine treated as control group ($n = 3$); 1 mM caffeine group ($n = 3$); 5 mM caffeine group

(n = 3); and 10 mM caffeine group (n = 3). In the other, 12 neonatal SD rats were divided into four groups, as shown in **Figure 6C**: no caffeine treated as control group (n = 3); 10 μM GSK650394 group (n = 3); 10 mM caffeine group (n = 3); and 10 μM GSK650394 + 10 mM caffeine group (n = 3).

Cell culture and drug treatment

The House Ear Institute-Organ of Corti 1 (HEI-OC1) cell line has been extensively used in many previous reports (Guan et al., 2016; He et al., 2016; Yu et al., 2017) and was a gift from professor Hao Xiong in the Sun Yat-sen University (Xiong et al., 2019). HEI-OC1 cells were cultured under permissive conditions (33°C, 10% CO_2) in DMEM (Servicebio, Wuhan, China) supplemented with 10% fetal bovine serum (Gibco, Sydney, Australia). Caffeine was added to the culture medium at a concentration of 1, 5, 10, and 20 mM. In order to confirm the role of SGK1 (serum and glucocorticoid-induced protein kinase 1) in HEI-OC1 cells after caffeine treatment, GSK650394, a SGK1 inhibitor, was used (Peng et al., 2012): no caffeine treated as control group; 10 μM GSK650394 group; 10 mM caffeine group; and 10 μM GSK650394 + 10 mM caffeine group. In order to confirm the role of HIF-1α (hypoxia inducible factor-1) in HEI-OC1 cells, we divided HEI-OC1 cells into four groups (**Figure 5F**): no caffeine treated as control group; 100 μM $CoCl_2$ group; 10 mM caffeine group; and 100 μM $CoCl_2$ + 10 mM caffeine group (Zhao et al., 2020). In order to verify whether autophagy leads to apoptosis, we divided HEI-OC1 cells into four groups (**Supplementary Figure S3**): no caffeine treated as control group; 5 mM 3-MA group; 10 mM caffeine group; and 5 mM 3-MA + 10 mM caffeine group.

Auditory brainstem response

Tests were performed under general anesthesia induced through injection of 100 mg/kg ketamine. ABR tests were conducted using a Tucker-Davis Technology System hardware and software (Alachua, NY, USA). C57BL/6 mice were subcutaneously inserted with subdermal needle electrodes at the vertex, below the left ear (reference), and on the right ear (ground) after being anesthetized. ABR tests were measured at frequencies of 8, 16, and 32 kHz. In order to obtain the average response to 1,024 stimuli, the stimulus sound was decreased from 90 to 10 dB SPL, whose intensity was reduced by 10 dB at intervals near the threshold. As soon as the electrophysiological response to the stimulus sound disappeared, we measured the minimum stimulus sound that evoked a response as the hearing threshold of the mouse tested at this frequency.

Immunofluorescence

Basilar membranes and cells were isolated and fixed in 4% paraformaldehyde. Basilar membranes were divided into three segments (apex, middle, and base) and mounted on glass slides. Then, they were incubated in 0.5% Triton X-100 for 20 min at room temperature. After incubation in 10% goat serum for blocking nonspecific antibody binding for 30 min at room temperature, the samples were incubated with the primary antibody (information in **Table1**) overnight at 4°C. After washing three times (5 min each), the tissues were incubated with the secondary antibody (Jackson, West Grove, PA, USA, 1: 100) at room temperature for 1 h. Basilar membranes needed to be incubated with phalloidin (Yeasen, Shanghai, China, 1:100) containing fluorescein isothiocyanate at room temperature for another 1 h. The nuclei were stained by DAPI (Biosharp, Shanghai, China) for 5 min. Images were captured by using Zeiss LSM800.

Immunohistochemistry

The sections were dewaxed and deparaffinized in xylene and rehydrated in graded alcohol solutions. Then, the sections were heated for 30 min in Tris–EDTA buffer by microwave oven. Subsequently, the slides were stained with hematoxylin and eosin (HE) or primary antibodies for SGK1 (information in **Table 1**) and their respective secondary antibodies. Before dehydration and mounting, the sections were counter-stained with hematoxylin. Images were performed with an Olympus microscope camera (Tokyo, Japan). The stria vascularis thickness of cochlea was measured by Olympus cellSens Standard software (Olympus life science, Tokyo, Japan).

RNA-Seq

Total RNA was extracted using TRIzol reagent kit (Invitrogen, Carlsbad, CA, USA) according to the manufacturer's protocol. RNA quality was assessed on an Agilent 2100 Bioanalyzer (Agilent Technologies, Palo Alto, CA, USA) and checked using RNase free agarose gel electrophoresis. After total RNA was extracted, mRNA was enriched by Oligo (dT) beads, while prokaryotic mRNA was enriched by removing rRNA by Ribo-Zero™ Magnetic Kit (Epicentre, Madison, WI, USA). Then the enriched mRNA was fragmented into short fragments using fragmentation buffer and reverse transcripted into cDNA with random primers. Second-strand cDNA were synthesized by DNA polymerase I, RNase H, dNTP, and buffer. Then the cDNA fragments were purified with the QIAquick PCR extraction kit (Qiagen, Venlo, Netherlands), end repaired, poly(A) added, and ligated to Illumina sequencing adapters. The ligation products were size selected by agarose gel electrophoresis, PCR amplified, and sequenced using Illumina HiSeq 2500 by Gene Denovo Biotechnology Co. (Guangzhou, China).

CCK-8

Cell viability was detected using CCK-8 kits (Topscience, Shanghai, China) according to the manufacturer's protocols. Briefly, 5,000 cells were plated into a 96-well flat-bottom plate and incubated overnight under permissive conditions. After drug treatment in 100 μl culture medium, 10 μl CCK-8 was added for 1 h at 37°C. The optical density (OD) values were measured at 450 nm by an ELISA reader (Thermo Multiskan Mk3, Waltham, MA, USA). The blank underwent the same procedure, but without cell seeding, whereas the negative control was just treated without drugs. The relative viability was calculated as (OD experiment–OD blank)/(OD control–OD blank) × 100%.

Flow cytometry

HEI-OC1 cells (5×10^3 cells/well) were seeded into six-well plates overnight. Cells were collected after being digested with trypsin. An Annexin FITC/PI Apoptosis Detection Kit (Yeasen, Shanghai,

TABLE 1 | Primers in this study.

Gene	Forward	Reserve
GAPDH	GGCATTGTGGAAGGGCTCAT	TGTCATCATACTTGGCAGGTTTC
SGK1	GCCAAGTCCCTCTCAACAAATCA	GTGCCTAGCCAGAAGAAGAACCTTT
p62	CCTCAGCCCTCTAGGCATTG	TTCTGGGGTAGTGGGTGTCA
Caspase3	GAGCTTGGAACGGTACGCTA	GCGAGATGACATTCCAGTGC
LC3B	AGAGCGATACAAGGGGGAGA	TGCAAGCGCCGTCTGATTA
Bcl-2	CAGCCTGAGAGCAACCCAAT	TATAGTTCCACAAAGGCATCCCAG
Bax	TGGAGCTGCAGAGGATGATT	TCTTGGATCCAGACAAGCAGC

China) was used to examine the rate of apoptosis. Data analysis was performed by using NovoCyte (Agilent, Santa Clara, CA, USA).

TUNEL assay

The experiment was conducted with the One Step TUNEL Apoptosis Assay Kit (Beyotime, Shanghai, China) according to the manufacturer's instructions. After being fixed in 4% paraformaldehyde for 20 min, HEI-OC1 cells were then incubated in 0.5% Triton X-100 for 5 min. Next, samples were labeled with 50 μl TUNEL reaction mixture and incubated at room temperature for 1 h in the dark. After washing, slides were immediately examined under a Leica microscope (DMi8). The percentage of apoptotic cells was calculated as (TUNEL-positive cells/total cells) × 100%. All assays were performed in triplicate.

Electron microscopy

HEI-OC1 cells were fixed in TEM fixative (Servicebio, Wuhan, China) for 24 h and then fixed at 4°C for preservation and transportation. The 1% agarose solution was prepared by heating and dissolving in advance. Before agarose solidification, the precipitation was suspended with forceps and wrapped in the agarose. Agarose blocks with samples avoid light post fixed with 1% OsO_4 (Ted Pella Inc., CA, USA) for 2 h at room temperature. An ethanol dehydration process (series of 30%, 50%, 70%, 80%, 95% and two changes of 100% ethanol) followed by a 20-min immersion in acetone was performed before the final EPON resin. The resin blocks were cut to 60–80 nm thin on an ultramicrotome (Leica, Germany), and the tissues were fished out onto 150 mesh cuprum grids with formvar film. Two percent of uranium acetate was saturated with alcohol solution to avoid light staining for 8 min, then 2.6% lead citrate to avoid CO_2 staining for 8 min. The cuprum grids are observed under TEM (Hitachi, HT7800), and images were taken.

Quantitative real-time polymerase chain reaction analysis

Total RNA was isolated from cells by using TRIzol reagent (Takara Bio, Tokyo, Japan). On the basis of the instructions of the reverse transcriptase kit (Takara, Tokyo, Japan), cDNA was synthesized using 2 μg of the total RNA in TProfessional Thermocycler (Biometra, Berlin, Germany). Then, cDNA samples were subjected to qRT-PCR for 40 cycles by using TB Green™ Premix Ex Taq™ II (Takara, Tokyo, Japan) in Roche LightCycler 96 (Roche, Basel, Switzerland). Primers (**Table 1**)

TABLE 2 | Antibodies in this study.

	Ratio	Brand	Art.NO
WB antibody			
GAPDH	1:1000	CST	5174
HIF-1α	1:1000	CST	36169
SGK1	1:500	Beyotime	AF1909
p62	1:1000	Boster	PB0458
Cleaved-Caspase3	1:1000	CST	9664
LC3B	1:1000	Proteintech	18725
Bcl-2	1:1000	Abcam	ab194583
Bax	1:1000	Abcam	ab182734
IF antibody			
SGK1	1:100	Abcam	ab43606
TUBB3	1:100	Proteintech	CL488-66240
p62	1:100	Boster	PB0458
IHC antibody			
SGK1	1:100	Beyotime	AF1909

were designed with the approval of the Sango Biotech Co. Ltd. (Shanghai, China). GAPDH was used as an internal control. The results were calculated using the comparative cycle threshold ($\Delta\Delta Ct$) method.

Western blot analysis

First, total protein was extracted from HEI-OC1 cells and basilar membrane by using RIPA buffer (Beyotime, Shanghai, China). Almost 10 μg of crude protein was denatured and electrophoresed on 12.5% SDS-PAGE gels. Proteins were transferred onto PVDF membranes by electro-blotting after electrophoretic separation, followed by blocking for 15 min at room temperature in Protein Free Rapid Blocking Buffer (Epizyme, Shanghai, China). The blots were incubated with SGK1, HIF-1α, P62, Bcl-2, Bax, Cleaved-Caspase3, and LC3B (information in **Table 2**) primary antibodies at 4°C overnight. After washing with PBS-T, membranes were hybridized with an appropriate secondary antibody (Abmart, Shanghai, China) at room temperature for 1 h. Lastly, images of the Western blot bands were performed with chemi Capture (Clinx, Shanghai, China) and the intensity in each group was measured with ImageJ. GAPDH was used as an internal control.

Statistical analysis

Data are shown as the mean ± SD, and all experiments were repeated at least three times. Statistical analysis was conducted using GraphPad Prism 6. Two-tailed, unpaired Student's t-tests were used to determine statistical significance when comparing

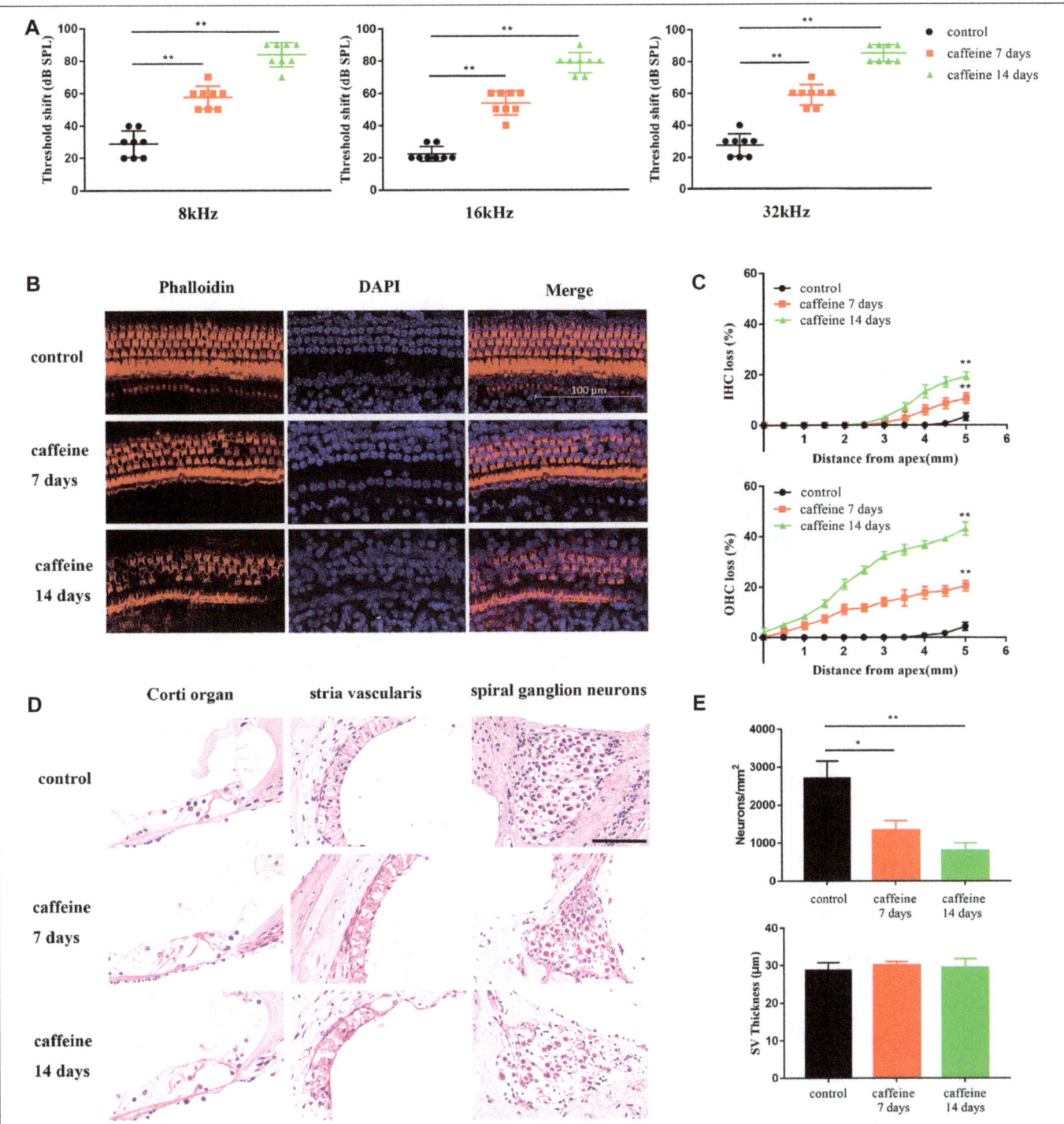

FIGURE 1 | Caffeine destroys cochlear hair cells, stria vascularis, and spiral ganglion neurons in C57BL/6 mice. **(A)** ABR threshold shifts measured in C57BL/6 mice treated with 120 mg/kg caffeine for 7 or 14 days. The control mice were treated with the same volume of normal saline. Data are presented as individual points and means ± SD, **$p < 0.01$. **(B)** Images of middle membrane stained with phalloidin (red). DAPI (blue) was used to stain the nuclei. Scale bar: 100 μm. **(C)** Hair cell counts in C57BL/6 mice treated with 120 mg/kg caffeine at 7 and 14 days and control mice treated with normal saline. N = 3 in each group. Data are presented as individual points and means ± SD, **$p < 0.01$. **(D)** Images of Corti organ, spiral ganglion neuron, and stria vascularis stained with HE. Scale bar: 100 μm. **(E)** Spiral ganglion neuron counts at the middle cochlear turn in each group. N = 3 in each group. Data are presented as individual points and means ± SD, **$p < 0.01$, *$p < 0.05$.

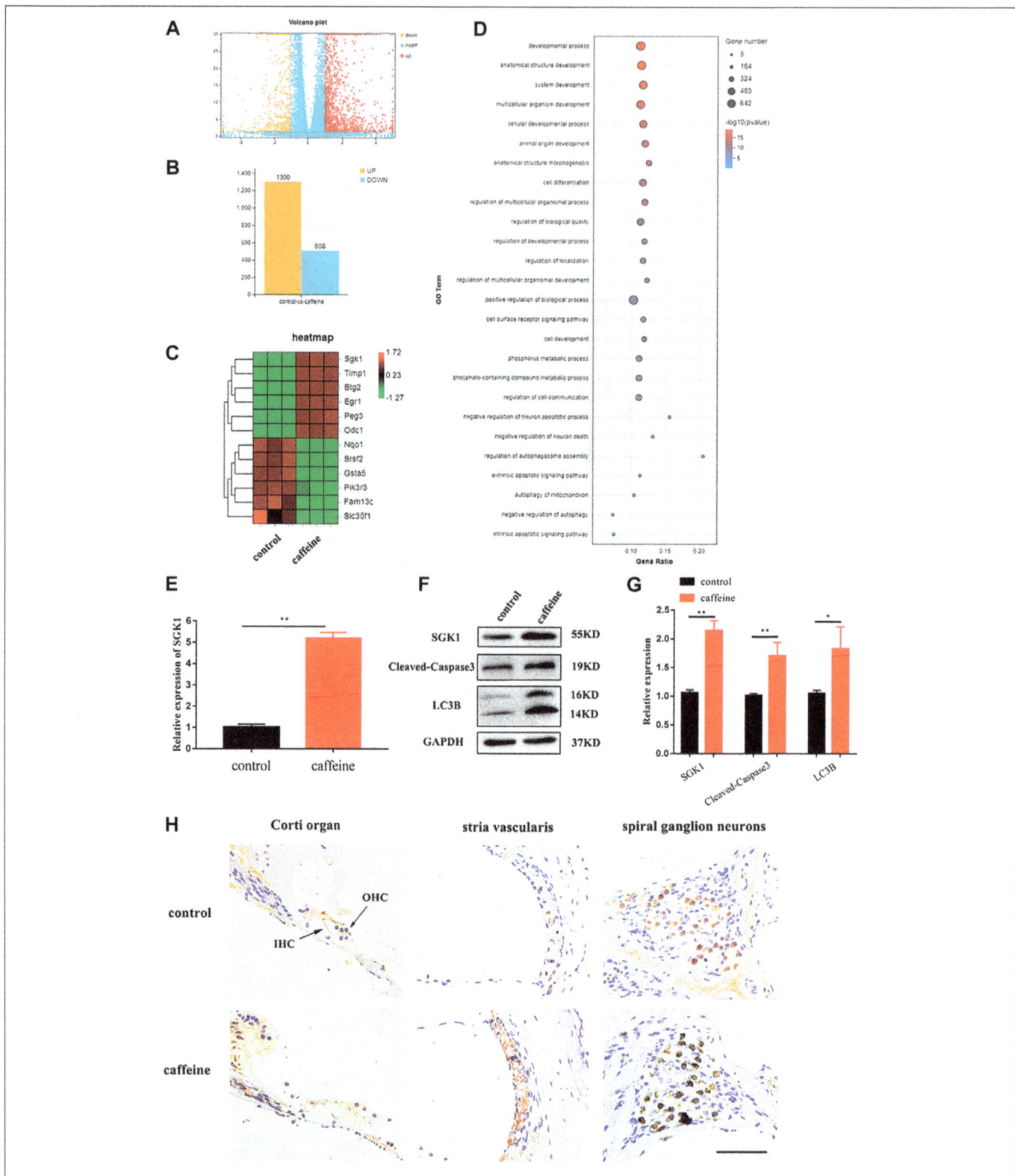

FIGURE 2 | Differentially expressed mRNA in the cochlea of C57BL/6 mice with 120 mg/kg caffeine and control. (A) Volcano plot showing the differentially expressed mRNAs in caffeine (120 mg/kg/day, continuous injection for 14 days) treatment and control group (normal saline, continuous injection for 14 days). (B) The number of differentially expressed mRNAs. (C) Heat map showing hierarchical clustering of differentially expressed mRNAs. Red indicates high relative expression, and green represents low relative expression. (D) Functional enrichment of differentially expressed mRNAs. (E) Different mRNA levels of SGK1 in the caffeine and control groups were confirmed by qRT-PCR. Data are shown as means ± SD, **$p < 0.01$. (F–G) Western blot analysis the expression of SGK1, Cleaved-Caspase3, LC3B, and GAPDH in cochlea. Data are shown as means ± SD, **$p < 0.01$, *$p < 0.05$. (H) Immunohistochemistry (IHC) for SGK1 in the organ of Corti, spiral ganglion neuron, and stria vascularis of C57BL/6 mice. Scale bar, 100 μm.

two groups, and one-way ANOVA followed by a Dunnett multiple-comparison test was used when comparing more than two groups. A value of $p < 0.05$ was considered statistically significant.

RESULTS

Caffeine destroys cochlear hair cells, stria vascularis, and spiral ganglion neurons in C57BL/6 mice

Two-month-old C57BL/6 mice were intraperitoneally injected with caffeine 120 mg/kg/day caffeine for 7 and 14 days, while mice in the control group were treated with normal saline. After 7 and 14 days of injection, auditory threshold shifts in the caffeine group significantly increased at 8, 16, and 32 kHz (**Figure 1A**). However, compared to the control group, auditory threshold shifts were not significantly difference after 20 mg/kg caffeine injection (**Supplementary Figure S1**). These results suggested that the effect of caffeine on hearing might be dose-dependent. To explore the position of caffeine damage, basilar membranes were stained with TRITC-phalloidin (**Figure 1B**), and paraffin sections of cochlea were stained with HE (**Figure 1D**). According to these results, caffeine caused disorder of the Corti organ and the loss of spiral ganglion neurons and hair cells (**Figures 1C,E**). Moreover, we also found that caffeine did not lead to significant stria vascularis damage.

Caffeine induces autophagy and apoptosis and increases the expression of SGK1 in the cochlea of C57BL/6 mice

To identify the mechanism of caffeine on hearing loss, cochlear tissues from the control and caffeine-treated C57BL/6 mice were collected for RNA sequencing, and a volcano plot (**Figure 2A**) was constructed to show all the molecules detected. Transcriptome analysis showed 1,300 upregulated and 508 downregulated mRNAs in caffeine-treated mice compared to the control group (**Figure 2B**). Heat maps (**Figure 2C**) were generated using the differentially expressed mRNAs. Bubble showed enrichments of various functional categories (**Figure 2D**). The expression change of SGK1, the most differentially expressed gene, was further confirmed by qRT-PCR (**Figure 2E**), which was consistent with the RNA-seq analysis. Additionally, the protein expression of SGK1, Cleaved-Caspase3, and LC3B was evaluated by Western blot analysis. The results showed that the expression of SGK1, Cleaved-Caspase3, and LC3B II/I markedly increased in the cochlea after caffeine injection (**Figures 2F,G**). To evaluate the major expression location of SGK1, we investigated the expression levels of SGK1 in C57BL/6 mouse cochlea through immunohistochemical staining. SGK1 was mainly expressed in the Corti organ, stria vascularis, and spiral ganglia (**Figure 2H**), which indicated that the expression of SGK1 increased in the cochlea after caffeine injection, suggesting that caffeine may induce autophagy and apoptosis in the cochlea.

Caffeine induces apoptosis and autophagy in HEI-OC1 cells

HEI-OC1 cells were used to investigate the effect of caffeine. Cells were treated with different caffeine concentrations (0, 0.1, 1, 5, 10, and 20 mM) for different times (12, 24, 48, and 72 h), and the results showed that caffeine inhibited HEI-OC1 cell viability in a time- and dose-dependent manner. When the concentration was greater than 1 mM, the inhibitory effect of caffeine on HEI-OC1 cells was markedly increased (**Figure 3A**). Moreover, the cell viability inhibition of HEI-OC1 at 10 mM was similar to that of 20 mM when treated for 72 h. Based on these results, treatments with 0, 1, 5, and 10 mM caffeine for 24 h were selected as the conditions in subsequent experiments. Dead cells were labeled by PI, and the cells undergoing apoptosis were labeled by Annexin V (**Figures 3B,C**). The rate of apoptosis in HEI-OC1 cells treated with 1 mM (14.25 ± 0.55%), 5 mM (36.38 ± 2.30%), and 10 mM (49.40 ± 3.34%) caffeine was significantly higher than that in the control group (1.20 ± 0.57%). HEI-OC1 cells in each group were examined by TUNEL assays in order to confirm the apoptosis effect. The percentage of TUNEL-positive cells was positively correlated with the concentration of caffeine (**Figures 3D,E**). Transmission electron microscope imaging showed that the caffeine-treated cells had more autophagic vacuoles (double membrane-bound autophagosomes) than the control cells, indicating that autophagy levels increase after caffeine treatment (**Figures 3F,G**). Taken together, these results suggested that caffeine induces apoptosis and autophagy in HEI-OC1 cells.

Caffeine induces apoptosis and autophagy via SGK1/HIF-1α pathway in HEI-OC1 cells

We next investigated the role of SGK1 in HEI-OC1 cells by detecting the expression of SGK1 and p62 in HEI-OC1 cells by immunofluorescence. As the concentration of caffeine increased, the fluorescence intensity of SGK1 increased and the fluorescence intensity of p62 decreased, which suggested that the expression of SGK1 and p62 had a consistent trend (**Figure 4A**). Furthermore, we analyzed the mRNA and protein levels of apoptotic and autophagic markers to explore the involved signaling pathway. After caffeine treatment, qRT-PCR (**Figures 4B,C**) and Western blot analyses (**Figures 5A,B**) showed that the expressions of SGK1, LC3B, and caspase3 significantly increased, while the expressions of p62 and the Bcl-2/Bax ratio decreased. Thus, these findings suggested that caffeine may induce apoptosis, induce autophagy, and increase the expression of SGK1. Next, we verified the interaction between SGK1 and HIF-1α by co-IP (**Figure 5C**). GSK650394 is a known SGK1 inhibitor. To further confirm the role of SGK1, we generated a control group, a GSK650394-treated group, a caffeine-treated group, and a GSK650394 + caffeine-treated group. Compared to caffeine treatment alone, Western blot analyses demonstrated that GSK650394 + caffeine treatment increased the expression of HIF-1α and p62 as well as the Bcl-2/Bax ratio but inhibited the expression of SGK1, Cleaved-Caspase3, and LC3B II/I (**Figures 5D,E**). Next, we took advantage of $CoCl_2$, an inducer

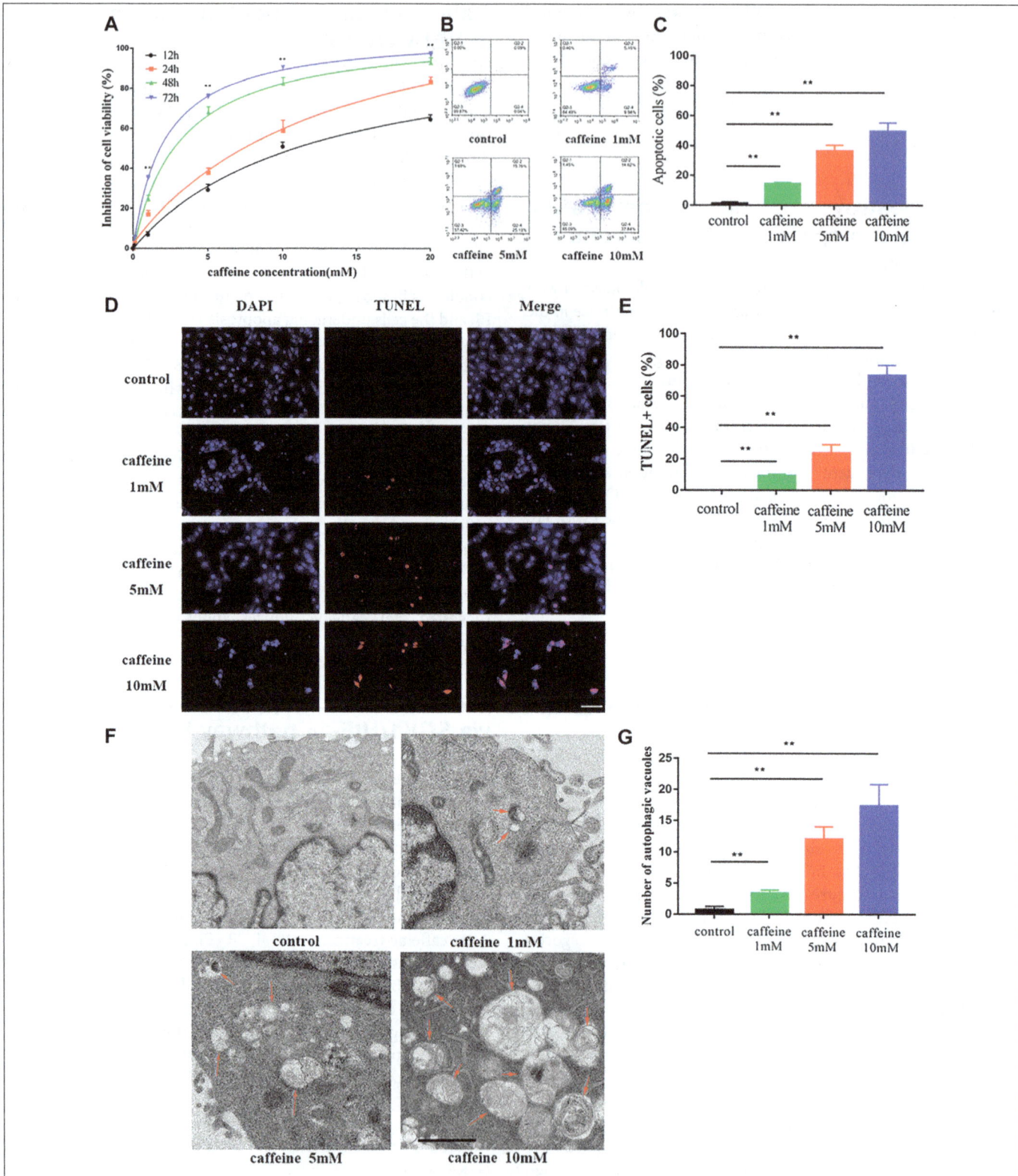

FIGURE 3 | Caffeine induced autophagy and apoptosis in HEI-OC1. **(A)** CCK-8 kit was used to measure cell viability in HEI-OC1 cells after different incubation times with varying concentrations of caffeine (from 0 to 20 mM). **(B–C)** The percent of apoptosis after 24 h of caffeine treatment with different concentrations was measured by flow cytometry. Data are shown as means ± SD, **$p < 0.01$. **(D–E)** TUNEL (red) and DAPI (blue) double staining showing the apoptotic HEI-OC-1 cells after different treatments. Scale bar: 100 μm. Data are shown as means ± SD, **$p < 0.01$. **(F–G)** Electron microscope analysis for evaluating autophagy in HEI-OC1 cells. Scale bar: 1 μm. Data are shown as means ± SD, **$p < 0.01$.

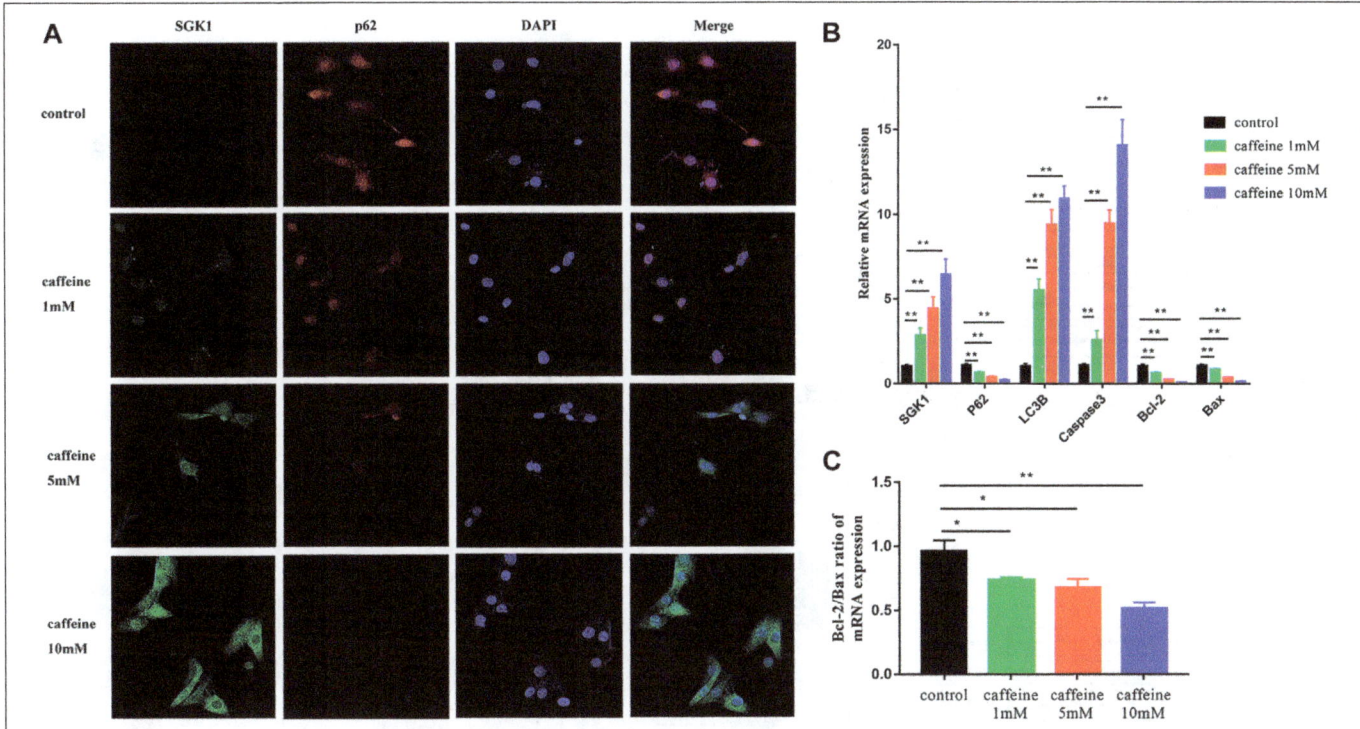

FIGURE 4 | Caffeine affected the expression of SGK1, autophagy, and apoptosis-related genes. **(A)** Immunofluorescence of p62 (red) and SGK1 (green) in HEI-OC1 cells after 24 h of caffeine treatment with different concentrations (0, 1, 5, 10 mM). DAPI (blue) was used to stain the nuclei. Scale bar: 100 µm. **(B)** qRT-PCR was used to analyze the mRNA expression of SGK1, p62, LC3B, and Caspase3 in HEI-OC1 cell lines after 24 h caffeine treatment with different concentrations (0, 1, 5, 10 mM), and GAPDH was used as the internal control. Experiments were repeated three times, and data are shown as the means ± SD, **$p < 0.01$. **(C)** Bcl-2/Bax ratio of mRNA expression in HEI-OC1 cells. Data are shown as means ± SD, **$p < 0.01$.

of HIF-1α, to explore the role of HIF-1α in HEI-OC1 cells after caffeine treatment. The Western blot data showed that $CoCl_2$ increased the expression of p62 and the Bcl-2/Bax ratio after caffeine treatment, while it inhibited the expression of SGK1, Cleaved-Caspase3, and LC3B II/I (**Figures 5F,G**). Additionally, we also found that $CoCl_2$ did not mediate the expression of SGK1 (**Supplementary Figure S2**), indicating that HIF-1α might be a downstream signaling molecule of SGK1. To explore the relationship between autophagy and apoptosis, 3-methyladenine (3-MA) was used as an autophagy inhibitor. After treatment with 3-MA and caffeine, the expression of Cleaved-Caspase3 decreased and the ratio of Bcl-2/Bax increased, suggesting that autophagy may lead to apoptosis when HEI-OC1 cells are treated with caffeine (**Supplementary Figure S3**).

Caffeine activates SGK1 to destroy hair cells and nerve fibers in P3 SD rats

Cultured neonatal rat basilar membrane *in vitro* is an important hearing research model. Cochlear basilar membranes were gently isolated from P3 SD rats and used for experiments after 24 h in culture. After treatment with different concentrations of caffeine, hair cells were labeled with TRITC–phalloidin and labeled auditory nerve fibers were labeled with the 488-TUBB3 antibody. Microscopic analysis showed that caffeine caused disorder and loss of hair cells, especially inner hair cells (**Figures 6A,B**). However, we also found that caffeine caused disorder of auditory nerve fibers. Additionally, we confirmed the role of SGK1 in the basilar membrane of neonatal SD rats (**Figure 6C**). GSK650394 effectively protected hair cells from caffeine damage. These results indicated that inhibition of SGK1 might be a potential target for protecting hair cell loss, especially inner hair cells (**Figure 6D**).

DISCUSSION

Absorption of caffeine is nearly complete within 45 min after ingestion, with caffeine blood levels peaking after 15 min to 2 h (Nehlig, 2018). The half-life of caffeine in humans ranges from 2 to 12 h, mainly due to interindividual differences in absorption and metabolism (Benowitz, 1990). Caffeine metabolism is greatly reduced during pregnancy, particularly in the third trimester, when the half-life can be as long as 15 h (van Dam et al., 2020). In addition, caffeine penetrates throughout the body and crosses the blood–brain barrier. Thus, caffeine is closely related to neurologic disease. Previous studies have found that caffeine might reduce the risk of Parkinson's disease and contribute to insomnia (Lara, 2010; Qi and Li, 2014). Hair cells function to transform the sound wave into electric signals (Wang Y. et al., 2017; Liu et al., 2019b; Qi et al., 2019; Fuping Qian and Chai, 2020; Jieyu Qi, 2020; Lv

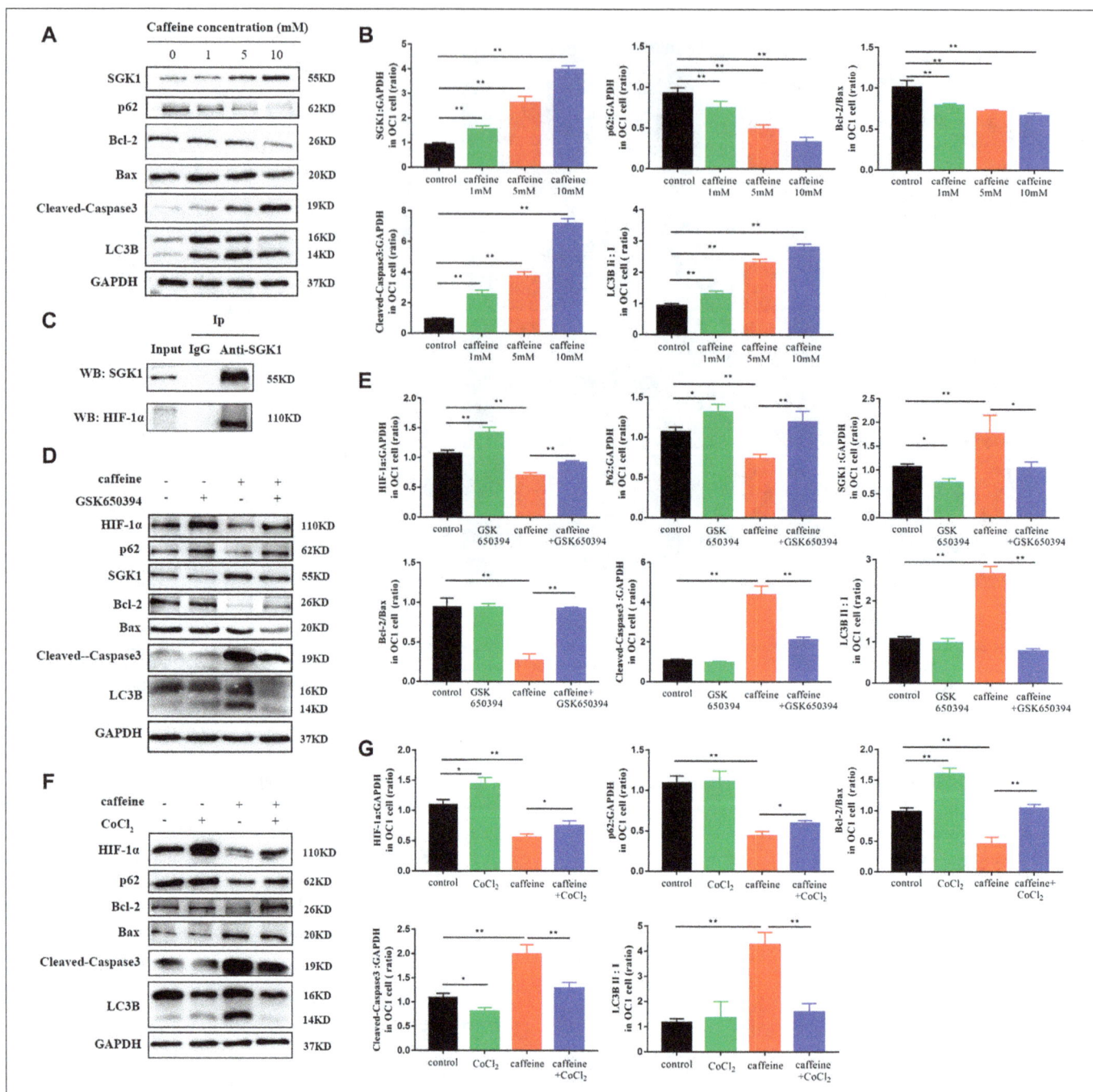

FIGURE 5 | Caffeine induced autophagy and apoptosis via the SGK1/HIF-1α signaling pathway. **(A)** Western blotting showed changes of SGK1, p62, LC3B, Bcl-2, Bax, and Cleaved-Caspase3 in HEI-OC1 cell lines after a 24-h caffeine treatment with different concentrations, and GAPDH was used as the internal control. **(B)** Quantification of the Western blot in SGK1, p62, LC3B, Bcl-2, Bax, and Cleaved-Caspase3. Experiments were repeated three times, and data are shown as the mean ± SD, **$p < 0.01$. **(C)** Co-immunoprecipitation (Co-IP) analysis of SGK1 and HIF-1α protein interaction. **(D)** Western blot assay was employed to investigate the expressions of HIF-1α, SGK1, P62, LC3B, and Cleaved-Caspase3 in HEI-OC1 cells after 24 h treatment with or without caffeine and GSK650394. GAPDH was used as the internal control. **(E)** Quantification of the Western blot in HIF-1α, SGK1, P62, LC3B, Bcl-2, Bax, and Cleaved-Caspase3. Experiments were repeated three times. Data are shown as means ± SD, **$p < 0.01$, *$p < 0.05$. **(F)** Western blot assay was employed to investigate the expression of HIF-1α, P62, LC3B, and Cleaved-Caspase3 in HEI-OC1 cells after a 24-h treatment with or without caffeine and $CoCl_2$. GAPDH was used as the internal control. **(G)** Quantification of the Western blot in **(F)**. Experiments were repeated three times. Data are shown as means ± SD, **$p < 0.01$, *$p < 0.05$.

et al., 2021) and are the most critical cells in the inner ear. Once damaged, hair cells have only very limited regeneration ability in mammals (Wang T. et al., 2015; Cheng et al., 2019; Tan et al., 2019; Zhang et al., 2020a; Zhang et al., 2020b; Chen et al., 2021). In the present study, we explored the effect of caffeine on hair cell damage and hearing loss. We first selected 20 and 120 mg/kg as

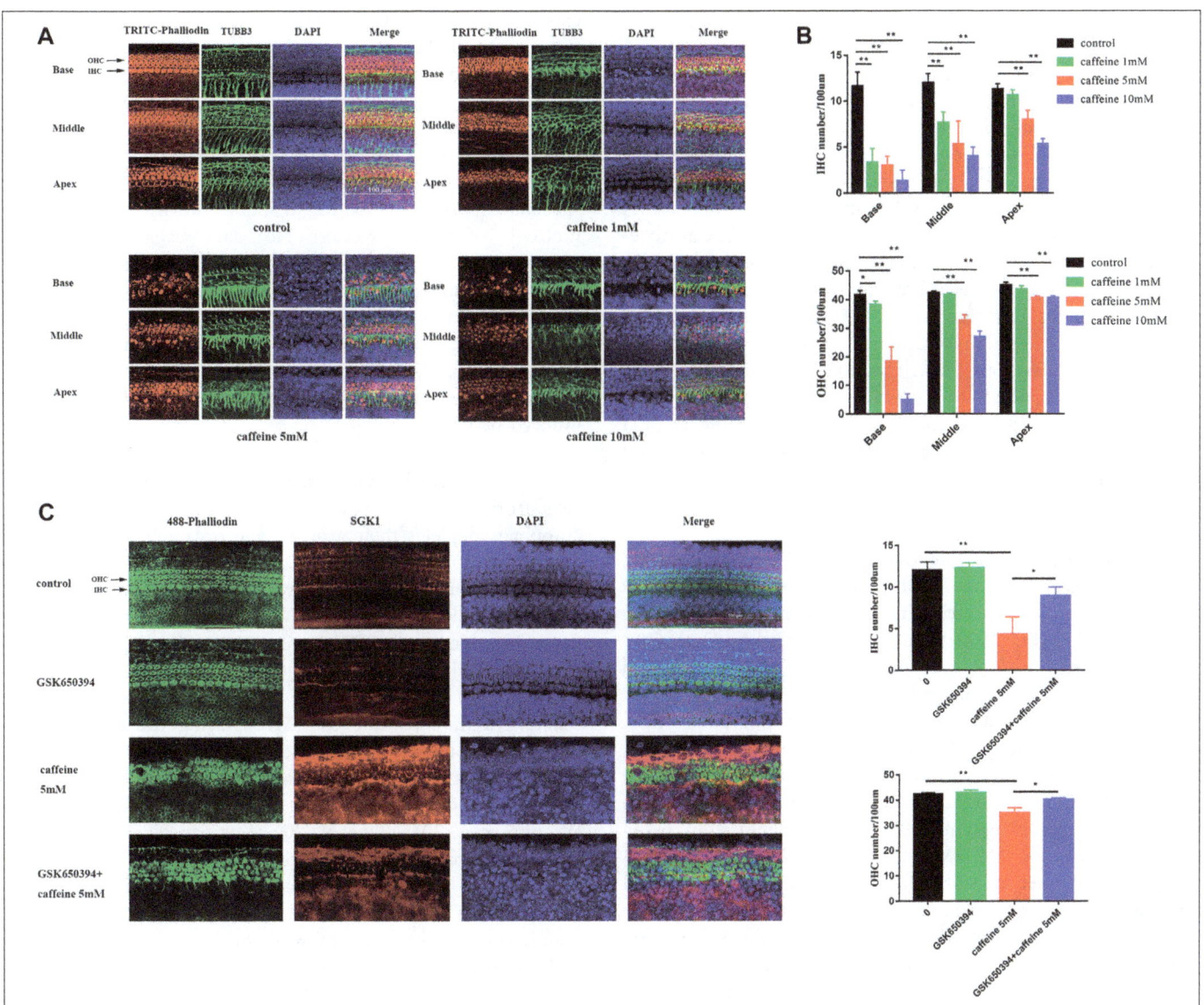

FIGURE 6 | Caffeine activates SGK1 to destroy hair cells and nerve fibers in P3 SD rats. (A–B) The basilar membranes of SD newborn mouse were stained with fluorescent phalloidin (red) and TUBB3 (green). DAPI (blue) was used to stain the nuclei. Scale bar: 100 μm. Data are shown as means ± SD, **$p < 0.01$, *$p < 0.05$. (C–D) The middle turn of basilar membranes was stained with fluorescent phalloidin (green) and SGK1 (red). DAPI (blue) was used to stain the nuclei. Scale bar: 100 μm. Data are shown as means ± SD, **$p < 0.01$, *$p < 0.05$.

the concentrations for two experimental groups (Mujica-Mota et al., 2014). The threshold shifts of mice treated with 20 mg/kg caffeine were not different from those of the control group (**Supplementary Figure S1**). However, the threshold shifts of mice in the 120-mg/kg caffeine group were higher than those of the control group. We also focused on the effect of caffeine duration on hearing. The 14-day injection caused more damage to hair cells than the 7-day injection, which indicated that hearing loss caused by caffeine was time-dependent. Western blot analyses of the cochlea verified that caffeine could induce autophagy and apoptosis in C57BL/6 mice. We also treated HEI-OC1 cells with different concentrations of caffeine (0, 0.1, 1, 5, 10, and 20 mM) for various time points (12, 24, 48, and 72 h). While treatment with 0.1 mM caffeine had no effect, treatments with caffeine concentrations greater than 1 mM caffeine significantly inhibited cell viability. In addition, 20 mM caffeine had little difference from 10 mM caffeine. Thus, we selected caffeine concentrations of 0, 1, 5, and 10 mM for 24 h for the conditions of the subsequent experiments. We cultured basilar membranes to investigate the effect of different concentrations of caffeine, and we evaluated several genes related to autophagy and apoptosis by RT-PCR and Western blot analyses. The results indicated that caffeine mainly destroyed inner hair cells. A recent study has found that coffee consumption is associated with a lower risk of disabling hearing impairment in men but not in women (Machado-Fragua et al., 2021). Moreover, previous studies have found that caffeine has definite neuroprotection in neurologic disease (Bagga and Patel, 2016; Xu et al., 2016). These differences may be due to differences in caffeine concentration and intake methods. Another review has indicated that the effect of caffeine occurs almost solely at the level of the central nervous system, suggesting that the effect of caffeine on the auditory and vestibular systems should be examined in future studies in a dose-dependent manner (Ghahraman et al., 2021). Our research revealed that the harmful effect of caffeine on cochlear hair cells was dose-dependent. Caffeine at 120 mg/kg increased auditory threshold shifts and caused hair cell loss in C57BL/6 mice, while 20 mg/kg caffeine did not cause hearing loss. Furthermore, we hypothesized that a caffeine concentration less than 1 mM may play a protective role in HEI-OC1 cells against apoptosis. It will be more difficult to find a certain protective concentration of caffeine against hearing loss, due to the large range of concentrations and diversity of hearing loss. In future studies, we will explore the possible protective effects of caffeine in the auditory system and central nervous system.

In the present research, we found that caffeine could activate the expression of SGK1 in C57BL/6 mice. SGK1 is a member of the AGC subfamily of protein kinases, a subfamily that includes proteins A, G, and C. As a ubiquitously expressed protein, SGK1 is involved in a wide variety of physiological processes and contributes to a variety of pathological conditions (Liu et al., 2017). There is a wide range of stimuli that regulate SGK expression, including dehydration, saline consumption, neuronal excitotoxicity, and DNA damage (You et al., 2004; Tang et al., 2011). In addition, SGK1 has been found to act as a switch for autophagy modulation and apoptosis in many diseases (Liu et al., 2017; Maestro et al., 2020). In our study, we utilized RNA-seq to identify different genes, and we confirmed that the expression of SGK1 increased in the cochlea after caffeine treatment both *in vitro* and *in vivo*. GSK650394 has been demonstrated *in vitro* and *in vivo* to be a specific inhibitor of SGK1, which mediates autophagy and apoptosis (Shanmugam et al., 2007; Sherk et al., 2008; Liu et al., 2017). We utilized GSK650394 and verified that caffeine induced autophagy and apoptosis by activating SGK1. Furthermore, we verified that GSK650394 protected hair cells against caffeine damage in neonatal SD rats. Thus, these findings suggested that GSK650394 might be a potential hearing protection drug, but additional experiments in different species are required in the future. According to experiments *in vitro*, we demonstrated that caffeine induced autophagy and apoptosis *via* the SGK1/HIF-1α pathway in hair cells.

HIF-1 is composed of HIF-1α and HIF-1β subunits, which are well known as oxygen-sensitive transcription factors. HIF-1α degradation is inhibited under hypoxic conditions, which facilitates the transcription of numerous genes involved in cellular adaptation to oxygen deprivation (Semenza, 2007). Importantly, a previous study has shown that the SGK1/HIF-1α signaling pathway plays a vital role in protecting renal cells from apoptosis by promoting autophagy, indicating that HIF-1α transcriptional activity is regulated by SGK1 (Xie et al., 2018). In addition, hypoxic conditions confer a great benefit to expanding cochlear stem/progenitor cells by stimulating HIF-1α (Chen et al., 2011). We verified the interaction between SGK1 and HIF-1α by co-IP. $CoCl_2$ is known as a chemical-specific inducer of HIF-1α *via* simulating hypoxia (Wang M. et al., 2017; Mikami et al., 2017; Rana et al., 2019). Our results showed that GSK650394 could increase the expression of HIF-1α, while $CoCl_2$ did not mediate the expression of SGK1. We speculated that HIF-1α might be a downstream signaling molecule of SGK1. Western blot data revealed that $CoCl_2$ reduced the expression of Cleaved-Caspase3 and LC3B II/I after treatment with 10 mM caffeine, while $CoCl_2$ increased the expression of p62 and the Bcl-2/Bax ratio. These results indicated that $CoCl_2$ relieves caffeine-induced autophagy and apoptosis caused by caffeine, suggesting that HIF-1α might play an important role in mediating autophagy and apoptosis induced by caffeine.

In most normal situations, the autophagic process protects cells from apoptosis. However, cells convert to apoptosis if autophagy depletes their proteins and organelles in the case of overstimulation (Maiuri et al., 2007). As a result, apoptosis and autophagy share similar pathways at the molecular level. Many previous studies have suggested that SGK1 inhibits autophagy-dependent apoptosis (Conza et al., 2017; Liu et al., 2017; Zuleger et al., 2018). However, we found that caffeine induced autophagy and apoptosis *via* the SGK1/HIF-1α pathway in our study. These differences may be due to SGK1 playing different roles in different organisms or different diseases. Furthermore, we utilized 3-MA to explore the relationship between autophagy and apoptosis. 3-MA, which is a specific autophagy inhibitor (Wang S. et al., 2015; Shi et al., 2020; Sugawara et al., 2020), could reduce apoptosis caused by caffeine (**Supplementary Figure S3**). These results indicated that autophagy may lead to apoptosis when HEI-OC1 cells are treated with caffeine. In this study, we mainly confirmed the role of SGK1 in the process of autophagy and apoptosis caused by caffeine *in vitro*. For future research, we will explore the role of SGK1 in the cochlea by using knockout mice.

In summary, the present study showed that caffeine induces autophagy and apoptosis in auditory hair cells *via* the SGK1/HIF-1a pathway. Our findings provided new insights into ototoxic drugs and suggested potential therapeutic targets for the amelioration of caffeine-induced ototoxicity.

ETHICS STATEMENT

The animal study was reviewed and approved by the Ethics Board of the first affiliated hospital of USTC.

AUTHOR CONTRIBUTIONS

CP and JS2 conceived and designed the study. XT, CX, and YS performed the cells and animal experiments. XT, XG, and CP performed the statistical analysis and drafted the manuscript. JS1 and JS2 reviewed and edited the manuscript. XT performed the additional experiments of the revised manuscript. All authors read and approved the final manuscript.

ACKNOWLEDGMENTS

We would like to thank the reviewers for their helpful comments, which significantly contributed to improve the paper.

REFERENCES

Bagga, P., and Patel, A. (2016). Pretreatment of Caffeine Leads to Partial Neuroprotection in MPTP Model of Parkinson's Disease. *Neural Regen. Res.* 11, 1750–1751. doi:10.4103/1673-5374.194716

Benowitz, N. L. (1990). Clinical Pharmacology of Caffeine. *Annu. Rev. Med.* 41, 277–288. doi:10.1146/annurev.me.41.020190.001425

Brice, C., and Smith, A. (2001). The Effects of Caffeine on Simulated Driving, Subjective Alertness and Sustained Attention. *Hum. Psychopharmacol. Clin. Exp.* 16, 523–531. doi:10.1002/hup.327

Brown, C. S., Emmett, S. D., Robler, S. K., and Tucci, D. L. (2018). Global Hearing Loss Prevention. *Otolaryngologic Clin. North America* 51, 575–592. doi:10.1016/j.otc.2018.01.006

Chen, H.-C., Sytwu, H.-K., Chang, J.-L., Wang, H.-W., Chen, H.-K., Kang, B.-H., et al. (2011). Hypoxia Enhances the Stemness Markers of Cochlear Stem/progenitor Cells and Expands Sphere Formation through Activation of Hypoxia-Inducible Factor-1alpha. *Hearing Res.* 275, 43–52. doi:10.1016/j.heares.2010.12.004

Chen, Y., Gu, Y., Li, Y., Li, G.-L., Chai, R., Li, W., et al. (2021). Generation of Mature and Functional Hair Cells by Co-expression of Gfi1, Pou4f3, and Atoh1 in the Postnatal Mouse Cochlea. *Cel Rep.* 35, 109016. doi:10.1016/j.celrep.2021.109016

Cheng, C., Hou, Y., Zhang, Z., Wang, Y., Lu, L., Zhang, L., et al. (2021). Disruption of the Autism-Related Gene Pak1 Causes Stereocilia Disorganization, Hair Cell Loss, and Deafness in Mice. *J. Genet. Genomics* 48, 324–332. doi:10.1016/j.jgg.2021.03.010

Cheng, C., Wang, Y., Guo, L., Lu, X., Zhu, W., Muhammad, W., et al. (2019). Age-related Transcriptome Changes in Sox2+ Supporting Cells in the Mouse Cochlea. *Stem Cel Res Ther* 10, 365. doi:10.1186/s13287-019-1437-0

Ding, Y., Meng, W., Kong, W., He, Z., and Chai, R. (2020). The Role of FoxG1 in the Inner Ear. *Front. Cel Dev. Biol.* 8, 614954. doi:10.3389/fcell.2020.614954

Fu, X., An, Y., Wang, H., Li, P., Lin, J., Yuan, J., et al. (2021a). Deficiency of Klc2 Induces Low-Frequency Sensorineural Hearing Loss in C57BL/6 J Mice and Human. *Mol. Neurobiol.* 58, 4376–4391. doi:10.1007/s12035-021-02422-w

Fu, X., Wan, P., Li, P., Wang, J., Guo, S., Zhang, Y., et al. (2021b). Mechanism and Prevention of Ototoxicity Induced by Aminoglycosides. *Front. Cel. Neurosci.* 15, 692762. doi:10.3389/fncel.2021.692762

Fuping Qian, X. W., Yin, Zhenhua., Xie, Gangcai., Yuan, Huijun., Dong, Liu., and Chai, Renjie. (2020). The Slc4a2b Gene Is Required for Hair Cell Development in Zebrafish. *Aging* 12, 18804–18821. doi:10.18632/aging.103840

Gao, D., Yu, H., Li, B., Chen, L., Li, X., and Gu, W. (2019a). Cisplatin Toxicology: The Role of Pro-inflammatory Cytokines and GABA Transporters in Cochlear Spiral Ganglion. *Curr. Pharm. Des.* 25, 4820–4826. doi:10.2174/1381612825666191106143743

Gao, S., Cheng, C., Wang, M., Jiang, P., Zhang, L., Wang, Y., et al. (2019b). Blebbistatin Inhibits Neomycin-Induced Apoptosis in Hair Cell-like HEI-OC-1 Cells and in Cochlear Hair Cells. *Front Cel Neurosci* 13, 590. doi:10.3389/fncel.2019.00590

Ghahraman, M. A., Farahani, S., and Tavanai, E. (2021). A Comprehensive Review of the Effects of Caffeine on the Auditory and Vestibular Systems. *Nutr. Neurosci.*, 1–14. doi:10.1080/1028415x.2021.1918984

Guan, M., Fang, Q., He, Z., Li, Y., Qian, F., Qian, X., et al. (2016). Inhibition of ARC Decreases the Survival of HEI-OC-1 Cells after Neomycin Damage In Vitro. *Oncotarget* 7, 66647–66659. doi:10.18632/oncotarget.11336

Guo, J., Chai, R., Li, H., and Sun, S. (2019). Protection of Hair Cells from Ototoxic Drug-Induced Hearing Loss. *Adv. Exp. Med. Biol.* 1130, 17–36. doi:10.1007/978-981-13-6123-4_2

Hartley, T. R., Lovallo, W. R., and Whitsett, T. L. (2004). Cardiovascular Effects of Caffeine in Men and Women. *Am. J. Cardiol.* 93, 1022–1026. doi:10.1016/j.amjcard.2003.12.057

He, Y., Yu, H., Cai, C., Sun, S., Chai, R., and Li, H. (2015). Inhibition of H3K4me2 Demethylation Protects Auditory Hair Cells from Neomycin-Induced Apoptosis. *Mol. Neurobiol.* 52, 196–205. doi:10.1007/s12035-014-8841-3

He, Z.-H., Li, M., Fang, Q.-J., Liao, F.-L., Zou, S.-Y., Wu, X., et al. (2021). FOXG1 Promotes Aging Inner Ear Hair Cell Survival through Activation of the Autophagy Pathway. *Autophagy*, 1–22. doi:10.1080/15548627.2021.1916194

He, Z.-h., Zou, S.-y., Li, M., Liao, F.-l., Wu, X., Sun, H.-y., et al. (2020). The Nuclear Transcription Factor FoxG1 Affects the Sensitivity of Mimetic Aging Hair Cells to Inflammation by Regulating Autophagy Pathways. *Redox Biol.* 28, 101364. doi:10.1016/j.redox.2019.101364

He, Z., Fang, Q., Li, H., Shao, B., Zhang, Y., Zhang, Y., et al. (2019). The Role of FOXG1 in the Postnatal Development and Survival of Mouse Cochlear Hair Cells. *Neuropharmacology* 144, 43–57. doi:10.1016/j.neuropharm.2018.10.021

He, Z., Guo, L., Shu, Y., Fang, Q., Zhou, H., Liu, Y., et al. (2017). Autophagy Protects Auditory Hair Cells against Neomycin-Induced Damage. *Autophagy* 13, 1884–1904. doi:10.1080/15548627.2017.1359449

He, Z., Sun, S., Waqas, M., Zhang, X., Qian, F., Cheng, C., et al. (2016). Reduced TRMU Expression Increases the Sensitivity of Hair-cell-like HEI-OC-1 Cells to Neomycin Damage In Vitro. *Sci. Rep.* 6, 29621. doi:10.1038/srep29621

Hussain, K., Murdin, L., and Schilder, A. G. (2018). Restriction of Salt, Caffeine and Alcohol Intake for the Treatment of Ménière's Disease or Syndrome. *Cochrane Database Syst. Rev.* 12, CD012173. doi:10.1002/14651858.CD012173.pub2

Jieyu Qi, L. Z., Tan, Fangzhi., Liu, Yan., Chu, Cenfeng., Zhu, Weijie., Wang, Yunfeng., et al. (2020). Espin Distribution as Revealed by Super-resolution Microscopy of Stereocilia. *Am. J. Translational Res.* 12, 130–141.

Kasala, S., Briyal, S., Prazad, P., Ranjan, A. K., Stefanov, G., Donovan, R., et al. (2020). Exposure to Morphine and Caffeine Induces Apoptosis and Mitochondrial Dysfunction in a Neonatal Rat Brain. *Front. Pediatr.* 8, 593. doi:10.3389/fped.2020.00593

Kwiecien, S., and Konturek, S. J. (2003). Gastric Analysis with Fractional Test Meals (Ethanol, Caffeine, and Peptone Meal), Augmented Histamine or Pentagastrin Tests, and Gastric pH Recording. *J. Physiol. Pharmacol.* 54 (3), 69–82.

Lara, D. R. (2010). Caffeine, Mental Health, and Psychiatric Disorders. *J. Alzheimers Dis.* 20 (1), S239–S248. doi:10.3233/JAD-2010-1378

Lasak, J. M., Allen, P., Mcvay, T., and Lewis, D. (2014). Hearing Loss. *Prim. Care Clin. Off. Pract.* 41, 19–31. doi:10.1016/j.pop.2013.10.003

Lee, J. W., and Bance, M. L. (2019). Hearing Loss. *Pract. Neurol.* 19, 28–35. doi:10.1136/practneurol-2018-001926

Li, A., You, D., Li, W., Cui, Y., He, Y., Li, W., et al. (2018). Novel Compounds Protect Auditory Hair Cells against Gentamycin-Induced Apoptosis by Maintaining the Expression Level of H3K4me2. *Drug Deliv.* 25, 1033–1043. doi:10.1080/10717544.2018.1461277

Li, Y., Chen, Y., Huang, H., Shi, M., Yang, W., Kuang, J., et al. (2017). Autophagy Mediated by Endoplasmic Reticulum Stress Enhances the Caffeine-Induced Apoptosis of Hepatic Stellate Cells. *Int. J. Mol. Med.* 40, 1405–1414. doi:10.3892/ijmm.2017.3145

Liszt, K. I., Ley, J. P., Lieder, B., Behrens, M., Stöger, V., Reiner, A., et al. (2017). Caffeine Induces Gastric Acid Secretion via Bitter Taste Signaling in Gastric Parietal Cells. *Proc. Natl. Acad. Sci. USA* 114, E6260–E6269. doi:10.1073/pnas.1703728114

Liu, L., Chen, Y., Qi, J., Zhang, Y., He, Y., Ni, W., et al. (2016). Wnt Activation Protects against Neomycin-Induced Hair Cell Damage in the Mouse Cochlea. *Cell Death Dis* 7, e2136. doi:10.1038/cddis.2016.35

Liu, W., Wang, X., Liu, Z., Wang, Y., Yin, B., Yu, P., et al. (2017). SGK1 Inhibition Induces Autophagy-dependent Apoptosis via the mTOR-Foxo3a Pathway. *Br. J. Cancer* 117, 1139–1153. doi:10.1038/bjc.2017.293

Liu, W., Xu, L., Wang, X., Zhang, D., Sun, G., Wang, M., et al. (2021). PRDX1 Activates Autophagy via the PTEN-AKT Signaling Pathway to Protect against

Cisplatin-Induced Spiral Ganglion Neuron Damage. *Autophagy*, 1–23. doi:10.1080/15548627.2021.1905466

Liu, W., Xu, X., Fan, Z., Sun, G., Han, Y., Zhang, D., et al. (2019a). Wnt Signaling Activates TP53-Induced Glycolysis and Apoptosis Regulator and Protects against Cisplatin-Induced Spiral Ganglion Neuron Damage in the Mouse Cochlea. *Antioxid. Redox Signaling* 30, 1389–1410. doi:10.1089/ars.2017.7288

Liu, Y., Qi, J., Chen, X., Tang, M., Chu, C., Zhu, W., et al. (2019b). Critical Role of Spectrin in Hearing Development and Deafness. *Sci. Adv.* 5, eaav7803. doi:10.1126/sciadv.aav7803

Lv, J., Fu, X., Li, Y., Hong, G., Li, P., Lin, J., et al. (2021). Deletion of Kcnj16 in Mice Does Not Alter Auditory Function. *Front. Cel Dev. Biol.* 9, 630361. doi:10.3389/fcell.2021.630361

Machado-Fragua, M. D., Struijk, E. A., Yévenes-Briones, H., Caballero, F. F., Rodríguez-Artalejo, F., and Lopez-Garcia, E. (2021). Coffee Consumption and Risk of Hearing Impairment in Men and Women. *Clin. Nutr.* 40, 3429–3435. doi:10.1016/j.clnu.2020.11.022

Maestro, I., Boya, P., and Martinez, A. (2020). Serum- and Glucocorticoid-Induced Kinase 1, a New Therapeutic Target for Autophagy Modulation in Chronic Diseases. *Expert Opin. Ther. Targets* 24, 231–243. doi:10.1080/14728222.2020.1730328

Maiuri, M. C., Zalckvar, E., Kimchi, A., and Kroemer, G. (2007). Self-eating and Self-Killing: Crosstalk between Autophagy and Apoptosis. *Nat. Rev. Mol. Cel Biol* 8, 741–752. doi:10.1038/nrm2239

Mielgo-Ayuso, J., Calleja-Gonzalez, J., Del Coso, J., Urdampilleta, A., Leon-Guereno, P., and Fernandez-Lazaro, D. (2019). Caffeine Supplementation and Physical Performance, Muscle Damage and Perception of Fatigue in Soccer Players: A Systematic Review. *Nutrients* 11, 440. doi:10.3390/nu11020440

Mikami, H., Saito, Y., Okamoto, N., Kakihana, A., Kuga, T., and Nakayama, Y. (2017). Requirement of Hsp105 in CoCl 2 -induced HIF-1α Accumulation and Transcriptional Activation. *Exp. Cel Res.* 352, 225–233. doi:10.1016/j.yexcr.2017.02.004

Mizushima, N., Yamamoto, A., Hatano, M., Kobayashi, Y., Kabeya, Y., Suzuki, K., et al. (2001). Dissection of Autophagosome Formation Using Apg5-Deficient Mouse Embryonic Stem Cells. *J. Cel Biol* 152, 657–668. doi:10.1083/jcb.152.4.657

Mujica-Mota, M. A., Gasbarrino, K., Rappaport, J. M., Shapiro, R. S., and Daniel, S. J. (2014). The Effect of Caffeine on Hearing in a guinea Pig Model of Acoustic Trauma. *Am. J. Otolaryngol.* 35, 99–105. doi:10.1016/j.amjoto.2013.11.009

Nehlig, A. (2018). Interindividual Differences in Caffeine Metabolism and Factors Driving Caffeine Consumption. *Pharmacol. Rev.* 70, 384–411. doi:10.1124/pr.117.014407

Paul, K. C., Chuang, Y. H., Shih, I. F., Keener, A., Bordelon, Y., Bronstein, J. M., et al. (2019). The Association between Lifestyle Factors and Parkinson's Disease Progression and Mortality. *Mov Disord.* 34, 58–66. doi:10.1002/mds.27577

Peng, H.-Y., Chen, G.-D., Hsieh, M.-C., Lai, C.-Y., Huang, Y.-P., and Lin, T.-B. (2012). Spinal SGK1/GRASP-1/Rab4 Is Involved in Complete Freund's Adjuvant-Induced Inflammatory Pain via Regulating Dorsal Horn GluR1-Containing AMPA Receptor Trafficking in Rats. *Pain* 153, 2380–2392. doi:10.1016/j.pain.2012.08.004

Qi, H., and Li, S. (2014). Dose-response Meta-Analysis on Coffee, tea and Caffeine Consumption with Risk of Parkinson's Disease. *Geriatr. Gerontol. Int.* 14, 430–439. doi:10.1111/ggi.12123

Qi, J., Liu, Y., Chu, C., Chen, X., Zhu, W., Shu, Y., et al. (2019). A Cytoskeleton Structure Revealed by Super-resolution Fluorescence Imaging in Inner Ear Hair Cells. *Cell Discov* 5, 12. doi:10.1038/s41421-018-0076-4

Rana, N. K., Singh, P., and Koch, B. (2019). CoCl2 Simulated Hypoxia Induce Cell Proliferation and Alter the Expression Pattern of Hypoxia Associated Genes Involved in Angiogenesis and Apoptosis. *Biol. Res.* 52, 12. doi:10.1186/s40659-019-0221-z

Salazar-Martinez, E., Willett, W. C., Ascherio, A., Manson, J. E., Leitzmann, M. F., Stampfer, M. J., et al. (2004). Coffee Consumption and Risk for Type 2 Diabetes Mellitus. *Ann. Intern. Med.* 140, 1–8. doi:10.7326/0003-4819-140-1-200401060-00005

Semenza, G. L. (2007). Life with Oxygen. *Science* 318, 62–64. doi:10.1126/science.1147949

Shi, Y., Tao, M., Ma, X., Hu, Y., Huang, G., Qiu, A., et al. (2020). Delayed Treatment with an Autophagy Inhibitor 3-MA Alleviates the Progression of Hyperuricemic Nephropathy. *Cel Death Dis* 11, 467. doi:10.1038/s41419-020-2673-z

Sinha, R. A., Farah, B. L., Singh, B. K., Siddique, M. M., Li, Y., Wu, Y., et al. (2014). Caffeine Stimulates Hepatic Lipid Metabolism by the Autophagy-Lysosomal Pathway in Mice. *Hepatology* 59, 1366–1380. doi:10.1002/hep.26667

Sugawara, E., Kato, M., Kudo, Y., Lee, W., Hisada, R., Fujieda, Y., et al. (2020). Autophagy Promotes Citrullination of VIM (Vimentin) and its Interaction with Major Histocompatibility Complex Class II in Synovial Fibroblasts. *Autophagy* 16, 946–955. doi:10.1080/15548627.2019.1664144

Sun, S., Sun, M., Zhang, Y., Cheng, C., Waqas, M., Yu, H., et al. (2014). *In Vivo* overexpression of X-Linked Inhibitor of Apoptosis Protein Protects against Neomycin-Induced Hair Cell Loss in the Apical Turn of the Cochlea during the Ototoxic-Sensitive Period. *Front. Cel. Neurosci.* 8, 248. doi:10.3389/fncel.2014.00248

Tan, F., Chu, C., Qi, J., Li, W., You, D., Li, K., et al. (2019). AAV-ie Enables Safe and Efficient Gene Transfer to Inner Ear Cells. *Nat. Commun.* 10, 3733. doi:10.1038/s41467-019-11687-8

Tang, C., Zelenak, C., Völkl, J., Eichenmüller, M., Regel, I., Fröhlich, H., et al. (2011). Hydration-sensitive Gene Expression in Brain. *Cell Physiol Biochem* 27, 757–768. doi:10.1159/000330084

Van Dam, R. M., Hu, F. B., and Willett, W. C. (2020). Coffee, Caffeine, and Health. *N. Engl. J. Med.* 383, 369–378. doi:10.1056/nejmra1816604

Wang, M., Zhao, X., Zhu, D., Liu, T., Liang, X., Liu, F., et al. (2017a). HIF-1α Promoted Vasculogenic Mimicry Formation in Hepatocellular Carcinoma through LOXL2 Up-Regulation in Hypoxic Tumor Microenvironment. *J. Exp. Clin. Cancer Res.* 36, 60. doi:10.1186/s13046-017-0533-1

Wang, S., Livingston, M. J., Su, Y., and Dong, Z. (2015a). Reciprocal Regulation of Cilia and Autophagy via the MTOR and Proteasome Pathways. *Autophagy* 11, 607–616. doi:10.1080/15548627.2015.1023983

Wang, T., Chai, R., Kim, G. S., Pham, N., Jansson, L., Nguyen, D.-H., et al. (2015b). Lgr5+ Cells Regenerate Hair Cells via Proliferation and Direct Transdifferentiation in Damaged Neonatal Mouse Utricle. *Nat. Commun.* 6, 6613. doi:10.1038/ncomms7613

Wang, Y., Li, J., Yao, X., Li, W., Du, H., Tang, M., et al. (2017b). Loss of CIB2 Causes Profound Hearing Loss and Abolishes Mechanoelectrical Transduction in Mice. *Front. Mol. Neurosci.* 10, 401. doi:10.3389/fnmol.2017.00401

Xie, Y., Jiang, D., Xiao, J., Fu, C., Zhang, Z., Ye, Z., et al. (2018). Ischemic Preconditioning Attenuates Ischemia/reperfusion-Induced Kidney Injury by Activating Autophagy via the SGK1 Signaling Pathway. *Cel Death Dis* 9, 338. doi:10.1038/s41419-018-0358-7

Xiong, H., Chen, S., Lai, L., Yang, H., Xu, Y., Pang, J., et al. (2019). Modulation of miR-34a/SIRT1 Signaling Protects Cochlear Hair Cells against Oxidative Stress and Delays Age-Related Hearing Loss through Coordinated Regulation of Mitophagy and Mitochondrial Biogenesis. *Neurobiol. Aging* 79, 30–42. doi:10.1016/j.neurobiolaging.2019.03.013

Xu, K., Di Luca, D. G., Orrú, M., Xu, Y., Chen, J.-F., and Schwarzschild, M. A. (2016). Neuroprotection by Caffeine in the MPTP Model of Parkinson's Disease and its Dependence on Adenosine A2A Receptors. *Neuroscience* 322, 129–137. doi:10.1016/j.neuroscience.2016.02.035

Yan, W., Liu, W., Qi, J., Fang, Q., Fan, Z., Sun, G., et al. (2018). A Three-Dimensional Culture System with Matrigel Promotes Purified Spiral Ganglion Neuron Survival and Function *In Vitro*. *Mol. Neurobiol.* 55, 2070–2084. doi:10.1007/s12035-017-0471-0

You, H., Jang, Y., You-Ten, A. I., Okada, H., Liepa, J., Wakeham, A., et al. (2004). p53-dependent Inhibition of FKHRL1 in Response to DNA Damage through Protein Kinase SGK1. *Proc. Natl. Acad. Sci.* 101, 14057–14062. doi:10.1073/pnas.0406286101

Yu, X., Liu, W., Fan, Z., Qian, F., Zhang, D., Han, Y., et al. (2017). c-Myb Knockdown Increases the Neomycin-Induced Damage to Hair-cell-like HEI-OC1 Cells *In Vitro*. *Sci. Rep.* 7, 41094. doi:10.1038/srep41094

Zhang, S., Qiang, R., Dong, Y., Zhang, Y., Chen, Y., Zhou, H., et al. (2020a). Hair Cell Regeneration from Inner Ear Progenitors in the Mammalian Cochlea. *Am. J. Stem Cell* 9, 25–35.

Zhang, S., Zhang, Y., Dong, Y., Guo, L., Zhang, Z., Shao, B., et al. (2020b). Knockdown of Foxg1 in Supporting Cells Increases the Trans-differentiation of Supporting Cells into Hair Cells in the Neonatal Mouse Cochlea. *Cell. Mol. Life Sci.* 77, 1401–1419. doi:10.1007/s00018-019-03291-2

Zhang, S., Zhang, Y., Yu, P., Hu, Y., Zhou, H., Guo, L., et al. (2017). Characterization of Lgr5+ Progenitor Cell Transcriptomes after Neomycin Injury in the Neonatal Mouse Cochlea. *Front. Mol. Neurosci.* 10, 213. doi:10.3389/fnmol.2017.00213

Zhang, Y., Li, W., He, Z., Wang, Y., Shao, B., Cheng, C., et al. (2019). Pre-treatment with Fasudil Prevents Neomycin-Induced Hair Cell Damage by Reducing the Accumulation of Reactive Oxygen Species. *Front. Mol. Neurosci.* 12, 264. doi:10.3389/fnmol.2019.00264

Zhao, J., Qi, X., Bai, J., Gao, X., and Cheng, L. (2020). A circRNA Derived from Linear HIPK3 Relieves the Neuronal Cell Apoptosis in Spinal Cord Injury via ceRNA Pattern. *Biochem. Biophysical Res. Commun.* 528, 359–367. doi:10.1016/j.bbrc.2020.02.108

Zhong, Z., Fu, X., Li, H., Chen, J., Wang, M., Gao, S., et al. (2020). Citicoline Protects Auditory Hair Cells against Neomycin-Induced Damage. *Front. Cel Dev. Biol.* 8, 712. doi:10.3389/fcell.2020.00712

Zhou, H., Qian, X., Xu, N., Zhang, S., Zhu, G., Zhang, Y., et al. (2020). Disruption of Atg7-dependent Autophagy Causes Electromotility Disturbances, Outer Hair Cell Loss, and Deafness in Mice. *Cel Death Dis* 11, 913. doi:10.1038/s41419-020-03110-8

Zulli, A., Smith, R. M., Kubatka, P., Novak, J., Uehara, Y., Loftus, H., et al. (2016). Caffeine and Cardiovascular Diseases: Critical Review of Current Research. *Eur. J. Nutr.* 55, 1331–1343. doi:10.1007/s00394-016-1179-z

Gpr125 Marks Distinct Cochlear Cell Types and is Dispensable for Cochlear Development and Hearing

Haiying Sun[1,2], Tian Wang[1], Patrick J. Atkinson[1], Sara E. Billings[1], Wuxing Dong[1] and Alan G. Cheng[1]*

[1] Department of Otolaryngology-Head and Neck Surgery, Stanford University School of Medicine, Stanford, CA, United States,
[2] Department of Otorhinolaryngology, Union Hospital, Tongji Medical College, Huazhong University of Science and Technology, Wuhan, China

*Correspondence:
Alan G. Cheng
aglcheng@stanford.edu

The G protein-coupled receptor (GPR) family critically regulates development and homeostasis of multiple organs. As a member of the GPR adhesion family, Gpr125 (Adgra3) modulates Wnt/PCP signaling and convergent extension in developing zebrafish, but whether it is essential for cochlear development in mammals is unknown. Here, we examined the $Gpr125^{lacZ/+}$ knock-in mice and show that Gpr125 is dynamically expressed in the developing and mature cochleae. From embryonic day (E) 15.5 to postnatal day (P) 30, Gpr125-β-Gal is consistently expressed in the lesser epithelial ridge and its presumed progenies, the supporting cell subtypes Claudius cells and Hensen's cells. In contrast, Gpr125-β-Gal is expressed transiently in outer hair cells, epithelial cells in the lateral cochlear wall, interdental cells, and spiral ganglion neurons in the late embryonic and early postnatal cochlea. In situ hybridization for Gpr125 mRNA confirmed Gpr125 expression and validated loss of expression in $Gpr125^{lacZ/lacZ}$ cochleae. Lastly, $Gpr125^{lacZ/+}$ and $Gpr125^{lacZ/lacZ}$ cochleae displayed no detectable loss or disorganization of either sensory or non-sensory cells in the embryonic and postnatal ages and exhibited normal auditory physiology. Together, our study reveals that Gpr125 is dynamically expressed in multiple cell types in the developing and mature cochlea and is dispensable for cochlear development and hearing.

Keywords: Gpr125, cochlea, lesser epithelial ridge, hair cell, spiral ganglion neurons

INTRODUCTION

G protein-coupled receptors (GPRs) form one of the largest gene families in the human genomes and serve critical functions across multiple organs (Pickering et al., 2008). Among the five subfamilies of mammalian GPRs, the adhesion family represents the second largest and consists of nine distinct subfamilies and 33 members, 10 of which have defined biological functions (Hamann et al., 2015; Vizurraga et al., 2020). For example, Gpr56 deficiency causes brain malformation and myelination defects (Ganesh et al., 2020) and disrupts seminiferous tubule remodeling in the developing testis in mice (Chen et al., 2010). Gpr124 knockout mice display abnormal angiogenesis in the developing forebrain and spinal cord, leading to hemorrhage and embryonic lethality (Cullen et al., 2011). Conditional deletion of Gpr124 in adult mice disrupts the blood–brain barrier in ischemic conditions, underscoring its role in the mature organ (Chang et al., 2017). Another member of the GPR adhesion family, Gpr126, is required for myelination by Schwann cells in the mouse peripheral nerve system (Monk et al., 2011). Lastly, *Celsr1*-deficient mice demonstrate neural tube closure defects, abnormal skin hair patterning, and deformities (Curtin et al., 2003; Doudney and Stanier, 2005; Aw et al., 2016; Boucherie et al., 2018). These findings implicate significant roles for adhesion GPRs during development and homeostasis.

Several adhesion GPRs have been shown to be important for cochlear development. First, mutation of *Gpr98* causes moderate to severe congenital hearing loss in humans (Moteki et al., 2015; Bousfiha et al., 2017). In mice, *Gpr98* (or Very Large G-protein coupled receptor 1, Vlgr1) is required for the assembly of the ankle link complex and in the subsequent bundle development and survival of cochlear hair cells (McGee et al., 2006; Zou et al., 2015). As another adhesion GPR, Celsr1 is a planar cell polarity core protein expressed in cochlear and vestibular hair cells in mice (Curtin et al., 2003; Duncan et al., 2017). Its deficiency causes planar cell polarity defects of vestibular and cochlear hair cells and aberrant turning of axons in Type II spiral ganglion neurons (SGNs) (Curtin et al., 2003; Duncan et al., 2017; Ghimire et al., 2018). While these studies underscore the roles of adhesion GPRs in the inner ear, whether other adhesion GPRs also play similar roles is currently unknown.

As a member of the adhesion family, Gpr125 is a 57-kDa transmembrane signal transducer (Hamann et al., 2015; Wu et al., 2018). Gpr125 was originally described as a marker of spermatogonia stem cells (Seandel et al., 2007). More recently, Gpr125 has also been shown to be required for gastrulation and convergent extension movements by interacting with Disheveled proteins in zebrafish (Li et al., 2013). Here, we examined the $Gpr125^{lacZ/+}$ reporter mice and show that Gpr125 is dynamically expressed in the embryonic and postnatal cochlea. We demonstrate that Gpr125-β-Gal is highly expressed in the LER and its derivatives in both the embryonic and postnatal cochleae. In addition, we found that Gpr125-β-Gal is transiently expressed in multiple other cell types in the late embryonic and early postnatal cochleae, including outer hair cells (OHCs), epithelial cells lining the lateral cochlear wall, interdental cells, and SGNs. Despite germline deletion of *Gpr125*, the embryonic and postnatal $Gpr125^{lacZ/lacZ}$ cochleae show normal specification and organization of hair cell and supporting cell subtypes with no detectable convergent extension or hair cell polarity defects. The adult $Gpr125^{lacZ/lacZ}$ mice also show normal auditory physiology. In summary, our study reveals that Gpr125 is dynamically expressed in multiple sensory and non-sensory cell types in the developing and mature cochlea, and is dispensable for the development and maintenance of the organ.

RESULTS

Gpr125 Marks the Lesser Epithelial Ridge in the Early Embryonic Cochlea

In mice, the cochlear duct arises as a ventral out-pocketing of the developing otocyst around E11 (Driver et al., 2017). The prosensory region marked by Sox2 is flanked medially by the greater epithelial ridge and laterally by the lesser epithelial ridge (LER). At E15.5, prosensory cells are specified to become hair cells first in the mid-basal region, extending as a wave toward the apical turn over the next 2–3 days (Chen et al., 2002). Coinciding with this wave of cell specification, the cochlear duct lengthens with sensory and non-sensory cells precisely oriented, in processes called convergent extension and planar polarization.

In the embryonic (E) 15.5 cochlea, prosensory cells are specified to become hair cells (Driver and Kelley, 2020). The prosensory domain resides in the floor of the cochlear duct between the greater and lesser epithelial ridges. Hair cell specification first occurs in the basal turn and then extends in a wave toward the apex (Chen et al., 2002). To study the expression pattern of *Gpr125* at this developmental stage, we examined the $Gpr125^{lacZ/+}$ knock-in mouse, in which a lacZ-neomycin cassette was inserted into exon 15 (see *Materials and Methods* for details). The cochleae were immunostained for lacZ [β-galactoside (β-Gal)], Myosin7a, and CD44 (**Figure 1A**). At E15.5, Myosin7a marks outer and inner hair cells, and CD44 marks the LER only in the basal turn and occasionally expressed in the periotic mesenchyme surrounding the cochlear duct (**Figures 1A,A'**; Hasson et al., 1995; Hertzano et al., 2010). As controls, no Gpr125-β-Gal-positive cells were observed in wild-type cochleae (**Figures 1B–D**). In each turn of $Gpr125^{lacZ/+}$ cochleae, robust nuclear Gpr125-β-Gal expression was detected in the LER and outer sulcus in the lateral cochlear ductal floor and in the SGNs in the modiolus (**Figures 1E–G, Supplementary Figures 1A–D**). Expression in the apical turn is noticeably less intense than the middle and basal turns in both the cochlear duct and SGNs, suggesting an increasing apical–basal gradient. In the basal turn where specification of Myosin7a$^+$ hair cells has occurred, we found CD44 expression overlapping with β-Gal expression in the LER (**Figure 1G**). We also observed a relatively weaker Gpr125-β-Gal signal in the outer sulcus extending to the lower half of the lateral cochlear wall (**Figures 1E–G**). Taken together, these results indicate that Gpr125 is expressed in the LER, preceding the onset of CD44 expression and sensory cell specification in the early embryonic cochlea.

Gpr125 Expression Broadens in the Late Embryonic Cochlea

At E18.5, both outer and inner hair cells and most support cell subtypes are specified in all three cochlear turns (Kolla et al., 2020). In the $Gpr125^{lacZ/+}$ cochlea, strong β-Gal signal was detected in the LER, lateral cochlear wall, and weak signal in the modiolus (**Figure 2A**). No Gpr125-β-Gal expression was detected in the wild-type cochlea (**Figures 2B,C,F,G,J,K**). In the lateral cochlear wall, Gpr125-β-Gal is strongly expressed in cells spanning from the LER to the lateral cochlear wall (**Figures 2D,H,L**). This expression is broader and more intense than that of E15.5, when Gpr125-β-Gal expression is restricted to the lower half of the lateral wall. Within the LER domain, cells located in the lateral two-thirds strongly express Gpr125-β-Gal, whereas the two rows of cells residing in the medial portion show weaker but detectable expression in all three cochlear turns (**Figures 2D,E,H,I,L,M**). We immunostained for CD44 and found that CD44 marks the LER, inner phalangeal

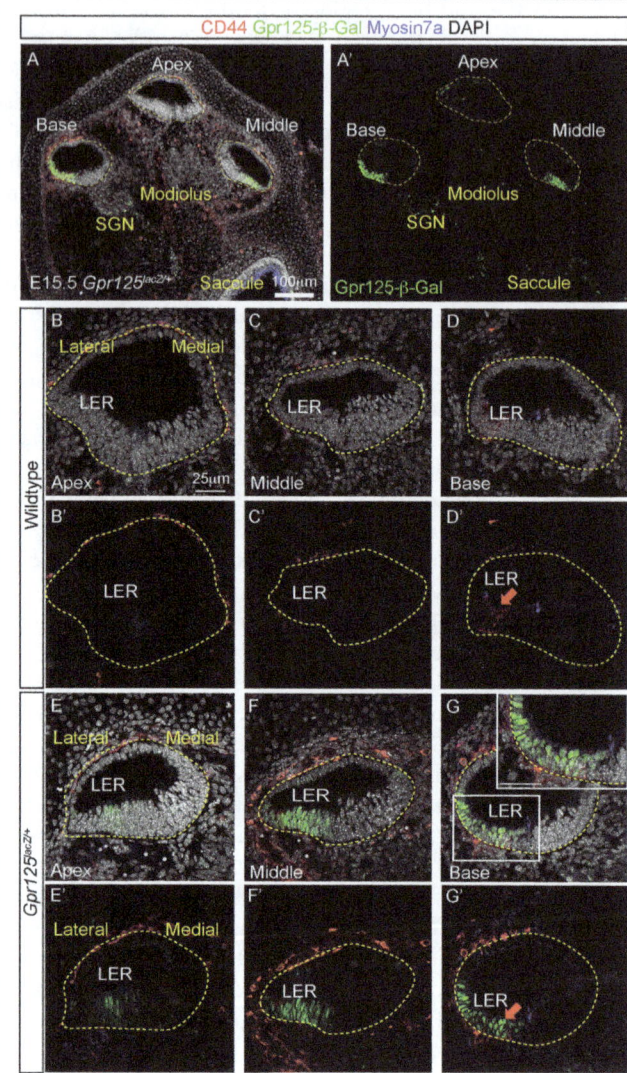

FIGURE 1 | Expression patterns of Gpr125 in E15.5 $Gpr125^{lacZ}/+$ mice. **(A,A')** Low-magnification images of midmodiolar cochlear sections of E15.5 $Gpr125^{lacZ}/+$ mice. Co-immunostaining of Gpr125-β-Gal (green), CD44 (red), and Myosin 7a (blue) shown in each cochlear turn. Gpr125-β-Gal-positive cells primarily occupied the floor throughout the entire cochlear duct. **(B–D')** No Gpr125-β-Gal-positive cells were found in the wild-type cochleae. **(E–G')** In the $Gpr125^{lacZ}/+$ cochleae, Gpr125-β-Gal expression was detected in the floor and SGNs of each cochlear turn. Expression is spatially restricted to the LER and outer sulcus, and more robust in the middle and base turn relative to the apex. Gpr125-β-Gal signal in the outer sulcus extends to the lower half of the lateral cochlear wall. Gpr125-β-Gal expression overlapped with CD44, which marks the LER only in the basal turn at this age. Inset in panel **(G)** shows high-magnification image. CD44 is also occasionally expressed in the periotic mesenchyme surrounding the cochlear duct. Red arrow marks CD44-positive cells in panels **(D',G')**. $n = 4$ for wild type, $n = 3$ for $Gpr125^{lacZ}/+$.

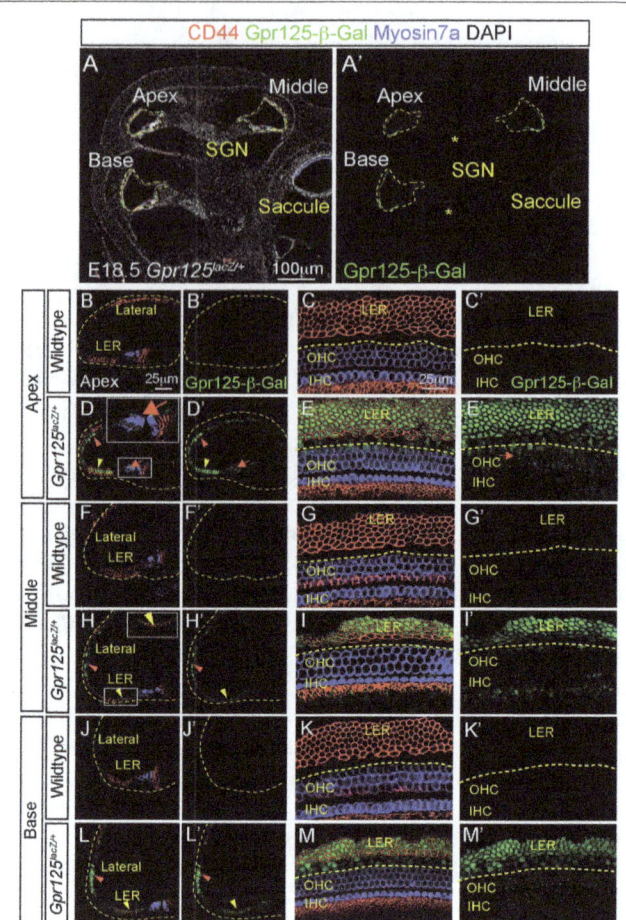

FIGURE 2 | Expression patterns of Gpr125 in E18.5 $Gpr125^{lacZ}/+$ mice. **(A,A')** Representative images of midmodiolar cochlear sections of E18.5 $Gpr125^{lacZ}/+$ mice immunostained for Gpr125-β-Gal (green), CD44 (red), and Myosin7a (blue). Gpr125-β-Gal expression located in the LER, lateral cochlear wall, OHCs and SGNs (asterisks). **(B–C')** CD44 marks the LER and inner phalangeal cells inside the cochlear duct and also the mesenchymal cells outside the roof. No Gpr125-β-Gal expression was observed in the wild-type cochleae. **(D,D')** Gpr125-β-Gal expression was detected at the LER (yellow arrowhead) extending to the lateral cochlear wall (red arrowhead) at the apical turn of $Gpr125^{lacZ}/+$ cochlea. Low expression was also noted in outer hair cells (red arrows). **(E,E')** Confocal images of whole mount cochlea (apical turn shown) from E18.5 $Gpr125^{lacZ}/+$ mice showing co-expression of Gpr125-β-Gal and CD44 in the LER. Gpr125-β-Gal expression was also detected in the CD44-negative Hensen's cells and OHCs (red arrows). **(F–G')** No Gpr125-β-Gal signal was detected at the middle turns of the wild-type cochlea. **(H–I')** Like the apical turn, Gpr125-β-Gal was detected in the lateral cochlear wall and LER in the middle turn of $Gpr125^{lacZ}/+$ cochlea (red and yellow arrowheads, respectively). Gpr125-β-Gal was not detected in hair cells. **(J–K')** No Gpr125-β-Gal signal was detected at the base of the wild-type cochlea. **(L–M')** Gpr125-β-Gal is expressed in the LER and lateral cochlear wall in the base turn of $Gpr125^{lacZ}/+$ cochlea. High-magnification images shown in inset for panels **(D,H)**. GER, greater epithelial ridge; LER, lesser epithelial ridge; IHC, inner hair cells; OHC, outer hair cells; SGN, spiral ganglion neurons.

cells inside the cochlear duct, and also the mesenchymal cells outside the roof (**Figures 2B–D'**), and overlapped with Gpr125-β-Gal expression in the LER (**Figures 2D,H,L**). Medial LER cells, which presumably give rise to Hensen's cells, lack CD44 expression (**Figures 2D,H,L**). No apical–basal gradient was observed with Gpr125-β-Gal expression in the LER at this age (**Figures 2D,E,H,I,L,M**). On the other hand, Gpr125-β-Gal is weakly expressed among OHCs only in the apical turn

(**Figures 2D,E**) at this time point. As hair cells are more mature in the basal turn, these data suggest that Gpr125 is transiently expressed in OHCs and is rapidly downregulated as the hair cells mature. Relative to E15.5, Gpr125 expression at E18.5 is less restricted, labeling the LER, lateral cochlear wall, and modiolus.

Expression Pattern of Gpr125 in the Postnatal Cochlea

The postnatal cochlea undergoes several morphological changes, including opening of the tunnel of Corti around P5–P7 and the apoptosis of the GER between P7 and P10 (Peeters et al., 2015; Basch et al., 2016). To determine the expression of Gpr125 in the postnatal cochlea, we immunolabeled Gpr125-β-Gal in the $Gpr125^{lacZ/+}$ cochlea at P0, P4, and P30. We first analyzed the wild-type cochlea at P0, P4, and P30 and no Gpr125-β-Gal-positive cells were detected (not shown). Similar to E18.5, Gpr125-β-Gal-positive cells were primarily observed in the LER and lateral cochlear wall in the P0 $Gpr125^{lacZ/+}$ cochlea (**Figure 3A**). In contrast to E18.5, the Gpr125-β-Gal signal is absent in the OHCs in all turns at P0 (**Figures 3A,C**), supporting the observation that Gpr125 is transiently expressed in the embryonic OHCs. Relative to E18.5, Gpr125-β-Gal expression is more robust in the CD44-positive lateral LER (presumed Claudius cells) and outer sulcus (**Figure 3C**). At both P0 and P4, expression of Gpr125-β-Gal is more intense in the medial, CD44-negative LER (presumed Hensen's cells) than at E18.5. Moreover, the expression of β-Gal in the outer sulcus and LER is more intense at P4 compared to P0 (**Figures 3B,D**). In the lateral cochlear wall, Gpr125-β-Gal signal was detected

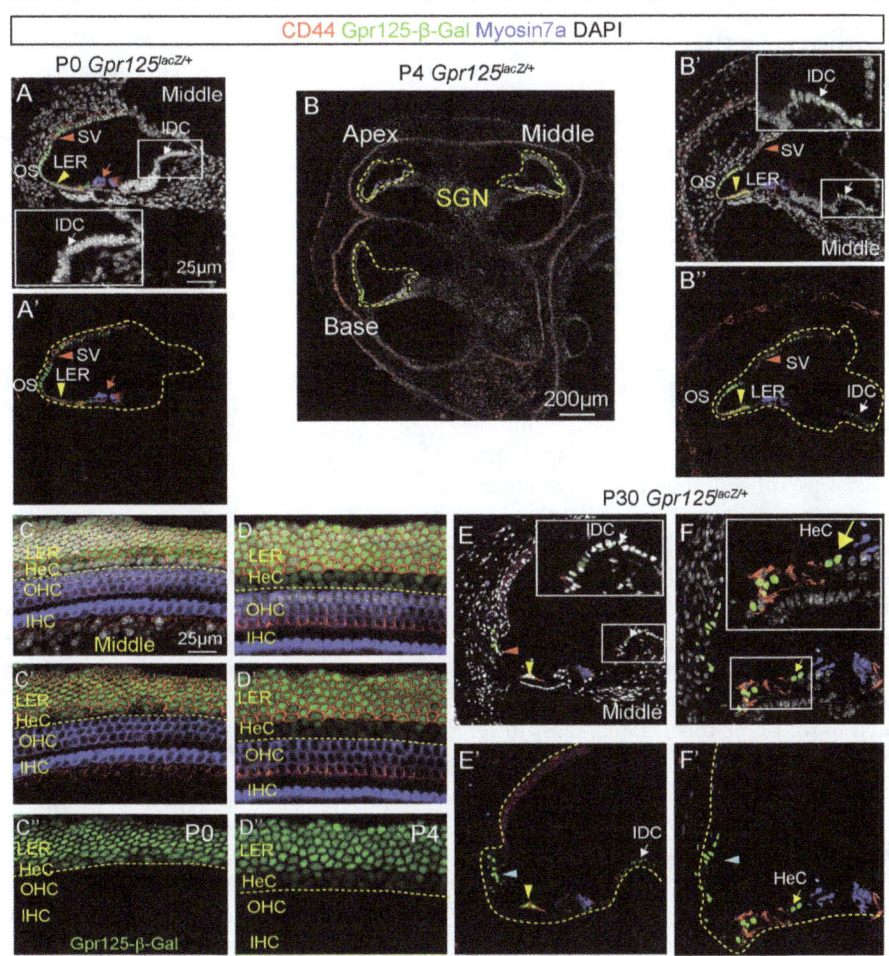

FIGURE 3 | Expression of Gpr125 in the postnatal cochlea. **(A,A')** Representative image of section of the middle turn of P0 $Gpr125^{lacZ/+}$ cochlea. Gpr125-β-Gal was detected in the lateral cochlear wall, stria vascularis (SV, red arrowheads), outer sulcus, SGNs, and LER (yellow arrowheads). CD44 marks Claudius cells. Inset demonstrates high magnification of interdental cells (IDC, white arrows) in panel **(A)**. No expression was detected in the IDCs or outer hair cells (red arrows). **(B)** Midmodiolar sections of P4 $Gpr125^{lacZ/+}$ cochlea showing Gpr125-β-Gal expression in the LER, SGNs, SV, and outer sulcus. **(B',B")** At P4, Gpr125-β-Gal expression was detected at the lateral cochlear wall, SV (red arrowheads), outer sulcus, IDCs (white arrows), and LER (yellow arrowheads). **(C–D")** Whole mount preparation of P0 and P4 $Gpr125^{lacZ/+}$ cochleae showing β-Gal and CD44 expression in LER, and Gpr125-β-Gal expression alone in Hensen's cells (HeC). **(E–F')** At P30, Gpr125-β-Gal expression was detected in Claudius cells (yellow arrowheads), Hensen's cells (yellow arrows), and outer sulcus (cyan arrowheads). Relative to P4, Gpr125-β-Gal expression in the IDC (white arrows) is more intense. Insets show magnification of boxed areas in A–E. SV, stria vascularis; LER, lesser epithelial ridge; OHC, outer hair cells; SGN, spiral ganglion neurons; IHC, inner hair cells.

in the stria vascularis, with signal appearing the highest in the epithelial layer at both P0 and P4 (**Figures 3A,B**). Compared to P0, Gpr125-β-Gal expression in the lateral wall is markedly lower at P4 (**Figure 3B**). Lastly, we detected Gpr125-β-Gal signal in interdental cells in P4 but not P0 $Gpr125^{lacZ/+}$ cochleae (**Figures 3A,B**).

In the mature, P30 cochlea, Gpr125-β-Gal expression is still robust in the outer sulcus, Claudius cells, and Hensen's cells. However, Gpr125-β-Gal signal is no longer detectable in the stria vascularis (**Figures 3E,F**). Furthermore, relative to P4, β-Gal expression in the interdental cells appears more intense at P30. There is no difference in the immunolabeling of β-Gal from the apical to basal turns (data not shown). Together, these data indicate that Gpr125 is dynamically expressed in multiple cell types in the postnatal cochlea, except in Claudius and Hensen's cells where expression is consistent.

Cochlear Development in the $Gpr125^{lacZ/lacZ}$ Mice

To validate Gpr125 deletion, *in situ* hybridization using probes specific for the Gpr125 exons 15–19 was performed in P0 wild-type and $Gpr125^{lacZ/lacZ}$ mice. As the lacZ cassette is inserted into exon 15, mRNA expression detected by these probes was expected to be lower in $Gpr125^{lacZ/lacZ}$ mice. After combining immunostaining for β-Gal and Myosin7a with *in situ* hybridization, we observed abundant *Gpr125* mRNA expression in multiple cochlear regions in wild-type mice and a notable absence of *Gpr125* transcripts in the same region in $Gpr125^{lacZ/lacZ}$ cochleae (**Figures 4A–C**). *Gpr125* mRNA signal is evident in several areas of the P0 wild-type cochleae, including hair cells, interdental cells, LER, Reissner's membrane, stria vascularis, tympanic border cells, spiral limbus, and the modiolus (presumed spiral ganglia neurons, SGNs) (**Figures 4B,D**). This pattern is noticeably broader than that of Gpr125-β-Gal. For example, *Gpr125 mRNA* was detected in P0 interdental cells and stria vascularis where no β-Gal signal was detected. No β-Gal signal was observed in the wild-type cochleae. In P0 $Gpr125^{lacZ/lacZ}$ cochleae, β-Gal signal was mainly noted in SGNs, LER, and stria vascularis similar to $Gpr125^{lacZ/+}$ cochleae (**Figures 4C,E**). Compared to wild-type cochlea, markedly lower *Gpr125* mRNA signal was detected in the stria vascularis and LER in the $Gpr125^{lacZ/lacZ}$ cochleae (**Figure 4E**), indicating that *Gpr125* transcripts are markedly reduced in the homozygous cochleae. The specificity of the signal was confirmed by the lack of signal in negative controls (using probes against *Dapb*) (**Figure 4F**). The signal intensity of each region was compared to positive controls (using probes against *Polr2*), which displayed robust staining (**Figure 4G**). Because some mRNA signal remained in the $Gpr125^{lacZ/lacZ}$ cochleae, we quantified the levels of β-Gal and *Gpr125* mRNA signal in defined regions of the cochlea. The *Gpr125* mRNA signal is the most intense in the LER and stria vascularis in the wild-type cochleae. Similarly, β-Gal expression in these two regions is the most intense in the $Gpr125^{lacZ/lacZ}$ cochleae (**Figure 4H**). Relatively lower *Gpr125* mRNA expression was detected in hair cells, interdental cells, Reissner's membrane, tympanic border cells, and spiral limbus of wild-type cochleae, whereas no *Gpr125* mRNA signal was detected in those regions in $Gpr125^{lacZ/lacZ}$ cochlea, suggesting that *Gpr125* is absent in these regions. Overall, *Gpr125* mRNA levels significantly correlated with the β-Gal signals ($R^2 = 0.82$, $p < 0.01$, Pearson's correlation, **Figure 4H**). Together, these data validate the $Gpr125^{lacZ/lacZ}$ cochlea as a model to assess *Gpr125* deficiency.

Dynamic Expression of Gpr125 in SGNs

We next characterized Gpr125 expression in the SGNs in the embryonic and postnatal cochlea. At E15.5 and E18.5, a relatively low expression of Gpr125-β-Gal was detected in Tuj1$^+$ (class III beta-tubulin) SGNs in $Gpr125^{lacZ/+}$ and $Gpr125^{lacZ/lacZ}$ cochleae (**Figures 5A–F**). In the modiolus, β-Gal expression is limited to SGNs in the modiolus at E15.5, E18.5, and P0. Relative to these ages, β-Gal expression is noticeably higher at P4 (**Figures 5G–L**). By P30, we could not detect any Gpr125-β-Gal signal in Tuj1-positive SGNs, while some Gpr125-β-Gal-positive, Tuj1-negative cells (presumably glial or satellite cells) were observed (**Figures 5M–O**). No apical-to-basal gradient of Gpr125-β-Gal expression was observed except for E15.5 (**Supplementary Figure 1**). Taken together, these findings demonstrate that Gpr125 expression in SGNs increases from embryonic to early postnatal ages, before becoming undetectable in the mature cochlea.

To investigate whether Gpr125 is required for SGN development and survival, we quantified the Tuj1-positive cells in middle turns of wild-type, $Gpr125^{lacZ/+}$, and $Gpr125^{lacZ/lacZ}$ cochleae. No significant differences were observed in the density of Tuj1-positive SGNs among all three groups (**Figure 5P**). Our results indicate that Gpr125 is not required for SGN development or survival in the embryonic, neonatal, or adult cochlea.

Normal Cochlear Development in the $Gpr125^{lacZ/lacZ}$ Mice

Gpr125 has been shown to modulate Wnt/PCP signaling and to be required for gastrulation in zebrafish (Li et al., 2013). Shortened cochlea as a result of defective convergent extension is a hallmark of PCP defects (Driver et al., 2017; Najarro et al., 2020). To test whether convergent extension was perturbed by *Gpr125* deficiency, we examined the otic capsule from P0 wild-type, $Gpr125^{lacZ/+}$, and $Gpr125^{lacZ/lacZ}$ mice and found them to be morphologically indistinguishable (**Figures 6A–C**). Moreover, length of the $Gpr125^{lacZ/lacZ}$ cochleae was comparable to those of wild-type and $Gpr125^{lacZ/+}$ littermates (**Figures 6D–F, Supplementary Figure 2A**), suggesting no obvious convergent extension defects. By immunostaining hair cells, bundles, and supporting cells, we found no hair cell or supporting cell loss or disorganization in the $Gpr125^{lacZ/lacZ}$ cochlea at any ages examined (**Figures 6G–P, Supplementary Figures 2B–N**). Phalloidin staining showed that stereociliary bundles are grossly intact in all ages of $Gpr125^{lacZ/lacZ}$ mice (**Figures 6G–P** and **Supplementary Figures 2B–K**). We also examined the stria vascularis, the lateral cochlear wall, and LER, where Gpr125 is robustly expressed, and found no cell loss or morphologic anomalies between E15.5

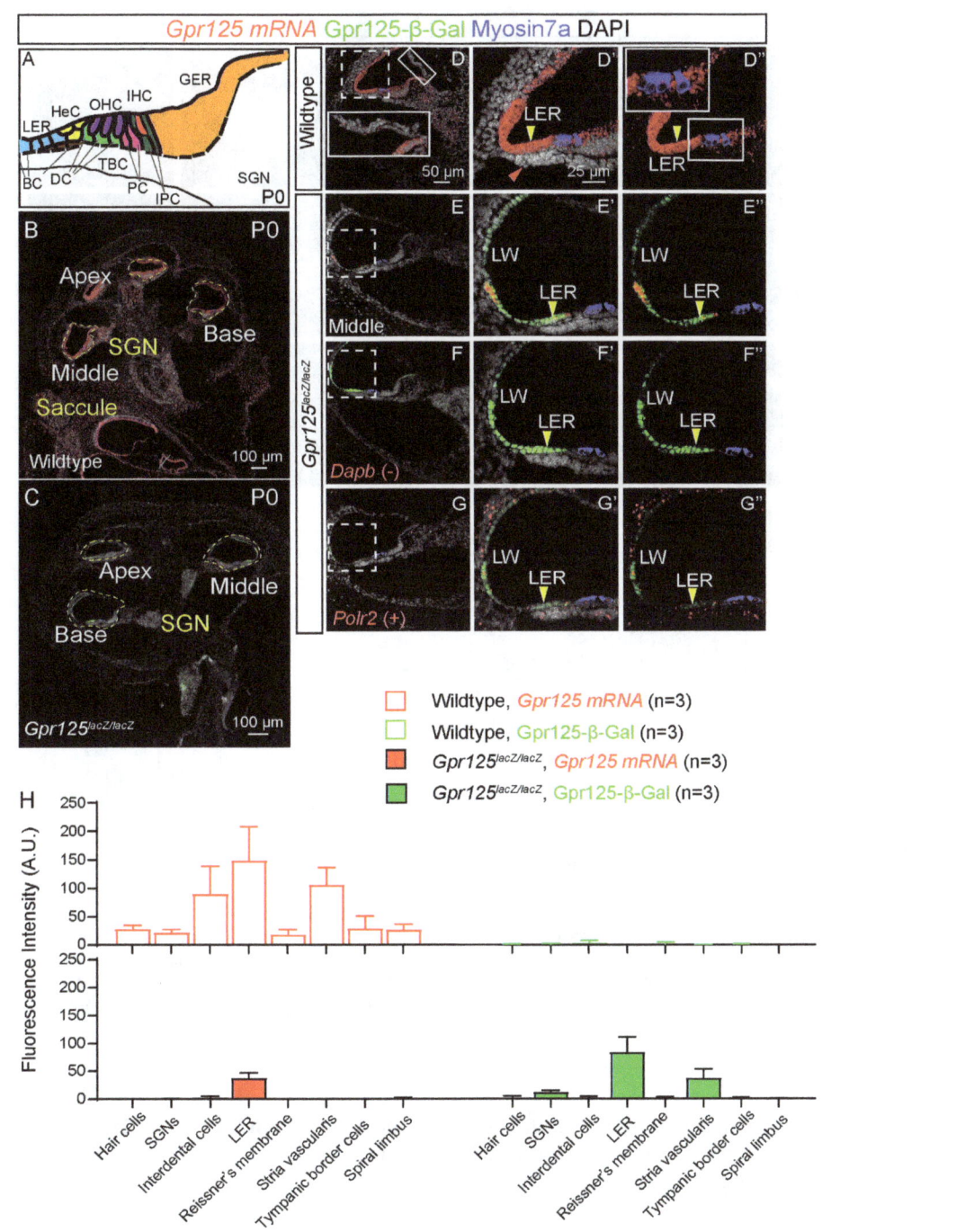

FIGURE 4 | *Gpr125* mRNA expression in wild-type and *Gpr125*[lacZ/lacZ] cochleae. **(A)** Schematic of P0 cochlea showing subtypes of hair cells and supporting cells. BC, Boettcher cells; DC, Deiters' cells; TBC, tympanic border cells; PC, pillar cells; IPC, inner phalangeal cells; LER, lesser epithelial ridge; HeC, Hensen's cells; OHC, outer hair cells; IHC, inner hair cells; GER, greater epithelial ridge; SGNs, spiral ganglion neurons. **(B,C)** Low-magnification image of cryosection demonstrates robust *Gpr125* mRNA expression in P0 wild-type cochlea. *Gpr125* mRNA expression is low or undetectable in most regions in the *Gpr125*[lacZ/lacZ] cochlea, with the exception of the lateral wall and LER where significant expression remained detectable. **(D–D")** High-magnification images of cochlear section showing robust *Gpr125* mRNA signals in the wild-type cochlea. Robust *Gpr125* mRNA signals were detected at the lateral cochlear wall (LW), outer sulcus, and lesser epithelial ridge, and at lower levels in the organ of Corti, Reissner's membrane, tympanic border cells (red arrow), spiral limbus, and greater epithelial ridge. No Gpr125-β-Gal-positive cells were detected in the wild-type cochlea. **(E–E")** Relative to the wild-type cochlea, *Gpr125* mRNA signal is dramatically lower in the *Gpr125*[lacZ/lacZ] cochlea. **(F–F")** Labeling for Dihydrodipicolinate reductase (*Dapb*) is used as a negative control. **(G–G")** Labeling for RNA polymerase II (*Polr2*) is used as a positive control. **(H)** Fluorescence intensity of *Gpr125* mRNA and Gpr125-β-Gal protein in cell types of interest. *Gpr125* mRNA signal is the highest in the LER in wild-type cochleae. Similarly, immunolabeling for β-Gal protein expression is the strongest in the LER in *Gpr125*[lacZ/lacZ] cochleae. The fluorescence of *Gpr125* mRNA correlated to β-Gal ($R^2 = 0.82$, $p < 0.01$, Pearson's correlation). Data are presented as mean ± SD.

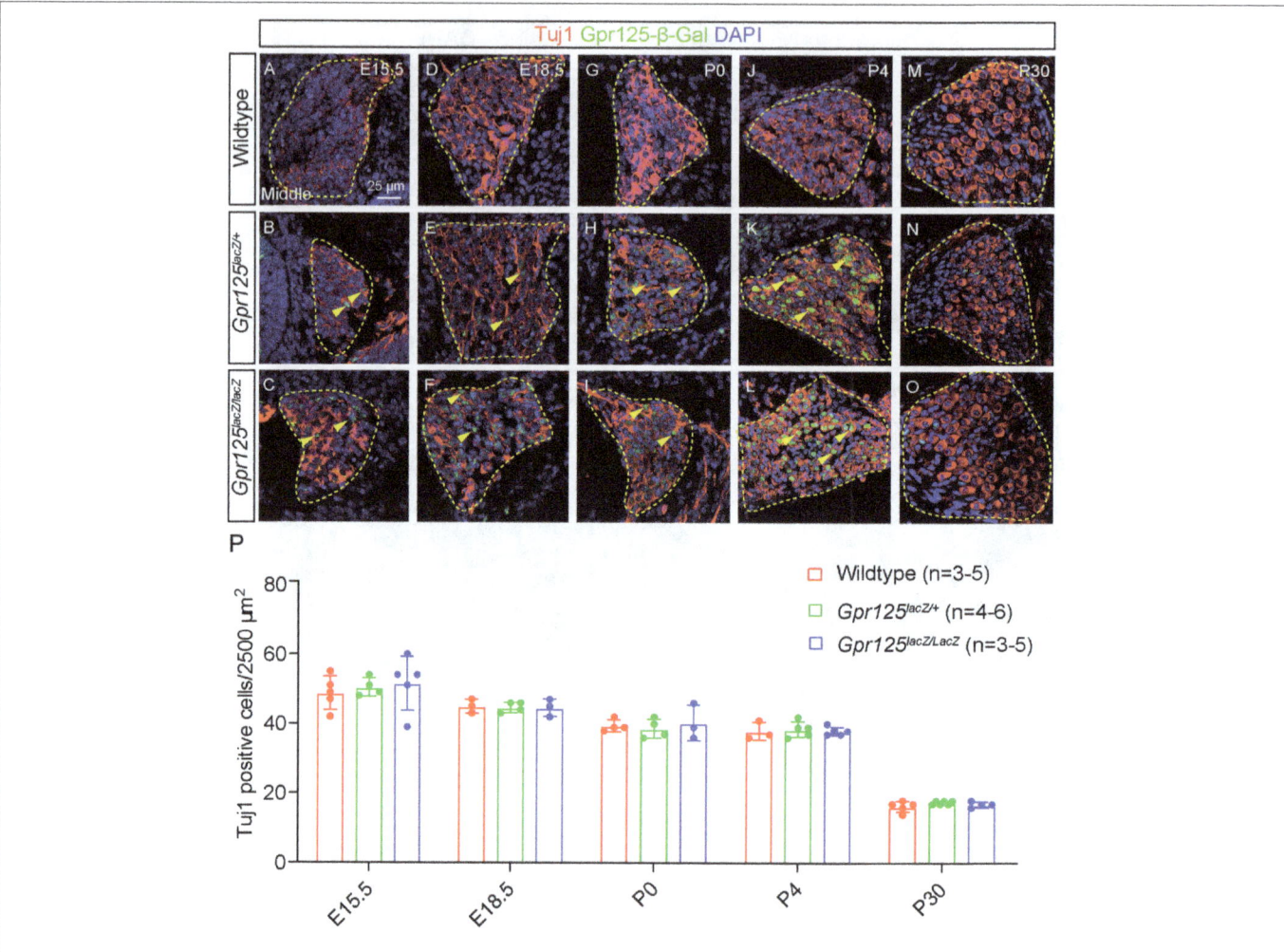

FIGURE 5 | Gpr125 deficiency does not impair spiral ganglion neuron development. Representative sections of Rosenthal's canal from the middle turn of wild-type, $Gpr125^{lacZ/+}$, and $Gpr125^{lacZ/lacZ}$ cochleae. All sections were co-stained for β-Gal (green), Tuj1 (red), and DAPI (blue). **(A–I)** Between E15.5 and P0, Gpr125-β-Gal expression is detected in a subset of Tuj1-positive SGNs in the $Gpr125^{lacZ/+}$ and $Gpr125^{lacZ/lacZ}$ cochleae (yellow arrowheads). **(J–L)** At P4, β-Gal expression is notably more intense in most Tuj1-positive SGNs. **(M–O)** At P30, Gpr125-β-Gal was undetectable in Tuj1-positive SGNs, but was noted in a few surrounding Tuj1-negative cells. Gpr125-β-Gal-positive signal was not observed in wild-type SGNs across ages. **(P)** Quantification of Tuj1-positive neurons showing no significant difference in counts among wild-type, $Gpr125^{lacZ/+}$, and $Gpr125^{lacZ/lacZ}$ cochleae in all ages examined ($p > 0.05$, one-way ANOVA). Data are presented as mean ± SD.

and P30 (**Figures 6Q–Z**). Collectively, these results suggest that Gpr125 is dispensable for cochlear development including specification and polarization of hair cells.

$Gpr125^{lacZ/lacZ}$ Mice Show No Hearing Loss

To explore whether Gpr125 is required for auditory function, ABR thresholds were examined from P30 and P120 $Gpr125^{lacZ/+}$, $Gpr125^{lacZ/lacZ}$, and wild-type littermate control mice (**Figures 7A–G**). ABR thresholds (4–45.3 kHz) showed no significant differences among three genotypes tested at P30 or P120 ($p > 0.05$, one-way ANOVA) (**Figures 7D,F**). We also measured the DPOAE responses of P30 and P120 $Gpr125^{lacZ/lacZ}$ mice and found no differences in thresholds compared with wild-type and $Gpr125^{lacZ/+}$ mice (**Figures 7E,G**). Together these results indicate Gpr125 is not required for auditory function in mice.

DISCUSSION

In this study, we systematically characterized the expression pattern and the role of Gpr125 during the cochlea development and maturation by employing the $Gpr125^{lacZ/+}$ knock-in mouse line. We found Gpr125 to be dynamically expressed in multiple cell types in the embryonic and postnatal cochlea, spanning the lateral cochlear wall, LER, organ of Corti, interdental cells, and modiolus (**Figure 8**). Gpr125 consistently marks the LER and its derivatives, Claudius and Hensen's cells, throughout the developmental stages examined. Lastly, $Gpr125^{lacZ/lacZ}$ mice display normal cochlear development and auditory function,

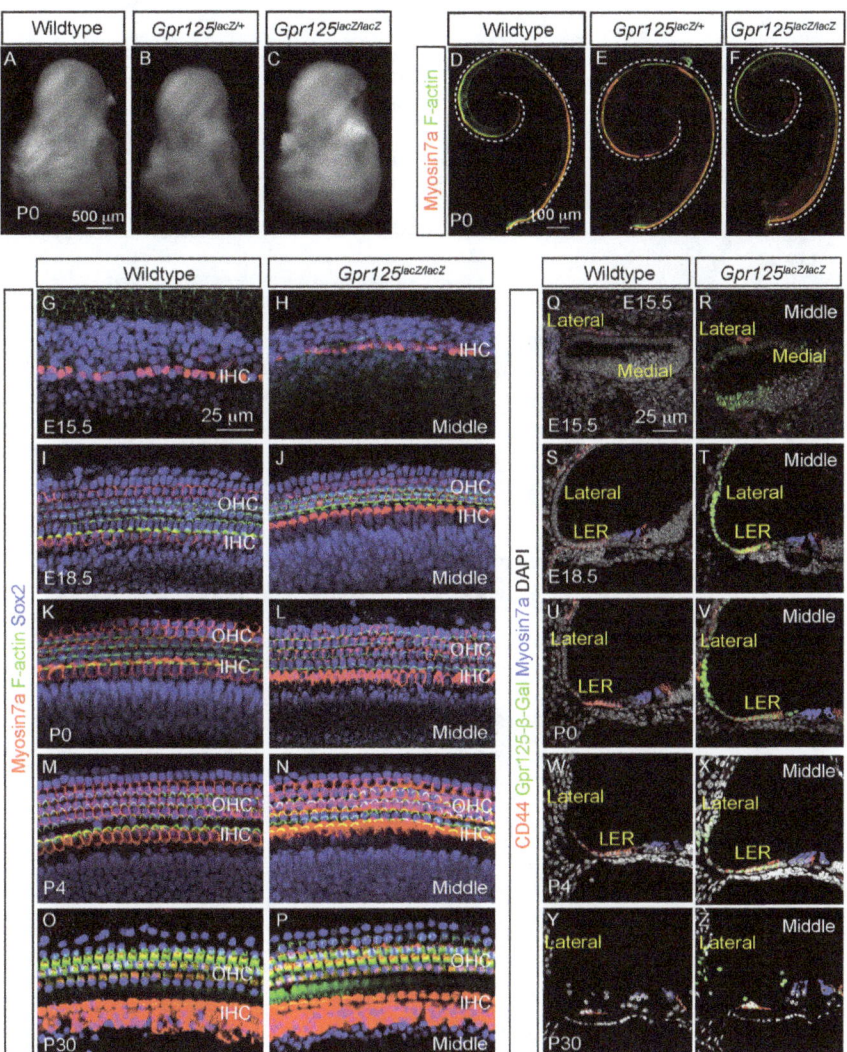

FIGURE 6 | Gpr125 is dispensable for cochlear development. **(A–C)** Otic capsule from P0 wild-type, Gpr125$^{lacZ/+}$, and Gpr125$^{lacZ/lacZ}$ mice. **(D–F)** Whole mount preparation of cochleae from the wild-type, Gpr125$^{lacZ/+}$, and Gpr125$^{lacZ/lacZ}$ mice showing no differences in length. **(G–P)** Whole mount preparation of E15.5, E18.5, P0, P4, and P30 cochleae immunostained for Myosin7a (red), F-actin (green), and Sox2 (blue), demonstrating no detectable loss of hair cells, hair bundles, or supporting cells in the Gpr125$^{lacZ/lacZ}$ cochleae. Images were taken from the middle turn. **(Q–Z)** Representative sections through the middle turn of E15.5, E18.5, P0, P4, and P30 cochleae from wild-type and Gpr125$^{lacZ/lacZ}$ mice. Gpr125$^{lacZ/lacZ}$ mutants demonstrate relatively normal cochlear morphology, including in the stria vascularis and LER that strongly express Gpr125-β-Gal.

suggesting that Gpr125 is dispensable for cochlear development and maintenance.

Markers of the Lesser Epithelial Ridge and Derivatives

The embryonic and postnatal cochlea is radially patterned in a manner perpendicular to the tonotopic gradient arranged longitudinally along the cochlea. By E11.0, the cochlear duct has already developed into five distinct structures: the prospective LER, the Reissner's membrane, the greater epithelial ridge (also known as Kölliker's organ), the stria vascularis, and the prosensory domain (Driver and Kelley, 2020). BMP4 marks the LER between E16 and P1 (Morsli et al., 1998), whereas CD44 marks the lateral LER in embryonic and neonatal cochlea (Hertzano et al., 2010). Unlike CD44, Gpr125 expression spans the lateral and medial LER and its derivatives in the embryonic, neonatal, and adult cochlea, consistent with recently published single-cell RNA-sequencing data (Kolla et al., 2020). The differential expression of CD44 and Gpr125 suggests that there are at least two distinct groups of LER cells, which likely give rise to Hensen's cells and Claudius cells in adult cochlea. Therefore, like the organ of Corti and GER, the LER is also radially patterned as the cochlea matures (Jansson et al., 2019; Munnamalai and Fekete, 2020).

While Hensen's cells and Claudius cells can be distinguished using molecular markers and spatially, whether they serve distinct functions in the cochlea is not known. A recent study

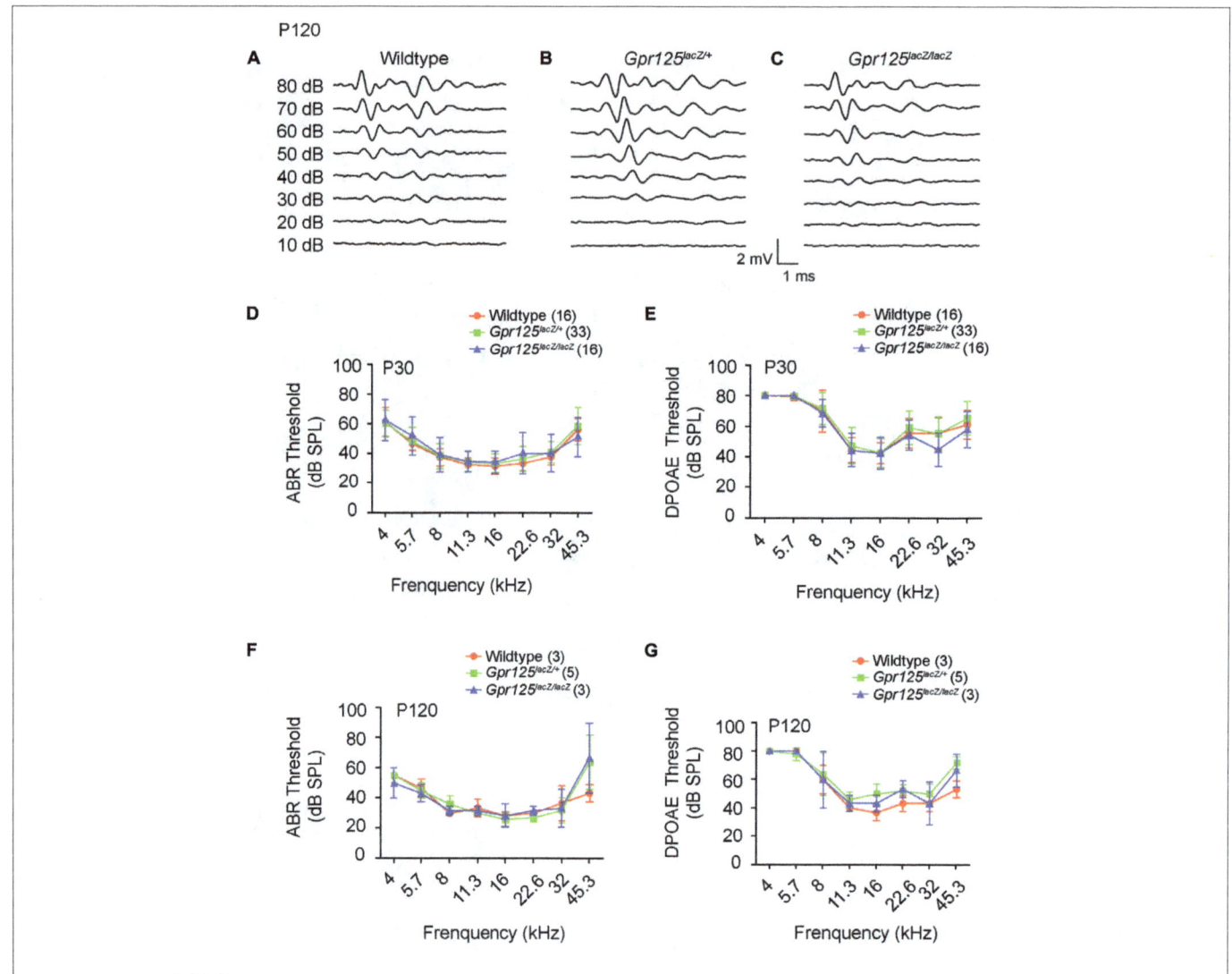

FIGURE 7 | $Gpr125^{lacZ/lacZ}$ mice exhibit normal auditory physiology. **(A–C)** Representative ABR waveforms of P120 wild-type, $Gpr125^{lacZ/+}$, and $Gpr125^{lacZ/lacZ}$ mice. **(D–G)** Comparable ABR and DPOAE thresholds of P30 and P120 wild-type, $Gpr125^{lacZ/+}$, and $Gpr125^{lacZ/lacZ}$ littermates. No significant differences were observed among wild-type, $Gpr125^{lacZ/+}$, and $Gpr125^{lacZ/lacZ}$ mice ($p > 0.05$, one-way ANOVA). Data are presented as mean ± SD.

characterized the requirement of the Notch ligand Jagged1 for the formation of Hensen's cells in the embryonic cochlea (Chrysostomou et al., 2020). Interestingly, LER cells formed Claudius cells instead of Hensen's cells in the absence of Jagged1. The use of Gpr125 as a marker can further facilitate studies of radial patterning of the LER and the functions of distinct cell populations therein. It is important, however, to note that the β-Gal signal in the P0 Gpr125-LacZ cochleae is noticeably less broad and intense than the Gpr125 mRNA signal in wild-type animals.

Gpr125 Is Dispensable for Cochlear Development and Function

Gpr125 has been shown to be required for gastrulation during development of zebrafish (Li et al., 2013). Given its role as a modulator of the Wnt/PCP signaling, we hypothesized that Gpr125 deficiency would perturb the development of the mouse cochlea. To our surprise, Gpr125 is dispensable for the cell survival, specification, and organization in all cochlear regions where it is expressed. More specifically, cochlear length is unaffected and organization of hair cells and supporting cells appear normal, suggesting no PCP defects.

In the P30 cochlea when the auditory system is functionally mature, we found that Gpr125 deletion does not lead to changes in thresholds of ABR and DPOAE. The endocochlear potential established by the stria vascularis, which was shown to express Gpr125-β-Gal at several developmental stages, is required for hair cell function. Since we did not detect any ABR/DPOAE changes in $Gpr125^{lacZ/lacZ}$ mice, we presume that endocochlear potential is not affected, but more studies are needed to confirm this interpretation. Our results also suggest that Gpr125 is not required for the maintenance and function of multiple other cochlear cell types. The lack of phenotype is possibly because

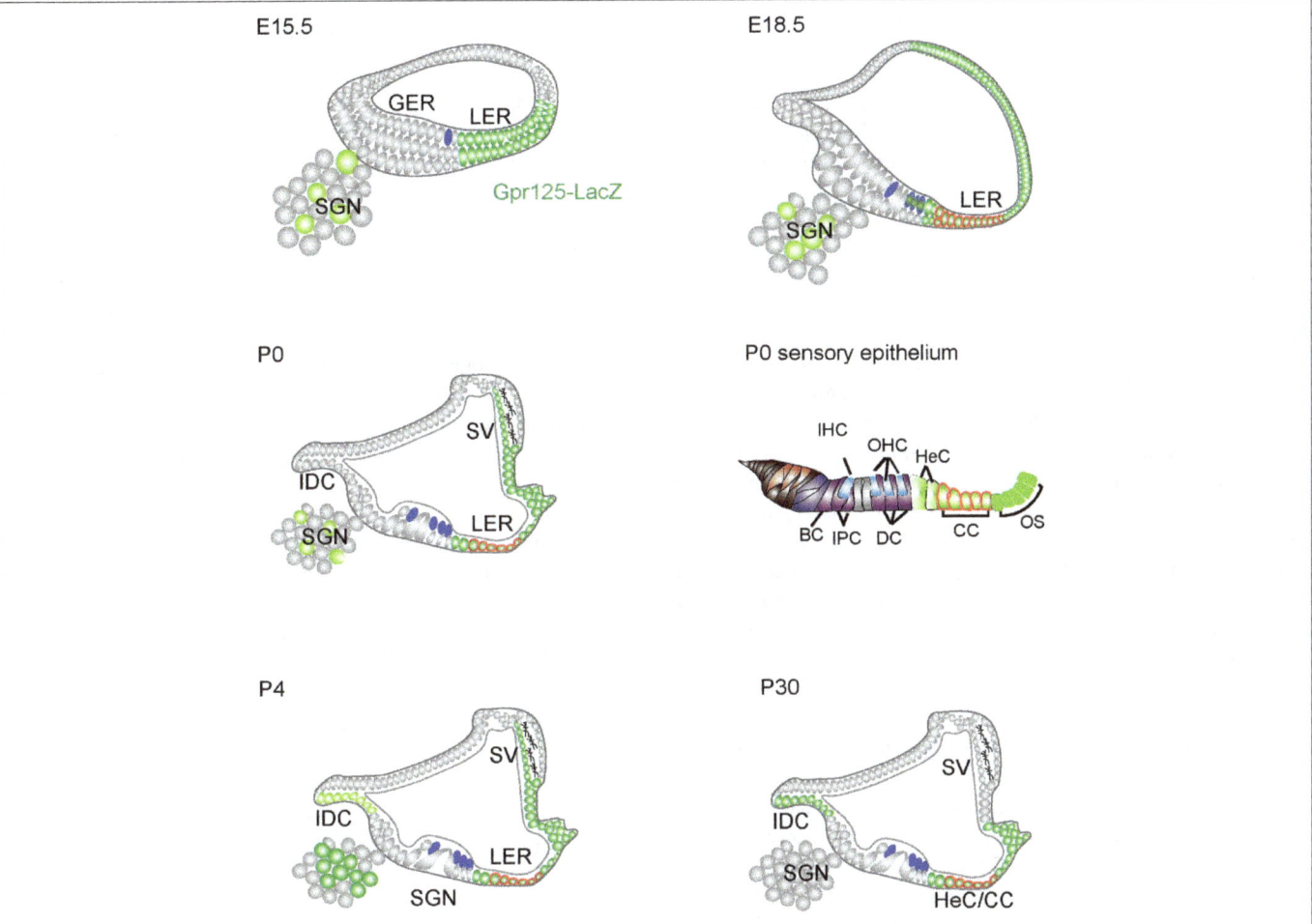

FIGURE 8 | Schematic depiction of Gpr125 expression in the developing and mature cochlea. At E15.5, Gpr125 is expressed in the LER, LW, and SGNs. At E18.5, Gpr125 is expressed broadly and strongly in the LER and lateral cochlear wall. It is expressed at lower levels in the OHCs and SGNs. At P0 and P4, Gpr125 is expressed in the LER, SV, and SGNs. The IDCs do not express Gpr125 at P0 and display robust expression later at P4 and P30. At P30, Gpr125 is expressed in the Claudius cells, Hensen's cells, and outer sulcus, but is no longer expressed in the SV and SGNs. SGN, spiral ganglion neurons; GER, greater epithelial ridge; LER, lesser epithelial ridge; SV, stria vascularis; OHC, outer hair cells; IHC, inner hair cells; HC, Hensen's cell, IDC, interdental cell; IPC, inner phalangeal cells; PC, pillar cells; DC, Deiters' cells; CC, Claudius's cells; OS, outer sulcus cells; BC, border cells.

of redundant regulatory elements of the PCP pathway or other adhesion GPR molecules. There are likely redundant PCP signals to direct and maintain hair cell orientation, evinced by recent studies on the interaction of Wnt secretion and PCP proteins (Landin Malt et al., 2020; Najarro et al., 2020).

Knockout mice of another adhesion GPR protein, Celsr1, has been shown to display PCP defects, including that of the cochlear and vestibular organs, and abnormal brain development (Curtin et al., 2003; Boutin et al., 2012; Duncan et al., 2017; Obara et al., 2017). Of note, development of type II SGNs, which make a distinctive 90° turn toward the cochlear base to synapse OHCs during cochlear development, was perturbed in Celsr1-deficent cochlea (Ghimire et al., 2018). In our study, we do not rule out more subtle defects such as type II SGNs neurite patterning in $Gpr125^{lacZ/lacZ}$ mice.

The second possible explanation for the lack of phenotype is due to compensation of Gpr125 by other adhesion GPR proteins that are not yet appreciated. Recent studies of Gpr56, Gpr124, and Gpr126 implicate adhesion GPRs in diverse development processes, including brain development, blood vessel formation, and myelination in mammals (Mogha et al., 2013; Chang et al., 2017; Sawal et al., 2018). According to published single-cell transcriptomic data, the embryonic and neonatal cochlear duct express several other adhesion GPRs (e.g., Gpr116, Gpr56, Gpr64, and Gpr126) but not others (e.g., Gpr123, Gpr124, Gpr110, Gpr97) (Kolla et al., 2020). Therefore, adhesion GPR members other than Gpr125 may serve redundant functions.

CONCLUSION

In summary, our study reveals that Gpr125 is dynamically expressed in the embryonic and postnatal cochlea. Gpr125 robustly and consistently labels the LER and its derivatives, whose function remains poorly understood. Since Gpr125 is dispensable for cochlear development and function, the

$Gpr125^{lacZ/+}$ reporter mice may be useful for cell sorting experiments to further interrogate LER cells, which have been shown to display progenitor cell characteristics (Zhai et al., 2005; Huang et al., 2009). Alternatively, a Gpr125-Cre knock-in mice can be generated for cell-specific manipulation. Thus, the current study may help further our understanding of cochlear development, function, and regeneration.

MATERIALS AND METHODS

Mice

$Gpr125^{lacZ/+}$ mice were generated by Deltagen (access number XM_1320, San Carlos, CA, United States) and were a kind gift from C.J. Kuo (Stanford University, CA, United States). To determine embryonic age, male $Gpr125^{lacZ/+}$ mouse was mated with female $Gpr125^{lacZ/+}$ mouse. The next morning, the vaginal plug was checked. The female was separated if a plug was present, and that noon was designated as embryonic age 0.5. Both male and female mice were examined. Animal care and all experimental procedures were carried out in accordance with institutional guidelines at Stanford University (protocol # 18606).

Genotyping

Genomic DNA extracted from mouse tails was digested in 1 M NaOH at 98°C for 1 h followed by the addition of 20 μl of 1 M Tris-HCl (pH 8.0). KAPA Taq PCR master mix was used to amplify DNA fragments. The primers used were as follows: Gpr125 Forward: 5′-GAwAGGCTGTGGGCAGTTGA CAGCAG-3′; Gpr125 Neo: 5′-GACGAGTTCTTCTGAGGGGA TCGATC-3′; Gpr125 Reverse: 5′-GCCCGTGACCATTTT TTGTCTCCTC-3′.

Immunofluorescence Staining

Immunofluorescence was performed as previously described (Atkinson et al., 2018). Whole mount cochleae were isolated and fixed in 4% paraformaldehyde for 40 min (in PBS, pH 7.4; Electron Microscopy Services) at room temperature. P30 otic capsules were decalcified in 500 mM EDTA for 2 days at 4°C. Cochlea from mice of different ages was dissected into three turns, with the Reissner's membrane, tectorial membrane, and stria vascularis removed. Then, tissues were washed with 0.1% Triton X-100 in PBS (PBST) three times for 5 to 10 min each and blocked with 5% donkey serum, 0.1% Triton X-100, 1% BSA, and 0.02% sodium azide (NaN_3) in PBS at pH 7.4 for 1 h at room temperature. Next, tissues were incubated with primary antibodies in the same blocking solution overnight at 4°C. The following day, tissues were washed with 0.1% Triton X-100 in PBS and incubated with secondary antibodies diluted in PBS containing 0.1% Triton X-100, 1% BSA, and 0.02% NaN_3 for 2 h at room temperature. After washing with PBS three times for 10 min, tissues were mounted in Antifade Fluorescence Mounting Medium (Dako, Agilent) and coverslipped.

For sections, cochleae were harvested on ice and fixed in 4% PFA overnight. Then, tissues were sequentially submerged in 10, 20, and 30% sucrose prior to being embedded in 100% OCT and frozen on dry ice. Serial sections were cut at 10 μm with a cryostat. Frozen slides were warmed for 30 min at room temperature and washed in PBS before incubating in PBST for 15 min to permeabilize the tissue. Sections were then treated the same as whole mount tissues.

The following primary antibodies were used: anti-Myosin7a (Rabbit, 1:1000, Proteus Bioscience, 25-6790), anti-Sox2 (Goat, 1:400, R&D, AF2018), anti-CD44 (Rat, 1:200, BD Pharmingen, 550538), anti-β-galactose (Chicken, 1:500, Abcam, ab9361), and anti-Tuj1 (Mouse, 1:500, Neuromics, 801201). Fluorescence-conjugated phalloidin (1:1,000, Invitrogen, Thermo Fisher Scientific, A22283), DAPI (1:10,000, Invitrogen, Thermo Fisher Scientific, D1306), Alexa Fluor donkey anti-goat 647 (1:200, Thermo Fisher Scientific, A21447), Fluor donkey anti-mouse 546 (1:200, Thermo Fisher Scientific, A10036), Alexa Fluor donkey anti-rabbit 546 (1:500, Thermo Fisher Scientific, A10040), Alexa Fluor donkey anti-rabbit 647 (1:200, Thermo Fisher Scientific, A31573), Alexa Fluor donkey anti-chicken 488 (1:500, Thermo Fisher Scientific, A10040), and Alexa Fluor donkey anti-rat 647 secondary antibodies (1:200; Thermo Fisher Scientific) were also used.

In situ Hybridization

In situ hybridization was performed as previously described (Jansson et al., 2019). Briefly, tissues were fixed and processed as for immunohistochemistry. The red chromogenic RNAscope kit (Red V2.5 HD, ACDBio, Newark, CA, 322350) was used following the manufacturer's instructions. Probes used were as follows: Mm-Adgra3-O1 (ACDBio, 827281), which was designed to detect exons 15–19 of *Gpr125* (also known as *Adgra3*), *Dapb* as negative control (ACDBio, 310043), and *Polr2a* as positive control (ACDBio, 312471).

Auditory Measurements

Auditory brainstem responses (ABRs) and distortion product otoacoustic emission (DPOAE) responses were performed in a sound-isolated and electrically shielded chamber (Atkinson et al., 2018). Mice at P30 ± 2 and P120 ± 2 were anesthetized with a mixture of xylazine (10 mg/kg) and ketamine (100 mg/kg). Body temperature was maintained near 37°C with a heating pad. ABR signals were measured from a needle electrode inserted inferior to the left ear, referenced to an electrode inserted at the vertex of the skull, and a ground electrode was inserted at the hind leg. Tone burst stimuli were delivered at frequencies 4, 5.7, 8, 11.3, 16, 22.6, 32, and 45.3 kHz and sound intensities were raised from 10 to 80 dB sound pressure level (SPL) in 10-dB steps. Up to 512 trials were averaged at each sound level and frequency.

DPOAEs were measured by a probe tip microphone in the external auditory canal. The sound stimuli were two 1-s sine wave tones of differing frequencies (F2 = 1.22 × F1). F2 was varied from 4 to 45.3 kHz, and the intensities of two tones were from 20 to 80 dB SPL with 10-dB steps. The amplitude of the cubic distortion product was measured at 2 × F1-F2. The threshold at each frequency was calculated when the DPOAE was > 5 dB SPL and 2 SDs above the noise level. For statistical analyses of both ABR and DPOAE responses, a lack of response is designated 80 dB SPL.

Image Analyses, Quantification, and Statistics

Cell quantification and measurements were performed using Fiji ImageJ (NIH). Whole mount preparation or sections of one cochlea from each animal were used for cell counting. The samples were scanned in z-stack mode at 1-μm intervals using confocal microscopy (Zeiss LSM700 confocal microscope, Oberkochen, Germany).

For quantification, Tuj1$^+$ SGNs were measured in one to three representative 50 μm^2 grids for each cochlea. For comparisons of immunofluorescence intensity from *Gpr125 mRNA in situ* hybridization, images were acquired using identical settings for all experimental groups. Immunofluorescence intensity was measured in regions of interest using Fiji ImageJ (NIH). All cell numbers and measurements were presented as mean ± SD. Cell counts, ABR, and DPOAE were compared by a one-way ANOVA (SPSS 20, IBM Armonk, NY). $p < 0.05$ is considered statistically significant.

ETHICS STATEMENT

The animal study was reviewed and approved by the Stanford University.

AUTHOR CONTRIBUTIONS

HS and AC conceived and designed the experiments. HS, PA, SB, and WD performed the experiments. HS, TW, SB, and AC analyzed the data. HS, TW, and AC wrote the manuscript. All authors contributed to the article and approved the submitted version.

ACKNOWLEDGMENTS

We are deeply grateful to our laboratory for insightful comments and fruitful discussion on the manuscript. We thank E. Huarcaya Najarro and K. Yuki for excellent technical support, and C. Kuo for sharing $Gpr125^{lacZ/+}$ mice. The imaging core was supported by the Stanford Initiative to Cure Hearing Loss through generous gifts from the Bill and Susan Oberndorf Foundation.

SUPPLEMENTARY MATERIAL

Supplementary Figure 1 | Expression of Gpr125-β-Gal in spiral ganglion neurons in E15.5 $Gpr125^{lacZ/+}$ mice. **(A,A')** Representative low magnification images of cochlear sections of E15.5 $Gpr125^{lacZ/+}$ mice immunostained for Gpr125-β-Gal (green) and Tuj1 (red). Gpr125-β-Gal was detected in Tuj1$^+$ spiral ganglion neurons (SGN) (dashed line), albeit at lower level than the cochlear duct. **(B–D)** High-magnification images of SGNs from each turn shown in panel **(A)**. There were few β-Gal$^+$, Tuj1$^+$ cells in the apical turn and many β-Gal$^+$, Tuj1$^+$ cells (arrowheads) in the middle and basal turns, respectively.

Supplementary Figure 2 | Gpr125 is dispensable for cochlear development. **(A)** No significant differences were seen among the lengths of wild-type, $Gpr125^{+/lacZ}$ and $Gpr125^{lacZ/lacZ}$ cochleae. **(B–J")** Whole mount preparation of wild-type and $Gpr125^{lacZ/lacZ}$ at E15.5, E18.5, P0, P4 and P30. Immunostaining for Myosin7a, F-actin and Sox2, demonstrated no loss of hair cells, hair bundles, or supporting cells in the $Gpr125^{lacZ/lacZ}$ cochleae. Images were taken from the middle turn. **(L–N)** Hair cells and supporting cell subtypes were quantified, showing no differences in cell counts among wild-type, $Gpr125^{+/lacZ}$ and $Gpr125^{lacZ/lacZ}$ cochleae ($p > 0.05$, One-way ANOVA). Data are presented as mean ± SD.

REFERENCES

Atkinson, P. J., Dong, Y., Gu, S., Liu, W., Najarro, E. H., Udagawa, T., et al. (2018). Sox2 haploinsufficiency primes regeneration and Wnt responsiveness in the mouse cochlea. *J. Clin. Invest.* 128, 1641–1656. doi: 10.1172/jci97248

Aw, W. Y., Heck, B. W., Joyce, B., and Devenport, D. (2016). Transient tissue-scale deformation coordinates alignment of planar cell polarity junctions in the mammalian skin. *Curr. Biol.* 26, 2090–2100. doi: 10.1016/j.cub.2016.06.030

Basch, M. L., Brown, R. M. II, Jen, H. I., and Groves, A. K. (2016). Where hearing starts: the development of the mammalian cochlea. *J. Anat.* 228, 233–254. doi: 10.1111/joa.12314

Boucherie, C., Boutin, C., Jossin, Y., Schakman, O., Goffinet, A. M., Ris, L., et al. (2018). Neural progenitor fate decision defects, cortical hypoplasia and behavioral impairment in Celsr1-deficient mice. *Mol. Psychiatry* 23, 723–734. doi: 10.1038/mp.2017.236

Bousfiha, A., Bakhchane, A., Charoute, H., Detsouli, M., Rouba, H., Charif, M., et al. (2017). Novel compound heterozygous mutations in the GPR98 (USH2C) gene identified by whole exome sequencing in a Moroccan deaf family. *Mol. Biol. Rep.* 44, 429–434. doi: 10.1007/s11033-017-4129-9

Boutin, C., Goffinet, A. M., and Tissir, F. (2012). Celsr1-3 cadherins in PCP and brain development. *Curr. Top. Dev. Biol.* 101, 161–183. doi: 10.1016/b978-0-12-394592-1.00010-7

Chang, J., Mancuso, M. R., Maier, C., Liang, X., Yuki, K., Yang, L., et al. (2017). Gpr124 is essential for blood-brain barrier integrity in central nervous system disease. *Nat. Med.* 23, 450–460.

Chen, G., Yang, L., Begum, S., and Xu, L. (2010). GPR56 is essential for testis development and male fertility in mice. *Dev. Dyn.* 239, 3358–3367. doi: 10.1002/dvdy.22468

Chen, P., Johnson, J. E., Zoghbi, H. Y., and Segil, N. (2002). The role of Math1 in inner ear development: uncoupling the establishment of the sensory primordium from hair cell fate determination. *Development* 129, 2495–2505. doi: 10.1242/dev.129.10.2495

Chrysostomou, E., Zhou, L., Darcy, Y. L., Graves, K. A., Doetzlhofer, A., and Cox, B. C. (2020). The notch ligand Jagged1 is required for the formation, maintenance and survival of hensen's cells in the mouse cochlea. *J. Neurosci.* 40, 9401–9413. doi: 10.1523/jneurosci.1192-20.2020

Cullen, M., Elzarrad, M. K., Seaman, S., Zudaire, E., Stevens, J., Yang, M. Y., et al. (2011). GPR124, an orphan G protein-coupled receptor, is required for CNS-specific vascularization and establishment of the blood-brain barrier. *Proc. Natl. Acad. Sci. U. S. A.* 108, 5759–5764. doi: 10.1073/pnas.1017192108

Curtin, J. A., Quint, E., Tsipouri, V., Arkell, R. M., Cattanach, B., Copp, A. J., et al. (2003). Mutation of Celsr1 disrupts planar polarity of inner ear hair cells and causes severe neural tube defects in the mouse. *Curr. Biol.* 13, 1129–1133. doi: 10.1016/s0960-9822(03)00374-9

Doudney, K., and Stanier, P. (2005). Epithelial cell polarity genes are required for neural tube closure. *Am. J. Med. Genet. C Semin. Med. Genet.* 135C, 42–47. doi: 10.1002/ajmg.c.30052

Driver, E. C., and Kelley, M. W. (2020). Development of the cochlea. *Development* 147:dev162263.

Driver, E. C., Northrop, A., and Kelley, M. W. (2017). Cell migration, intercalation and growth regulate mammalian cochlear extension. *Development* 144, 3766–3776.

Duncan, J. S., Stoller, M. L., Francl, A. F., Tissir, F., Devenport, D., and Deans, M. R. (2017). Celsr1 coordinates the planar polarity of vestibular hair cells during inner ear development. *Dev. Biol.* 423, 126–137. doi: 10.1016/j.ydbio.2017.01.020

Ganesh, R. A., Venkataraman, K., and Sirdeshmukh, R. (2020). GPR56: an adhesion GPCR involved in brain development, neurological disorders and cancer. *Brain Res.* 1747:147055. doi: 10.1016/j.brainres.2020.147055

Ghimire, S. R., Ratzan, E. M., and Deans, M. R. (2018). A non-autonomous function of the core PCP protein VANGL2 directs peripheral axon turning in the developing cochlea. *Development* 145:dev159012.

Hamann, J., Aust, G., Arac, D., Engel, F. B., Formstone, C., Fredriksson, R., et al. (2015). International union of basic and clinical pharmacology. XCIV. adhesion G protein-coupled receptors. *Pharmacol. Rev.* 67, 338–367.

Hasson, T., Heintzelman, M. B., Santos-Sacchi, J., Corey, D. P., and Mooseker, M. S. (1995). Expression in cochlea and retina of myosin VIIa, the gene product defective in Usher syndrome type 1B. *Proc. Natl. Acad. Sci. U. S. A.* 92, 9815–9819. doi: 10.1073/pnas.92.21.9815

Hertzano, R., Puligilla, C., Chan, S. L., Timothy, C., Depireux, D. A., Ahmed, Z., et al. (2010). CD44 is a marker for the outer pillar cells in the early postnatal mouse inner ear. *J. Assoc. Res. Otolaryngol.* 11, 407–418. doi: 10.1007/s10162-010-0211-x

Huang, Y., Chi, F., Han, Z., Yang, J., Gao, W., and Li, Y. (2009). New ectopic vestibular hair cell-like cells induced by Math1 gene transfer in postnatal rats. *Brain Res.* 1276, 31–38. doi: 10.1016/j.brainres.2009.04.036

Jansson, L., Ebeid, M., Shen, J. W., Mokhtari, T. E., Quiruz, L. A., Ornitz, D. M., et al. (2019). beta-Catenin is required for radial cell patterning and identity in the developing mouse cochlea. *Proc. Natl. Acad. Sci. U. S. A.* 116, 21054–21060. doi: 10.1073/pnas.1910223116

Kolla, L., Kelly, M. C., Mann, Z. F., Anaya-Rocha, A., Ellis, K., Lemons, A., et al. (2020). Characterization of the development of the mouse cochlear epithelium at the single cell level. *Nat. Commun.* 11:2389.

Landin Malt, A., Hogan, A. K., Smith, C. D., Madani, M. S., and Lu, X. (2020). Wnts regulate planar cell polarity via heterotrimeric G protein and PI3K signaling. *J. Cell Biol.* 219:e201912071.

Li, X., Roszko, I., Sepich, D. S., Ni, M., Hamm, H. E., Marlow, F. L., et al. (2013). Gpr125 modulates dishevelled distribution and planar cell polarity signaling. *Development* 140, 3028–3039. doi: 10.1242/dev.094839

McGee, J., Goodyear, R. J., McMillan, D. R., Stauffer, E. A., Holt, J. R., Locke, K. G., et al. (2006). The very large G-protein-coupled receptor VLGR1: a component of the ankle link complex required for the normal development of auditory hair bundles. *J. Neurosci.* 26, 6543–6553. doi: 10.1523/jneurosci.0693-06.2006

Mogha, A., Benesh, A. E., Patra, C., Engel, F. B., Schoneberg, T., Liebscher, I., et al. (2013). Gpr126 functions in Schwann cells to control differentiation and myelination via G-protein activation. *J. Neurosci.* 33, 17976–17985. doi: 10.1523/jneurosci.1809-13.2013

Monk, K. R., Oshima, K., Jors, S., Heller, S., and Talbot, W. S. (2011). Gpr126 is essential for peripheral nerve development and myelination in mammals. *Development* 138, 2673–2680. doi: 10.1242/dev.062224

Morsli, H., Choo, D., Ryan, A., Johnson, R., and Wu, D. K. (1998). Development of the mouse inner ear and origin of its sensory organs. *J. Neurosci.* 18, 3327–3335. doi: 10.1523/jneurosci.18-09-03327.1998

Moteki, H., Yoshimura, H., Azaiez, H., Booth, K. T., Shearer, A. E., Sloan, C. M., et al. (2015). USH2 caused by GPR98 mutation diagnosed by massively parallel sequencing in advance of the occurrence of visual symptoms. *Ann. Otol. Rhinol. Laryngol.* 124 Suppl 1, 123S–128S.

Munnamalai, V., and Fekete, D. M. (2020). The acquisition of positional information across the radial axis of the cochlea. *Dev. Dyn.* 249, 281–297. doi: 10.1002/dvdy.118

Najarro, E. H., Huang, J., Jacobo, A., Quiruz, L. A., Grillet, N., and Cheng, A. G. (2020). Dual regulation of planar polarization by secreted Wnts and Vangl2 in the developing mouse cochlea. *Development* 147:dev191981.

Obara, N., Suzuki, Y., Irie, K., and Shibata, S. (2017). Expression of planar cell polarity genes during mouse tooth development. *Arch. Oral Biol.* 83, 85–91. doi: 10.1016/j.archoralbio.2017.07.008

Peeters, R. P., Ng, L., Ma, M., and Forrest, D. (2015). The timecourse of apoptotic cell death during postnatal remodeling of the mouse cochlea and its premature onset by triiodothyronine (T3). *Mol. Cell Endocrinol.* 407, 1–8. doi: 10.1016/j.mce.2015.02.025

Pickering, C., Hagglund, M., Szmydynger-Chodobska, J., Marques, F., Palha, J. A., Waller, L., et al. (2008). The adhesion GPCR GPR125 is specifically expressed in the choroid plexus and is upregulated following brain injury. *BMC Neurosci.* 9:97.

Sawal, H. A., Harripaul, R., Mikhailov, A., Vleuten, K., Naeem, F., Nasr, T., et al. (2018). Three mutations in the bilateral frontoparietal polymicrogyria gene GPR56 in Pakistani intellectual disability families. *J. Pediatr. Genet.* 7, 60–66.

Seandel, M., James, D., Shmelkov, S. V., Falciatori, I., Kim, J., Chavala, S., et al. (2007). Generation of functional multipotent adult stem cells from GPR125+ germline progenitors. *Nature* 449, 346–350. doi: 10.1038/nature06129

Vizurraga, A., Adhikari, R., Yeung, J., Yu, M., and Tall, G. G. (2020). Mechanisms of adhesion G protein-coupled receptor activation. *J. Biol. Chem.* 295, 14065–14083. doi: 10.1074/jbc.rev120.007423

Wu, Y., Chen, W., Gong, L., Ke, C., Wang, H., and Cai, Y. (2018). Elevated G-protein receptor 125 (GPR125) expression predicts good outcomes in colorectal cancer and inhibits Wnt/beta-catenin signaling pathway. *Med. Sci. Monit.* 24, 6608–6616. doi: 10.12659/msm.910105

Zhai, S., Shi, L., Wang, B. E., Zheng, G., Song, W., Hu, Y., et al. (2005). Isolation and culture of hair cell progenitors from postnatal rat cochleae. *J. Neurobiol.* 65, 282–293. doi: 10.1002/neu.20190

Zou, J., Mathur, P. D., Zheng, T., Wang, Y., Almishaal, A., Park, A. H., et al. (2015). Individual USH2 proteins make distinct contributions to the ankle link complex during development of the mouse cochlear stereociliary bundle. *Hum. Mol. Genet.* 24, 6944–6957.

Generation of a Spiral Ganglion Neuron Degeneration Mouse Model

Zhengqing Hu[1,2]*, Fnu Komal[2], Aditi Singh[2] and Meng Deng[2]

[1] John D. Dingell VA Medical Center, Detroit, MI, United States,
[2] Department of Otolaryngology-HNS, Wayne State University School of Medicine, Detroit, MI, United States

*Correspondence:
Zhengqing Hu
zh@med.wayne.edu;
Zhengqing.hu@va.gov

Spiral ganglion neurons (SGNs) can be injured by a wide variety of insults. However, there still is a lack of degeneration models to specifically damage the SGNs without disturbing other types of cells in the inner ear. This study aims to generate an SGN-specific damage model using the Cre-LoxP transgenic mouse strains. The Cre-inducible diphtheria toxin receptor ($iDTR^{+/+}$) knock-in mouse strain was crossed with a mouse strain with Cre activity specific to neurons ($Nefl^{CreER/CreER}$). Expression of the Cre-recombinase activity was evaluated using the reporter mouse strain Ai9 at pre-hearing, hearing onset, and post-hearing stages. Accordingly, heterozygous $Nefl^{CreER/+}$;$iDTR^{+/-}$ mice were treated with tamoxifen on postnatal days 1–5 (P1–5), followed by diphtheria toxin (DT) or vehicle injection on P7, P14, and P21 to evaluate the SGN loss. Robust tamoxifen-induced Cre-mediated Ai9 tdTomato fluorescence was observed in the SGN area of heterozygous $Nefl^{CreER/+}$;$Ai9^{+/-}$ mice treated with tamoxifen, whereas vehicle-treated heterozygote mice did not show tdTomato fluorescence. Compared to vehicle-treated $Nefl^{CreER/+}$;$iDTR^{+/-}$ mice, DT-treated $Nefl^{CreER/+}$;$iDTR^{+/-}$ mice showed significant auditory brainstem response (ABR) threshold shifts and SGN cell loss. Hair cell count and functional study did not show significant changes. These results demonstrate that the $Nefl^{CreER/CreER}$ mouse strain exhibits inducible SGN-specific Cre activity in the inner ear, which may serve as a valuable SGN damage model for regeneration research of the inner ear.

Keywords: auditory brainstem response, degeneration, iDTR, neurofilament, spiral ganglion, Cre-LoxP

INTRODUCTION

In the auditory system, spiral ganglion neurons (SGNs) are bipolar neurons that transfer auditory signals from auditory hair cells to the cochlear nucleus in the brainstem (Echteler, 1992; Nayagam et al., 2011). SGNs are sensitive to a variety of insults, including sound overstimulation, genetic disorders, aging, ototoxic drugs, and trauma (Ylikoski et al., 1998; Carignano et al., 2019; Wu et al., 2021). Degeneration of SGNs usually causes irreversible sensorineural hearing loss, in which the auditory signals perceived by hair cells are not able to transfer to the cochlear nucleus. It is essential to establish an SGN damage model to understand the degeneration of SGNs. This would provide fundamental knowledge to guide the prevention of SGN damage and the regeneration of SGNs to conduct auditory signals from the inner ear to the brainstem. Currently, knowledge on the SGN degeneration model is very limited.

SGNs receive auditory signals from hair cells; therefore, injuries to hair cells often cause secondary damage to SGNs (Johnsson, 1974; Pan et al., 2017). For instance, ototoxic drugs, including aminoglycoside and cisplatin, cause hair cell damage, which leads to secondary damage to SGNs (Dallos and Harris, 1978; Breglio et al., 2017). In other circumstances, aging can cause progressive hair cell degeneration, which subsequently injures SGNs as a secondary degeneration (Carignano et al., 2019; Wu et al., 2021). Additionally, some ototoxic drugs (e.g., neomycin), aging, and other insults can directly damage SGNs (Majumder et al., 2017; Zhong et al., 2020). The combination of primary and secondary patterns complicates the mechanisms of SGN degeneration. Therefore, it is necessary to develop an approach only targeting SGNs without interfering with hair cells.

The Cre-LoxP system provides the opportunity to target cell types expressing a tissue-specific gene (Nakamura et al., 2006; Rotheneichner et al., 2017; Jahn et al., 2018). In a previous study, $Bhlhb5^{Cre/+}$ mice that showed Cre activity in SGNs were bred with mice expressing the Cre-inducible diphtheria toxin receptor (iDTR; $iDTR^{+/+}$ mice) (Pan et al., 2017). It was found that diphtheria toxin (DT) injection caused 30–40% SGN damage in $Bhlhb5^{Cre/+}$;$iDTR^{+/-}$ offspring. It is known that SGN development continues during the postnatal period up to postnatal day 28 (P28) (Shrestha et al., 2018; Sun et al., 2018). However, in the aforementioned study, DT was injected on P21. It remains unclear whether an early postnatal or pre-hearing DT injection would damage SGNs and whether SGN damage is consistent or recovered during postnatal development. Moreover, significant auditory brainstem response (ABR) threshold changes were not observed in DT-treated $Bhlhb5^{Cre/+}$;$iDTR^{+/-}$ offspring. Therefore, the generation of an SGN loss model with significant functional ABR threshold shifts remains a challenge.

In this study, a mouse strain with the estrogen receptor tamoxifen 2-inducible Cre cassette knocked into the Nefl gene ($Nefl^{CreER/CreER}$) was bred with the iDTR mouse strain. Nefl encodes neurofilament light chain (Nefl), which is a major neuronal cytoskeleton component expressed in the soma, dendrites, and axon of developing and mature neurons, including the neurons along the auditory pathway (Liem, 1993; Illing, 2001; Liu et al., 2004). In the cochlea, Nefl is expressed in SGNs, but not in other types of cells such as hair cells (Torkos et al., 2008; Sun et al., 2018). When bred with mice expressing the Cre-inducible iDTR, the SGNs of $Nefl^{Cre/+}$;$iDTR^{+/-}$ offspring were expected to be specifically damaged following DT treatment without interfering with hair cells. To determine whether SGN damage occurred before, around, or after hearing onset, DT was administered on postnatal days 7, 14, and 21, respectively. Functional, morphological, and protein expression assays were used to evaluate SGN damage following DT treatment.

MATERIALS AND METHODS

Animals and Genotyping

The experimental procedures on animals were approved by the Institutional Animal Care and Use Committee (IACUC) at Wayne State University. The $Nefl^{CreER/CreER}$ (stock no. 008363), iDTR (stock no. 007900), and the reporter Ai9 (stock no. 007909) mouse strains were obtained from Jackson Laboratories (Bar Harbor, ME, United States) (Buch et al., 2005; Rotolo et al., 2008; Madisen et al., 2010). They were maintained and bred following the guidelines of the local Division of Laboratory Animal Resources. $Nefl^{CreER/CreER}$ mice were crossed with iDTR or Ai9 mice, followed by genotyping. Heterozygous $Nefl^{CreER/+}$;$iDTR^{+/-}$ and $Nefl^{CreER/+}$;$Ai9^{+/-}$ mice were used in this study. The homozygous animals were used for breeding and maintenance of the strains.

A tail snip-based genotyping was performed to determine the genotypes of the mice (Fang et al., 2012). Two millimeters of the tail was snipped and placed in alkaline lysis buffer (25 mM NaOH and 0.2 mM ethylenediaminetetraacetic acid (EDTA; E5134, Sigma, St. Louis, MO, United States) for the hotshot procedure of 98°C for 1 h, followed by neutralization (40 mM Tris-HCl; Sigma) for 5 min at room temperature to harvest gDNA in the supernatant. Allele-specific PCR was used to determine the genotypes of the mice using the vendor's protocols. The primers included: $Nefl^{CreER/CreER}$: common, ATT ATT ATT GTA AAC ATC TGT GTG ATT CA; mutant forward, CGC ATA GAA ATT GCA TCA ACG CAT; and wild type reverse, AGA GGA GCA GGT GGC TAA GAA GAA AGA; Ai9: wild type forward, AAG GGA GCT GCA GTG GAG TA; wild type reverse, CCG AAA ATC TGT GGG AAG TC; mutant forward, CTG TTC CTG TAC GGC ATG G; and mutant reverse, GGC ATT AAA GCA GCG TAT CC; iDTR: common, AAA GTC GCT CTG AGT TGT TAT; mutant, GCG AAG AGT TTG TCC TCA ACC; and wild type reverse, GGA GCG GGA GAA ATG GAT ATG.

Tamoxifen and Diphtheria Toxin Treatment

$Nefl^{CreER/CreER}$ mice were crossed with the reporter strain Ai9 to obtain heterozygous $Nefl^{CreER/+}$;$Ai9^{+/-}$ offspring for the characterization of Cre activity in the cochlea. Tamoxifen or vehicle was administered to the dam *via* gavage on P1 for 4–5 days, and the pups received treatment *via* feeding. Tamoxifen (T5648, Sigma) was dissolved in corn oil (C8267, Sigma) at 10 mg/ml. Either tamoxifen (4 mg/40 g body weight) or corn oil was administered daily *via* oral gavage for 4–5 consecutive days (Koundakjian et al., 2007; Fang et al., 2012). Treated mice were followed up and euthanized on P10, P14, P21, and P28 for histology and immunofluorescence study to determine the Cre activity. $Nefl^{CreER/CreER}$ mice were crossed with iDTR mice to obtain heterozygous $Nefl^{CreER/+}$;$iDTR^{+/-}$ mice in order to determine the SGN degeneration. For the DT treatment, $Nefl^{CreER/+}$;$iDTR^{+/-}$ mice were treated with tamoxifen as above, and a single dose of DT (List Biology Laboratories #150, 10 ng/g body weight, i.p.) was administered on P7, P14, or P21 (**Figure 1**).

Hearing Tests

Animals received hearing tests at 4 and 5 weeks old prior to euthanasia. Distortion product otoacoustic emission (DPOAE) and ABR tests were used to study the function of outer hair cells and the auditory system using the RP2.1 and RZ6 systems [Tucker-Davis Technology (TDT), Alachua, FL, United States] (Hu et al., 2009; Zhang et al., 2011; Deng et al., 2019). The TDT System 3 software was applied for signal generation and auditory response collection. The ABR stimulation level ranged from 5 to 90 dB sound pressure level (SPL) in 5-dB steps using 8, 16, 24, and 32 kHz pure tone and click sound. The threshold was determined as the lowest stimulation decibel SPL that generated a wave II amplitude larger than 0.2 mV. At 16 and 24 kHz, the

Generation of a Spiral Ganglion Neuron Degeneration Mouse Model

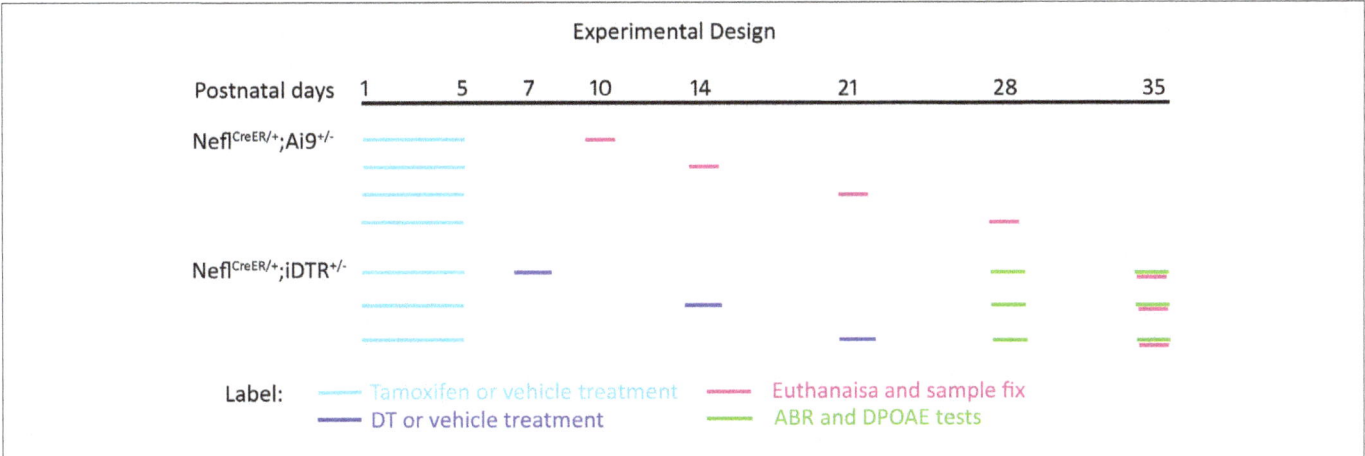

FIGURE 1 | Schematic diagram of the experimental design. $Nefl^{CreER/+};Ai9^{+/-}$ mice were treated with tamoxifen or vehicle on postnatal day 1 (P1) for 4–5 consecutive days. The pups were followed up and euthanized on P10, P14, P21, and P28. $Nefl^{CreER/+};iDTR^{+/-}$ mice were treated with tamoxifen on P1–P5, followed by either vehicle or diphtheria toxin (DT) treatment on P7, P14, and P21. Hearing tests, including auditory brainstem response (ABR) and distortion product otoacoustic emission (DPOAE), were conducted on P28 and P35, and mice were euthanized on P35.

configuration of DPOAE was set as F2/F1 = 1.2 and L1 = L2 + 10 dB. L1 ranged from 10 to 80 dB SPL in 5-dB SPL steps. The DPOAE threshold was determined as the lowest level of DPOAE responses (dp) of at least 10 dB above the noise floor.

Immunofluorescence and Imaging

Mice were anesthetized with CO_2, followed by heart perfusion using saline (0.9% NaCl) and 4% paraformaldehyde (PFA; 158127, Sigma). The cochlear tissues were rapidly dissected and perfused with PFA. The dissected cochlear tissue was decalcified in 0.1 M EDTA for 1–2 weeks until the tissues softened, followed by surface preparation or cryosection at 10-μm thickness using our published methods (Hu et al., 2004; Zhang et al., 2011; Deng et al., 2019; Deng and Hu, 2020). Immunofluorescence was used for the detection of neuronal and hair cell proteins using our published methods (Hu et al., 2004; Zhang et al., 2011; Deng et al., 2019; Deng and Hu, 2020). The primary antibodies included anti-Nefl (1:200; sc-20012, Santa Cruz Biotechnology, Dallas, TX, United States), anti-beta III tubulin (TUJ1, 1:1,000; ab-2313564, Aves Labs, Tigard, OR, United States), and anti-myosin VIIa [1:200; 138-1-C, Developmental Studies Hybridoma Bank (DSHB), Iowa, City, IA, United States, and 25-6790, Proteus, Ramona, CA, United States]. Secondary antibodies were Alexa Fluor-488 (715-546-150), Cy3 (711-165-152), or Alexa Fluor-647 (703-606-155) conjugated antibodies (1:500; all from Jackson ImmunoResearch, West Grove, PA, United States). Leica SPE confocal microscope and DM2500 upright epifluorescence microscopes were used for observation and imaging.

Quantitative Study and Statistical Analysis

In the quantitative study, the ABR and DPOAE data were analyzed using two-way analysis of variance (ANOVA) with *post-hoc* tests. The two factors were treatment type (DT and vehicle) and treatment time (P7, P14, and P21). *Post-hoc* tests were used to compare the vehicle and DT treatments in the P7, P14, and P21 groups. For cell counting, the cells and the area were calculated using the cell count and measurement modules of ImageJ software (NIH) using our published methods (Li et al., 2016; Hu et al., 2017, 2019, 2021; Liu et al., 2018). For SGN cell counting, the SGN area was determined, and *Nefl*-positive cells were calculated for the P7, P14, and P21 groups. The average cell number per 10^4 μm^2 was calculated for data analysis. All three cochlear turns were analyzed for the generation of data. For hair cell counting, surface preparation was performed to expose the hair cell epithelium, and myosin VIIa-positive cells were calculated at 100-μm distance for each animal using our published methods (Liu et al., 2018; Deng et al., 2019). Six animals were included in each group for statistical analysis of the ABR, DPOAE, and SGN cell counts, and five cochlear basilar membranes were dissected per group for analysis of the number of hair cells. A *p*-value of 0.05 was considered as the criterion of statistical significance.

RESULTS

Characterization of the Cre Activity of $Nefl^{CreER/CreER}$ Mouse Spiral Ganglion Neurons

Nefl is expressed in developing and mature neurons, including SGNs (Sun et al., 2018). The $Nefl^{CreER/CreER}$ mouse strain possessing a tamoxifen-inducible Cre cassette knocked into the *Nefl* gene was used in this study (Rotolo et al., 2008). To determine the *Nefl*-mediated CreER activity, the Cre reporter transgenic mouse strain Ai9 that has a LoxP-flanked STOP cassette preventing the transcription of a ubiquitous CAG promoter-driven tdTomato fluorescence was used. Tamoxifen or vehicle was administered to the dam *via* gavage on P1 for 4–5 days (**Figure 1**). The heterozygous $Nefl^{CreER/+};Ai9^{+/-}$ pups received treatment *via* feeding and were followed up and euthanized on P10. It was observed that SGNs expressed both CreER-mediated tdTomato fluorescence and Nefl immunofluorescence, suggesting the CreER activity of $Nefl^{CreER/+}$ at the neonatal stage (**Figure 2A**). It is known that SGNs develop during the postnatal period and mature around P21–28 (Shrestha et al., 2018; Sun et al., 2018), so we opted to determine the CreER activity during postnatal development. The dam was treated with tamoxifen or vehicle by gavage from P1 to P5 for 4–5 days, and the offspring received tamoxifen *via* feeding, followed by euthanasia on P14, P21, and P28. Robust tdTomato fluorescence was observed in SGNs from P14 to P28 in tamoxifen-treated $Nefl^{CreER/+}$;Ai9$^{+/-}$ offspring, which overlapped with the Nefl immunofluorescence (**Figures 2B–D**). In vehicle-treated $Nefl^{CreER/+}$;Ai9$^{+/-}$ offspring, only Nefl immunofluorescence was observed without tdTomato fluorescence (**Figures 2B–D**). This experiment suggests that $Nefl^{CreER/+}$ mouse SGNs possess the inducible CreER activity during the postnatal development period.

Functional Evaluation of the Spiral Ganglion Neuron Loss by Click and Pure Tone Auditory Brainstem Response

To generate an SGN damage model, the iDTR knock-in mouse strain was used. iDTR mice had the simian DTR insertion at the ROSA26 locus that is blocked by an upstream LoxP-flanked STOP sequence (Buch et al., 2005). When bred with Cre-recombinase-expressing $Nefl^{CreER/CreER}$ mice, the STOP sequence was deleted in *Nefl*-Cre-expressing SGNs to allow DTR expression. Following DT treatment, iDTR-expressing SGNs were susceptible to ablation.

Homozygous $Nefl^{CreER/CreER}$ and iDTR mice were crossbred to obtain heterozygous $Nefl^{CreER/+}$;iDTR$^{+/-}$ offspring, which were treated with tamoxifen on P1–P5, followed by DT or vehicle injection on P7, P14, and P21 (**Figure 1**). Click and pure tone ABR tests were performed at 4 and 5 weeks old (**Figure 3**). It was found in the P7 treatment group that all DT-treated mice did not have an ABR response waveform following 90-dB SPL click stimulation (> 90 dB SPL) at 4 weeks old, whereas the threshold of vehicle-treated mice was 22.5 ± 4.2 dB SPL (mean ± SD) (**Figure 3E**). The click ABR threshold was similar a week later, at 5 weeks old: no response at 90 dB SPL in the DT group and remained normal (24.1 ± 3.8 dB SPL) in the vehicle group (**Figure 3E1**). In the P14 treatment group, the click ABR thresholds were 23.3 ± 6.1 and 85.8 ± 8.0 dB SPL for the vehicle and DT groups at 4 weeks old and were 22.5 ± 4.2 and > 90 dB SPL at 5 weeks old, respectively. In the P21 group, the click ABR thresholds for the vehicle and DT groups were 25.8 ± 11.1 and 76.3 ± 16.0 dB SPL at 4 weeks old and were 28.3 ± 9.3 and 83.8 ± 9.5 dB SPL at 5 weeks old, respectively (**Figures 3E,E1**). In the statistical analysis, two-way ANOVA and *post-hoc* tests were performed with two factors: treatment types (vehicle and DT) and treatment ages (P7, P14, and P21; n = 6 mice per group). In the test at 4 weeks old, the overall effects of treatment type and treatment age were not statistically significant [$F_{(2,30)}$ = 1.595, p = 0.2196]. The effect of treatment age was also not statistically significant [$F_{(2,30)}$ = 0.3451, p = 0.7109]. However, the effect of treatment type (vehicle vs. DT) was statistically significant [$F_{(1,30)}$ = 459.7, p < 0.0001]. In the *post-hoc* test of the comparison of the vehicle and DT groups, significant differences were observed in the P7, P14, and P21 groups (p < 0.0001 for all three groups). In the test at 5 weeks old, the overall effects of treatment type and treatment age were not statistically significant [$F_{(2,30)}$ = 2.831, p = 0.0748]. The effect of treatment age was also statistically insignificant [$F_{(2,30)}$ = 0.09132, p = 0.9130]. However, the effect of treatment type was statistically significant [$F_{(1,30)}$ = 1197, p < 0.0001]. In the *post-hoc* test of the comparison of the vehicle and DT groups, P7, P14, and P21 groups had significant differences (p < 0.0001 for all three groups).

In pure tone ABR, responses to the 16-kHz stimulation were analyzed (**Figures 3F,F1**). In the P7 group, the thresholds of the vehicle and DT groups were 29.2 ± 4.9 and 88.3 ± 2.6 dB SPL at 4 weeks old and were 34.2 ± 5.8 and > 90 dB SPL at 5 weeks old, respectively. For the P14 group, these thresholds became 32.5 ± 8.2 and 83.3 ± 5.2 dB SPL at 4 weeks old and 38.3 ± 13.3 and > 90 dB SPL at 5 weeks old, respectively. For the P21 group, the threshold values were 32.5 ± 7.6 and 82.5 ± 9.6 dB SPL at 4 weeks old and were 35.0 ± 5.5 and 86.3 ± 4.8 dB SPL at 5 weeks old, respectively. In the statistical analysis, two-way ANOVA and *post-hoc* tests were performed with the two factors: treatment type (vehicle and DT) and treatment age (P7, P14, and P21; n = 6 mice per group). In the test at 4 weeks old, the overall effects of treatment type and treatment age were not statistically significant [$F_{(2,30)}$ = 2.500, p = 0.0990]. The effect of treatment age was also statistically insignificant [$F_{(2,30)}$ = 0.2880, p = 0.7518]. However, the effect of treatment type (vehicle vs. DT) was statistically significant [$F_{(1,30)}$ = 407.2, p < 0.0001]. In the *post-hoc* test of the vehicle and DT groups, significant differences were observed in the P7, P14, and P21 groups (p < 0.0001 for the three groups). In the test at 5 weeks old, the overall effects of treatment type and age were not statistically significant [$F_{(2,30)}$ = 0.3387, p = 0.7154]. The effect of treatment age was statistically insignificant [$F_{(2,30)}$ = 0.6290, p = 0.5400]. However, the effect of treatment type was statistically significant [$F_{(1,30)}$ = 594.6, p < 0.0001]. In the *post-hoc* comparison of the vehicle and DT groups, the P7, P14, and P21 groups showed significant differences (p < 0.0001).

Neuronal Protein Expression Changes

Immunofluorescence using anti-Nefl and anti-TUJ1 antibodies was conducted to study the morphology and protein expressions of SGNs for the $Nefl^{CreER/+}$;iDTR$^{+/-}$ offspring at the end of the experiment. It was observed that SGNs expressed neuronal proteins Nefl and TUJ1 in the P7, P14, and P21 groups (**Figures 4A–C**). In the quantitative study, the number of Nefl-expressing cells was consistent in vehicle-treated groups, whereas it decreased in the P7, P14, and P21 groups treated with DT (**Figure 4D**). In vehicle-treated mice, the average numbers of Nefl-expressing cells per 10^4 μm^2 were 30.6 ± 5.0, 31.1 ± 4.3, and 31.4 ± 5.0 for the P7, P14, and P21 groups, respectively. In DT-treated groups, the average numbers of Nefl-expressing cells per 10^4 μm^2 were 12.9 ± 3.0, 19.0 ± 3.1, and 17.9 ± 2.8 for the P7, P14, and P21 groups, respectively. In the statistical analysis, two-way ANOVA and *post-hoc* tests were performed with two factors: treatment type (vehicle and DT) and treatment age (P7, P14, and

Generation of a Spiral Ganglion Neuron Degeneration Mouse Model

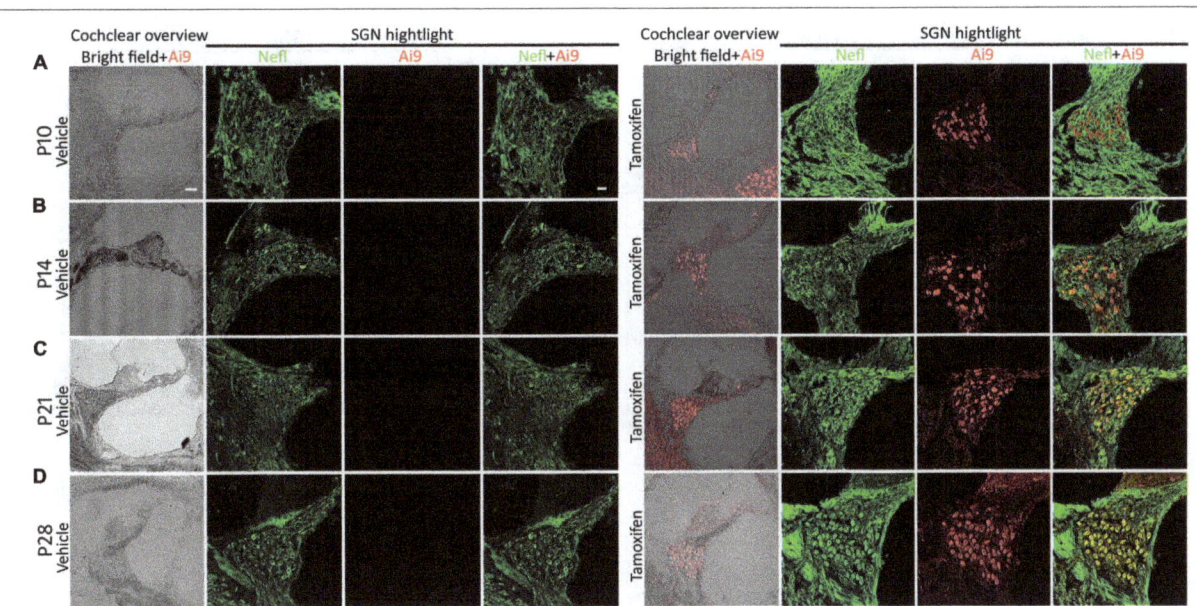

FIGURE 2 | Cre activity of $Nefl^{CreER/+}$ mice. $Nefl^{CreER/CreER}$ mice were crossed with a reporter strain, Ai9, to obtain heterozygous $Nefl^{CreER/+}$;Ai9$^{+/-}$ mice, which were treated with tamoxifen or vehicle on postnatal day 1 (P1) for 4–5 consecutive days. The pups were euthanized on P10 **(A)**, P14 **(B)**, P21 **(C)**, and P28 **(D)**. In the vehicle group, no significant Ai9 tdTomato fluorescence was observed in the cochlear overview or spiral ganglion neuron (SGN) area highlight. However, robust Ai9 tdTomato fluorescence was identified in the cochlear overview and SGN area highlight in heterozygote mice treated with tamoxifen. In the SGN area, Ai9 tdTomato fluorescence was co-labeled with Nefl immunofluorescence in the tamoxifen groups, whereas only Nefl immunofluorescence was observed in the vehicle groups **(A–D)**, suggesting tamoxifen-induced Cre activity of $Nefl^{CreER/+}$;Ai9$^{+/-}$ mouse SGNs. *Scale*, 50 μm in cochlear overview and 20 μm in SGN highlight.

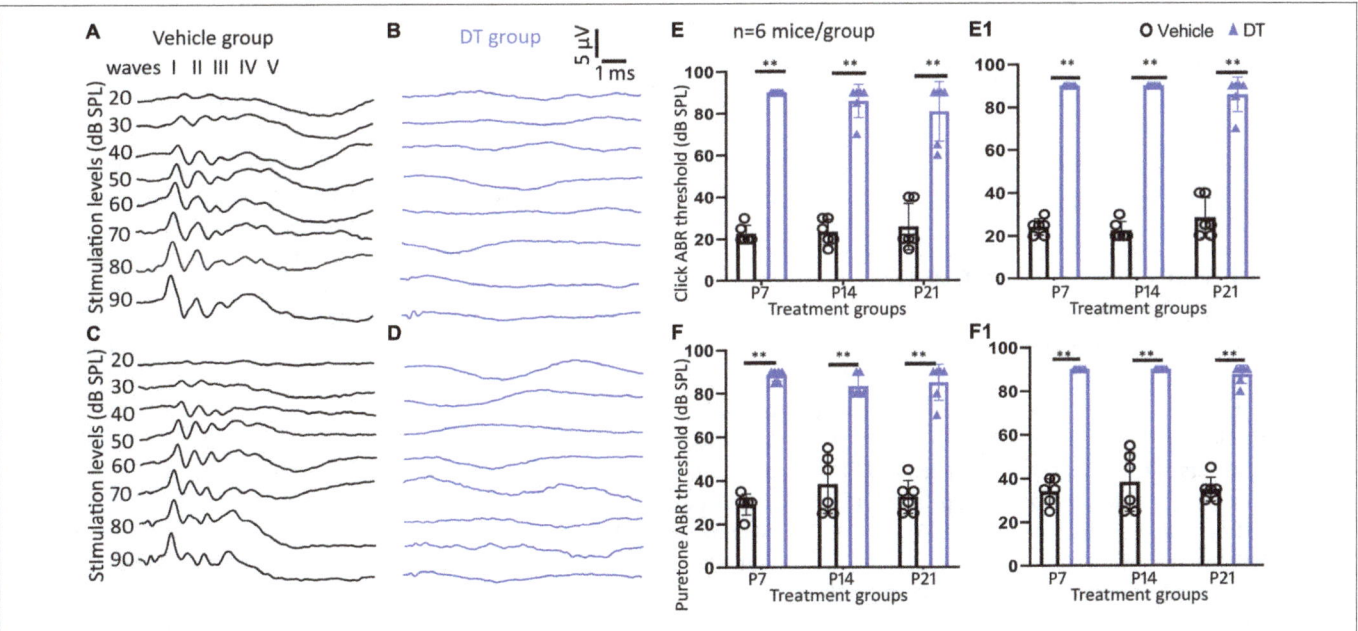

FIGURE 3 | Auditory brainstem response (ABR) measurement study. Representative ABR waveforms of the vehicle and diphtheria toxin (DT) groups are shown in **(A–D)**. ABR was tested on 4- **(A,B)** and 5-week-old **(C,D)** $Nefl^{CreER/+}$;iDTR$^{+/-}$ mice that were treated with tamoxifen on P1–P5, followed by either vehicle **(A,C)** or DT **(B,D)** treatment. Quantitative analysis shows significant differences in click **(E,E1)** and pure tone (16 kHz) **(F,F1)** between the DT and vehicle groups in the P7, P14, and P21 treatment groups in the measurements at both 4 **(E,F)** and 5 weeks old **(E1,F1)**. **$p < 0.01$ (ANOVA, $n = 6$ mice per group).

P21; $n = 6$ mice per group). The overall and the treatment age effects were not statistically significant [$F_{(2,30)} = 3.065, p = 0.0916$, and $F_{(2,30)} = 1.677, p = 0.2355$, respectively]. However, the effect of treatment type (vehicle vs. DT) was statistically significant [$F_{(1,30)} = 80.64, p = 0.0003$]. In the *post-hoc* comparison of the vehicle and DT groups, significant differences were observed

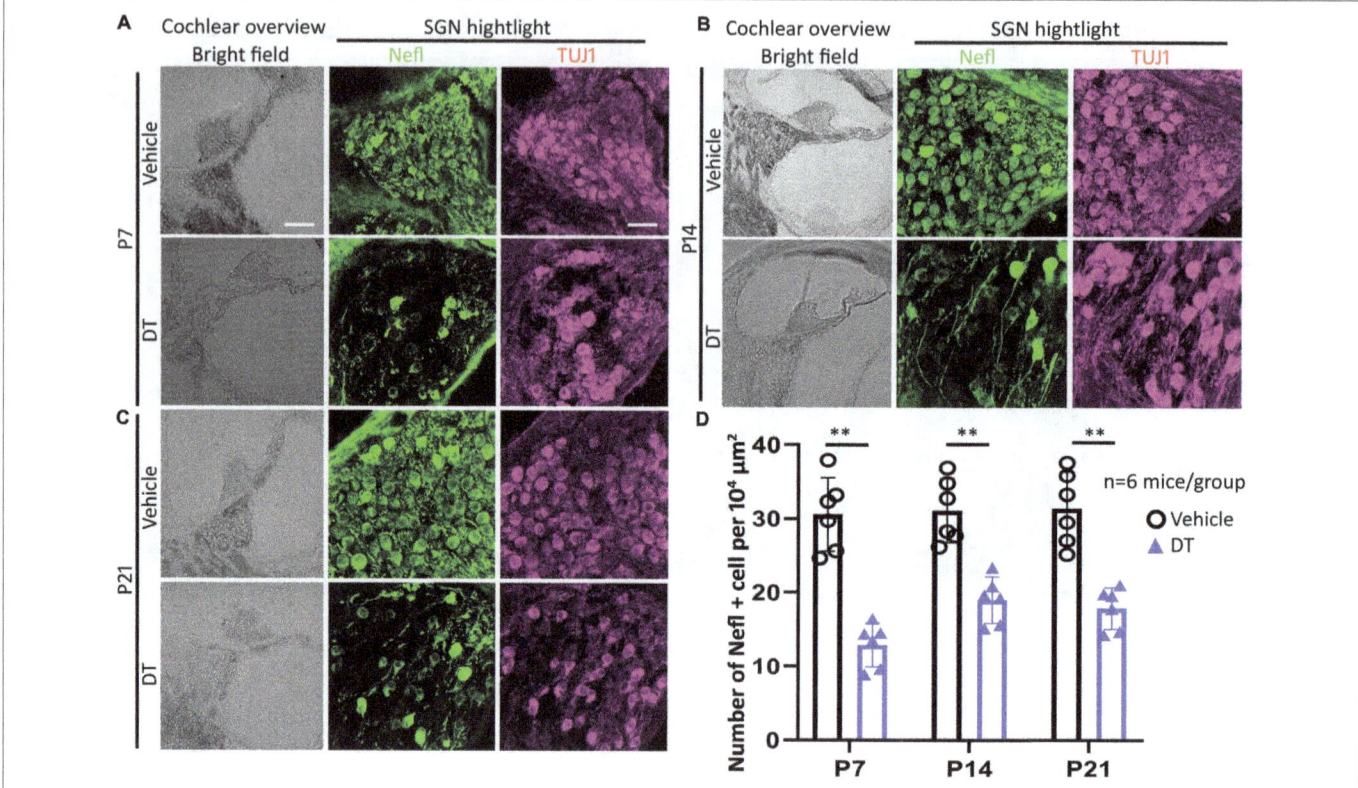

FIGURE 4 | Spiral ganglion neuron (SGN) study of $Nefl^{CreER/+}$;iDTR$^{+/-}$ mice. $Nefl^{CreER/+}$;iDTR$^{+/-}$ mice were treated with tamoxifen, followed by diphtheria toxin (DT) or vehicle treatment on P7 **(A)**, P14 **(B)**, and P21 **(C)**. Nefl and TUJ1 immunofluorescence was used to identify SGNs. In the quantitative study **(D)**, significantly decreased numbers of Nefl-expressing SGNs were observed in the DT treatment groups, including the P7, P14, and P21 groups. **$p < 0.01$ (ANOVA, $n = 6$ mice per group). *Scale*, 100 μm in cochlear overview and 25 μm in SGN highlight.

($p = 0.0002$, 0.0042, and 0.0018 for the P7, P14, and P21 groups, respectively) (**Figure 4**).

Hair Cell Function and Protein Expression Study

To evaluate the hair cell function of the $Nefl^{CreER/+}$;iDTR$^{+/-}$ offspring, DPOAE was performed. The DPOAE thresholds were determined in the P14 and P21 groups at 4 weeks old (**Figure 5A**). In the statistical analysis using two-way ANOVA, the overall and individual effects of treatment type (vehicle vs. DT) and treatment age (P14 vs. P21; $n = 6$ mice per group) at 16-kHz stimulation were not statistically significant ($p > 0.05$): $p = 0.9108$, 0.6062, and 0.1360 for the overall, treatment type, and treatment age effects, respectively (**Figure 5A1**). In the analysis of the 24-kHz stimulation, these numbers became $p = 0.2640$, 0.1601, and 0.9175, respectively (**Figure 5A2**). These data suggest that the DPOAE thresholds were not significantly different between the DT and vehicle groups.

In the hair cell protein expression study, anti-myosin VIIa antibodies were used to identify hair cells using the basilar membrane surface preparation for the P14 group (**Figure 5B**). In the quantification study, the average numbers of inner hair cells were 11.9 ± 0.96 and 11.1 ± 1.5 per 100 μm for the vehicle and DT groups, whereas the numbers for outer hair cells were 35.4 ± 2.87 and 33.4 ± 4.42, respectively (**Figure 5B1**). Statistical analysis showed no significant difference between the vehicle and DT groups (ANOVA, $n = 5$ mice per group): the p-values were 0.9138 and 0.4626 for inner and outer hair cells, respectively.

These data show that hair cell number and function were not statistically different between the DT and vehicle groups, suggesting no hair cell damage was observed in this animal model.

DISCUSSION

In this study, it was found that $Nefl^{CreER/CreER}$ mice exhibited Cre activity during the postnatal period from P1 to P28. When bred with iDTR mouse, the offspring $Nefl^{CreER/+}$;iDTR$^{+/-}$ were responsive to DT treatment and demonstrated damage specific to SGNs in the cochlea on P7–P21, which was indicated by the functional ABR test and SGN cell counts. DPOAE and cell counting suggest that hair cells were not affected following DT treatment. These data indicate that the SGNs of $Nefl^{CreER/+}$;iDTR$^{+/-}$ mice could be specifically damaged by DT treatment in the cochlea.

Nefl encodes Nefl, which is expressed in developing and mature neurons, including SGNs (Torkos et al., 2008; Sun et al., 2018). A previous study has shown that the $Nefl^{CreER/+}$ mouse

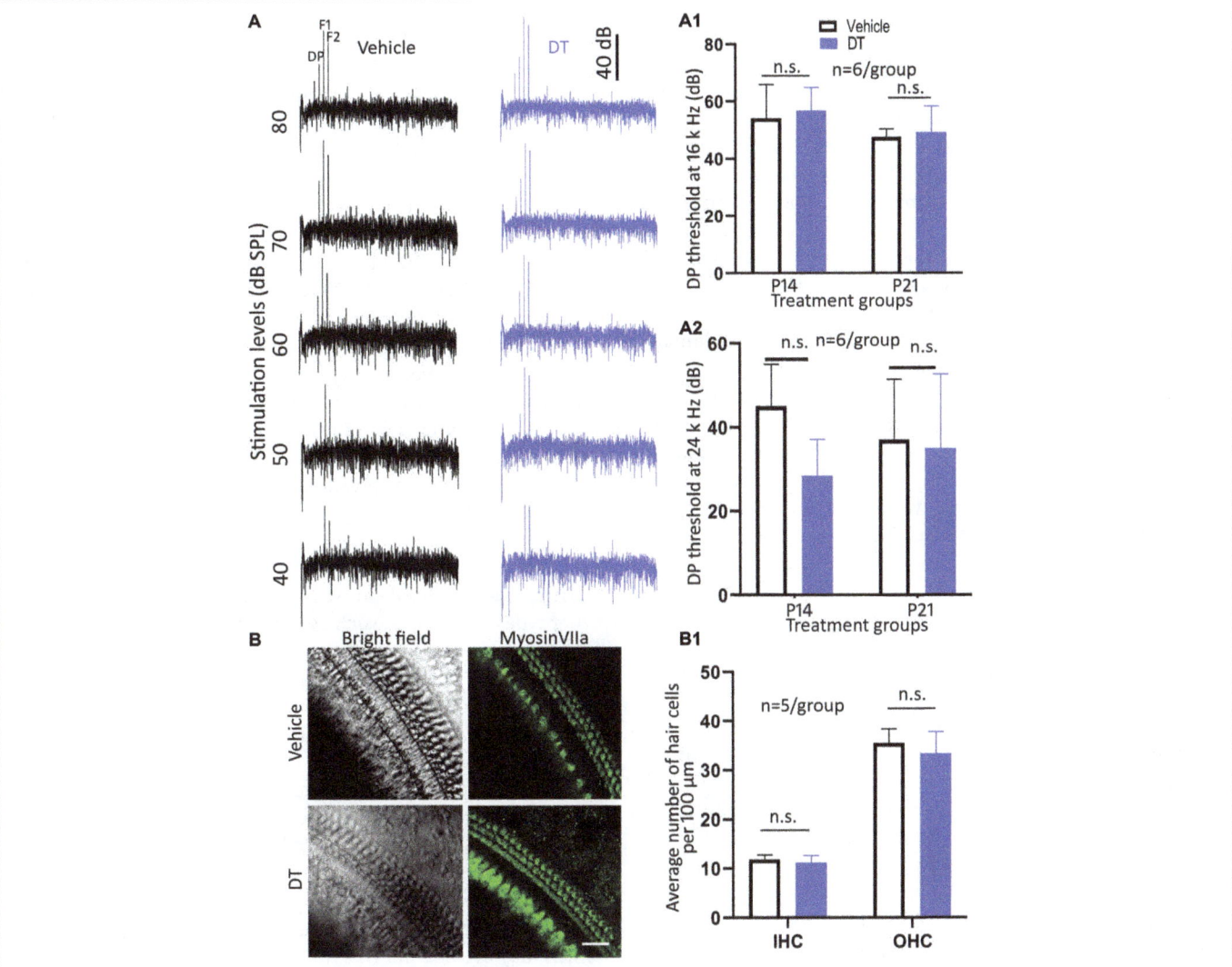

FIGURE 5 | Hair cell protein expression and distortion product otoacoustic emission (DPOAE) study. Representative DPOAE waveforms of $Nefl^{CreER/+}$;$iDTR^{+/-}$ mice treated with either diphtheria toxin (DT) or vehicle are shown in **(A)**. In the quantitative study, DPOAE measurements at 4 weeks old did not show a significant difference between the DT and vehicle treatments at 16 **(A1)** or 24 kHz **(A2)** in the P14 or P21 groups (two-way ANOVA: $p > 0.05$, $n = 6$ mice/group). In the surface preparation of $Nefl^{CreER/+}$;$iDTR^{+/-}$ mice treated with either DT or vehicle on P14, the numbers of myosin VIIa-expressing cells are statistically insignificant (**B,B1**; ANOVA: $p > 0.05$, $n = 5$ mice/group). n.s. statistically insignificant. Scale, 25 μm in **(B)**.

strain shows neuronal-specific Cre activity in the central nervous system (Rotolo et al., 2008). However, the auditory system Cre activity of this mouse strain has not been determined. In this study, $Nefl^{CreER/CreER}$ mice were crossed with a reporter mouse strain, the Ai9 mouse, to obtain $Nefl^{CreER/+}$;$Ai9^{+/-}$ offspring in order to determine the Cre activity in the auditory system. Tamoxifen was administered to the offspring via feeding from dams that had been gavaged with tamoxifen. It was found that tamoxifen-treated $Nefl^{CreER/+}$;$Ai9^{+/-}$ pups showed robust Ai9 tdTomato fluorescence in the SGN area and the nerve projections, whereas vehicle-treated $Nefl^{CreER/+}$;$Ai9^{+/-}$ pups did not show Ai9 fluorescence. The Ai9 fluorescence totally overlapped with Nefl immunofluorescence. Additionally, tamoxifen-treated mice showed Cre activity during the postnatal period, from P1 to P28. These data are consistent with previous reports of Cre activity in central nervous system neurons (Rotolo et al., 2008). Importantly, the Cre activity is robustly inducible for at least 28 days after birth, which is useful for the generation of a postnatal and young adult SGN damage model using the iDTR transgenic mouse model.

It is known that the hearing onset of mouse is around postnatal days 12–14 (Ehret, 1976; Kamiya et al., 2001; Romand, 2003) and SGN development and subtype characterization progress during the postnatal period up to P28 (Shrestha et al., 2018; Sun et al., 2018). A previous study has reported on an SGN damage model following DT treatment on P21 (Pan et al., 2017). Whether SGNs respond to damage in the pre-hearing and hearing onset periods remains unclear. To generate a specific SGN damage model, in the present study, homozygous $Nefl^{CreER/CreER}$ mice were crossed with iDTR mice, and the heterozygous offspring were exposed to either DT or vehicle on P7, P14, and P21. Nefl and TUJ1 immunostaining was used to evaluate the expressions of the neuronal proteins of SGNs, and Nefl-expressing cells were used to quantitatively examine the number of surviving SGNs. It was found that approximately 58, 39, and 43% SGNs were damaged in the P7, P14, and P21 groups, respectively. In a previous study, roughly 30–40% of SGN loss was observed 7 days post-DT injection in the SGN-damaged Cre-positive group (Pan et al., 2017). In the present study, the SGN loss at 2–3 weeks post-DT treatment in the P14 and P21 groups was similar to that in the previous study using a different Cre mouse strain, the $Bhlhb5^{CreER/+}$ mouse strain. However, the SGN loss at 4 weeks post-DT treatment in the P7 group was approximately 58%, which was significantly larger than that in the P14 and P21 groups. The difference may be related to the treatment time, and the pre-hearing damage to the SGN on P7 may have caused more severe neuronal degeneration than did post-hearing insults. The follow-up time post-DT treatment may have also contributed to the different damage levels, which may require additional experiments in our future studies. These data suggest that DT treatment on P7 at the pre-hearing stage may cause a more significant SGN loss.

In the functional assays, click and pure tone ABR tests were performed to evaluate the function of the auditory system at 4 and 5 weeks old. Compared to vehicle-treated groups, significant click ABR threshold shifts (>50–60 dB SPL) were observed in DT-treated animals in the P7, P14, and P21 groups. In the pure tone ABR test at 16 kHz, the threshold shifts between the DT- and vehicle-treated animals were around 50–55 dB SPL in the P7, P14, and P21 groups. These results were different from those of a previous study, in which the ABR thresholds largely overlapped in the presence and absence of Cre activity following DT treatment using $Bhlhb5^{CreER/+}$;iDTR mice. The reason for this discrepancy is unclear. One possibility might be attributed to the neuronal gene that mediates the Cre activity. The $Bhlhb5$ gene was used to mediate Cre activity in the previous report, whereas the $Nefl$ gene was selected for the current study. $Nefl$ is robustly expressed along the nerve projections of bipolar SGNs, and Cre-mediated iDTR-positive nerve projections may have been significantly damaged in response to DT treatment, which may have caused SGN–hair cell disconnection and subsequent hearing threshold changes. Further research may be required to understand the ABR threshold shifts in this mouse strain. In the meantime, these functional data show that significant hearing function changes can be achieved following DT treatment using the $Nefl^{CreER/CreER}$ mouse strain, which may serve as a useful animal model for SGN degeneration study.

Hair cell protein expression and DPOAE tests were used to evaluate whether hair cells are affected in the $Nefl^{CreER/+}$;iDTR$^{+/-}$ mouse strain in this study. It was found that the DPOAE thresholds were statistically insignificant between the DT and vehicle groups, suggesting that the outer hair cell function is not compromised following DT treatment. In hair cell protein expression and hair cell counting using basilar membrane surface preparation, both inner and outer hair cells expressed the hair cell protein myosin VIIa in the DT and vehicle groups. In cell counting, no significant difference was identified between the vehicle and DT groups, suggesting that hair cell loss was not observed. These functional, protein expression, and morphology data suggest that hair cells were not affected post-DT treatment in the $Nefl^{CreER/+}$;iDTR$^{+/-}$ mouse model.

In summary, inducible $Nefl$-CreER-mediated Cre activity was identified in $Nefl^{CreER/+}$;Ai9$^{+/-}$ mouse SGNs for at least 28 days after birth. When crossed with an iDTR mouse strain, the offspring $Nefl^{CreER/+}$;iDTR$^{+/-}$ showed SGN loss following a single dose of DT injection. Compared to vehicle-treated mice, both SGN number and ABR thresholds were significantly changed in DT-injected $Nefl^{CreER/+}$;iDTR$^{+/-}$ mice. The inner and outer hair cell numbers and the DPOAE thresholds were not significantly changed between the DT- and vehicle-treated groups. These data suggest that DT treatment can specifically target SGNs of the postnatal $Nefl^{CreER/+}$;iDTR$^{+/-}$ mouse model in the cochlea.

There are some limitations to this SGN damage model. The present study focused on SGN evaluation, whereas damage to other types of neurons, such as the central auditory neurons, has not been determined. Additionally, this report focused on SGN damage assays before, around, and after hearing onset, while SGN damage of mature mice has not been identified. These limitations should be addressed in future independent experiments. Taken together, this report identified a mouse model with inducible damage specific to the neuronal lineage in the cochlea, which can be used to further characterize primary SGN degeneration without interfering with hair cells. The mouse model reported in this study may prove to be a powerful mammalian model to investigate the development of postnatal SGNs, degeneration of SGNs, prevention of SGN damage, and regeneration of SGNs, which may provide insights into SGN research in the future.

ETHICS STATEMENT

The animal study was reviewed and approved by the Institutional Animal Care and Use Committee (IACUC) at Wayne State University.

AUTHOR CONTRIBUTIONS

ZH designed the project. ZH, FK, AS, and MD performed the experiment, analyzed the data, and wrote the manuscript. All authors contributed to the article and approved the submitted version.

ACKNOWLEDGMENTS

We thank Li Tian and Janice Gibbons for technical support and for the myosin VIIa antibody from the Developmental Studies Hybridoma Bank (DSHB).

REFERENCES

Breglio, A. M., Rusheen, A. E., Shide, E. D., Fernandez, K. A., Spielbauer, K. K., McLachlin, K. M., et al. (2017). Cisplatin is retained in the cochlea indefinitely following chemotherapy. *Nat. Commun.* 8:1654. doi: 10.1038/s41467-017-01837-1

Buch, T., Heppner, F. L., Tertilt, C., Heinen, T. J., Kremer, M., Wunderlich, F. T., et al. (2005). A Cre-inducible diphtheria toxin receptor mediates cell lineage ablation after toxin administration. *Nat. Methods* 2, 419–426. doi: 10.1038/nmeth762

Carignano, C., Barila, E. P., Rías, E. I., Dionisio, L., Aztiria, E., and Spitzmaul, G. (2019). Inner hair cell and neuron degeneration contribute to hearing loss in a DFNA2-like mouse model. *Neuroscience* 410, 202–216. doi: 10.1016/j.neuroscience.2019.05.012

Dallos, P., and Harris, D. (1978). Properties of auditory nerve responses in absence of outer hair cells. *J. Neurophysiol.* 41, 365–383. doi: 10.1152/jn.1978.41.2.365

Deng, X., and Hu, Z. (2020). Generation of cochlear hair cells from Sox2 positive supporting cells via DNA demethylation. *Int. J. Mol. Sci.* 21:8649. doi: 10.3390/ijms21228649

Deng, X., Liu, Z., Li, X., Zhou, Y., and Hu, Z. (2019). Generation of new hair cells by DNA methyltransferase (Dnmt) inhibitor 5-azacytidine in a chemically-deafened mouse model. *Sci. Rep.* 9:7997. doi: 10.1038/s41598-019-44313-0

Echteler, S. M. (1992). Developmental segregation in the afferent projections to mammalian auditory hair cells. *Proc. Natl. Acad. Sci. U.S.A.* 89, 6324–6327. doi: 10.1073/pnas.89.14.6324

Ehret, G. (1976). Development of absolute auditory thresholds in the house mouse (*Mus musculus*). *J. Am. Audiol. Soc.* 1, 179–184.

Fang, J., Zhang, W. C., Yamashita, T., Gao, J., Zhu, M. S., and Zuo, J. (2012). Outer hair cell-specific prestin-CreERT2 knockin mouse lines. *Genesis* 50, 124–131. doi: 10.1002/dvg.20810

Hu, Z., Liu, Z., Li, X., and Deng, X. (2017). Stimulation of synapse formation between stem cell-derived neurons and native brainstem auditory neurons. *Sci. Rep.* 7:13843. doi: 10.1038/s41598-017-13764-8

Hu, Z., Tao, L., and Deng, M. (2021). Postnatal changes of neural stem cells in the mammalian auditory cortex. *Int. J. Mol. Sci.* 22:1550. doi: 10.3390/ijms22041550

Hu, Z., Tao, L., Liu, Z., Jiang, Y., and Deng, X. (2019). Identification of neural stem cells from postnatal mouse auditory cortex in vitro. *Stem Cells Dev.* 28, 860–870. doi: 10.1089/scd.2018.0247

Hu, Z., Ulfendahl, M., and Olivius, N. P. (2004). Central migration of neuronal tissue and embryonic stem cells following transplantation along the adult auditory nerve. *Brain Res.* 1026, 68–73. doi: 10.1016/j.brainres.2004.08.013

Hu, Z., Ulfendahl, M., Prieskorn, D. M., Olivius, P., and Miller, J. M. (2009). Functional evaluation of a cell replacement therapy in the inner ear. *Otol. Neurotol.* 30, 551–558. doi: 10.1097/MAO.0b013e31819fe70a

Illing, R. B. (2001). Activity-dependent plasticity in the adult auditory brainstem. *Audiol. Neurootol.* 6, 319–345. doi: 10.1159/000046844

Jahn, H. M., Kasakow, C. V., Helfer, A., Michely, J., Verkhratsky, A., Maurer, H. H., et al. (2018). Refined protocols of tamoxifen injection for inducible DNA recombination in mouse astroglia. *Sci. Rep.* 8:5913. doi: 10.1038/s41598-018-24085-9

Johnsson, L. G. (1974). Sequence of degeneration of Corti's organ and its first-order neurons. *Ann. Otol. Rhinol. Laryngol.* 83, 294–303. doi: 10.1177/000348947408300303

Kamiya, K., Takahashi, K., Kitamura, K., Momoi, T., and Yoshikawa, Y. (2001). Mitosis and apoptosis in postnatal auditory system of the C3H/He strain. *Brain Res.* 901, 296–302. doi: 10.1016/S0006-8993(01)02300-9

Koundakjian, E. J., Appler, J. L., and Goodrich, L. V. (2007). Auditory neurons make stereotyped wiring decisions before maturation of their targets. *J. Neurosci.* 27, 14078–14088. doi: 10.1523/JNEUROSCI.3765-07.2007

Li, X., Aleardi, A., Wang, J., Zhou, Y., Andrade, R., and Hu, Z. (2016). Differentiation of spiral ganglion-derived neural stem cells into functional synaptogenetic neurons. *Stem Cells Dev.* 25, 803–813. doi: 10.1089/scd.2015.0345

Liem, R. K. (1993). Molecular biology of neuronal intermediate filaments. *Curr. Opin. Cell Biol.* 5, 12–16. doi: 10.1016/S0955-0674(05)80003-1

Liu, Q., Xie, F., Siedlak, S. L., Nunomura, A., Honda, K., Moreira, P. I., et al. (2004). Neurofilament proteins in neurodegenerative diseases. *Cell. Mol. Life Sci.* 61, 3057–3075. doi: 10.1007/s00018-004-4268-8

Liu, Z., Jiang, Y., Li, X., and Hu, Z. (2018). Embryonic stem cell-derived peripheral auditory neurons form neural connections with mouse central auditory neurons in vitro via the alpha2delta1 receptor. *Stem Cell Rep.* 11, 157–170. doi: 10.1016/j.stemcr.2018.05.006

Madisen, L., Zwingman, T. A., Sunkin, S. M., Oh, S. W., Zariwala, H. A., Gu, H., et al. (2010). A robust and high-throughput Cre reporting and characterization system for the whole mouse brain. *Nat. Neurosci.* 13, 133–140. doi: 10.1038/nn.2467

Majumder, P., Moore, P. A., Richardson, G. P., and Gale, J. E. (2017). Protecting mammalian hair cells from aminoglycoside-toxicity: assessing phenoxybenzamine's potential. *Front. Cell. Neurosci.* 11:94. doi: 10.3389/fncel.2017.00094

Nakamura, E., Nguyen, M. T., and Mackem, S. (2006). Kinetics of tamoxifen-regulated Cre activity in mice using a cartilage-specific CreER(T) to assay temporal activity windows along the proximodistal limb skeleton. *Dev. Dyn.* 235, 2603–2612. doi: 10.1002/dvdy.20892

Nayagam, B. A., Muniak, M. A., and Ryugo, D. K. (2011). The spiral ganglion: connecting the peripheral and central auditory systems. *Hear. Res.* 278, 2–20. doi: 10.1016/j.heares.2011.04.003

Pan, H., Song, Q., Huang, Y., Wang, J., Chai, R., Yin, S., et al. (2017). Auditory neuropathy after damage to cochlear spiral ganglion neurons in mice resulting from conditional expression of diphtheria toxin receptors. *Sci. Rep.* 7:6409. doi: 10.1038/s41598-017-06600-6

Romand, R. (2003). The roles of retinoic acid during inner ear development. *Curr. Top. Dev. Biol.* 57, 261–291. doi: 10.1016/S0070-2153(03)57009-0

Rotheneichner, P., Romanelli, P., Bieler, L., Pagitsch, S., Zaunmair, P., Kreutzer, C., et al. (2017). Tamoxifen activation of cre-recombinase has no persisting effects on adult neurogenesis or learning and anxiety. *Front. Neurosci.* 11:27. doi: 10.3389/fnins.2017.00027

Rotolo, T., Smallwood, P. M., Williams, J., and Nathans, J. (2008). Genetically-directed, cell type-specific sparse labeling for the analysis of neuronal morphology. *PLoS One* 3:e4099. doi: 10.1371/journal.pone.0004099

Shrestha, B. R., Chia, C., Wu, L., Kujawa, S. G., Liberman, M. C., and Goodrich, L. V. (2018). Sensory neuron diversity in the inner ear is shaped by activity. *Cell* 174, 1229–1246.e17. doi: 10.1016/j.cell.2018.07.007

Sun, S., Babola, T., Pregernig, G., So, K. S., Nguyen, M., Su, S. M., et al. (2018). Hair cell mechanotransduction regulates spontaneous activity and spiral ganglion subtype specification in the auditory system. *Cell* 174, 1247–1263.e15. doi: 10.1016/j.cell.2018.07.008

Torkos, A., Wissel, K., Warnecke, A., Lenarz, T., and Stöver, T. (2008). Technical report: laser microdissection and pressure catapulting is superior to conventional manual dissection for isolating pure spiral ganglion fractions from the cochlea. *Hear. Res.* 235, 8–14. doi: 10.1016/j.heares.2007.09.004

Wu, P. Z., O'Malley, J. T., de Gruttola, V., and Liberman, M. C. (2021). Primary neural degeneration in noise-exposed human cochleas: correlations with outer hair cell loss and word-discrimination scores. *J. Neurosci.* 41, 4439–4447. doi: 10.1523/JNEUROSCI.3238-20.2021

Ylikoski, J., Pirvola, U., Virkkala, J., Suvanto, P., Liang, X. Q., Magal, E., et al. (1998). Guinea pig auditory neurons are protected by glial cell line-derived growth factor from degeneration after noise trauma. *Hear. Res.* 124, 17–26. doi: 10.1016/S0378-5955(98)00095-1

Zhang, L., Jiang, H., and Hu, Z. (2011). Concentration-dependent effect of nerve growth factor on cell fate determination of neural progenitors. *Stem Cells Dev.* 20, 1723–1731. doi: 10.1089/scd.2010.0370

Zhong, Z., Fu, X., Li, H., Chen, J., Wang, M., Gao, S., et al. (2020). Citicoline protects auditory hair cells against neomycin-induced damage. *Front. Cell. Dev. Biol.* 8:712. doi: 10.3389/fcell.2020.00712

Cochlear Sox2+ Glial Cells are Potent Progenitors for Spiral Ganglion Neuron Reprogramming Induced by Small Molecules

Zhen Chen[1], Yuhang Huang[1], Chaorong Yu[1], Qing Liu[1], Cui Qiu[1] and Guoqiang Wan[1,2,3,4]*

[1] MOE Key Laboratory of Model Animal for Disease Study, Department of Otorhinolaryngology Head and Neck Surgery, The Affiliated Drum Tower Hospital of Medical School, Model Animal Research Center of Medical School, Nanjing University, Nanjing, China, [2] Research Institute of Otolaryngology, Nanjing, China, [3] Jiangsu Key Laboratory of Molecular Medicine, Medical School of Nanjing University, Nanjing, China, [4] Institute for Brain Sciences, Nanjing University, Nanjing, China

*Correspondence:
Guoqiang Wan
guoqiangwan@nju.edu.cn

In the mammalian cochlea, spiral ganglion neurons (SGNs) relay the acoustic information to the central auditory circuits. Degeneration of SGNs is a major cause of sensorineural hearing loss and severely affects the effectiveness of cochlear implant therapy. Cochlear glial cells are able to form spheres and differentiate into neurons *in vitro*. However, the identity of these progenitor cells is elusive, and it is unclear how to differentiate these cells toward functional SGNs. In this study, we found that Sox2+ subpopulation of cochlear glial cells preserves high potency of neuronal differentiation. Interestingly, Sox2 expression was downregulated during neuronal differentiation and Sox2 overexpression paradoxically inhibited neuronal differentiation. Our data suggest that Sox2+ glial cells are potent SGN progenitor cells, a phenotype independent of Sox2 expression. Furthermore, we identified a combination of small molecules that not only promoted neuronal differentiation of Sox2− glial cells, but also removed glial cell identity and promoted the maturation of the induced neurons (iNs) toward SGN fate. In summary, we identified Sox2+ glial subpopulation with high neuronal potency and small molecules inducing neuronal differentiation toward SGNs.

Keywords: Sox2+ glial cells, glia-to-neuron conversion, small molecules reprogramming, SGN regeneration, lineage tracing

INTRODUCTION

In the mammalian cochlea, the spiral ganglion neurons (SGNs) relay the acoustic information from inner hair cells (IHCs) to the central auditory circuits (Fettiplace, 2017). SGNs are essential for normal hearing and communication, and degeneration causes sensorineural hearing loss (Sun et al., 2016; Liu et al., 2019; Zhao et al., 2019). Degeneration of SGN nerve terminals or cell bodies can be caused by ototoxicity, noise, or aging (Lang et al., 2005; Bao and Ohlemiller, 2010; Fryatt et al., 2011; Liberman, 2017; Vlajkovic et al., 2017). Because the SGNs lack the ability to regenerate in mammals, damages to the SGNs lead to permanent hearing impairment (Guo et al., 2016, 2020, 2021; Yan et al., 2018; Liu et al., 2021). In addition, the effectiveness of hearing aids and cochlear implants relies on the health and numbers of intact SGNs (Muller and Barr-Gillespie, 2015). If SGNs could be replaced or regenerated, it might be possible to restore the hearing of patients with severely damaged SGNs (Meas et al., 2018b) and benefit individuals treated with hearing aids and cochlear implants.

At the early stage of SGN damage which precedes neuronal cell body degeneration, neurotrophic factors such as neurotrophin 3 (NT3), brain-derived neurotrophic factor (BDNF), and glial-derived neurotrophic factor (GDNF) are used to support the survival of SGNs and their neurite outgrowth to the sensory HCs (Wise et al., 2011; Suzuki et al., 2016; Akil et al., 2019). However, therapeutic strategies are limited to generate induced neurons (iNs) to replace the SGNs once they are lost and SGN regeneration remains a major challenge.

Multiple attempts have been made to replace and regenerate SGNs, including transplantations of iNs differentiated from embryonic stem cells (ESC) or iPSC-derived progenitors (Chen et al., 2012; Koehler et al., 2013; Perny et al., 2017), or neuronal differentiation of cochlear-resident multipotent stem cells/progenitor cells to SGNs (Oshima et al., 2007; Zhang et al., 2011; Diensthuber et al., 2014a,b; Li et al., 2016; McLean et al., 2016; Noda et al., 2018). For induced differentiation of ESC or iPSC-derived progenitors, three-dimensional culture systems have been used to convert mouse ESC into hair cells, supporting cells, and neuronal cells (Koehler et al., 2013; Perny et al., 2017). hESC differentiated into neuronal cells expressed specific neuronal markers with electrophysiological properties characteristic of auditory neurons (Chen et al., 2012). However, transplantation of ESC-derived iNs is hampered by immuno-rejection, tumorigenesis, SGN maturation and functional integration (Lee et al., 2013; Lukovic et al., 2014).

Alternatively, inner ear-resident cells, such as progenitor cells within the utricle (Li et al., 2003) or in the spiral ganglion region (Oshima et al., 2007; Zhang et al., 2011; Li et al., 2016; McLean et al., 2016), could also be induced to neuron-like cells, forming neurites, developing synapses and expressing neuronal markers *in vitro*. It has been reported that $Plp1^+$ glial cells were cochlear-resident multipotent stem cells/progenitor cells (McLean et al., 2016). Induced neuronal reprogramming of these cochlear-resident progenitors have several advantages over cell transplantations such as enhanced cell survival, physiological relevance of cellular localization and ease of maturation due to lineage similarities. However, $Plp1^+$ glial cells may include heterogenous cell subpopulation. The identity of these progenitor cells is elusive, and it is unclear how to induce these cells to functional SGNs post-injury both *in vitro* and *in vivo*.

In this study, we found that $Sox2^+$ subpopulation of cochlear glial cells preserves high potency of neuronal differentiation and identified a combination of small molecules promoted the maturation of the iNs toward SGNs fate. Together, we found that cochlear $Sox2^+$ glial cells subpopulation is highly potent in neuronal differentiation and identified small molecules promoting both neuronal differentiation efficiency and maturity toward the SGN fate.

MATERIALS AND METHODS

Animals
$Plp1^{CreERT}$ (stock number 005975), $Sox2^{CreERT}$, (stock number 017593) lines were obtained from Jackson laboratory and crossed with Rosa26-LSL-Cas9-tdTomato (NBRI T002249) mice obtained from Gempharmatech Inc., China. Scrt2-P2A-tdTomato mice were generated as previously reported (Li C. et al., 2020). Mice were injected i.p. with Tamoxifen (Sigma, T5648) at 33 mg/kg for postnatal mice (P1–P3) and 50 mg/kg for juvenile mice (P17–P20). Tamoxifen was dissolved in corn oil.

All mice used in this work were on a mixed background containing C57BL6 and FVB/N strains. Both male and female mice were used. All animal procedures were approved by the Institutional Animal Care and Use Committee of Model Animal Research Center of Nanjing University.

Cell Culture
Both sexes of the 6–8 postnatal 4–21 days (P4–P21) mice spiral ganglia were dissected in HBSS (Invitrogen 14065056) at pH 7.4 on ice for tissue harvesting. The stria vascularis, vestibule and the organ of Corti were removed carefully with forceps (Dumont) to dissect the modiolus. The modiolus were digested with Trypsin/EDTA (Sigma 59418C) and DNase I (20 U/ml) at 37°C in a total volume of 50 μl for ~15 min with shaking at 300 rpm/min (Thermo) in 1.5 ml EP tube. Dissociation was terminated by adding 0.4 ml SCM media containing DMEM/F12 (HyClone 36254) supplemented with B27 (Thermo 17504044) and N2 (Thermo 17502048) supplement, 20 ng/ml EGF (Peprotech 315-09), 10 ng/ml bFGF (Peprotech 450-33), 50 ng/ml IGF (Peprotech 250-19), and 50 ng/ml heparan sulfate (MCE HY-101916). The samples were then carefully triturated with 1 ml pipette tips and next with 200 μl tips, followed by suspension with 1 ml SCM medium.

The cell suspension was then passed through a 70-μm cell strainer, and spun at 300 g for 5–10 min. A small white cell pellet should be observed at the bottom and then carefully aspirate the supernatant. SCM medium were added to resuspend and count cells, and then 200,000–240,000 cells were plated in each well of the six-well dish (Corning 3471). For propagation, the cochlear glial spheres were harvested after 5–7 days and passaged for 3–4 generations.

For P21 mice, the modiolus were calcified and the cochlear glial cells decrease the potential to form spheres. P21 modiolus were digested with Trypsin/EDTA (Sigma 59418C) and DNase I (20 U/ml) at 37°C in a total volume of 50–100 μl for ~20 min with shaking 300 rpm/min (Thermo) in 1.5 ml EP tube. We used culture media contains DMEM/F12, 10% FBS, B27 in 2D dish (Lang et al., 2011). Firstly, culture media was added to stop trypsin reaction. Tissues were triturated with pipet tips and centrifuged at 300 × *g* for 5–10 min. The pellet was resuspended in culture media and filtered through a 70 μm cell strainer. Cells were counted, plated and grown to full confluency (5–7 days). Media was then removed and replaced with SCM media for suspension culture.

Neuronal Differentiation
To induce neuronal differentiation, cochlear glial spheres were plated on 96-well plate (Thermo 310109008) or glass slides (Thermo Fisher 12-545-80) coated with Poly-L-ornithine (Sigma P4957) and 10 ng/ml Laminin (Corning 354232) in SCM for 12–24 h, and then replaced with SCDM containing DMEM/F12 (HyClone 36254) supplemented with B27 (Thermo 17504044)

and N2 (Thermo 17502048) supplement, 50 ng/ml BDNF (Stemcell 78005), 50 ng/ml NT3 (Stemcell 78074). Half of the medium was replaced every 2–3 days. Differentiated cells were analyzed after 9 days or more for immunocytochemistry and qPCR. Additional control SCDM/FGF referred to SCDM supplemented with bFGF (100 ng/ml).

The induction media (IM) for small molecule reprogramming contains Neurobasal Medium (Thermo 21103049), supplemented with B27 and N2, GlutaMax (Thermo 35050061), penicillin-streptomycin and bFGF (100 ng/ml), with or without small molecules Forskolin (20 μM), ISX9 (20 μM), I-BET (1–2 μM), Chir99021 (10 μM) (all from Selleck), and LIF (1000 U/ml) (Novus Biologicals).

Real-Time Quantitative PCR

RNA was isolated using Trizol (Takara 9108) and reverse transcription of total RNA was performed with the Primescript RT reagent kit (Takara RR047A) according to the manufacturer's protocol. The Quantitative PCR reactions were performed with the Hieff UNICON® qPCR SYBR Green Master Mix (YEASEN 11198ES03) on LightCycler 96 (Roche LightCycler® 96 Instrument). Details of the primers were in **Table 1**. Data are normalized to GAPDH, and fold changes are calculated by using $2^{-\Delta\Delta CT}$ method.

Immunofluorescence

Cells were fixed in 4% paraformaldehyde in PBS for 15 min with shaking at room temperature. Inner ear tissues were dissected and fixed in 4% paraformaldehyde in PBS for 2 h with shaking at room temperature, followed by decalcification in 5% EDTA for 4–5 days. Then cells were blocked with 5% heat inactivated horse serum with 0.3% Triton X-100 in PBS for 1 h.

Cells were incubated with primary antibody overnight at 4°C. The primary antibodies used in this study were as follows: anti-Sox2 (goat anti-Sox2;sc-17320, Santa Cruz Biotechnologies; 1:200); anti-Sox10 (rabit anti-Sox10; 69661, Cell Signaling Technology; 1:200); anti-TUJ1 (mouse anti-TUJ1; MMS 435P, Biolegend; 1:2,000); anti-Prox1 (goat anti-Prox1; AF2727, R&D; 1:250); anti-Gata3 (Rabbit anti-Gata3; 5852T, Cell Signaling Technology; 1:1500); anti-Map2 (Mouse anti-Map2; M4403, Sigma-Aldrich; 1:250); anti-Syp (mouse anti-Syp; MA5-14532, Thermofisher; 1:300), and anti-GFP (Rabbit anti-GFP; 31002, Yeasen; 1:400).

Then cells or tissues were incubated with Alexa 488-, Alexa 568-, and/or Alexa 647-labeled secondary antibodies for 1–2 h with shaking at room temperature. Nuclei were visualized with DAPI.

Confocal z-stacks (0.5 μm step size) of cochlear tissues were taken using Leica SP5 microscope equipped with 40× and 63× oil-immersion lens. ImageJ software (version 1.52i, NIH, Bethesda, MD, United States) was used for image processing and three-dimensional reconstruction of z-stacks. All immunofluorescence images shown are representative of at least three individual results. Efficiency of conversion was measured by the number of TUJ1$^+$ cells divided by the total number of plated cells from random 6–10 fields. Axon length was measured with NeuronJ, a plugin of ImageJ to facilitate the tracing and quantification of elongated image structures (Ho et al., 2011).

Molecular Cloning and Lentiviral Infections

cDNAs for Sox2 was cloned into lentiviral constructs of pLKO.1 vector (Addgene 10879). We modified the plasmid to replace the PuroR with Sox2-P2A-EGFP. Lentiviruses were produced by transfection of lentiviral backbones containing the indicated transgenes together with packaging plasmids pSPAX2 (Addgene 12260) and pMD2G (Addgene 12259) into HEK293T cells (ATCC® CRL-3216™). Viruses were concentrated from culture supernatant by ultra-centrifugation (25,000 rpm, 2 h, 4°C). After 24–48 h infection of spheres with 10 μg/ml polybrene in suspension culture, virus-containing medium was replaced with fresh SCM media.

RNA-seq Analyses

Total RNA was extracted from the tissue using TRIzol® Reagent according the manufacturer's instructions (TaKara) and genomic DNA was removed using DNase I (TaKara). Then RNA quality was determined by 2100 Bioanalyzer (Agilent) and quantified using the ND-2000 (NanoDrop Technologies). RNA-seq transcriptome library was prepared following TruSeq™ RNA sample preparation Kit from Illumina (San Diego, CA, United States) using 1 μg of total RNA. Libraries were size selected for cDNA target fragments of 200–300 bp on 2% Low Range Ultra Agarose followed by PCR amplified using Phusion DNA polymerase (NEB) for 15 PCR cycles. After quantified by TBS380, paired-end RNA-seq sequencing library was sequenced with the Illumina HiSeq x ten/NovaSeq 6000 sequencer (2 × 150 bp read length). The raw paired end reads were trimmed and quality controlled by SeqPrep and Sickle with default parameters. Then clean reads were separately

TABLE 1 | Primers used for real-time qPCR.

Gene ID	Forward (5′–3′)	Reverse (5′–3′)
GAPDH	ACCACGAGAAATATGACAACTCAC	CCAAAGTTGTCATGGATGACC
Tubb3	TAGACCCCAGCGGCAACTAT	GTTCCAGGTTCCAAGTCCACC
Nestin	ACAGTGAGGCAGATGAGTTAGG	GAGGCAGGAGACTTCAGGTAG
Prox1	TCTCAGCCAAACCCTCTC	CCGTTGACTGCGAATCTG
Sox2	GCGGAGTGGAAACTTTTGTCC	CGGGAAGCGTGTACTTATCCTT
Vglut1	GTTCTGGCTTCTGGTGTCTTATG	CTCTCCAATGCTCTCCTCTATGT
Islet1	CTTGCGGACCTGCTATGC	AACCACACTCGGATGACTCT
Scrt2	GTCCTCTGCCTGTCCATTCCT	GCTGCCTCCCAAGTCTGTTC
Sox10	CCAGGTGAAGACAGAGAC	AGACTGAGGGAGGTGTAG
Sox9	GCAATACGACTACGCTGAC	ATGTAAGTGAAGGTGGAGTAGA
Pou3f4	CTGGAGGAGGCTGATTCAT	GATGGAGGTTCGCTTCTTG
Pou4f1	AAACAAATAACCCACACCAAACAG	CTTCCTCAGAGCACCAGTTC
Ntrk3	GTGACGAGCGAGGACAATG	GGTAGTAGACAGTGAGCAACA
S100a4	TGGTCTGGTCTCAACGGTTA	TGGAAGGTGGACACAATTACATC

aligned to reference genome with orientation mode using TopHat (Langmead and Salzberg, 2012) software.

To identify differential expression genes (DEGs) between two different samples, the expression level of each transcript was calculated according to the fragments per kilobase of exon per million mapped reads (FRKM) method. RSEM (Li and Dewey, 2011) was used to quantify gene abundances. R statistical package software EdgeR (Empirical analysis of Digital Gene Expression in R (Robinson et al., 2010) was utilized for differential expression analysis. In addition, functional-enrichment analysis including GO and KEGG were performed to identify which DEGs were significantly enriched in GO terms and metabolic pathways at Bonferroni-corrected P-value ≤ 0.05 compared with the whole-transcriptome background.

The transcription data of primary SGN were obtained from previous study (Noda et al., 2018). Raw RNA-seq data have been deposited in the NCBI Gene Expression Omnibus (GEO) under accession number GSE169042.

Statistical Analysis

Statistical tests were performed using Graphpad Prism 8 (Graphpad Software Inc., La Jolla, CA, United States). Results were reported as mean $\pm$ SD. Specific statistical tests used in each experiment were described in figure legends. Results were analyzed using Student's t-test or one-way ANOVA, followed by Bonferroni's multiple comparisons test.

RESULTS

Postnatal Cochlear Spheres Proliferate and Differentiate Into Neuron-Like Cells

To expand the population of progenitor cells, we dissociated cochlear modiolus from the postnatal 3–4 days (P3–P4) mice and digested into single cells for 3D suspension culture. The cells grew spheres *in vitro* and were able to proliferate for more than five generations (**Figures 1A,B**). We then optimized the growth media by evaluating the sphere numbers with diameters larger than 50 μm. The result showed that bFGF is the primary factor for spheres growth, consistent with the previous report (Diensthuber et al., 2014a). Heparan sulfate has been reported to promote the binding and activation of FGF (Loo and Salmivirta, 2002). Therefore, we cultured the spheres with serum-free media containing IGF, EGF, FGF, and heparan sulfate (**Figure 1C**). Real-time quantitative PCR (RT-qPCR) results showed increased expression of neuronal stem cell markers such as *Sox2* and *Nestin* in spheres compared to cochlear modiolus (**Figure 1D**). These results indicated that postnatal cochlear spheres were able to proliferate and preserve the stemness following passages *in vitro*.

To investigate the neuronal potential of the spheres, we induced the spheres for neuronal differentiation. After induction for 8–9 days, the differentiated cells showed typical bipolar neuronal morphology and neuronal marker TUJ1 expression (**Figure 1E**, top panels). Brain-derived neurotrophic factor and NT3 are important neurotrophic factors for SGN development and function, and are able to promote neuronal differentiation *in vitro* (Wise et al., 2011; Li et al., 2016; Suzuki et al., 2016; Akil et al., 2019). We found that BDNF and NT3 treatment not only increased the differentiation efficiency (**Figures 1E,F**) but also promoted neurite extension (**Figures 1E,G**) during induced differentiation of the spheres. Therefore, BDNF and NT3 were added in the subsequent differentiation experiments. RT-qPCR results also showed that neuronal markers *Tubb3*, *Vglut1* expression were increased, while neuronal stemness markers *Nestin* and *Sox2* were decreased after induced neuronal differentiation (**Figure 1H**). These results indicate that postnatal cochlear spheres are able to differentiate into neuron-like cells.

Sox2 Expression Identifies a Subpopulation of Cochlear Glial Cells

Previous studies show the glial cells in association with the SGNs may serve as the source of neuronal progenitors (McLean et al., 2016). Based on the function and localization, cochlear glial cells consist of two major populations including Schwann cells (SCs) and satellite glial cells (SGCs) (Jessen and Mirsky, 2005; Wan and Corfas, 2017). The SCs wrap the axons of SGNs with myelin sheaths and are primarily localized to the osseous spiral lamina (OSL) of the cochlea; while the SGCs are in close association with the SGN cell bodies exclusively localized to the Rosenthal's canal (RC) of the cochlea (Wan and Corfas, 2017). Despite these differences, the two glial populations share same developmental origin and both serve important roles in survival and function of the SGNs.

It has been reported proteolipid protein 1 (Plp1) was widely expressed in cochlear glial cells, including SCs and SGCs (Jessen and Mirsky, 2005; McLean et al., 2016; Meas et al., 2018b), while Sox2 was expressed in a cochlear glial subpopulation (Zuchero and Barres, 2015; Meas et al., 2018b). To label the cochlear glial cells and the Sox2$^+$ subpopulation of glial cells in mice, we crossed the Plp1^{CreERT} and Sox2^{CreERT} with Rosa26-tdTomato line for lineage tracing. After induction with tamoxifen from P1 to P3, majority of the Sox2$^+$ cells were labeled with tdTomato (70.6 $\pm$ 4.3% of the total Sox2$^+$ cells) (**Figure 2A**). Importantly, Sox2^{CreERT}/tdTomato (Sox2-tdT) positive cells all expressed Sox2 in the cochlea, suggesting the inducible Sox2-tdT specifically labels the Sox2$^+$ subpopulation of glial cells in mice (**Figure 2A**).

The results of the immunofluorescence showed that Plp1^{CreERT}/tdTomato (Plp1-td) not only labels the Sox2$^+$ glial cells, but also Sox2$^-$ glial cells at both P4 and P21 (**Figures 2B,C**), indicating that Sox2 positive cells are a subpopulation of Plp1 positive cochlear glial cells. Thus, Plp1-tdT labels both SCs and SGCs while Sox2-tdT positive glial cells represents a lineage population of cochlear glial cells.

Cochlear Sox2$^+$ Glial Cells Are Primary Progenitors for Neuronal Differentiation

To directly compare the potency of Plp1$^+$ and Sox2$^+$ glial cells as neuronal progenitors, the lineage-traced cells (Plp1-tdT and Sox2-tdT) were subjected to sphere formation and neuronal differentiation assays (**Figure 3A**). Although both Plp1-tdT and Sox2-tdT cells were able to form spheres, >95% of the spheres were Plp1-positive while only about 60% of the spheres were Sox2-positive (**Figures 3B,C**), suggesting that both Plp1$^+$/Sox2$^+$ and Plp1$^+$/Sox2$^-$ glial cells were able to proliferate as spheres.

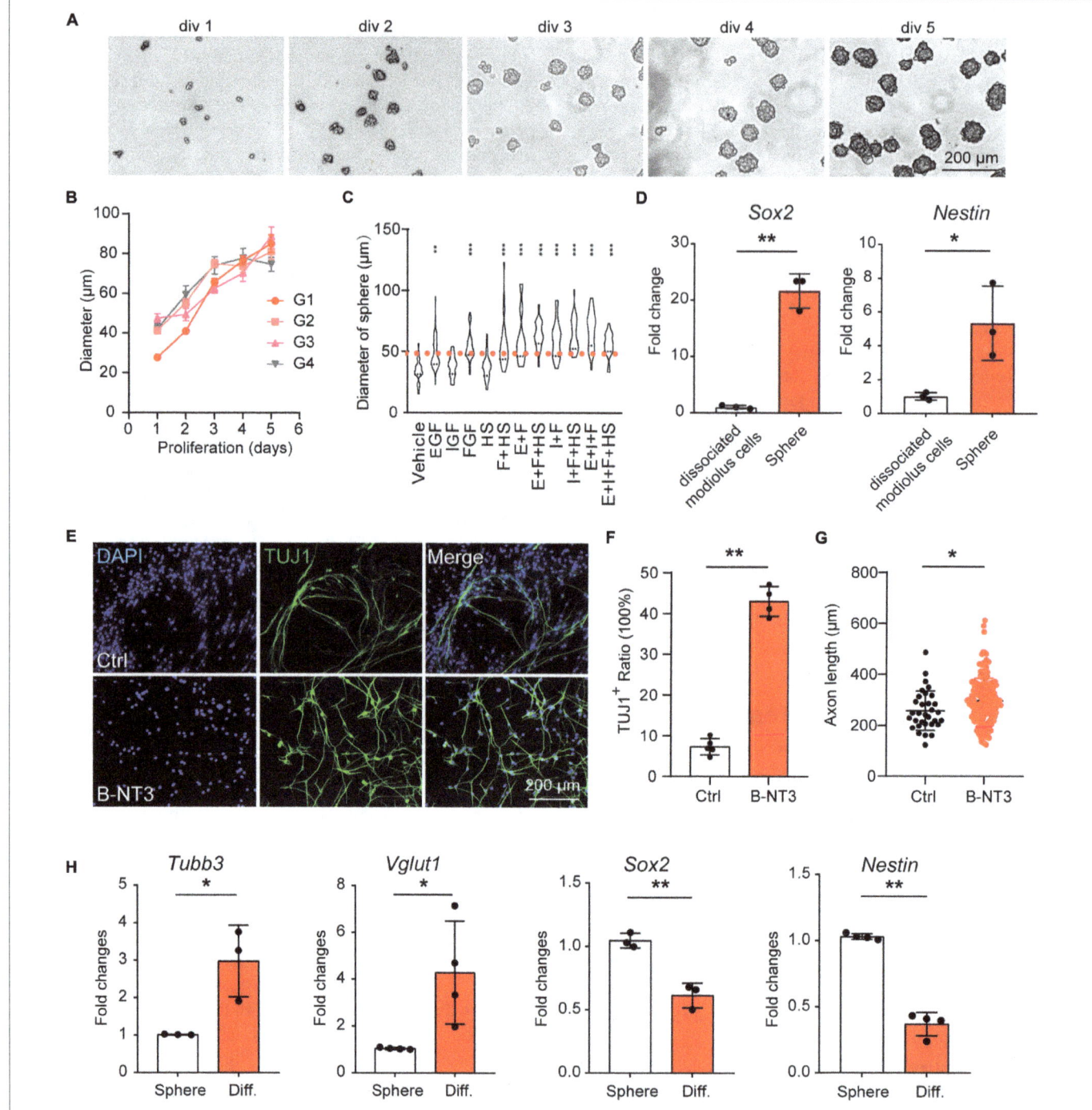

FIGURE 1 | Postnatal cochlear glial cells proliferate as neurospheres and differentiate into neuron-like cells. **(A)** Bright-field images of the proliferating generation 1 (G1) spheres at 1–5 days *in vitro* (div). **(B)** Diameters of G1–G4 spheres during propagation. **(C)** Quantification of sphere diameters at 5 div with supplementations of E, I, F, H. E, EGF; I, IGF; F, FGF, and H, heparan sulfate. N = 21–48. P-values were calculated against vehicle control. **(D)** mRNA expression of *Sox2* and *Nestin* in cochlear spheres compared to controls (dissociate modiolus cells). N = 3, error bars represent mean ± SD. **(E)** Representative TUJ1-positive cells after differentiation at 18 div with BDNF and NT3 (B-NT3). **(F)** The ratio of TUJ1 positive cells. N = 5 and 4, error bars represent mean ± SD. **(G)** Axon lengths of the induced neuron-like cells. N = 35 and 220, error bars represent mean ± SD. **(H)** mRNA expression of *Tubb3*, *Vglut1*, *Sox2*, and *Nestin* of either spheres or differentiated neuron-like cells (Diff). N = 3 or 4, error bars represent mean ± SD. $*p < 0.05$, $**p < 0.01$, $***p < 0.001$ by one-way ANOVA **(C)** or unpaired student's *t*-test **(D,F–H)**.

Interestingly, Plp1-tdT$^+$ or Sox2-tdT$^+$ cells were clustered at the periphery of the spheres with the non-glial cells proliferating at the center of spheres (**Figure 3B**). These non-glial cells were also highly proliferative and Plp1-tdT or Sox2-tdT cells contribute to only about 20 or 12% of the total cells after sphere culture, respectively (**Supplementary Figure 1A**). To investigate the

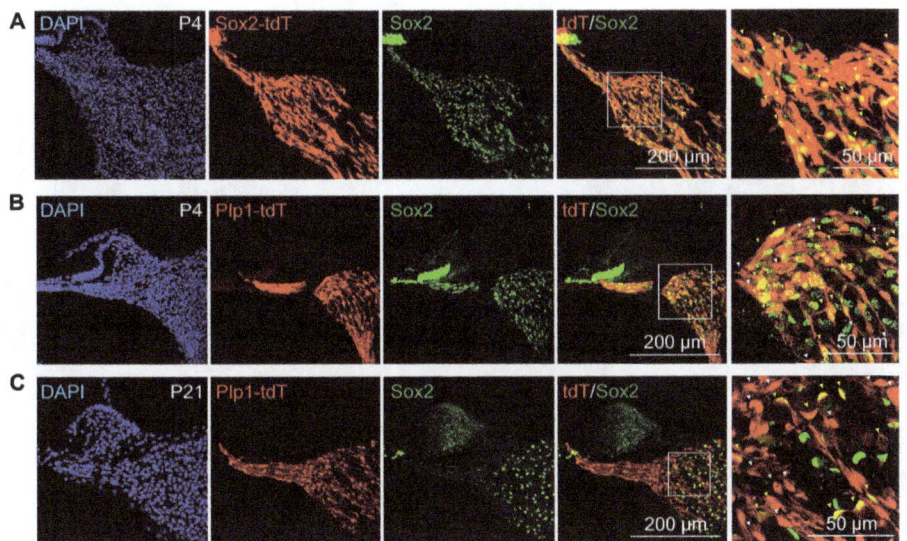

FIGURE 2 | Sox2 labels a subpopulation of cochlear glial cells. **(A)** Immunocytochemical staining of Sox2-tdT cochlea for Sox2, showed Sox2-Cre:tdTomato labeled the Sox2 positive cochlear glial cells in P4 mice. The yellow arrowheads represent Sox2-tdT$^+$/Sox2$^+$ cells. **(B,C)** Sox2 were expressed in a subpopulation of Plp1-tdT positive cells in both P4 **(B)** and P21 **(C)** cochlea. The white arrowheads represent Plp1-tdT$^+$/Sox2$^-$ cells, and the yellow arrows represent Plp1-tdT$^+$/Sox2$^+$ cells. tdTomato expression was induced by tamoxifen from P1 to P3.

identity of these non-glial cells, Plp1-tdT$^-$ cells were separated from Plp1-tdT$^+$ cells by FACS followed by continuous sphere culture (**Supplementary Figure 1B**). While the non-glial markers failed to express Sox10 or Sox2 as expected, they expressed high levels of Sox9 and Pou3f4 (**Supplementary Figure 1C**), both of which are enriched in otic mesenchyme cells (Coate et al., 2012; Brooks et al., 2020).

To address if Plp1$^+$/Sox2$^+$ and Plp1$^+$/Sox2$^-$ glial cells display different potential for neuronal differentiation, spheres from Plp1-tdT and Sox2-tdT mice were induced to neuronal differentiation for 8–9 days. Firstly, both Plp1-tdT and Sox2-tdT positive cells developed typical bipolar neuronal morphology and expressed neuronal marker TUJ1 (**Figure 3D**). Intriguingly, while only ~68% Plp1-tdT cells expressed TUJ1, more than 90% Sox2-tdT cells were co-labeled with TUJ1 (**Figure 3E**). Further analyses indicated that almost all TUJ1$^+$ neurons were derived from Plp1$^+$ glial cells but a large proportion of Plp1$^+$ cells were unable to differentiate (**Figure 3F**, left). In contrast, although Sox2$^+$ glial cells only contributed to ~70% of total iNs, almost all Sox2$^+$ cells were successfully differentiated (**Figure 3F**, right). These results indicate that Plp1$^+$ cochlear glial cells are the major source of neuronal differentiation *in vitro*, and that Plp1$^+$/Sox2$^+$ glial subpopulation displays much higher potency/efficiency in neuronal differentiation compared to the Plp1$^+$/Sox2$^-$ glial cells (**Figure 3G**).

P21 Cochlear Sox2$^+$ Glial Cells Preserve High Potency of Neuronal Differentiation

As Sox2 expression marks a subpopulation of cochlear glial cells with high neuronal differentiation potency, we next examined the expression of Sox2 at different postnatal ages. The ratio of Sox2$^+$ glial cells were calculated based on co-labeling with Sox10, a generic marker of cochlear glial cells similar to Plp1 (Jessen and Mirsky, 2005). We found that the percentage of Sox2$^+$ glial cells gradually declined after birth (**Figures 4A,B**). Specifically, at P4, ~70% glial cells were Sox2$^+$, and the Sox2$^+$ ratio decreased to ~47 and ~38% at P7 and P10. At hearing onset (P14), the percentage of Sox2$^+$ glial cells reduced further to ~30%, which was maintained at P21 (**Figure 4C**).

We next examined if the Sox2$^+$ glial population remains highly efficient in neuronal differentiation at P21. Due to difficulties in obtaining sufficient cochlear glial cells in the calcified modiolus of P21 cochlea, the P21 cochlear glial cells were initially cultured 2D in SCM-FBS medium (Lang et al., 2011) and then transferred to 3D sphere suspension culture. We used the same inducible Plp1^{CreERT} and Sox2^{CreERT} to cross with Rosa26-tdTomato line to specific label the total glial cell population and Sox2$^+$ glial cell subpopulation, respectively (**Figure 3A**). Lineage tracing was induced by tamoxifen injection from P17 to P20, and the cochlear glial cells isolated at P21. Both P21 Plp1-tdT and Sox2-tdT positive cells distributed at the periphery of spheres (**Figure 5A**), similar to the observation from the P4 spheres (**Figure 3B**). Followed by induction of neuronal differentiation, ~55% Plp1$^+$ glial cells were TUJ1 positive and ~90% Sox2$^+$ glial cells were TUJ1 positive (**Figures 5B,C**). In summary, the cochlear Sox2$^+$ glial cell subpopulation preserves high potency of neuronal differentiation in both neonatal (P4) and P21 mice.

Sox2 Downregulation Is Required for Efficient Neuronal Differentiation

To further investigate if the Sox2 expression contributes to the high neuronal differentiation potential of the Sox2$^+$ glial cells, we overexpressed Sox2 in both Sox2$^+$ and Sox2$^-$ glial cells during 3D suspension culture of the spheres. Spheres were infected with lentivirus encoding Sox2-GFP or GFP control and

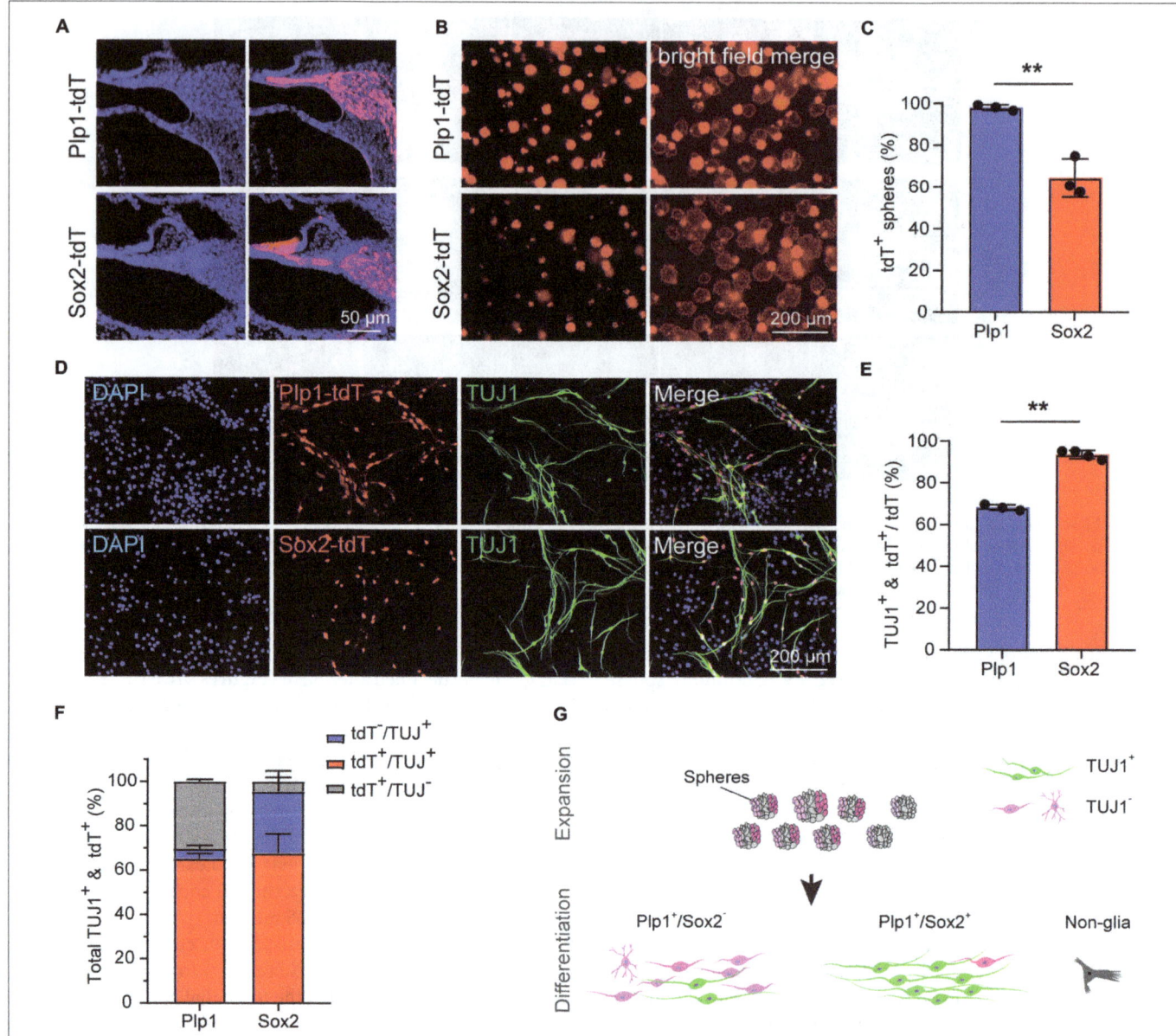

FIGURE 3 | The Sox2+ cochlear glial cells were highly efficient in neuronal differentiation. **(A)** Distributions of Sox2-tdT and Plp1-tdT positive cochlear glial cells in P4 cochlea. tdTomato expression was induced by tamoxifen from P1 to P3. **(B,C)** Representative images and quantification of the Sox2-tdT and Plp1-tdT positive spheres at 5 div. N = 3, error bars represent mean ± SD. **(D,E)** Representative images and ratios of TUJ1+ neurons differentiated from Sox2-tdT and Plp1-tdT positive cells at 8–9 div. N = 3 or 4, error bars represent mean ± SD. Data from 3 to 4 independent experiments. **(F)** Percentages of TUJ1+ neurons derived from Sox2-tdT or Plp1-tdT positive cells relative to the total amount of TUJ1+ plus tdT+ cells. **(G)** A model showing Sox2+ glial cells exhibit high potential for neuronal differentiation. **p < 0.01 by unpaired student's t-test.

the Sox2 overexpression was validated by both RT-qPCR and immunofluorescence (**Figures 6A,B**).

Next, the spheres were induced to neuronal differentiation for 8–9 days and were immuno-stained with TUJ1 antibody. We first evaluated the effect of Sox2 overexpression on neuronal differentiation of Sox2$^-$ glial cells. Neuronal differentiation of Sox2$^-$ glial cells, as marked by TUJ1$^+$/Sox2-tdT$^-$ cells, was not affect by Sox2 overexpression compared to GFP controls (**Figures 6C,D**). This result suggest that the incompetence of Sox2$^-$ glial cells in neuronal differentiation is not due to lack of Sox2 expression. To our surprise, neuronal differentiation of the Sox2-tdT (Sox2$^+$) glial cells was significantly reduced after Sox2 overexpression (**Figures 6C,E**). Consistently, *Sox2* expression was decreased dramatically from the proliferative stage in 3D culture to the differentiation stage in 2D culture, and then maintained at a stably low level during the entire process of neuronal differentiation (**Figure 6F**). These results suggest that Sox2$^+$ glial cells exhibit high potential for

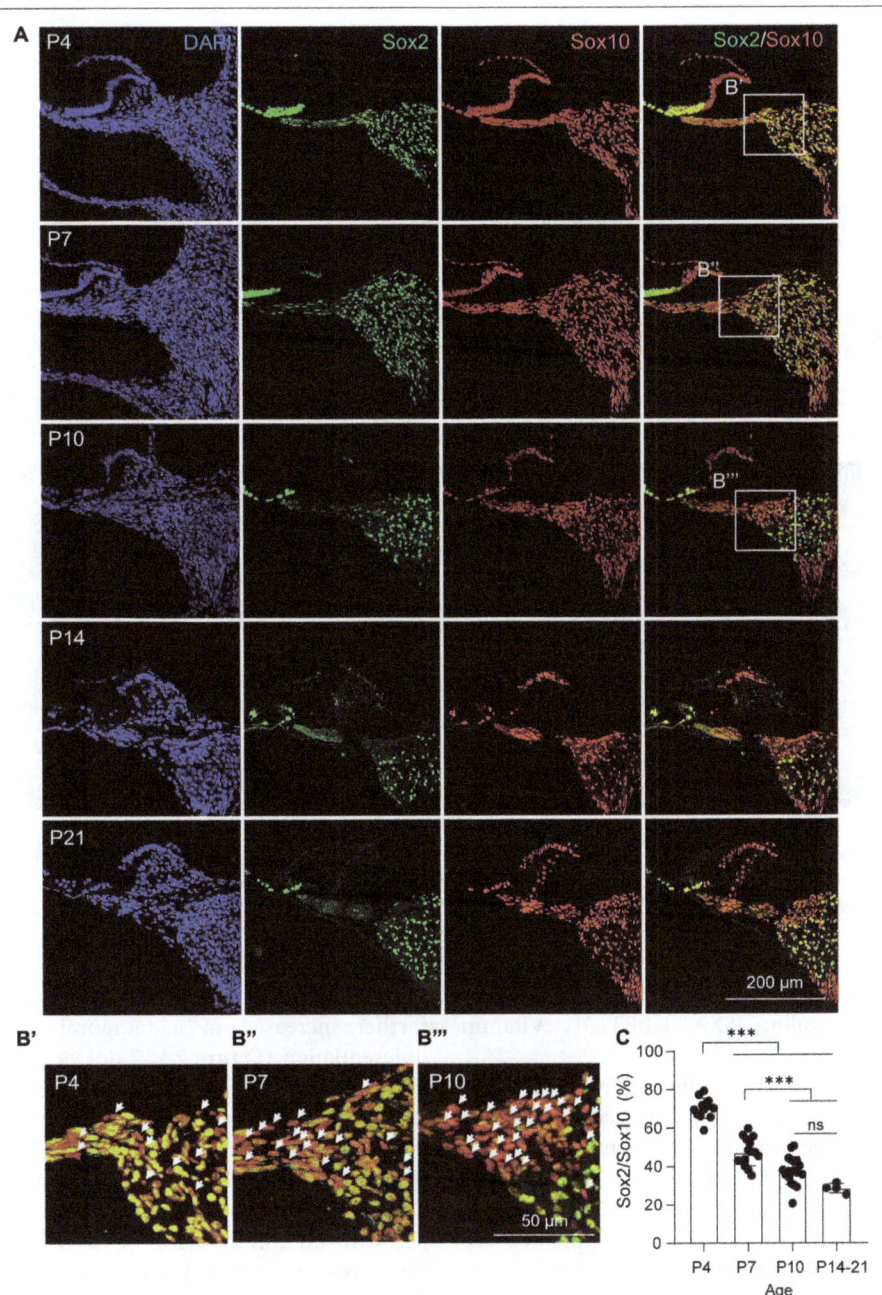

FIGURE 4 | Dynamic changes of Sox2+ cochlear glial cells during postnatal development. **(A,B)** Immunocytochemical staining of Sox2 and Sox10 from P4, P7, P10, P14, and P21 cochleae. The white arrow represents the Sox2−/Sox10+ cell. **(C)** Percentages of Sox2+/Sox10+ cells from P4, P7, P10, and P14 to P21 cochleae. N = 4–13 sections from 3 cochleae, error bars represent mean ± SD. ***p < 0.001 by one-way ANOVA.

neuronal differentiation independent of Sox2 expression, and that downregulation of Sox2 is required for efficient neuronal differentiation.

Small Molecules Promote Neuronal Differentiation and Maturation Toward Spiral Ganglion Neuron Fate

Although cochlear glial cells can be differentiated into iNs, the specific markers for SGNs were rarely detected, indicative of a major huddle in SGN fate conversion and maturation. Small molecules have been reported to promote neuronal reprogramming from somatic and glial cells (Hu et al., 2015; He et al., 2017; Belin-Rauscent et al., 2018). To promote the neuronal differentiation and maturation to SGNs from cochlear glial cells, we next screened 10 neurogenic small molecules that were shown to activate neuronal signaling pathways, inhibit glial signaling pathways, or modulate epigenetics to promote neuronal reprogramming. Small molecules selected for our initial screening were as

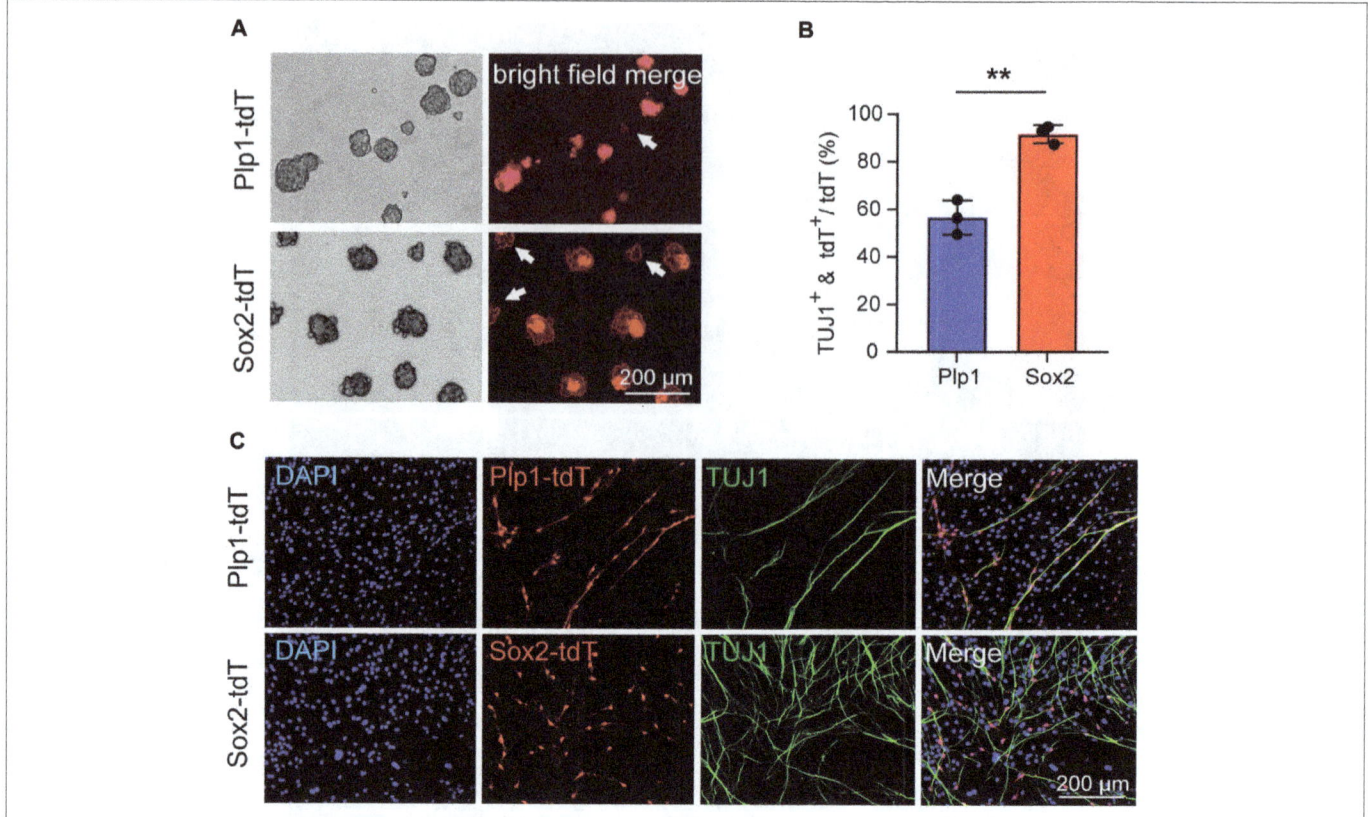

FIGURE 5 | Cochlear Sox2+ glial subpopulation preserves high potency of neuronal differentiation in P21 mice. **(A)** Representative images of the Sox2-tdT and Plp1-tdT positive spheres culture 5 div. The white arrow represents the Plp1-tdT or Sox2-tdT negative spheres. **(B,C)** Representative images **(C)** and ratios **(B)** of TUJ1+ neurons differentiated from Sox2-tdT or Plp1-tdT positive cells. $N = 3$, error bars represent mean ± SD. **$p < 0.01$ by unpaired student's t-test.

follows: SB431542, CHIR99021, Y27632, retinoic acid (RA), valproic acid (VPA), Forskolin, ISX9, I-BET151, Vitamin C (Vc), and LIF.

It has been reported that Forskolin, ISX9, I-BET151, and CHIR99021 (FIBC) combination induced neuronal differentiation from mouse embryonic fibroblasts (MEFs) and astrocytes efficiently (Hu et al., 2015; He et al., 2017). Firstly, we used the FIBC combination to test the concentration for neuronal differentiation from cochlear glial cells (**Supplementary Figure 2A**). Based on the bipolar neuronal morphology of TUJ1$^+$ cells and minimal cytotoxicity, we identified the optimal concentrations of Forskolin (20 μM), ISX9 (20 μM), I-BET151 (2 μM), and CHIR99021 (10 μM). Next, we induced the neuronal differentiation with FIBC in the presence of SB431542, Y27632 (Y), RA, VPA, Vc, or LIF (L). The results showed FIBC and Y27632 (FIBCY) and FIBC and LIF (FIBCL) increased the expression of Prox1 (**Supplementary Figure 3E**), an SGN marker, compared with other small molecules (**Supplementary Figure 2B**). Thus, we used FIBCY and FIBCL as the small molecules cocktail for neuronal induction and maturation.

RT-qPCR results also showed increased expression of generic neuronal markers such as *Tubb3* (**Supplementary Figures 3A,B**), and SGN-specific markers including *Prox1*, *Islet1*, and *Scrt2* (**Supplementary Figure 3G**) of the iNs by small molecules FIBCL compared with SCDM or IM control medium (**Figure 7A**).

Furthermore, the expression of *Tubb3*, *Scrt2*, and *Islet1* were further increased in a temporal manner during neuronal differentiation (**Figure 7A**, 7 dpi vs. 18 dpi). FIBCY and FIBCL increased the number of TUJ1$^+$ cells and induced both co-labeling of TUJ1 and Prox1 (**Figure 7B**). Quantitative analyses indicate that FIBCY and FIBCL significantly increased the percentage of overall TUJ1$^+$ cells (**Figure 7C**) and percentage of TUJ1$^+$ cells co-expressing Prox1 (**Figure 7D**). FIBCL appeared to perform better in inducing TUJ1$^+$ iNs than FIBCY (**Figure 7C**). These results suggested that FIBCY/FIBCL promoted neuronal differentiation and maturation toward SGNs from neonatal cochlear glial cells.

We then induced neuronal differentiation of P21 Plp1-tdT glial cells in the presence or absence of FIBCL. For P21 glial cells, FIBCL also promoted the expression of SGN markers *Scrt2*, *Islet1* (**Figure 7E**). Remarkably, FIBCL treatment resulted in a significant increase in the percentage of TUJ1$^+$/Plp1-tdT$^+$ cells (∼90%) compared to the control group (∼55%) (**Figures 7F,G**). As Plp1$^+$/Sox2$^+$ but not Plp1$^+$/Sox2$^-$ cells showed potent neuronal differentiation in control condition, FIBCL treatment may have also promoted neuronal differentiation of Plp1$^+$/Sox2$^-$ glial cells. Together, these results highlight the effectiveness of small molecule combinations FIBCY and FIBCL in promoting neuronal differentiation and SGN maturation of neonatal and P21 cochlear glial cells.

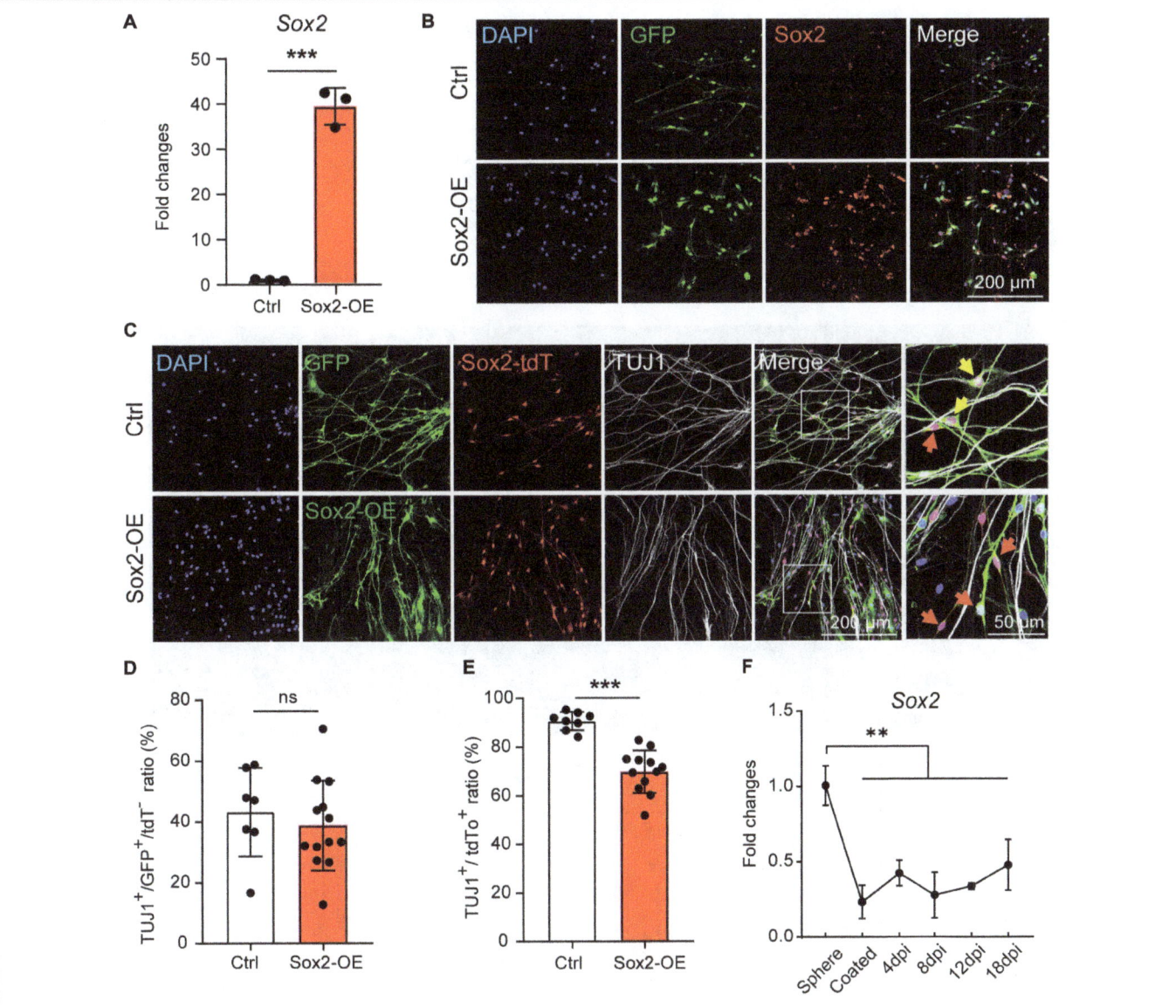

FIGURE 6 | Sox2 overexpression inhibits the neuronal differentiation of Sox2+ glial cells. **(A,B)** mRNA expression **(A)** and immunocytochemical staining **(B)** of Sox2 overexpressed in cochlear glial cells. $N = 3$, error bars represent mean ± SD. **(C)** Immunocytochemical staining of TUJ1+ neurons differentiated from cochlear glial cells of Sox2-tdT mice. The yellow arrows represent TUJ1+/GFP+/tdT− cells, and the red arrows represent TUJ1−/GFP+/tdT+ glial cells. **(D)** Quantification of TUJ1+/GFP+ cells from Sox2-tdT negative glial cells. $N = 8$–13 images from 3 coverslips, error bars represent mean ± SD. **(E)** Quantification of TUJ1+/Sox2-tdT+ cells from glial cells overexpressing either GFP or Sox2. $N = 7$–11 images from 3 coverslips, error bars represent mean ± SD. **(F)** mRNA expression of Sox2 during induced neuronal differentiation of the cochlear glial cells at different conditions and time points. $N = 3$, error bars represent mean ± SD. **$p < 0.01$, ***$p < 0.001$ by one-way ANOVA **(F)** or unpaired student's t-test **(A,E)**.

FIBCL-Induced Neurons Display Similar Transcriptomic Profile as the Primary Spiral Ganglion Neurons

To evaluate the maturity under different induction conditions of iNs, we performed transcriptome sequencing analyses. Pearson correlation analyses showed that the expression profiles of neurons induced by SCDM and SCDM/FGF were relatively closer to that of the spheres (**Figure 8A**). However, the overall expression profile of FIBCL-iNs was distinct from those of the spheres, SCDM or SCDM/FGF, and was more similar to that of the primary SGNs (**Figure 8A**). In addition, the results of principal component analyses (PCA) showed that FIBCL-iNs were similar to the SGNs (**Figure 8B**). Comparing the differentially expressed genes between SCDM and FIBCL-iNs, we found about 3200 genes in the FIBCL group were significantly upregulated and 3000 genes were significantly downregulated (**Figure 8C**). The GO and KEGG enrichment analyses of these genes, respectively showed that the upregulated genes were mainly enriched in neuron development, neurotransmitter, synapse and calcium ion channels; while the downregulated genes contained glial cell migration and myelination, as well as GPCR and cytokine signaling pathways (**Figures 8D–G**).

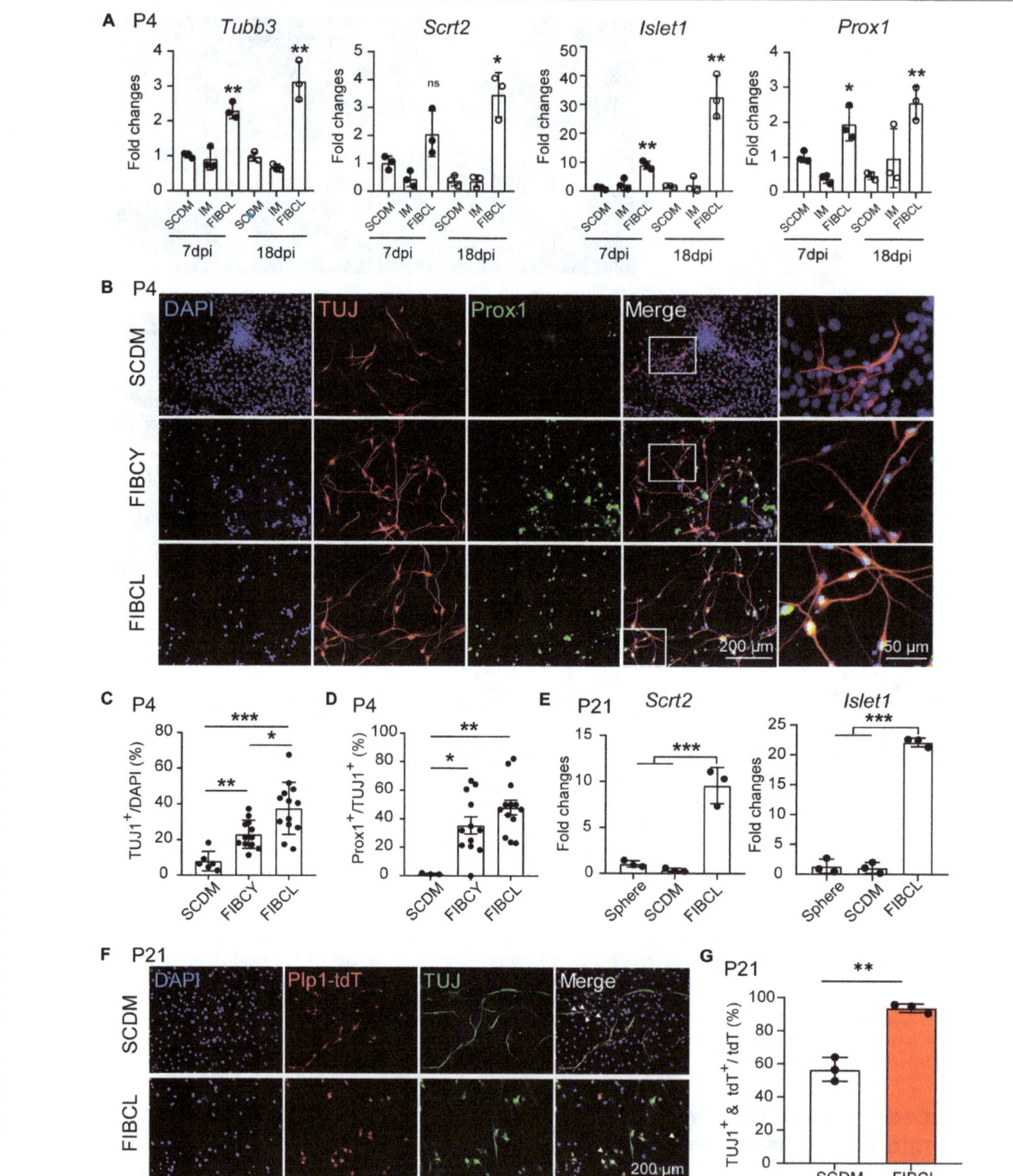

FIGURE 7 | Small molecules promote neuronal differentiation and maturation of cochlear glial cells. (A) RT-qPCR gene expression analyses of P4 cochlear glial cells differentiated in SCDM, IM or FIBCL at 7 and 18 div. FIBCL, Forskolin, ISX9, I-BET151, CHIR99021, and LIF. $N = 3$, error bars represent mean ± SD.
(B) Immunocytochemical stainings of TUJ1 and Prox1 in neurons induced from P4 cochlear glial cells at different conditions. (C,D) Percentages of TUJ1 positive cells (C) and TUJ1/Prox1 double positive cells (D) differentiated in SCDM, FIBCY, or FIBCL. $N = 3–13$ images from 2 wells of each condition, error bars represent mean ± SD. (E) mRNA expression of SGN markers Scrt2 and Islet1. $N = 3$, error bars represent mean ± SD. (F) Immunocytochemical staining of TUJ1 of induced neurons from P21 Plp1-tdT cochlear glial cells. The white arrowheads represent the Plp1-tdT$^+$/TUJ1$^−$ cells. (G) Percentages of TUJ1 positive cells differentiated from P21 Plp1-tdT$^+$ cochlear glial cells. $N = 3$, error bars represent mean ± SD. *$p < 0.05$, **$p < 0.01$, ***$p < 0.001$ by one-way ANOVA (A,C–E) or unpaired student's t-test (G).

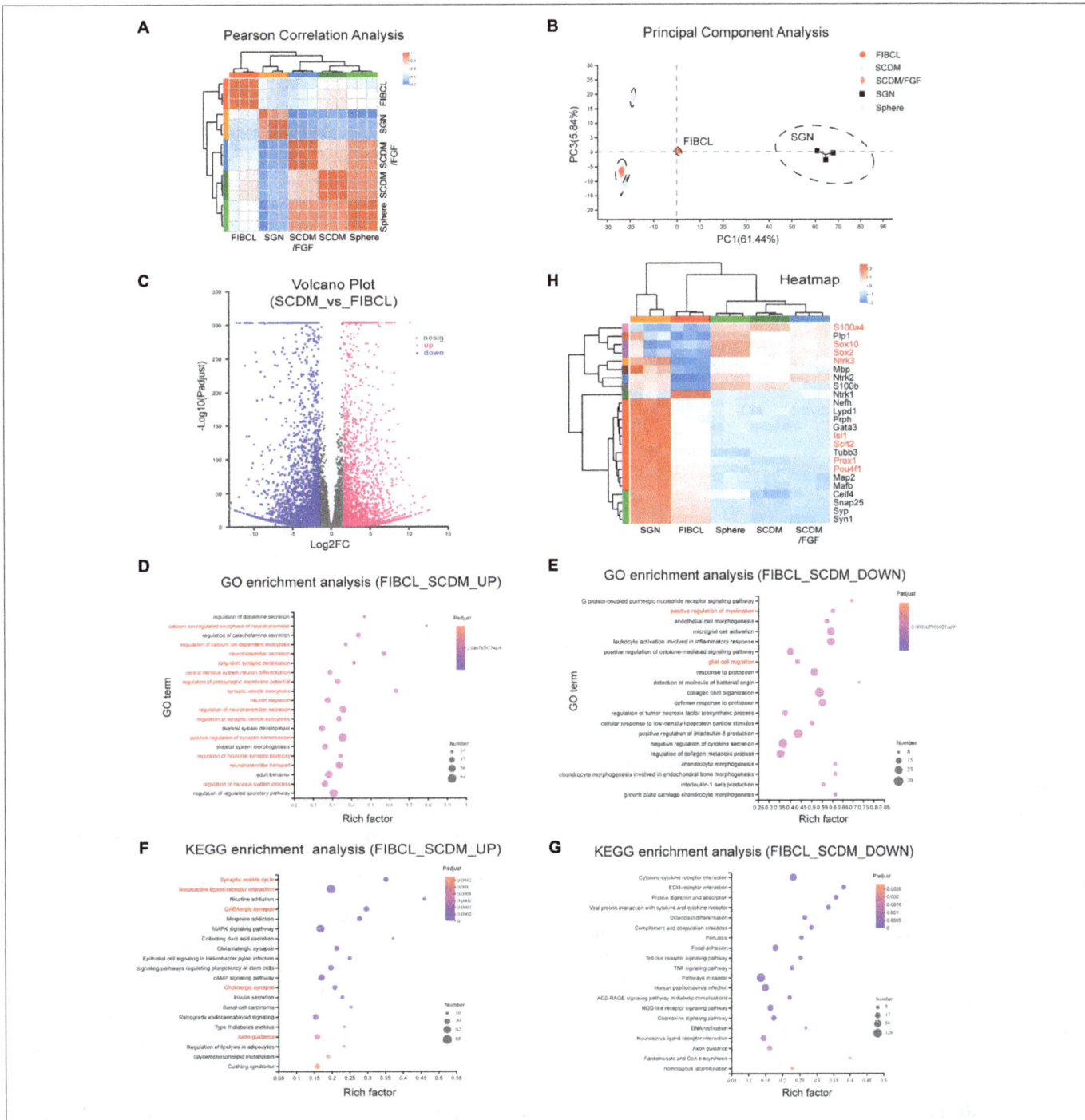

FIGURE 8 | Transcriptomic analyses of the induced neurons. **(A,B)** Pearson correlation analysis **(A)** and principal component analysis **(B)** of neurospheres, differentiated culture in SCDM, SCDM/FGF, FIBCL media, and primary SGNs. **(C)** Volcano graph of the genes upregulated and downregulated in the FIBCL-induced neurons compared to the SCDM media. **(D,E)** GO enrichment analysis of upregulated **(D)** and downregulated **(E)** functional pathways in the FIBCL-induced neurons compared to the SCDM media. **(F,G)** KEGG enrichment analysis of upregulated **(D)** and downregulated **(E)** cellular processes in the FIBCL-induced neurons compared to the SCDM media. **(H)** Heatmap graph of specific glial and neuronal genes expressed in spheres, differentiated culture in SCDM, SCDM/FGF, FIBCL media, and primary SGNs. Changes in expression of selected genes (gene symbol highlighted in red) were validated by RT-qPCR in **Supplementary Figure 4**.

Analyses of specific gene expression revealed that glial cell-specific genes such as *Plp1*, *Sox10*, *S100β*, and *MBP* still maintained high expression in sphere, SCDM and SCDM/FGF groups, but the expression levels of these genes were significantly downregulated in FIBCL-iNs group (**Figure 8H**). Interestingly, Sox2 expression was also further reduced after FIBCL treatment (**Figure 8H**), consistent with an inhibitory role of Sox2 in neuronal differentiation (**Figure 6**). In addition, expression

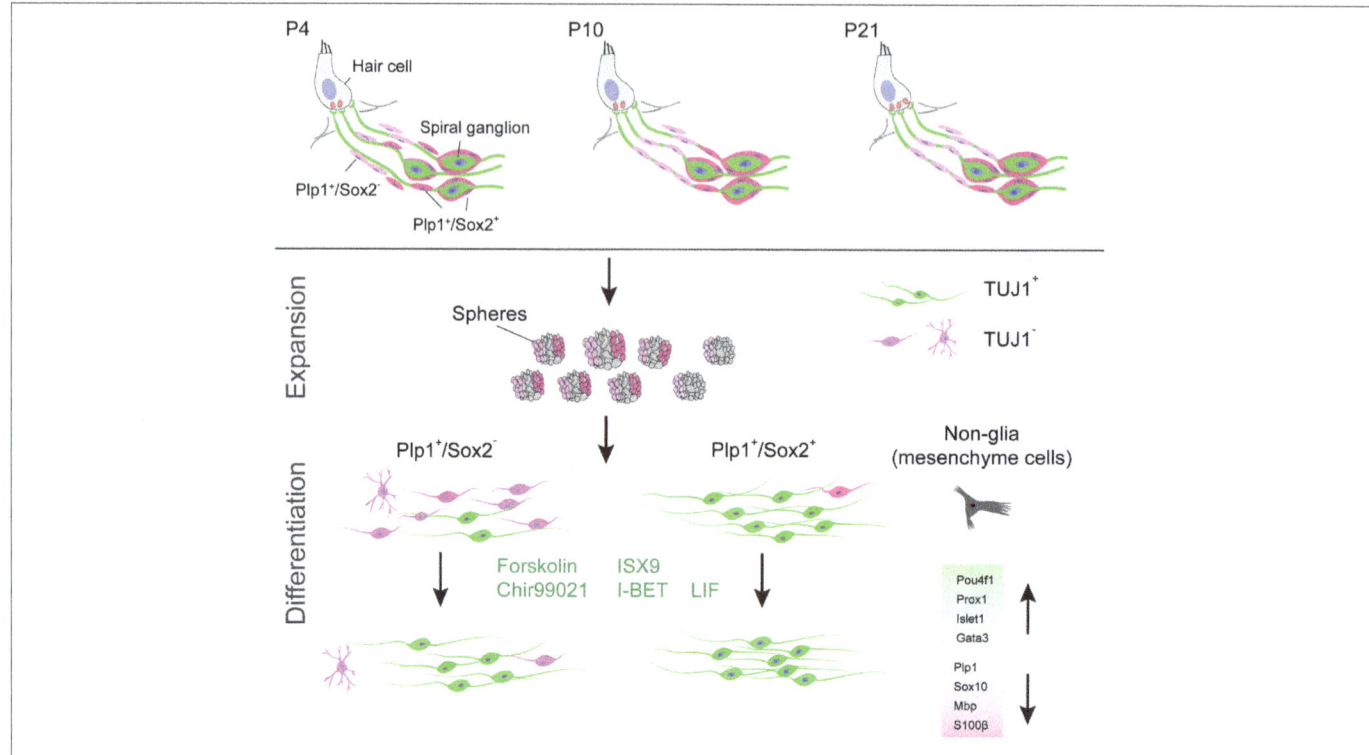

FIGURE 9 | Graphic summary of cochlear Sox2+ glial cells as potent progenitors for spiral ganglion neuron reprogramming induced by small molecules. Sox2+ cells are a subpopulation of Plp1+ cochlear glial cells. Although both Sox2+ and Sox2− glial cells can form neurospheres, Plp1+/Sox2+ spheres are more neurogenic compared to Plp1+/Sox2− spheres. Efficiency and maturity of the induced neurons can be further improved by a small molecule cocktail.

levels of neuron-specific genes such as *Tubb3*, *Nefh*, *Snap25*, *Syp* (**Supplementary Figure 3D**), and *Map2* (**Supplementary Figure 3F**) were induced in SCDM and SCDM/FGF groups compared to the spheres, which were further upregulated in the FIBCL group (**Figure 8H**). Finally, the expression levels of SGN-specific genes such as *Isl1*, *Pou4f1*, *Prox1*, *Gata3* (**Supplementary Figure 3C**), and *Mafb* were also significantly upregulated, while cochlear glial genes such as *Sox10*, *Sox2*, and *S100a4* were downregulated in the FIBCL-iNs (**Figure 8H** and **Supplementary Figure 4**). Overall, the RNA-seq results indicate that iNs in control medium were at the immature state, retaining some of the glial cell characteristics; while small molecules FIBCL removed glial cell barriers and further promoted neuronal maturation.

DISCUSSION

Spiral ganglion neurons lack the ability to regenerate after damage in the mammalian cochlea, which is a major cause of auditory neuropathy and may compromise the therapeutic effects of cochlear implants (Guo et al., 2019). Extensive studies have been performed using neural stem cells for regeneration of neurons and the SGNs (Fang et al., 2019; Li et al., 2019; Tang et al., 2019; Han et al., 2020; Xia et al., 2020; Yang et al., 2020, 2021; Yuan et al., 2021). Yet, functional regeneration of SGNs from the resident glial cells may represent a novel strategy for hearing restoration caused by SGN damages. In this study, we found that the cochlear Sox2+ glial cell subpopulation exhibits high potency of neuronal differentiation, and the efficiency of neuronal differentiation requires Sox2 downregulation. Furthermore, we identified a small molecule combination that promotes neuronal differentiation and maturation toward SGN fate (**Figure 9**).

Cochlear Sox2+ Glial Cell Subpopulation as Potent Neuronal Progenitors

The starting progenitor population is one of the key considerations for successful cell fate reprogramming (Gascon et al., 2017). In the brain and retina, astrocytes (Guo et al., 2014; Qian et al., 2020) and Müller glial cells (Qian et al., 2020) have been shown to convert to new neurons and retinal ganglion cells under specific conditions. Cochlear glial cells were regarded as specialized cells and exhibited characteristics as well as corresponding functions of glial cells. Similar to the central glial cells, cochlear glial cells can also proliferate and regenerate themselves upon injury *in vivo* (Lang et al., 2015; Wan and Corfas, 2017), suggesting that these glial cells may also function as progenitors for SGNs.

Cochlear glial cells are heterogeneous and include SCs and Satellite cells (Wan and Corfas, 2017). While Plp1 and Sox10 are generic markers for cochlear glial cells, Sox2 is only expressed in a subset of glial cells. Sox2+ glial cells are mainly located around the SGN cell body, which overlapped with SGCs. A few Sox2+ glial cells are also located along SGN axons at OSL after P14 in mice. In this study, we identified Sox2+ glial cells sub-population as potent neuronal progenitors compared to Sox2⁻ glial cells, suggesting that Sox2⁺ glial cells may be the target progenitor population for SGN regeneration in future studies.

In recent years, mechanisms of proliferation and neuronal differentiation of the cochlear glial progenitor has been under close investigation. The Plp1⁺ cochlear glial cells serve as potent progenitors for neurons, astrocytes and oligodendrocytes, but not hair cells *in vitro* (McLean et al., 2016). Cochlear glial cells isolated from Sox2-eGFP reporter mice also displayed potent neurogenic potential *in vitro* (Lang et al., 2015; Meas et al., 2018a). However, a direct comparison of glial subpopulations is lacking and the iNs did not appear to mature as SGNs. Importantly, two groups recently reported that iNs can be generated from Plp1⁺ glial cell by Ng1/Nd1 or Lin28 overexpression *in vivo* post-SGN injury, and that iNs expressed both pan-neuronal and SGN markers (Kempfle et al., 2020; Li X. et al., 2020). However, the efficiency of neuronal conversion and neuronal maturity is still limited. Based on our findings, we believe that direct reprogramming of the Sox2⁺ glial cells may be key to enhance functional glia-to-neuron conversion *in vivo*.

Role of Sox2 Expression in Neuronal Differentiation From Cochlear Glial Cells

Developmentally, Sox2 is generally expressed in a variety of cells types including neuronal stem cells (Graham et al., 2003; Zhang and Cui, 2014; Cui et al., 2018) and tissue specific cells, such as DRG satellite cells and cochlear supporting cells (Kiernan et al., 2005; Koike et al., 2015). Our finding on higher potential of Sox2⁺ glial cells poses a question on whether Sox2 expression is required for efficient neuronal induction or merely serves as a marker for progenitors with high neurogenic potential. Our results point to the later scenario and may also suggest that Sox2 serves as an inhibitory signal for efficient neuronal induction. This notion is consistent with the observations in CNS, whereby Sox2 was highly expressed in neuronal progenitor cells (NPCs) and inhibited the neuronal differentiation of these progenitor cells (Graham et al., 2003; Cavallaro et al., 2008). Sox2 expression was gradually downregulated during the process of neuronal differentiation (Cavallaro et al., 2008; Cui et al., 2018; Mercurio et al., 2019). Knockdown of Sox2 partially rescued the impairment of neuronal differentiation induced by miR-145 downregulation (Morgado et al., 2016).

Intriguingly, although Sox2 was downregulated during neuronal differentiation of the cochlear glial cells, we observed that the iNs still maintained the expression of Sox2 at a specific level. Sox2 expression of iNs was higher than that of SGNs, which may present a barrier for further neuronal maturation. This is in congruence with our finding that the small molecule cocktail promoted further neuronal maturation while also significantly reduced the expression of Sox2.

Small Molecules Promote Efficiency and Maturity of Induced Neurons

Neuronal reprogramming may not be initiated due to the stable barriers of glial cells identity and lack of neuronal factors to regulate specific transcriptional program (Mertens et al., 2016; Black and Gersbach, 2018; Li et al., 2018). Small molecules that modulate specific signaling pathways have been shown to promote neuronal reprogramming. For example, small molecules CHIR99021, Forskolin, and ISX9 were shown to improve the neuronal conversion and differentiation (Schneider et al., 2008; Dworkin and Mantamadiotis, 2010; Liu et al., 2013; Li et al., 2015; Gao et al., 2017; Gascon et al., 2017; Yang et al., 2019). IBET151 serves to erase the initial cell-fate specific gene expression pattern (Di Micco et al., 2014; Li et al., 2015; Wu et al., 2015; Marazzi et al., 2018). VPA has been reported to enhanced neuronal induction of cochlear glial cells (Moon et al., 2018). However, more small molecules were hardly studied in cochlear glia-to-neuron induction.

In this study, the small molecule cocktail we identified can promote neuronal maturation and cell fate conversion toward SGNs. The results showed upregulation of generic neuronal genes and SGN specific genes such as *Prox1*, *Islet1*, *Pou4f1*, and *Scrt2*. Consistent with previous reports that Ng1/Nd1 or Lin28 induced glial cells-to-auditory neuron conversion in the cochlea (Kempfle et al., 2020; Li X. et al., 2020), the iNs also exhibited increased expression of both *Nd1* and *Lin28*. Furthermore, we observed the downregulation of glial cell markers such as Plp1, Sox10, S100β, and MBP. Thus, the small molecule cocktail induces neuron differentiation and maturation by removal of glial identity and establishment of neuronal identity.

Outlook Into Functional Maturation of the Induced Neurons

Although the small molecule cocktail greatly promoted neuronal induction toward SGN, expression levels of SGN-specific genes were still lower than those in primary SGNs and some key SGN markers, such as *Ntrk3*, were not upregulated. It is possible that means to upregulate these developmental and functional relevant genes may further promote the maturation of the iNs to functional SGNs *in vivo*.

Other challenges in functional maturation of the iNs remain to be addressed. For example, synaptic connections between the iNs and hair cells or cochlear nucleus are the fundamental elements of the cochlear neuronal circuitry *in vivo*. Previous studies showed synapse formation between ESC-derived iNs and sensory epithelium or cochlear nucleus *in vitro* with limited efficiency (Liu et al., 2018; Meas et al., 2018b) and the de novo synapses were not observed *in vivo* (Kempfle et al., 2020; Li X. et al., 2020). Secondly, SGNs are heterogenous in nature and display distinct molecular signature and spontaneous firing rates Petitpre et al., 2018). The determination of SGN identity is induced by interaction of different spontaneous activity from hair cells (Petitpre et al., 2018; Shrestha et al., 2018; Sun et al., 2018). How the iNs may adopt specific SGN subtype and integrate into the cochlear neuronal circuitry needs to be explored in future studies.

ETHICS STATEMENT

The animal study was reviewed and approved by Institutional Animal Care and Use Committee of Model Animal Research Center of Nanjing University.

AUTHOR CONTRIBUTIONS

GW conceived the study. ZC and GW designed the experiments, analyzed the results, and wrote the manuscript. ZC, YH, CY, QL, and CQ performed the experiments. All authors have read and agreed to the published version of the manuscript.

SUPPLEMENTARY MATERIAL

Supplementary Figure 1 | The non-glial cells in the spheres are likely derived from cochlear mesenchyme cells. **(A)** Percentage of Plp1-tdT$^+$ or Sox2-tdT$^+$ cells to the total number of cells after sphere culture. N = 8–10, error bars represent mean ± SD. **(B)** Representative images of Plp1-tdT$^+$ glial and Plp1-tdT$^-$ non-glial cells after FACS followed by sphere culture. **(C)** RT-qPCR analyses of the glial and non-glial spheres with glial markers (Sox10, Sox2) and mesenchymal markers (Sox9, Pou3f4). N = 3, error bars represent mean ± SD. ***p < 0.001 by unpaired student's t-test.

Supplementary Figure 2 | Small molecules screening and optimization. **(A)** Representative images of TUJ1 immunostaining of iNs treated with various concentrations of small molecules, I-BET, Forskolin, ISX9, Chir99021 at 15 div. **(B)** Representative images of Prox1 immunostaining of iNs treated with small molecules Y27632, SB431542, RA, LIF, Vitamin C, and VPA at 15 div. The white arrowheads represent Prox1$^+$ cells.

Supplementary Figure 3 | Specific expression of SGN markers. **(A)** Representative cartoon showing cochlear localization of SGNs and surrounding glial cells. **(B–G)** Specific expressions of TUJ1 **(B)**, Gata3 **(C)**, Syp **(D)**, Prox1 **(E)**, Map2 **(F)**, and Scrt2 **(G)** in P3–P42 cochlear SGNs.

Supplementary Figure 4 | RT-qPCR validations of glial and neuronal genes regulated during FIBCL-induced differentiation. mRNA expressions of *Islet1*, *Scrt2*, *Pou4f1*, *Prox1*, *Sox10*, *Sox2*, *Ntrk3*, and *S100a4* (as highlighted in **Figure 8H**) in non-differentiated spheres or differentiated cultures treated with SCDM, SCDM/FGF, or FIBCL were analyzed by RT-qPCR. N = 3, error bars represent mean ± SD. *p < 0.05, **p < 0.01, ***p < 0.001 by one-way ANOVA.

REFERENCES

Akil, O., Blits, B., Lustig, L. R., and Leake, P. A. (2019). Virally mediated overexpression of glial-derived neurotrophic factor elicits age- and dose-dependent neuronal toxicity and hearing loss. *Hum. Gene Ther.* 30, 88–105. doi: 10.1089/hum.2018.028

Bao, J., and Ohlemiller, K. K. (2010). Age-related loss of spiral ganglion neurons. *Hear Res.* 264, 93–97. doi: 10.1016/j.heares.2009.10.009

Belin-Rauscent, A., Lacoste, J., Hermine, O., Moussy, A., Everitt, B. J., and Belin, D. (2018). Decrease of cocaine, but not heroin, self-administration and relapse by the tyrosine kinase inhibitor masitinib in male Sprague Dawley rats. *Psychopharmacology* 235, 1545–1556. doi: 10.1007/s00213-018-4865-0

Black, J. B., and Gersbach, C. A. (2018). Synthetic transcription factors for cell fate reprogramming. *Curr. Opin. Genet. Dev.* 52, 13–21. doi: 10.1016/j.gde.2018.05.001

Brooks, P. M., Rose, K. P., MacRae, M. L., Rangoussis, K. M., Gurjar, M., Hertzano, R., et al. (2020). Pou3f4-expressing otic mesenchyme cells promote spiral ganglion neuron survival in the postnatal mouse cochlea. *J. Comp. Neurol.* 528, 1967–1985. doi: 10.1002/cne.24867

Cavallaro, M., Mariani, J., Lancini, C., Latorre, E., Caccia, R., Gullo, F., et al. (2008). Impaired generation of mature neurons by neural stem cells from hypomorphic Sox2 mutants. *Development* 135, 541–557. doi: 10.1242/dev.010801

Chen, W., Jongkamonwiwat, N., Abbas, L., Eshtan, S. J., Johnson, S. L., Kuhn, S., et al. (2012). Restoration of auditory evoked responses by human ES-cell-derived otic progenitors. *Nature* 490, 278–282. doi: 10.1038/nature11415

Coate, T. M., Raft, S., Zhao, X., Ryan, A. K., Crenshaw, E. B. III, and Kelley, M. W. (2012). Otic mesenchyme cells regulate spiral ganglion axon fasciculation through a Pou3f4/EphA4 signaling pathway. *Neuron* 73, 49–63. doi: 10.1016/j.neuron.2011.10.029

Cui, C. P., Zhang, Y., Wang, C., Yuan, F., Li, H., Yao, Y., et al. (2018). Dynamic ubiquitylation of Sox2 regulates proteostasis and governs neural progenitor cell differentiation. *Nat. Commun.* 9:4648. doi: 10.1038/s41467-018-07025-z

Di Micco, R., Fontanals-Cirera, B., Low, V., Ntziachristos, P., Yuen, S. K., Lovell, C. D., et al. (2014). Control of embryonic stem cell identity by BRD4-dependent transcriptional elongation of super-enhancer-associated pluripotency genes. *Cell Rep.* 9, 234–247. doi: 10.1016/j.celrep.2014.08.055

Diensthuber, M., Zecha, V., Wagenblast, J., Arnhold, S., Edge, A. S., and Stover, T. (2014a). Spiral ganglion stem cells can be propagated and differentiated into neurons and glia. *Biores. Open. Access* 3, 88–97. doi: 10.1089/biores.2014.0016

Diensthuber, M., Zecha, V., Wagenblast, J., Arnhold, S., and Stover, T. (2014b). Clonal colony formation from spiral ganglion stem cells. *Neuroreport* 25, 1129–1135. doi: 10.1097/WNR.0000000000000240

Dworkin, S., and Mantamadiotis, T. (2010). Targeting CREB signalling in neurogenesis. *Expert Opin. Ther. Targets* 14, 869–879. doi: 10.1517/14728222.2010.501332

Fang, Q., Zhang, Y., Chen, X., Li, H., Cheng, L., Zhu, W., et al. (2019). Three-dimensional graphene enhances neural stem cell proliferation through metabolic regulation. *Front. Bioeng. Biotechnol.* 7:436. doi: 10.3389/fbioe.2019.00436

Fettiplace, R. (2017). Hair cell transduction, tuning, and synaptic transmission in the mammalian cochlea. *Compr. Physiol.* 7, 1197–1227. doi: 10.1002/cphy.c160049

Fryatt, A. G., Mulheran, M., Egerton, J., Gunthorpe, M. J., and Grubb, B. D. (2011). Ototrauma induces sodium channel plasticity in auditory afferent neurons. *Mol. Cell Neurosci.* 48, 51–61. doi: 10.1016/j.mcn.2011.06.005

Gao, L., Guan, W., Wang, M., Wang, H., Yu, J., Liu, Q., et al. (2017). Direct generation of human neuronal cells from adult astrocytes by small molecules. *Stem Cell Rep.* 8, 538–547. doi: 10.1016/j.stemcr.2017.01.014

Gascon, S., Masserdotti, G., Russo, G. L., and Gotz, M. (2017). Direct neuronal reprogramming: achievements, hurdles, and new roads to success. *Cell Stem Cell* 21, 18–34. doi: 10.1016/j.stem.2017.06.011

Graham, V., Khudyakov, J., Ellis, P., and Pevny, L. (2003). SOX2 functions to maintain neural progenitor identity. *Neuron* 39, 749–765. doi: 10.1016/S0896-6273(03)00497-5

Guo, R., Li, J., Chen, C., Xiao, M., Liao, M., Hu, Y., et al. (2021). Biomimetic 3D bacterial cellulose-graphene foam hybrid scaffold regulates neural stem cell proliferation and differentiation. *Colloids Surf. B Biointerfaces* 200:111590. doi: 10.1016/j.colsurfb.2021.111590

Guo, R., Ma, X., Liao, M., Liu, Y., Hu, Y., Qian, X., et al. (2019). Development and application of cochlear implant-based electric-acoustic stimulation of spiral ganglion neurons. *ACS Biomater. Sci. Eng.* 5, 6735–6741. doi: 10.1021/acsbiomaterials.9b01265

Guo, R., Xiao, M., Zhao, W., Zhou, S., Hu, Y., Liao, M., et al. (2020). 2D Ti3C2TxMXene couples electrical stimulation to promote proliferation and neural differentiation of neural stem cells. *Acta Biomater.* S1742-7061, 30749–30752. doi: 10.1016/j.actbio.2020.12.035

Guo, R., Zhang, S., Xiao, M., Qian, F., He, Z., Li, D., et al. (2016). Accelerating bioelectric functional development of neural stem cells by graphene coupling: implications for neural interfacing with conductive materials. *Biomaterials* 106, 193–204. doi: 10.1016/j.biomaterials.2016.08.019

Guo, Z., Zhang, L., Wu, Z., Chen, Y., Wang, F., and Chen, G. (2014). In vivo direct reprogramming of reactive glial cells into functional neurons after brain injury and in an Alzheimer's disease model. *Cell Stem Cell* 14, 188–202. doi: 10.1016/j.stem.2013.12.001

Han, S., Xu, Y., Sun, J., Liu, Y., Zhao, Y., Tao, W., et al. (2020). Isolation and analysis of extracellular vesicles in a Morpho butterfly wing-integrated microvortex biochip. *Biosens. Bioelectron.* 154:112073. doi: 10.1016/j.bios.2020.11 2073

He, Z., Guo, L., Shu, Y., Fang, Q., Zhou, H., Liu, Y., et al. (2017). Autophagy protects auditory hair cells against neomycin-induced damage. *Autophagy* 13, 1884–1904. doi: 10.1080/15548627.2017.1359449

Ho, S.-Y., Chao, C.-Y., Huang, H.-L., Chiu, T.-W., Charoenkwan, P., and Hwang, E. (2011). NeurphologyJ: an automatic neuronal morphology quantification method and its application in pharmacological discovery. *BMC Bioinformatics* 12:230. doi: 10.1186/1471-2105-12-230

Hu, W., Qiu, B., Guan, W., Wang, Q., Wang, M., Li, W., et al. (2015). Direct conversion of normal and Alzheimer's disease human fibroblasts into neuronal cells by small molecules. *Cell Stem Cell* 17, 204–212. doi: 10.1016/j.stem.2015.07.006

Jessen, K. R., and Mirsky, R. (2005). The origin and development of glial cells in peripheral nerves. *Nat. Rev. Neurosci.* 6, 671–682. doi: 10.1038/nrn1746

Kempfle, J. S., Luu, N. C., Petrillo, M., Al-Asad, R., Zhang, A., and Edge, A. S. B. (2020). Lin28 reprograms inner ear glia to a neuronal fate. *Stem Cells* 38, 890–903. doi: 10.1002/stem.3181

Kiernan, A. E., Pelling, A. L., Leung, K. K. H., Tang, A. S. P., Bell, D. M., Tease, C., et al. (2005). Sox2 is required for sensory organ development in the mammalian inner ear. *Nature* 434, 1031–1035. doi: 10.1038/nature03487

Koehler, K. R., Mikosz, A. M., Molosh, A. I., Patel, D., and Hashino, E. (2013). Generation of inner ear sensory epithelia from pluripotent stem cells in 3D culture. *Nature* 500, 217–221. doi: 10.1038/nature12298

Koike, T., Wakabayashi, T., Mori, T., Hirahara, Y., and Yamada, H. (2015). Sox2 promotes survival of satellite glial cells in vitro. *Biochem. Biophys. Res. Commun.* 464, 269–274. doi: 10.1016/j.bbrc.2015.06.141

Lang, H., Li, M., Kilpatrick, L. A., Zhu, J., Samuvel, D. J., Krug, E. L., et al. (2011). Sox2 up-regulation and glial cell proliferation following degeneration of spiral ganglion neurons in the adult mouse inner ear. *J. Assoc. Res. Otolaryngol.* 12, 151–171. doi: 10.1007/s10162-010-0244-1

Lang, H., Schulte, B. A., and Schmiedt, R. A. (2005). Ouabain induces apoptotic cell death in type I spiral ganglion neurons, but not type II neurons. *J. Assoc. Res. Otolaryngol.* 6, 63–74. doi: 10.1007/s10162-004-5021-6

Lang, H., Xing, Y., Brown, L. N., Samuvel, D. J., Panganiban, C. H., Havens, L. T., et al. (2015). Neural stem/progenitor cell properties of glial cells in the adult mouse auditory nerve. *Sci. Rep.* 5:13383. doi: 10.1038/srep13 383

Langmead, B., and Salzberg, S. L. (2012). Fast gapped-read alignment with Bowtie 2. *Nat. Methods* 9, 357–359. doi: 10.1038/nmeth.1923

Lee, A. S., Tang, C., Rao, M. S., Weissman, I. L., and Wu, J. C. (2013). Tumorigenicity as a clinical hurdle for pluripotent stem cell therapies. *Nat. Med.* 19, 998–1004. doi: 10.1038/nm.3267

Li, B., and Dewey, C. N. (2011). RSEM: accurate transcript quantification from RNA-Seq data with or without a reference genome. *BMC Bioinformatics* 12:323. doi: 10.1186/1471-2105-12-323

Li, C., Li, X., Bi, Z., Sugino, K., Wang, G., Zhu, T., et al. (2020). Comprehensive transcriptome analysis of cochlear spiral ganglion neurons at multiple ages. *Elife* 9:e50491. doi: 10.7554/eLife.50491

Li, G., Chen, K., You, D., Xia, M., Li, W., Fan, S., et al. (2019). Laminin-coated electrospun regenerated silk fibroin mats promote neural progenitor cell proliferation, differentiation, and survival in vitro. *Front. Bioeng. Biotechnol.* 7:190. doi: 10.3389/fbioe.2019.00190

Li, H., Liu, H., and Heller, S. (2003). Pluripotent stem cells from the adult mouse inner ear. *Nat. Med.* 9, 1293–1299. doi: 10.1038/nm925

Li, X., Aleardi, A., Wang, J., Zhou, Y., Andrade, R., and Hu, Z. (2016). Differentiation of spiral ganglion-derived neural stem cells into functional synaptogenetic neurons. *Stem Cells Dev* 25, 803–813. doi: 10.1089/scd.2015.0345

Li, X., Bi, Z., Sun, Y., Li, C., Li, Y., and Liu, Z. (2020). In vivo ectopic Ngn1 and Neurod1 convert neonatal cochlear glial cells into spiral ganglion neurons. *FASEB J.* 34, 4764–4782. doi: 10.1096/fj.201902118R

Li, X., Xu, J., and Deng, H. (2018). Small molecule-induced cellular fate reprogramming: promising road leading to Rome. *Curr. Opin. Genet. Dev.* 52, 29–35. doi: 10.1016/j.gde.2018.05.004

Li, X., Zuo, X., Jing, J., Ma, Y., Wang, J., Liu, D., et al. (2015). Small-molecule-driven direct reprogramming of mouse fibroblasts into functional neurons. *Cell Stem Cell* 17, 195–203. doi: 10.1016/j.stem.2015.06.003

Liberman, M. C. (2017). Noise-induced and age-related hearing loss: new perspectives and potential therapies. *F1000Res.* 6:927. doi: 10.12688/f1000research.11310.1

Liu, M. L., Zang, T., Zou, Y., Chang, J. C., Gibson, J. R., Huber, K. M., et al. (2013). Small molecules enable neurogenin 2 to efficiently convert human fibroblasts into cholinergic neurons. *Nat. Commun.* 4:2183. doi: 10.1038/ncomms3183

Liu, W., Xu, L., Wang, X., Zhang, D., Sun, G., Wang, M., et al. (2021). PRDX1 activates autophagy via the PTEN-AKT signaling pathway to protect against cisplatin-induced spiral ganglion neuron damage. *Autophagy* 1–23. doi: 10.1080/15548627.2021.1905466

Liu, W., Xu, X., Fan, Z., Sun, G., Han, Y., Zhang, D., et al. (2019). Wnt signaling activates TP53-induced glycolysis and apoptosis regulator and protects against cisplatin-induced spiral ganglion neuron damage in the mouse cochlea. *Antioxid. Redox Signal.* 30, 1389–1410. doi: 10.1089/ars.2017.7288

Liu, Z., Jiang, Y., Li, X., and Hu, Z. (2018). Embryonic stem cell-derived peripheral auditory neurons form neural connections with mouse central auditory neurons in vitro via the alpha2delta1 receptor. *Stem Cell Rep.* 11, 157–170. doi: 10.1016/j.stemcr.2018.05.006

Loo, B.-M., and Salmivirta, M. (2002). Heparin/Heparan sulfate domains in binding and signaling of fibroblast growth factor 8b. *J. Biol. Chem.* 277, 32616–32623. doi: 10.1074/jbc.M204961200

Lukovic, D., Stojkovic, M., Moreno-Manzano, V., Bhattacharya, S. S., and Erceg, S. (2014). Perspectives and future directions of human pluripotent stem cell-based therapies: lessons from Geron's clinical trial for spinal cord injury. *Stem Cells Dev.* 23, 1–4. doi: 10.1089/scd.2013.0266

Marazzi, I., Greenbaum, B. D., Low, D. H. P., and Guccione, E. (2018). Chromatin dependencies in cancer and inflammation. *Nat. Rev. Mol. Cell Biol.* 19, 245–261. doi: 10.1038/nrm.2017.113

McLean, W. J., McLean, D. T., Eatock, R. A., and Edge, A. S. (2016). Distinct capacity for differentiation to inner ear cell types by progenitor cells of the cochlea and vestibular organs. *Development* 143, 4381–4393. doi: 10.1242/dev.139840

Meas, S. J., Nishimura, K., Scheibinger, M., and Dabdoub, A. (2018a). In vitro methods to cultivate spiral ganglion cells, and purification of cellular subtypes for induced neuronal reprogramming. *Front. Neurosci.* 12:822. doi: 10.3389/fnins.2018.00822

Meas, S. J., Zhang, C. L., and Dabdoub, A. (2018b). Reprogramming glia into neurons in the peripheral auditory system as a solution for sensorineural hearing loss: lessons from the central nervous system. *Front. Mol. Neurosci.* 11:77. doi: 10.3389/fnmol.2018.00077

Mercurio, S., Serra, L., and Nicolis, S. K. (2019). More than just stem cells: functional roles of the transcription factor Sox2 in differentiated glia and neurons. *Int. J. Mol. Sci.* 20:4540. doi: 10.3390/ijms20184540

Mertens, J., Marchetto, M. C., Bardy, C., and Gage, F. H. (2016). Evaluating cell reprogramming, differentiation and conversion technologies in neuroscience. *Nat. Rev. Neurosci.* 17, 424–437. doi: 10.1038/nrn.2016.46

Moon, B. S., Lu, W., and Park, H. J. (2018). Valproic acid promotes the neuronal differentiation of spiral ganglion neural stem cells with robust axonal growth. *Biochem. Biophys. Res. Commun.* 503, 2728–2735. doi: 10.1016/j.bbrc.2018.08.032

Morgado, A. L., Rodrigues, C. M., and Sola, S. (2016). MicroRNA-145 regulates neural stem cell differentiation through the Sox2-Lin28/let-7 signaling pathway. *Stem Cells* 34, 1386–1395. doi: 10.1002/stem.2309

Muller, U., and Barr-Gillespie, P. G. (2015). New treatment options for hearing loss. *Nat. Rev. Drug Discov.* 14, 346–365. doi: 10.1038/nrd4533

Noda, T., Meas, S. J., Nogami, J., Amemiya, Y., Uchi, R., Ohkawa, Y., et al. (2018). Direct reprogramming of spiral ganglion non-neuronal cells into neurons: toward ameliorating sensorineural hearing loss by gene therapy. *Front. Cell Dev. Biol.* 6:16. doi: 10.3389/fcell.2018.00016

Oshima, K., Grimm, C. M., Corrales, C. E., Senn, P., Martinez Monedero, R., Geleoc, G. S., et al. (2007). Differential distribution of stem cells in the auditory and vestibular organs of the inner ear. *J. Assoc. Res. Otolaryngol.* 8, 18–31. doi: 10.1007/s10162-006-0058-3

Perny, M., Ting, C. C., Kleinlogel, S., Senn, P., and Roccio, M. (2017). Generation of otic sensory neurons from mouse embryonic stem cells in 3D culture. *Front. Cell Neurosci.* 11:409. doi: 10.3389/fncel.2017.00409

Petitpre, C., Wu, H., Sharma, A., Tokarska, A., Fontanet, P., Wang, Y., et al. (2018). Neuronal heterogeneity and stereotyped connectivity in the auditory afferent system. *Nat. Commun.* 9:3691. doi: 10.1038/s41467-018-06033-3

Qian, H., Kang, X., Hu, J., Zhang, D., Liang, Z., Meng, F., et al. (2020). Reversing a model of Parkinson's disease with in situ converted nigral neurons. *Nature* 582, 550–556. doi: 10.1038/s41586-020-2388-4

Robinson, M. D., McCarthy, D. J., and Smyth, G. K. (2010). edgeR: a bioconductor package for differential expression analysis of digital gene expression data. *Bioinformatics* 26, 139–140. doi: 10.1093/bioinformatics/btp616

Schneider, J. W., Gao, Z., Li, S., Farooqi, M., Tang, T. S., Bezprozvanny, I., et al. (2008). Small-molecule activation of neuronal cell fate. *Nat. Chem. Biol.* 4, 408–410. doi: 10.1038/nchembio.95

Shrestha, B. R., Chia, C., Wu, L., Kujawa, S. G., Liberman, M. C., and Goodrich, L. V. (2018). Sensory neuron diversity in the inner ear is shaped by activity. *Cell* 174, 1229–1246.e17. doi: 10.1016/j.cell.2018.07.007

Sun, G., Liu, W., Fan, Z., Zhang, D., Han, Y., Xu, L., et al. (2016). The three-dimensional culture system with matrigel and neurotrophic factors preserves the structure and function of spiral ganglion neuron in vitro. *Neural Plast.* 2016:4280407. doi: 10.1155/2016/4280407

Sun, S., Babola, T., Pregernig, G., So, K. S., Nguyen, M., Su, S. M., et al. (2018). Hair cell mechanotransduction regulates spontaneous activity and spiral ganglion subtype specification in the auditory system. *Cell* 174, 1247–1263.e15. doi: 10.1016/j.cell.2018.07.008

Suzuki, J., Corfas, G., and Liberman, M. C. (2016). Round-window delivery of neurotrophin 3 regenerates cochlear synapses after acoustic overexposure. *Sci. Rep.* 6:24907. doi: 10.1038/srep24907

Tang, M., Li, J., He, L., Guo, R., Yan, X., Li, D., et al. (2019). Transcriptomic profiling of neural stem cell differentiation on graphene substrates. *Colloids Surf. B Biointerfaces* 182:110324. doi: 10.1016/j.colsurfb.2019.06.054

Vlajkovic, S. M., Ambepitiya, K., Barclay, M., Boison, D., Housley, G. D., and Thorne, P. R. (2017). Adenosine receptors regulate susceptibility to noise-induced neural injury in the mouse cochlea and hearing loss. *Hear Res.* 345, 43–51. doi: 10.1016/j.heares.2016.12.015

Wan, G., and Corfas, G. (2017). Transient auditory nerve demyelination as a new mechanism for hidden hearing loss. *Nat. Commun.* 8:14487. doi: 10.1038/ncomms14487

Wise, A. K., Tu, T., Atkinson, P. J., Flynn, B. O., Sgro, B. E., Hume, C., et al. (2011). The effect of deafness duration on neurotrophin gene therapy for spiral ganglion neuron protection. *Hear Res.* 278, 69–76. doi: 10.1016/j.heares.2011.04.010

Wu, T., Pinto, H. B., Kamikawa, Y. F., and Donohoe, M. E. (2015). The BET family member BRD4 interacts with OCT4 and regulates pluripotency gene expression. *Stem Cell Rep.* 4, 390–403. doi: 10.1016/j.stemcr.2015.01.012

Xia, L., Shang, Y., Chen, X., Li, H., Xu, X., Liu, W., et al. (2020). Oriented neural spheroid formation and differentiation of neural stem cells guided by anisotropic inverse opals. *Front. Bioeng. Biotechnol.* 8:848. doi: 10.3389/fbioe.2020.00848

Yan, W., Liu, W., Qi, J., Fang, Q., Fan, Z., Sun, G., et al. (2018). A three-dimensional culture system with matrigel promotes purified spiral ganglion neuron survival and function in vitro. *Mol. Neurobiol.* 55, 2070–2084. doi: 10.1007/s12035-017-0471-0

Yang, Y., Chen, R., Wu, X., Zhao, Y., Fan, Y., Xiao, Z., et al. (2019). Rapid and efficient conversion of human fibroblasts into functional neurons by small molecules. *Stem Cell Rep.* 13, 862–876. doi: 10.1016/j.stemcr.2019.09.007

Yang, Y., Gao, B., Hu, Y., Wei, H., Zhang, C., Chai, R., et al. (2021). Ordered inverse-opal scaffold based on bionic transpiration to create a biomimetic spine. *Nanoscale* 13, 8614–8622. doi: 10.1039/D1NR00731A

Yang, Y., Zhang, Y., Chai, R., and Gu, Z. (2020). A polydopamine-functionalized carbon microfibrous scaffold accelerates the development of neural stem cells. *Front. Bioeng. Biotechnol.* 8:616. doi: 10.3389/fbioe.2020.00616

Yuan, T. F., Dong, Y., Zhang, L., Qi, J., Yao, C., Wang, Y., et al. (2021). Neuromodulation-based stem cell therapy in brain repair: recent advances and future perspectives. *Neurosci. Bull.* 37, 735–745. doi: 10.1007/s12264-021-00667-y

Zhang, L., Jiang, H., and Hu, Z. (2011). Concentration-dependent effect of nerve growth factor on cell fate determination of neural progenitors. *Stem Cells Dev.* 20, 1723–1731. doi: 10.1089/scd.2010.0370

Zhang, S., and Cui, W. (2014). Sox2, a key factor in the regulation of pluripotency and neural differentiation. *World J. Stem Cells* 6, 305–311. doi: 10.4252/wjsc.v6.i3.305

Zhao, J., Tang, M., Cao, J., Ye, D., Guo, X., Xi, J., et al. (2019). Structurally tunable reduced graphene oxide substrate maintains mouse embryonic stem cell pluripotency. *Adv. Sci. (Weinh.)* 6:1802136. doi: 10.1002/advs.201802136

Zuchero, J. B., and Barres, B. A. (2015). Glia in mammalian development and disease. *Development* 142, 3805–3809. doi: 10.1242/dev.129304

Sirtuin-3 Protects Cochlear Hair Cells Against Noise-Induced Damage *via* the Superoxide Dismutase 2/Reactive Oxygen Species Signaling Pathway

Wenqi Liang, Chunli Zhao, Zhongrui Chen, Zijing Yang, Ke Liu* and Shusheng Gong*

Department of Otolaryngology Head and Neck Surgery, Beijing Friendship Hospital, Capital Medical University, Beijing, China

*Correspondence:
Ke Liu
liuke@ccmu.edu.cn
Shusheng Gong
gongss@ccmu.edu.cn

Mitochondrial oxidative stress is involved in hair cell damage caused by noise-induced hearing loss (NIHL). Sirtuin-3 (SIRT3) plays an important role in hair cell survival by regulating mitochondrial function; however, the role of SIRT3 in NIHL is unknown. In this study, we used 3-TYP to inhibit SIRT3 and found that this inhibition aggravated oxidative damage in the hair cells of mice with NIHL. Moreover, 3-TYP reduced the enzymatic activity and deacetylation levels of superoxide dismutase 2 (SOD2). Subsequently, we administered adeno-associated virus-SIRT3 to the posterior semicircular canals and found that SIRT3 overexpression significantly attenuated hair cell injury and that this protective effect of SIRT3 could be blocked by 2-methoxyestradiol, a SOD2 inhibitor. These findings suggest that insufficient SIRT3/SOD2 signaling leads to mitochondrial oxidative damage resulting in hair cell injury in NIHL. Thus, ameliorating noise-induced mitochondrial redox imbalance by intervening in the SIRT3/SOD2 signaling pathway may be a new therapeutic target for hair cell injury.

Keywords: SIRT3, SOD2, noise-induced hearing loss, viral transduction, oxidative stress

INTRODUCTION

Noise is a worldwide public health problem and an important risk factor for sensorineural hearing loss (SNHL). Oxidative stress-induced hair cell damage plays an important role in its development (Zhang et al., 2019). Noise exposure (NE) causes oxidative stress, elevates reactive oxygen species (ROS) levels, and causes hair cell damage, which further contributes to hearing loss (Delmaghani et al., 2015). Although several studies in the past decades have focused on countering noise-induced hair cell damage by interfering with ROS, there are no clinically relevant intervention targets to date. Therefore, key targets in the pathogenesis of noise-induced hearing loss (NIHL) should be explored.

Mitochondrial abnormalities caused by ROS accumulation play an important role in the pathogenesis of NIHL (Ding et al., 2020; Zhong et al., 2020). ROS are mainly produced in the mitochondrial oxidative respiratory chain; therefore, mitochondrial dysfunction can lead to cellular ROS accumulation (Gao et al., 2019; Zhao et al., 2019). Thus, mitochondrial dysfunction supposedly causes most oxidative damage (Tian et al., 2013). Sirtuin-3 (SIRT3), a member of the Sirtuin family, is a nicotinamide adenine dinucleotide (NAD$^+$)-dependent deacetylase that is localized in the mitochondria (Onyango et al., 2002); it is the major mitochondrial deacetylase (Lombard et al., 2007) and a key factor regulating autophagy pathways. Autophagy and apoptosis are often simultaneously triggered by similar stimuli, such as oxidative stress, in both hair cells and spiral ganglion neurons (SGNs) (He et al., 2021;

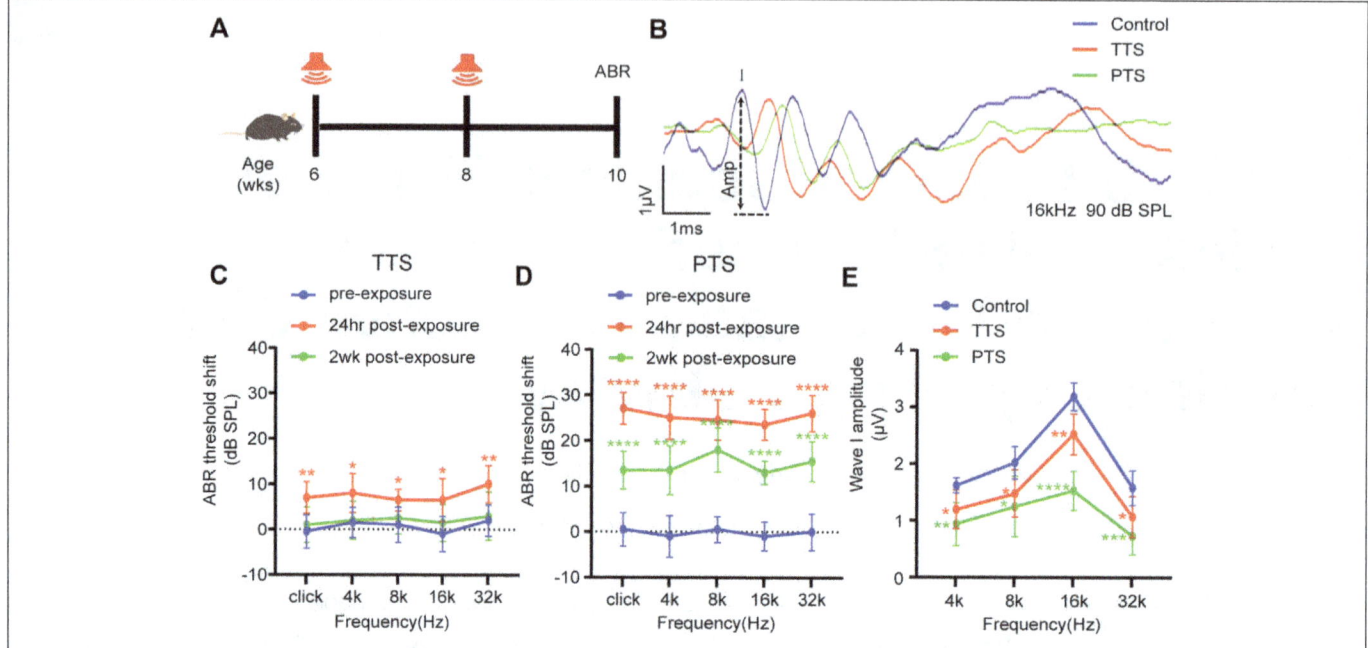

FIGURE 1 | Changes in ABR thresholds and I-wave amplitudes after one or two NEs. **(A)** Mice underwent NE at 6 and 8 weeks of age or only at 8 weeks of age, and ABR testing was performed at 10 weeks of age. **(B)** Overlapped ABR waves were recorded in response to 16 kHz 90 dB SPL stimuli in control, TTS and PTS mice. **(C)** ABR test showing changes in the hearing thresholds of mice in the TTS group before NE and at 24 h and 2 weeks after NE. **(D)** ABR test showing changes in hearing thresholds of mice in the PTS group before NE and at 24 h and 2 weeks after NE. **(E)** ABR test showing changes in I-wave amplitude after NE. (n = 10 per group). ABR, auditory brainstem response; NE, noise exposure; TTS, temporary threshold shift; PTS, permanent threshold shift. *p < 0.05; **p < 0.01; ***p < 0.001; ****p < 0.0001.

Liu et al., 2021). As the main site of cellular energy metabolism, mitochondria have various biological functions such as regulating cell proliferation, differentiation, apoptosis and senescence. SIRT3 regulates mitochondrial energy metabolism and biosynthesis; therefore, abnormal SIRT3 expression negatively affects mitochondrial function. Increased SIRT3 expression protects cells from oxidative stress-induced cell death and inhibits apoptosis in age-related SGNs and hair cells (Someya et al., 2010). Furthermore, SIRT3 overexpression reduces axonal degeneration induced by NE, thus making mice resistant to NIHL (Brown et al., 2014).

Superoxide dismutase 2 (SOD2) is a key antioxidant enzyme in mitochondria that reduces ROS production and protects cells from oxidative stress (Sarsour et al., 2014). Acetylation is one of the most important post-translational SOD2 modifications, leading to the downregulation of the SOD2 function (Dikalova et al., 2017). SIRT3 works by deacetylating proteins, particularly lysine of SOD2, to regulate its activity and thus maintain mitochondrial function (Yang et al., 2016).

Given the important role of mitochondrial function in the development of NIHL, we hypothesized that changes in SOD2 deacetylation levels due to SIRT3 activity are involved in the pathogenesis of NIHL. To test this hypothesis, we explored the protective effect of SIRT3 on hair cell injury in NIHL mice and its underlying mechanisms.

MATERIALS AND METHODS

Animals and Treatments

C57BL/6 J male mice were obtained from the Experimental Animal Center of Capital Medical University (Beijing, China). Experiments were performed on mice after abnormal hearing was excluded by audiometric testing. According to the different interventions strategies, mice were randomly divided into the following groups: 27 mice in the control group, 5 in the TTS group, 73 in the PTS group, 37 in the PTS+3-TYP group, 5 in the PTS + corn oil group, 5 in the PTS+2-ME group, 5 in the PTS + saline group, 9 in the PTS + AAV-SIRT3 group, 5 in the PTS + AAV-GFP group, and 5 in the PTS+2-ME + AAV-SIRT3 group. Mice in the PTS group received NE at 6 and 8 weeks old of mice, whereas mice in the TTS group received NE only at 8 weeks old, and both groups underwent auditory brainstem response (ABR) testing at 10 weeks (**Figure 1A**). For the intervention group mice received 3-TYP, 2-ME or AAV-SIRT3 in addition to NE. Both 3-TYP (MCE Chemicals & Equipment Co., Malta, NY) and 2-methoxyestradiol (2-ME; Selleck Chemicals, Houston, TX) were administered by intraperitoneal injection starting 1 week prior to NE for 7 days 3-TYP was administered at 50 mg/kg/day, and 2-ME was administered at 16 mg/kg/day. The control group mice were injected with equal amounts of either saline or corn oil. AAV-SIRT3 was surgically introduced into the inner ear at 4 weeks in the AAV-SIRT3 intervention group of mice, and an equal amount of empty virus was introduced into the control group mice. The animals were cared for and used in accordance with the Guideline for the Care and Use of Laboratory Animals of the National Institutes of Health. The experimental protocols were approved by the Committee on the Ethics of Animal Experiments of Capital Medical University.

Noise Exposure

Animals in the noise group were placed in wire mesh cages inside an anechoic chamber and exposed to 100 dB sound pressure level (SPL) broadband white noise for 2 h. Noise synthesis was performed using Cool Edit Pro software (Adobe Systems, San Jose, CA) and transmitted through XTi4002, CROWN amplifiers (Harman, Elkhart, IN) to two speakers (JBL KP6000, PROFESSIONAL, Harman) for noise release.

ABR Testing

We used the TDT system 3 evoked potential workstation (Tucker-Davis Technologies, Alachua, FL, United States) to record ABR. Prior to initiating the ABR test, mice were anesthetized by intraperitoneal injection of 100 mg/kg ketamine and 10 mg/kg xylazine. After anesthesia, the recording electrode was inserted in the subcutaneous area at the midpoint of the line connecting the anterior margins of the auricles on both sides of the mouse, the reference electrode was inserted into the subcutaneous area behind the tested ear, and the ground electrode was inserted into the subcutaneous area behind the contralateral ear. The tests were performed using click and tone bursts at frequencies of 4, 8, 16, and 32 kHz with the SigGenRZ software (Tucker-Davis Technologies). Sound intensity was attenuated from 90 to 0 dB in 5 dB intervals, and the responses were analyzed using BioSigRZ software (Tucker-Davis Technologies), digitized, and averaged for each frequency-level combination (1,024 samples/level). The threshold was defined as the lowest stimulus decibel that evoked a significant positive wave in the response trajectory. All ABR tests were performed by the same researchers.

Tissue Preparation

After ABR testing, mice were sacrificed under deep anesthesia, and the cochlea was removed and immersed in 4% paraformaldehyde at 4°C for overnight fixation. Parts of the cochlea were decalcified in 10% ethylenediaminetetraacetic acid (EDTA) for 12 h and subsequently dehydrated in 30% sucrose for 2 h. Afterward, the cochlea was immersed in an optimal cutting temperature compound. Frozen sections of 10 μm thickness were stored at −20°C for immunohistochemistry. Other cochleae were decalcified using 10% EDTA for 2 h; structures such as vascular striae, spiral ligaments and capping membranes were carefully excised under a microscope, and the remaining basilar membranes were divided into the apical, middle, and basal turns for immunofluorescence staining.

Immunostaining

Cochlear sections and spreads were incubated with 5% normal goat serum (ZSGB-BIO, Beijing, China) and 0.3% Triton X-100 (Sigma-Aldrich, St. Louis, MO) in phosphate-buffered saline (PBS) for 2 h at room temperature. After washing three times with PBS, the samples were incubated with primary antibody solution at 4°C overnight. After multiple washes, the samples were incubated with secondary antibodies at a ratio of 1:300 for 2 h at room temperature and protected from light. The primary antibodies used were anti-myosin-VIIa (1:300, *Proteus* BioSciences Inc. Ramona, CA), anti-CtBP2 (1:500, BD Biosciences, Franklin Lakes, NJ), anti-GluR2 (1:400, Millipore, Burlington, MA), anti-8-hydroxy-2′-deoxyguanosine (8-OHdG, 1:300, Abcam, Cambridge, United Kingdom), anti-green fluorescent protein (GFP) (1:100, Santa Cruz Biotechnology, Dallas, TX), and anti-4-HNE (1:500; Abcam). The secondary antibodies used were goat anti-mouse IgG1 Alexa Fluor 568, goat anti-mouse IgG2a Alexa Fluor 488, and goat anti-rabbit IgG (H + L) Alexa Fluor 647 (1:300, Invitrogen/Molecular Probes, Eugene, OR). 4, 6-diamidino-2-phe-nylindole (DAPI) was used for the final addition of coverslips. The expression of 8-OHdG and 4HNE was analyzed using Image-Pro Plus 6.0 software (Media Cybernetics, Inc. United States).

Hair Cells and Synapses Counting

Cochlear samples were observed and imaged using a Leica scanning confocal microscope (Leica Camera AG, Hessen, Germany). The basilar membrane was divided into apical, middle, and basal turns to count the hair cells separately. Lost hair cells were examined under a ×63 oil immersion objective lens and their numbers and proportions were statistically analyzed. Ten cochlear samples from each group were used for hair cell counts. Scans were taken at 0.35 μm/layer intervals from the top to the bottom of the inner hair cell (IHC) and subsequently superimposed. In each region, the total number of synapses was evaluated for a total of approximately 10 IHCs, and the average was subsequently calculated. The number of paired and unpaired synapses at the apical, middle, and basal turns were counted.

Viral Constructs and Posterior Semicircular Canal Transduction

Purified adeno-associated virus (AAV) eight vectors with SIRT3 and the GFP gene (AAV8-SIRT3-GFP) and AAV8-GFP vectors were obtained from Vigenebio Biosciences Co. (Jinan, China). The expression of carrier genes was driven by the cytomegalovirus promoter. Viral particles were purified using ion-exchange column chromatography; physical titers were 1.81×10^{12} vg/ml (AAV8-SIRT3-GFP) and 1.19×10^{12} vg/mL (AAV8-GFP). The vectors were stored at approximately −80°C. As previously described, the injection was administered through the semicircular canals (canalostomy) (Guo et al., 2018). A 2 μl volume of the virus was injected at a rate of 0.5 μl/min.

Western Blotting (WB)

Cochlear proteins were extracted and protein concentrations were measured using a BCA Protein Quantification Kit (Beyotime, China). Equal amounts of proteins were separated by 12% sodium dodecyl sulfate polyacrylamide gel electrophoresis and subsequently electrotransferred to polyvinylidene fluoride membranes. After blocking in 5% skim milk at room temperature for 1 h, samples were incubated with anti-SOD2 (Cell Signaling Technology), anti-ac-SOD2 (Abcam), anti-C-cas3 (Cell Signaling Technology), anti-Cyt c (Abcam), anti-COX IV (Abcam), and β-actin (Cell Signaling Technology) primary antibodies overnight at 4°C, followed by incubation with the appropriate secondary antibody at room temperature for 1 h. After washing with Tris-buffered saline with Tween, protein bands were observed using chemiluminescent reagents (Applygen Technologies Inc. China).

ROS Detection

The intracellular ROS assay was performed using the Reactive Oxygen Species Assay Kit (Beyotime, Shanghai, China). After collecting the cochlear cells, they were resuspended in 100 μL of diluted dichloro-dihydro-fluorescein diacetate and incubated for 20 min at 37°C in a cell culture incubator. Afterward, the cells were washed three times with a serum-free cell culture medium, and chemiluminescence was measured using an EnSpire enzyme marker (PerkinElmer, Waltham, MA).

A mitochondrial membrane potential assay kit with JC-1 (Beyotime, China) was used to analyze mitochondrial ROS production. The cochlea was cut and digested with trypsin, and the cells were collected by centrifugation. Cell pellets were then resuspended in a cell culture medium containing JC-1 staining working solution and incubated at 37°C for 20 min in the dark, washed with cold JC-1 staining buffer and analyzed by flow cytometry (FACS Aria IIu, BD Biosciences) within 1 h.

Measurement of SOD2 Activity

The SOD2 activity assay was performed using the Cu/Zn-SOD and Mn-SOD Assay Kit with WST-8 (Beyotime, China) according to the manufacturer's instructions. After the cochlear tissue was cut and digested with trypsin, the cells were extracted by centrifugation. Cells were incubated for 1 h at 37°C using Cu/Zn-SOD inhibitor A and for 15 min at 37°C using Cu/Zn-SOD inhibitor B. Consequently, samples were added to a 96-well plate and mixed with the assay solution. Chemiluminescence was measured using an EnSpire enzyme marker (PerkinElmer). SOD2 viability units were calculated using a standard curve.

Determination of NADPH Oxidase Activity

According to the manufacturer's instructions, NADPH oxidase activity was assayed using a NADP +/NADPH Assay Kit with WST-8 (Beyotime, China). Bilateral cochleae were dissected from eight mice (four per group) and homogenized in NADP +/NADPH extracts. The samples were centrifuged at 12,000 g for 10 min at 4 °C, and the supernatant was subsequently collected. For testing, 200 μl of the sample was aspirated and placed in a water bath at 60°C for 30 min. Afterward, they were centrifuged at 10,000 g for 5 min at 4°C, the supernatant was collected and mixed with G6PDH working solution and color development solution, and incubated for 20 min at 37°C protected from the light. Sample chemiluminescence was measured using an EnSpire enzyme marker (PerkinElmer). NADPH oxidase activity was calculated from the standard curve.

Statistical Analysis

Quantitative values are expressed as mean ± standard error of the mean (SEM) and statistically analyzed using GraphPad Prism software version 8.0 (GraphPad Software Inc., San Diego, CA). The statistical methods selected were two-way analysis of variance or unpaired t-test, as appropriate. For all analyses, values of $p < 0.05$ were considered statistically significant.

RESULTS

Noise Exposure Causes a Hearing Threshold Shift in Mice

Using the ABR test, we found that the hearing thresholds of mice receiving a single NE increased transiently after NE and then decreased, which were not significantly different from those of the control group mice at 2 weeks after NE, indicating that a single NE caused a hearing temporary threshold shift (TTS) (**Figure 1C**). The hearing thresholds in mice increased after two NEs, and although they decreased 2 weeks later, there was still a significant difference from the thresholds of the control group mice, indicating that two NEs caused a permanent threshold shift (PTS) in hearing in mice (**Figure 1D**). The amplitude of ABR wave I in both the PTS and TTS groups was significantly different from that in the control group (**Figures 1B,E**).

Noise Exposure Leads to Loss of Cochlear Outer Hair Cells and Reduced Inner Hair Cell Synapses

We examined changes in the number of hair cells and synapses after NE. We divided the cochlear Basilar membrane into the apical, middle, and basal turns in the PTS and TTS group mice for this study. Compared with the control group mice, the TTS group mice showed no significant loss of outer hair cells (OHCs) in either the apical, middle or basal turns, whereas the PTS group mice showed significant OHC loss (**Figures 2A,B**). We analyzed the synapses of the IHCs in two dimensions: paired and orphan synapses. Compared with the control group mice, both the PTS and TTS group mice had decreased number of paired synapses, with the PTS group mice showing a more significant decrease. Both the PTS and TTS groups showed an increased number of unpaired synapses compared to the control group, with a greater increase observed in the PTS group (**Figures 2C–E**). Regarding both audiology and morphology, the damage in the PTS group was more significant than that in the TTS group; therefore, we chose the PTS group to investigate the mechanism of SIRT3 in NIHL.

Noise Exposure Induces Oxidative Damage in Hair Cells

We analyzed the mitochondrial membrane potential in the inner ear cells of the PTS and control group mice. Compared with the control group mice, the PTS group mice showed decreased JC-1 aggregates and increased JC-1 monomers, indicating that the

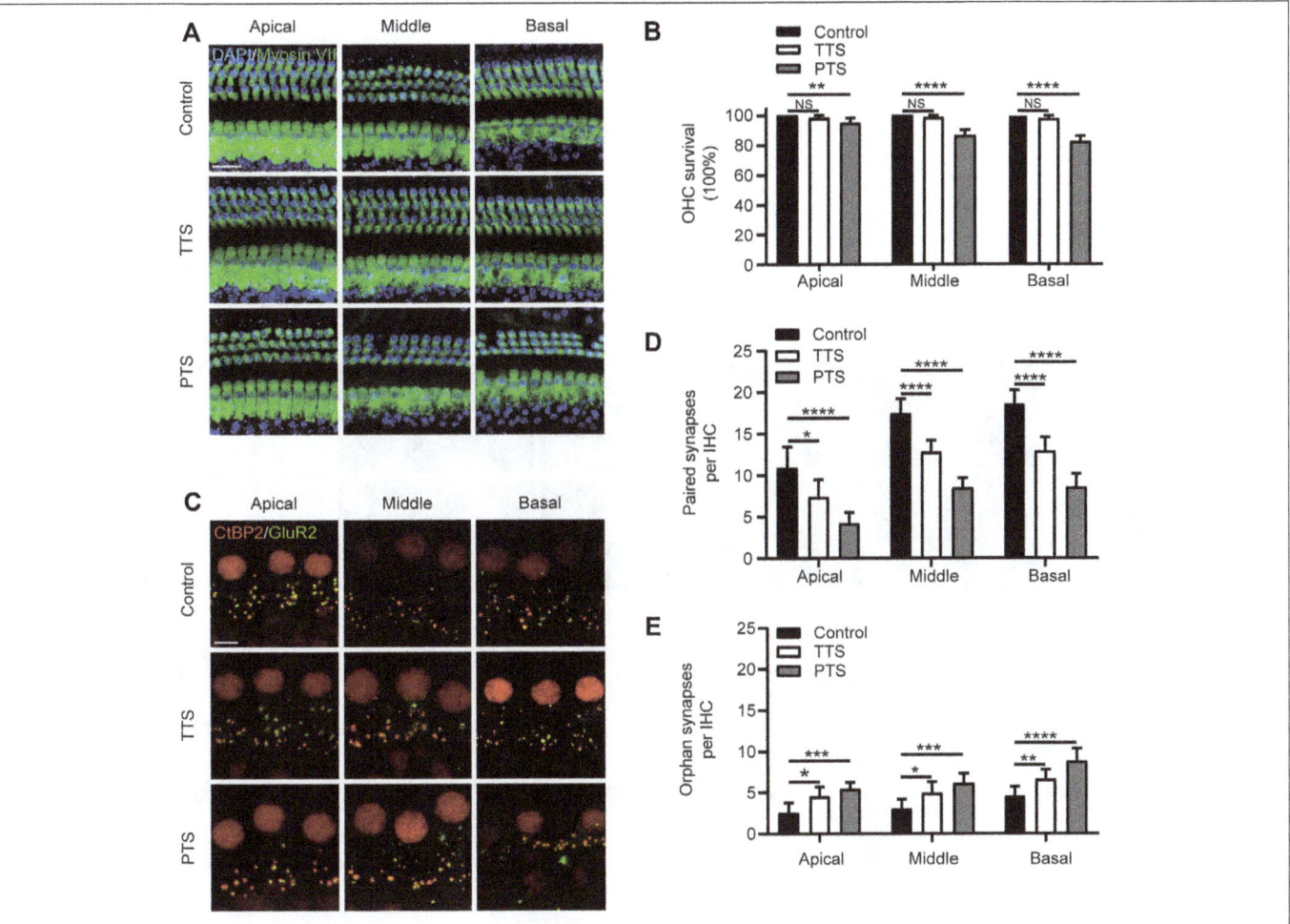

FIGURE 2 | Morphological alterations of mice in the PTS and TTS groups. The basilar membrane was divided into apical, middle, and basal turns for separate observation. (A) Immunohistochemical staining showing changes in the number of hair cells (Myosin VII, green; DAPI, blue) in the PTS and TTS groups. (B) Quantification of Myosin VII and DAPI-positive HCs. (C) Immunohistochemical staining showing changes in the number of presynaptic (CtBP2, red) and postsynaptic structures (GluR2, green) in the IHCs of the PTS and TTS groups. (D) Quantification of CtBP2 and GluR2 overlapping fluorescent spots. (E) Quantification of CtBP2 or GluR2 fluorescent spots alone. (n = 10 per group). TTS, temporary threshold shift; PTS, permanent threshold shift; DAPI, 4, 6-diamidino-2-phenylindole; OHC, outer hair cell; IHC, inner hair cell. NS, not significant; *$p < 0.05$; **$p < 0.01$; ***$p < 0.001$; ****$p < 0.0001$. Scale bars: A, 20 μm; C, 5 μm.

mitochondrial membrane potential was decreased in these mice (**Figures 3A,B**). Immunofluorescence staining of frozen sections of mouse cochlea revealed that 8-OH expression was elevated in the PTS group compared to that in the control group (**Figures 3C,D**). WB analysis on mouse cochleae revealed that Cytochrome c expression was decreased in the mitochondria and increased in the cytoplasm in the PTS group compared with that in the control group (**Figures 3E,F**). The level of NADPH oxidase activity in the PTS group was significantly higher than that in the control group (**Figure 3G**).

3-TYP Exacerbates Noise-Induced Hair Cell Damage

We used the SIRT3 inhibitor 3-TYP for the intervention, which was administered 1 week before each NE (**Figure 4A**). The ABR test results showed that the hearing threshold of the PTS+3-TYP group was significantly higher than that of the PTS group (**Figure 4B**). The OHC survival rate was significantly lower in the PTS+3-TYP group than in the PTS group (**Figures 4C,D**). The analysis of the number of paired synapses at the level of IHCs revealed no significant changes in the basolateral membrane in the PTS+3-TYP group compared with that in the PTS group, while this number was significantly reduced in the middle and basal turns. The number of unpaired synapses in the PTS+3-TYP and PTS groups was not significantly different in the apical and middle turns, whereas a significantly higher value was observed in the basal rotation (**Figures 4E–G**).

3-TYP Increases the Acetylation Level of SOD2 and Aggravates Oxidative Stress and Apoptosis

To explore the effect of 3-TYP on SOD2, we performed WB assays for both Ac-SOD2 and SOD2 in the cochlea and assayed SOD2 activity. We observed that the acetylation level of SOD2

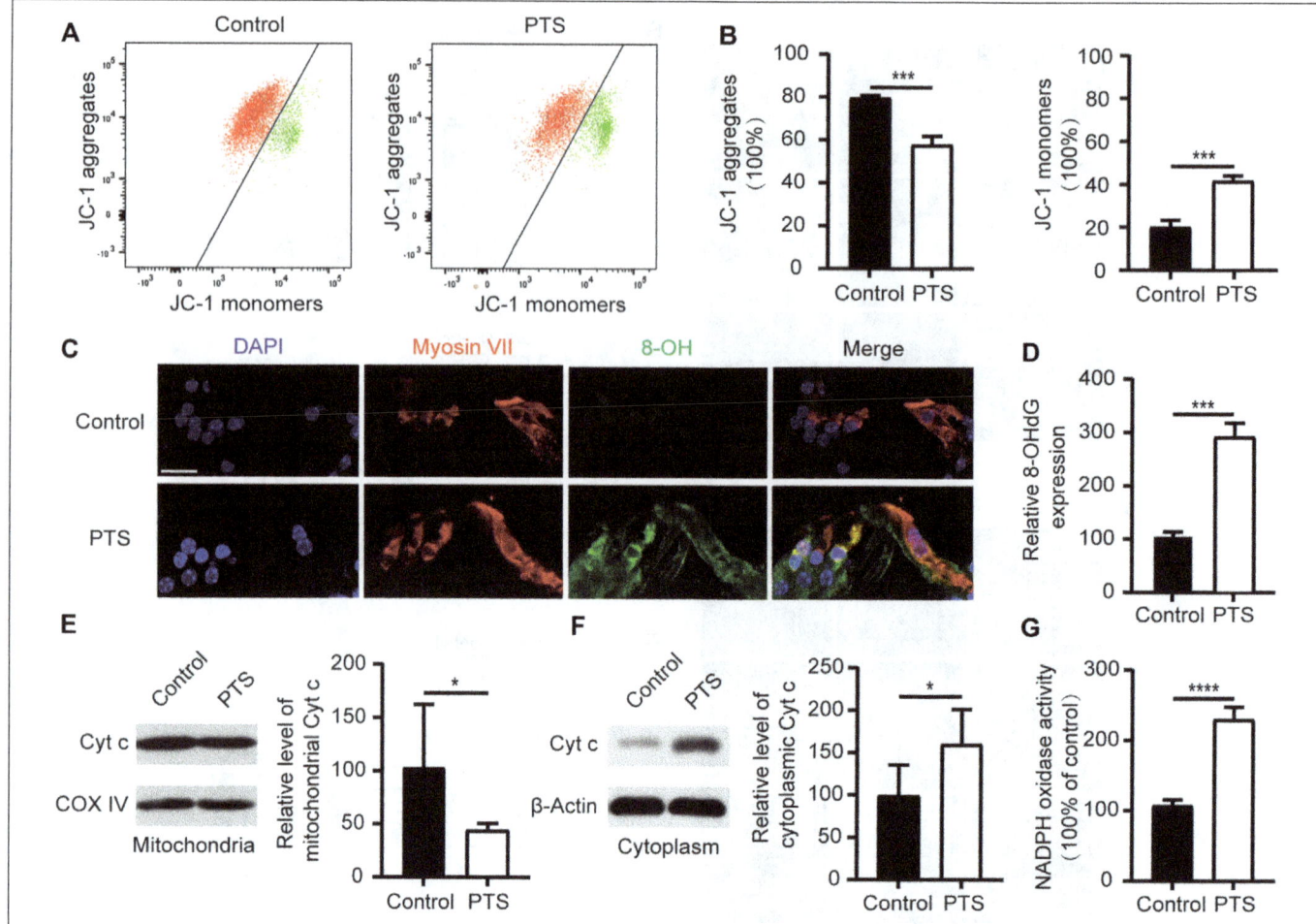

FIGURE 3 | Changes in mitochondrial membrane potential, ROS, apoptosis levels, and NADPH oxidase activity in the hair cells of mice in the PTS and control groups. (A) Detection of mitochondrial membrane potential in the PTS and control groups using flow cytometry. (B) Ratio of JC-1 aggregates and JC-1 monomers ($n = 3$ per group). (C) Immunohistochemical staining of frozen sections of the cochlea showing changes in 8-OH expression in the PTS and control groups. (D) Quantification of 8-OH fluorescence intensity ($n = 5$ per group). (E) WB showing changes in Cytochrome c expression in the mitochondria. (F) WB showing changes in Cytochrome c expression in the cell plasma ($n = 6$ per group). (G) Levels of NADPH oxidase activity in the different groups ($n = 4$ per group). ROS, reactive oxygen species; PTS, permanent threshold shift; WB, western blotting. $*p < 0.05$; $***p < 0.001$; $****p < 0.0001$. Scale bars: C, 20 μm.

was elevated in the PTS+3-TYP group compared to that in the PTS group (**Figure 5A**). SOD2 activity was significantly decreased in the PTS+3-TYP group compared with that in the PTS group (**Figure 5B**). 4-Hydroxynonenal (4HNE) was used to detect cellular oxidative stress levels, and we observed that 4HNE expression in IHCs was significantly higher in the PTS+3-TYP group than in the PTS group (**Figures 5C,D**). In the cochlea, intracellular ROS levels were significantly higher in the PTS+3-TYP group than in the PTS group (**Figure 5E**). Caspase 3 and Cytochrome c protein expression levels were significantly higher in the PTS+3-TYP group than in the PTS group (**Figures 5F,G**).

SIRT3 Overexpression Protects Hair Cells Against Noise Exposure in a SOD2 Dependent Manner

We induced SIRT3 overexpression by introducing AAV-SIRT3 in 4-week-old mice undergoing posterior semicircular canal surgery. The SOD2 inhibitor 2-ME was administered starting 1 week before each NE (**Figure 6A**). Most IHCs could be transfected with AAV-SIRT3, as observed on confocal microscopy (**Figure 6B**). WB results showed that SIRT3 expression was significantly higher in the PTS + AAV-SIRT3 group than in the PTS group (**Figure 6C**). These findings indicate that SIRT3 overexpression by the introduction of AAV-SIRT3 into the posterior semicircular canal is feasible. The ABR results showed no significant difference in hearing thresholds between the PTS and PTS+2-ME groups, and hearing thresholds were significantly lower in the PTS + AAV-SIRT3 group. The thresholds were significantly higher in the PTS+2-ME + AAV-SIRT3 group than in the PTS + AAV-SIRT3 group (**Figure 6D**). Immunofluorescence CtBP2 staining in the apical, middle, and basal turns revealed no significant difference in the number of synapses in the PTS+2-ME group compared with that in the PTS group, whereas the number of synapses in the PTS + AAV-SIRT3 group was significantly elevated. Compared with the PTS + AAV-

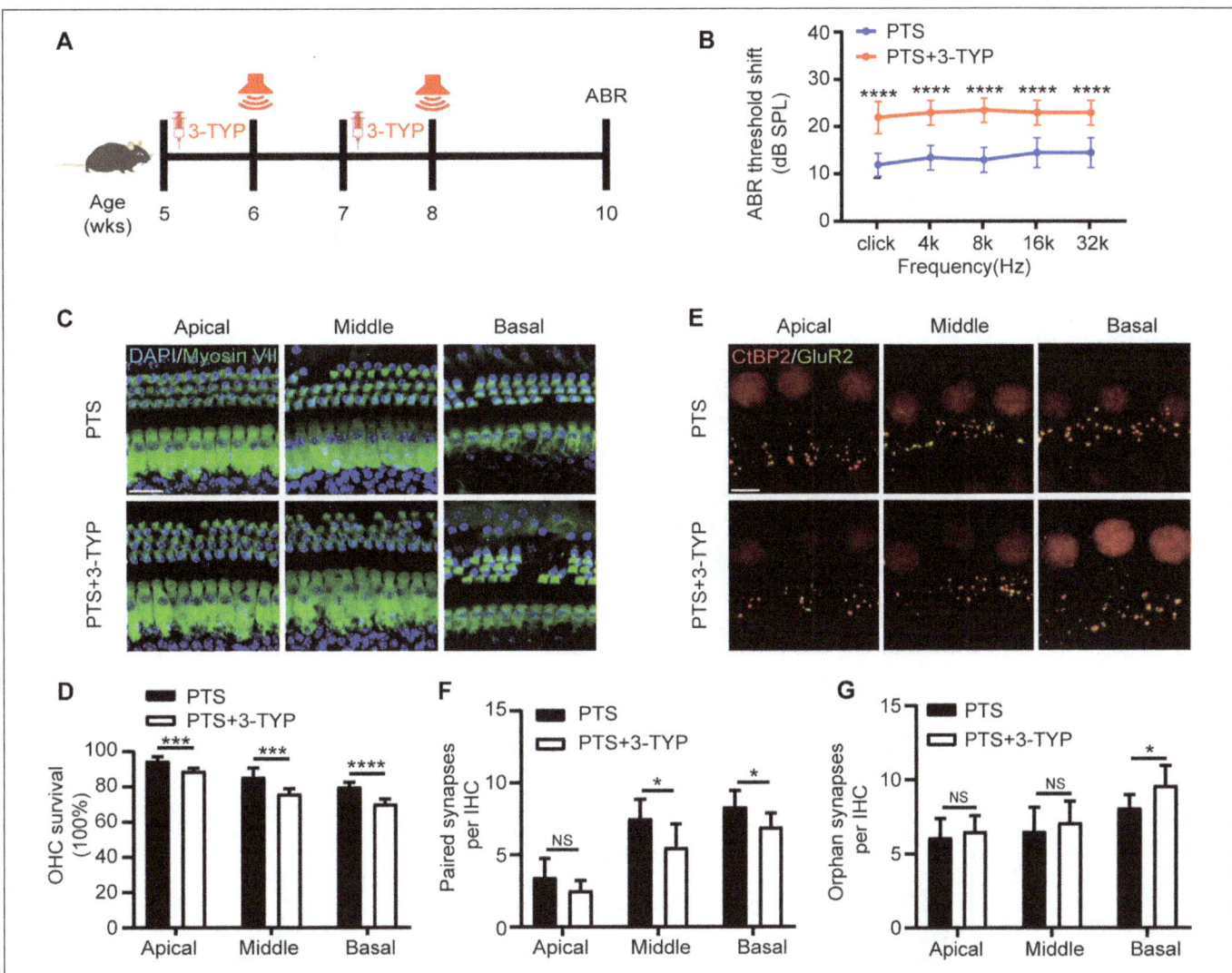

FIGURE 4 | Effect of SIRT3 inhibitors on hair cells in the PTS group. **(A)** Schedule of 3-TYP and NE administration to C57BL/6 J mice. **(B)** ABR findings showing the effect of 3-TYP on the hearing threshold in mice after NE. **(C)** Immunohistochemical staining showing 3-TYP-induced changes in the number of hair cells (Myosin VII, green; DAPI, blue) after NE. **(D)** Quantification of Myosin VII and DAPI-positive HCs. **(E)** Immunohistochemical staining showing the effect of 3-TYP on the number of presynaptic (CtBP2, red) and postsynaptic (GluR2, green) structures after NE. **(F)** Quantification of CtBP2 and GluR2 overlapping fluorescent spots. **(G)** Quantification of CtBP2 or GluR2 fluorescent spots alone. (n = 10 per group). PTS, permanent threshold shift; NE, noise exposure; ABR, auditory brainstem response; DAPI, 4, 6-diamidino-2-phenylindole; OHC, outer hair cell, IHC, inner hair cell. NS, not significant; *p < 0.05; ***p < 0.001; ****p < 0.0001. Scale bars: C, 20 μm; E, 5 μm.

SIRT3 group, the number of synapses in the PTS+2-ME + AAV-SIRT3 group was significantly decreased in the apical, middle, and basal turns (**Figures 6E,F**). The audiological and morphological levels were not significantly different between the PTS + AAV8-GFP and PTS group mice; therefore, these findings are not shown in this figure.

DISCUSSION

NIHL is a major occupational risk in industrialized countries and is estimated to affect approximately 5% of the world population (Basner et al., 2014). In the inner ear, the mechanical vibration of a sound wave is transduced into electrical signals by hair cells (Chen et al., 2021), and these electrical signals are transmitted to auditory cortex through the synapses of the SGNs (Guo et al., 2020). Loss of hair cells and SGNs is the main cause of hearing loss (Zhang et al., 2021). It is well documented that oxidative damage is a major cause of hearing loss cochlear and hair cells, which can be easily damaged by various insults, including mutations in deafness genes (Qian et al., 2020), aging (Qi et al., 2019), noise, drugs, infections and injuries (Liu et al., 2019), or lack of regenerative capacity (Chen et al., 2021). NE increases ROS level, which causes hearing loss through oxidative damage to hair cells and neurons (Delmaghani et al., 2015). Mitochondria are the main sites of intracellular ROS production. We found that mitochondrial SIRT3 plays an important role in NIHL by regulating redox imbalance through SOD2 activation.

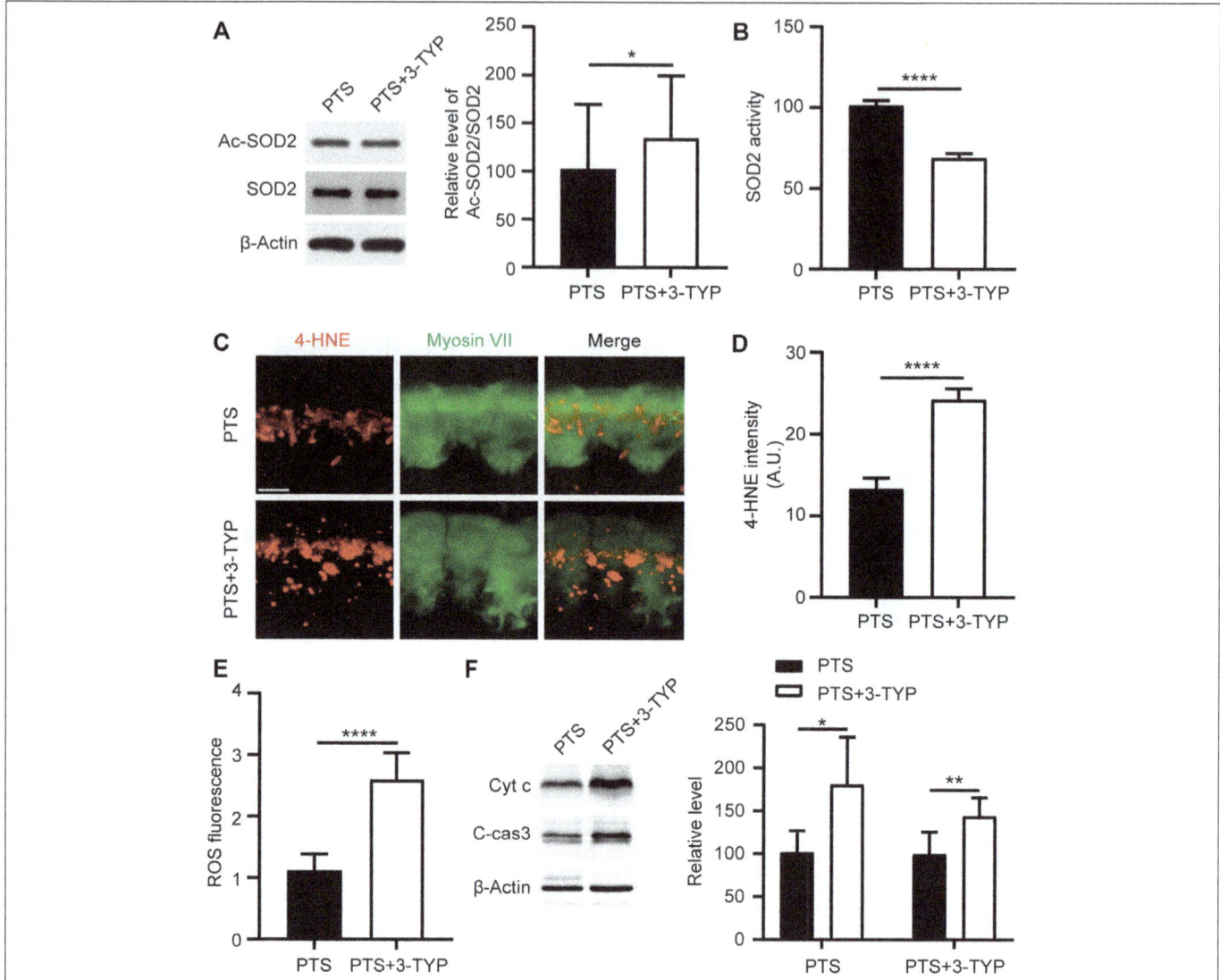

FIGURE 5 | Effect of 3-TYP on SOD2 acetylation, ROS and apoptosis-related protein levels in the hair cells of mice in the PTS group. (A) Western blotting showing the effect of 3-TYP on SOD2 acetylation levels in mice in the PTS group. The results are expressed as the percentage of the PTS group, which was set to 100% ($n = 3$ per group). (B) Effect of 3-TYP on SOD2 activity in the cochlear cells of PTS mice ($n = 10$ per group). (C) Immunohistochemical staining showing changes in 4-HNE fluorescence intensity in IHCs. (D) Quantification of 4-HNE fluorescence intensity ($n = 6$ per group). (E) Detection of ROS levels in the cochlear cells ($n = 10$ per group). (F) WB showing changes in caspase 3 and Cytochrome c expression ($n = 6$ per group). ROS, reactive oxygen species; PTS, permanent threshold shift; IHC, inner hair cell. $*p < 0.05$; $****p < 0.0001$. Scale bars: C, 5 μm.

In C57BL/6 J mice, repetitive noise-induced impairment of cochlear function and altered synaptic morphology have dose-dependent characteristics (Qian et al., 2021). Our previous study found that a single moderate NE caused TTS; however, repeated NE caused PTS (Luo et al., 2020). To select a suitable model for NIHL, we chose 2 h of 100 dB SPL white noise in one and two episodes of NE. One NE caused TTS, and two NEs caused PTS (**Figure 1**). Previous studies have shown that the main site of noise-induced inner ear damage is the ribbon synapse (Feng et al., 2020). Therefore, in addition to OHC count, we counted IHC ribbon synapses. In agreement with previous studies, we found that hair cell damage was more significant in the PTS group than in the TTS group, both at the audiological and morphological levels; therefore, we chose the PTS group for further study (**Figure 2**). Oxidative stress plays an important role in NIHL, and genetic variants of oxidative stress affect the susceptibility to noise (White, 2019). We found that, compared with the control group mice, the PTS group mice had significantly reduced mitochondrial membrane potential and significantly increased 8-OH expression, indicating that NE caused intracellular ROS accumulation by affecting mitochondrial function (**Figure 3**).

Studies have reported that SIRT3 can balance ROS levels by modifying post-translational levels and can activate long-term transcriptional programs to protect cells from oxidative damage (van de Ven et al., 2017). SIRT3 resists the ototoxicity of gentamicin (Han et al., 2020), and its upregulation protects

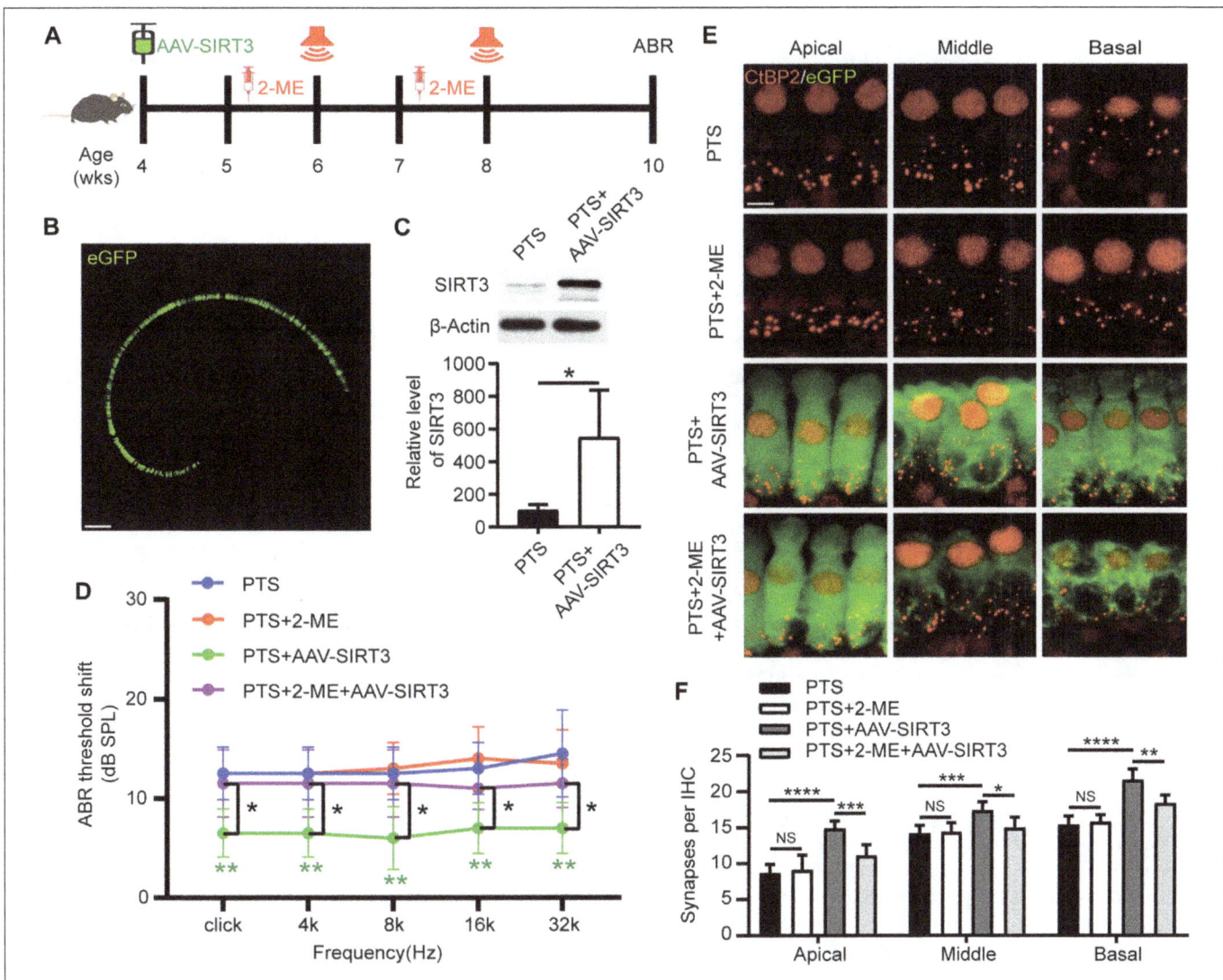

FIGURE 6 | Effect of AAV-SIRT3 and SOD2 inhibitors on the hair cells of mice in the PTS group. **(A)** Schedule of AAV-SIRT3 and SOD2 inhibitor 2-ME administration to C57BL/6 J mice. **(B)** Representative confocal images of the cochlear apical turn via the posterior semicircular canal after injecting 2 μL of AAV-SIRT3. **(C)** WB showing changes in SIRT3 expression after AAV-SIRT3 injection. (n = 4 per group). **(D)** ABR showing the effects of AAV-SIRT3 and 2-ME on hearing thresholds in PTS mice. **(E)** Immunohistochemical staining showing the effects of AAV-SIRT3 and 2-ME on the number of presynaptic structures (CtBP2, red) in mice after NE. **(F)** Quantification of CtBP2 fluorescent spots. (n = 10 per group). AAV, adeno-associated virus; PTS, permanent threshold shift; 2-ME, 2-methoxyestradiol; ABR, auditory brainstem response; NE, noise exposure. NS, not significant; $*p < 0.05$; $**p < 0.01$; $***p < 0.001$; $****p < 0.0001$. Scale bars: B, 100 μm; E, 5 μm.

mice against hearing loss caused by high-fat diet and aging (Miwa, 2021). SIRT3 is a major regulator of the mitochondrial oxidative stress response (Giblin et al., 2014). Nicotinamide riboside (NR), as a SIRT3 agonist, has a protective effect on hair cells and synapses in mice after NE by reducing cellular oxidative damage (Han et al., 2020). Further, supplementation with the NAD^+ precursor NR to elevate NAD levels can rescue animals from NIHL; however, animals lacking SIRT3 do not benefit from this effect (Brown et al., 2014). This is consistent with our findings. Using 3-TYP to suppress SIRT3, we found that SIRT3 inhibition significantly aggravated the damage to hair cells and worsened hearing loss in mice after NE (**Figure 4**). Consistent with previous studies, we suggest that SIRT3 plays a protective role against NE-induced hair cell damage.

SOD2, a SOD that is expressed only in the intracellular mitochondrial matrix (Slot et al., 1986), plays a crucial role in resisting oxidative damage caused by mitochondrial superoxide (Jowko et al., 2017). SOD2 serves as the first line of defense against mitochondrial oxidative damage and is the main mitochondrial ROS scavenger (Miao and St, 2009). SOD2 converts SOD to hydrogen peroxide, which is subsequently converted to water by catalase and other peroxidases (Fridovich, 1995). Diet-induced obese mice showed significant hearing loss due to reduced SOD2 levels, resulting in elevated ROS and increased hair cell mortality (Lee et al., 2020). SOD2 upregulation plays a protective role in acute acoustic injury in rats (Zhu et al., 2020). SOD2 is post-translationally regulated in several ways; however, acetylation is the major SOD2 active

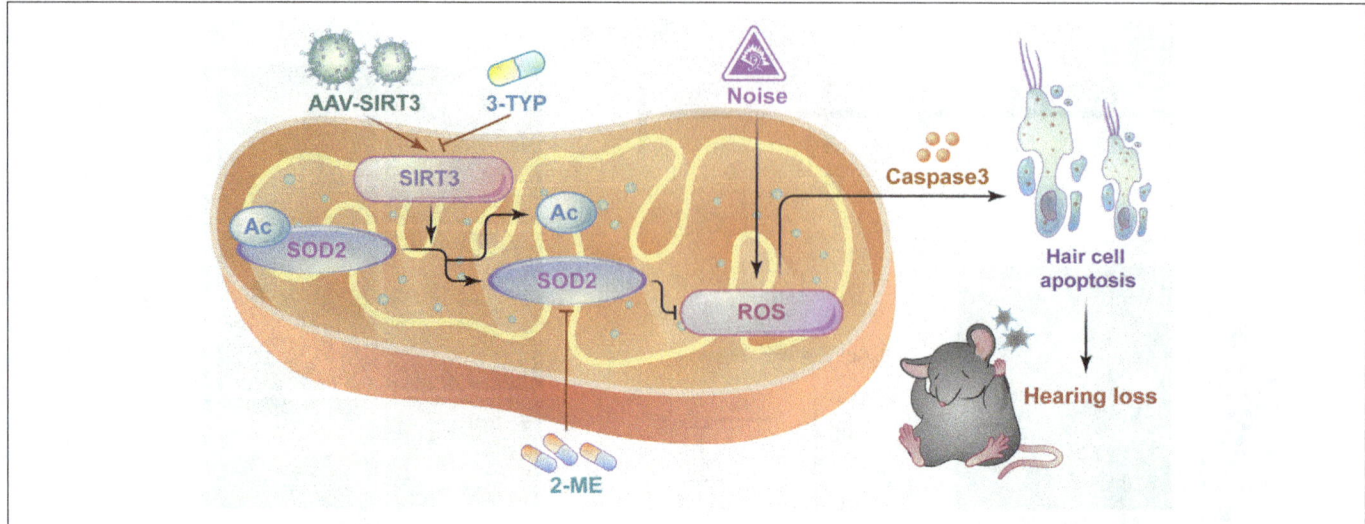

FIGURE 7 | Schematic model showing the critical role of mitochondrial oxidative stress in NIHL model hair cells and the protective role of SIRT3/SOD2 signaling. SIRT3 deacetylates and activates SOD2, reducing reactive oxygen species production and thereby ameliorating noise-induced hair cell damage.

modification (Zou et al., 2016). The reduced level of lysine acetylation in SOD2 increases its enzymatic activity (Candas and Li, 2014). The 4-HNE level reflects cellular membrane damage due to lipid peroxidation induced by ROS. We found that SIRT3 inhibition resulted in a significant increase in the acetylation level of SOD2, a decrease in SOD2 activity, a significant increase in ROS levels, and an increase in apoptosis (**Figure 5**).

SIRT3 maintains ROS homeostasis by activating SOD2 through deacetylation and converting harmful superoxide radicals to harmless oxygen or hydrogen peroxide (Shen et al., 2020). In multiple disease models, SIRT3 has been reported to play an important role in antioxidant damage by regulating its downstream molecule, SOD2. In a mouse model of acute kidney injury, SIRT3 reduced Ac-SOD2 and ROS levels and attenuated oxidative damage, thereby resisting apoptosis (Zhang et al., 2021). Activating the Akt-SIRT3-SOD2 signaling pathway ameliorates mitochondrial damage and attenuates brain ischemia-reperfusion injury in diabetic mice (Liu et al., 2021). In this study, we found that SIRT3 overexpression attenuated hearing loss by protecting hair cells, and this protective effect could be blocked by the SOD2 inhibitor 2-ME (**Figure 6**). Therefore, we conclude that SIRT3 overexpression reduces noise-induced hair cell damage by activating SOD2. Mitochondria, as a major source of ROS, play a key role in regulating cellular functions. It is widely believed that mitochondrial oxidative stress leads to NIHL. Our current work reveals innovative molecular mechanisms by which mitochondrial oxidative stress regulates noise-induced hair cell injury. Thus, the study results provide new potential therapeutic targets with important implications for intervention in the development of NIHL.

However, our study has some limitations. First, mitochondrial redox homeostasis is a complex system, and the linkage of SIRT3/SOD2 signaling with other antioxidant systems requires further investigation. Second, further investigations are warranted to evaluate SIRT3/SOD2-mediated alterations in the mitochondrial function of hair cells and determine the pathogenesis of TTS.

CONCLUSION

This study identified a critical role for the SIRT3/SOD2 signaling pathway in hearing protection by maintaining the redox state of mitochondria in hair cells after NE (**Figure 7**). Our findings reveal an interaction between SIRT3 and noise-induced oxidative stress in hair cells and suggest a potential therapeutic strategy to improve NIHL by activating SIRT3-mediated SOD2 deacetylation.

ETHICS STATEMENT

The animal study was reviewed and approved by the Committee on the Ethics of Animal Experiments of Capital Medical University.

AUTHOR CONTRIBUTIONS

KL and SG conceived and designed the research. WL, CZ, and ZC conducted the experiments. WL and ZY analyzed the generated data and wrote the manuscript. All authors have read and agreed to the published version of the manuscript.

REFERENCES

Basner, M., Babisch, W., Davis, A., Brink, M., Clark, C., Janssen, S., et al. (2014). Auditory and Non-auditory Effects of Noise on Health. *The Lancet* 383 (9925), 1325–1332. doi:10.1016/S0140-6736(13)61613-X

Brown, K. D., Maqsood, S., Huang, J.-Y., Pan, Y., Harkcom, W., Li, W., et al. (2014). Activation of SIRT3 by the NAD+ Precursor Nicotinamide Riboside Protects from Noise-Induced Hearing Loss. *Cel Metab.* 20 (6), 1059–1068. doi:10.1016/j.cmet.2014.11.003

Candas, D., and Li, J. J. (2014). MnSOD in Oxidative Stress Response-Potential

RegulationviaMitochondrial Protein Influx. *Antioxid. Redox Signaling* 20 (10), 1599–1617. doi:10.1089/ars.2013.5305

Chen, Y., Gu, Y., Li, Y., Li, G.-L., Chai, R., Li, W., et al. (2021). Generation of Mature and Functional Hair Cells by Co-expression of Gfi1, Pou4f3, and Atoh1 in the Postnatal Mouse Cochlea. *Cel Rep.* 35 (3), 109016. doi:10.1016/j.celrep.2021.109016

Delmaghani, S., Defourny, J., Aghaie, A., Beurg, M., Dulon, D., Thelen, N., et al. (2015). Hypervulnerability to Sound Exposure through Impaired Adaptive Proliferation of Peroxisomes. *Cell* 163 (4), 894–906. doi:10.1016/j.cell.2015.10.023

Dikalova, A. E., Itani, H. A., Nazarewicz, R. R., McMaster, W. G., Flynn, C. R., Uzhachenko, R., et al. (2017). Sirt3 Impairment and SOD2 Hyperacetylation in Vascular Oxidative Stress and Hypertension. *Circ. Res.* 121 (5), 564–574. doi:10.1161/CIRCRESAHA.117.310933

Ding, Y., Meng, W., Kong, W., He, Z., and Chai, R. (2020). The Role of FoxG1 in the Inner Ear. *Front. Cel Dev. Biol.* 8, 614954. doi:10.3389/fcell.2020.614954

Feng, S., Yang, L., Hui, L., Luo, Y., Du, Z., Xiong, W., et al. (2020). Long-term Exposure to Low-Intensity Environmental Noise Aggravates Age-Related Hearing Loss via Disruption of Cochlear Ribbon Synapses. *Am. J. Transl. Res.* 12 (7), 3674–3687.

Fridovich, I. (1995). Superoxide Radical and Superoxide Dismutases. *Annu. Rev. Biochem.* 64, 97–112. doi:10.1146/annurev.bi.64.070195.000525

Gao, S., Cheng, C., Wang, M., Jiang, P., Zhang, L., Wang, Y., et al. (2019). Blebbistatin Inhibits Neomycin-Induced Apoptosis in Hair Cell-like HEI-OC-1 Cells and in Cochlear Hair Cells. *Front. Cel. Neurosci.* 13, 590. doi:10.3389/fncel.2019.00590

Giblin, W., Skinner, M. E., and Lombard, D. B. (2014). Sirtuins: Guardians of Mammalian Healthspan. *Trends Genet.* 30 (7), 271–286. doi:10.1016/j.tig.2014.04.007

Guo, J.-Y., He, L., Qu, T.-F., Liu, Y.-Y., Liu, K., Wang, G.-P., et al. (2018). Canalostomy as a Surgical Approach to Local Drug Delivery into the Inner Ears of Adult and Neonatal Mice. *JoVE* 135. doi:10.3791/57351

Guo, R., Xiao, M., Zhao, W., Zhou, S., Hu, Y., Liao, M., et al. (2020). 2D Ti3C2TxMXene Couples Electrical Stimulation to Promote Proliferation and Neural Differentiation of Neural Stem Cells. *Acta Biomater.* S1742-7061, 30749–30752. doi:10.1016/j.actbio.2020.12.035

Han, H., Dong, Y., and Ma, X. (2020). Dihydromyricetin Protects against Gentamicin-Induced Ototoxicity via PGC-1α/SIRT3 Signaling In Vitro. *Front. Cel Dev. Biol.* 8, 702. doi:10.3389/fcell.2020.00702

Han, S., Du, Z., Liu, K., and Gong, S. (2020). Nicotinamide Riboside Protects Noise-Induced Hearing Loss by Recovering the Hair Cell Ribbon Synapses. *Neurosci. Lett.* 725, 134910. doi:10.1016/j.neulet.2020.134910

He, Z.-H., Li, M., Fang, Q.-J., Liao, F.-L., Zou, S.-Y., Wu, X., et al. (2021). FOXG1 Promotes Aging Inner Ear Hair Cell Survival through Activation of the Autophagy Pathway. *Autophagy* 19, 1–22. doi:10.1080/15548627.2021.1916194

Jówko, E., Gierczuk, D., Cieśliński, I., and Kotowska, J. (2017). SOD2gene Polymorphism and Response of Oxidative Stress Parameters in Young Wrestlers to a Three-Month Training. *Free Radic. Res.* 51 (5), 506–516. doi:10.1080/10715762.2017.1327716

Lee, Y. Y., Choo, O.-s., Kim, Y. J., Gil, E. S., Jang, J. H., Kang, Y., et al. (2020). Atorvastatin Prevents Hearing Impairment in the Presence of Hyperlipidemia. *Biochim. Biophys. Acta (Bba) - Mol. Cel Res.* 1867 (12), 118850. doi:10.1016/j.bbamcr.2020.118850

Liu, L., Cao, Q., Gao, W., Li, B., Xia, Z., and Zhao, B. (2021). Melatonin Protects against Focal Cerebral Ischemia-Reperfusion Injury in Diabetic Mice by Ameliorating Mitochondrial Impairments: Involvement of the Akt-SIRT3-SOD2 Signaling Pathway. *Aging* 13 (12), 16105–16123. doi:10.18632/aging.203137

Liu, W., Xu, L., Wang, X., Zhang, D., Sun, G., Wang, M., et al. (2021). PRDX1 Activates Autophagy via the PTEN-AKT Signaling Pathway to Protect against Cisplatin-Induced Spiral Ganglion Neuron Damage. *Autophagy* 12, 1–23. doi:10.1080/15548627.2021.1905466

Liu, Y., Qi, J., Chen, X., Tang, M., Chu, C., Zhu, W., et al. (2019). Critical Role of Spectrin in Hearing Development and Deafness. *Sci. Adv.* 5 (4), v7803. doi:10.1126/sciadv.aav7803

Lombard, D. B., Alt, F. W., Cheng, H.-L., Bunkenborg, J., Streeper, R. S., Mostoslavsky, R., et al. (2007). Mammalian Sir2 Homolog SIRT3 Regulates Global Mitochondrial Lysine Acetylation. *Mol. Cel. Biol.* 27 (24), 8807–8814. doi:10.1128/MCB.01636-07

Luo, Y., Qu, T., Song, Q., Qi, Y., Yu, S., Gong, S., et al. (2020). Repeated Moderate Sound Exposure Causes Accumulated Trauma to Cochlear Ribbon Synapses in Mice. *Neuroscience* 429, 173–184. doi:10.1016/j.neuroscience.2019.12.049

Miao, L., and St. Clair, D. K. (2009). Regulation of Superoxide Dismutase Genes: Implications in Disease. *Free Radic. Biol. Med.* 47 (4), 344–356. doi:10.1016/j.freeradbiomed.2009.05.018

Miwa, T. (2021). Protective Effects of N1-Methylnicotinamide against High-Fat Diet- and Age-Induced Hearing Loss via Moderate Overexpression of Sirtuin 1 Protein. *Front. Cel. Neurosci.* 15, 634868. doi:10.3389/fncel.2021.634868

Onyango, P., Celic, I., McCaffery, J. M., Boeke, J. D., and Feinberg, A. P. (2002). SIRT3, a Human SIR2 Homologue, Is an NAD- Dependent Deacetylase Localized to Mitochondria. *Proc. Natl. Acad. Sci.* 99 (21), 13653–13658. doi:10.1073/pnas.222538099

Qi, J., Liu, Y., Chu, C., Chen, X., Zhu, W., Shu, Y., et al. (2019). A Cytoskeleton Structure Revealed by Super-resolution Fluorescence Imaging in Inner Ear Hair Cells. *Cell Discov* 5, 12. doi:10.1038/s41421-018-0076-4

Qian, F., Wang, X., Yin, Z., Xie, G., Yuan, H., Liu, D., et al. (2020). The Slc4a2b Gene Is Required for Hair Cell Development in Zebrafish. *aging* 12 (19), 18804–18821. doi:10.18632/aging.103840

Qian, M., Wang, Q., Wang, Z., Ma, Q., Wang, X., Han, K., et al. (2021). Dose-Dependent Pattern of Cochlear Synaptic Degeneration in C57BL/6J Mice Induced by Repeated Noise Exposure. *Neural Plasticity* 2021, 1–12. doi:10.1155/2021/9919977

Sarsour, E. H., Kalen, A. L., and Goswami, P. C. (2014). Manganese Superoxide Dismutase Regulates a Redox Cycle within the Cell Cycle. *Antioxid. Redox Signaling* 20 (10), 1618–1627. doi:10.1089/ars.2013.5303

Shen, Y., Wu, Q., Shi, J., and Zhou, S. (2020). Regulation of SIRT3 on Mitochondrial Functions and Oxidative Stress in Parkinson's Disease. *Biomed. Pharmacother.* 132, 110928. doi:10.1016/j.biopha.2020.110928

Slot, J. W., Geuze, H. J., Freeman, B. A., and Crapo, J. D. (1986). Intracellular Localization of the Copper-Zinc and Manganese Superoxide Dismutases in Rat Liver Parenchymal Cells. *Lab. Invest.* 55 (3), 363–371.

Someya, S., Yu, W., Hallows, W. C., Xu, J., Vann, J. M., Leeuwenburgh, C., et al. (2010). Sirt3 Mediates Reduction of Oxidative Damage and Prevention of Age-Related Hearing Loss under Caloric Restriction. *Cell* 143 (5), 802–812. doi:10.1016/j.cell.2010.10.002

Tian, C. J., Kim, Y. J., Kim, S. W., Lim, H. J., Kim, Y. S., and Choung, Y.-H. (2013). A Combination of Cilostazol and Ginkgo Biloba Extract Protects against Cisplatin-Induced Cochleo-Vestibular Dysfunction by Inhibiting the Mitochondrial Apoptotic and ERK Pathways. *Cell Death Dis* 4, e509. doi:10.1038/cddis.2013.33

van de Ven, R. A. H., Santos, D., and Haigis, M. C. (2017). Mitochondrial Sirtuins and Molecular Mechanisms of Aging. *Trends Mol. Med.* 23 (4), 320–331. doi:10.1016/j.molmed.2017.02.005

White, P. M. (2019). Genetic Susceptibility to Hearing Loss from Noise Exposure. *Hearing J.* 72 (10), 8–9. doi:10.1097/01.HJ.0000602896.08600.65

Yang, W., Nagasawa, K., Münch, C., Xu, Y., Satterstrom, K., Jeong, S., et al. (2016). Mitochondrial Sirtuin Network Reveals Dynamic SIRT3-dependent Deacetylation in Response to Membrane Depolarization. *Cell* 167 (4), 985–1000. doi:10.1016/j.cell.2016.10.016

Zhang, C., Suo, M., Liu, L., Qi, Y., Zhang, C., Xie, L., et al. (2021). Melatonin Alleviates Contrast-Induced Acute Kidney Injury by Activation of Sirt3. *Oxidative Med. Cell Longevity* 2021, 1–21. doi:10.1155/2021/6668887

Zhang, Y., Li, W., He, Z., Wang, Y., Shao, B., Cheng, C., et al. (2019). Pre-treatment with Fasudil Prevents Neomycin-Induced Hair Cell Damage by Reducing the Accumulation of Reactive Oxygen Species. *Front. Mol. Neurosci.* 12, 264. doi:10.3389/fnmol.2019.00264

Zhang, Y., Li, Y., Fu, X., Wang, P., Wang, Q., Meng, W., et al. (2021). The Detrimental and Beneficial Functions of Macrophages after Cochlear Injury. *Front. Cel Dev. Biol.* 9, 631904. doi:10.3389/fcell.2021.631904

Zhao, J., Tang, M., Cao, J., Ye, D., Guo, X., Xi, J., et al. (2019). Structurally Tunable Reduced Graphene Oxide Substrate Maintains Mouse Embryonic Stem Cell Pluripotency. *Adv. Sci.* 6 (12), 1802136. doi:10.1002/advs.201802136

Zhong, Z., Fu, X., Li, H., Chen, J., Wang, M., Gao, S., et al. (2020). Citicoline Protects Auditory Hair Cells against Neomycin-Induced Damage. *Front. Cel Dev. Biol.* 8, 712. doi:10.3389/fcell.2020.00712

Zhu, G., Wu, Y., Qiu, Y., Tian, K., Mi, W., Liu, X., et al. (2020). Hsp70/Bmi1-FoxO1-SOD Signaling Pathway Contributes to the Protective Effect of Sound Conditioning against Acute Acoustic Trauma in a Rat Model. *Neural Plasticity* 2020, 1–22. doi:10.1155/2020/8823785

Zou, X., Santa-Maria, C. A., O'Brien, J., Gius, D., and Zhu, Y. (2016). Manganese Superoxide Dismutase Acetylation and Dysregulation, Due to Loss of SIRT3 Activity, Promote a Luminal B-like Breast Carcinogenic-Permissive Phenotype. *Antioxid. Redox Signaling* 25 (6), 326–336. doi:10.1089/ars.2016.6641

A Model of Waardenburg Syndrome Using Patient-Derived iPSCs With a *SOX10* Mutation Displays Compromised Maturation and Function of the Neural Crest That Involves Inner Ear Development

Jie Wen[1,2,3†], Jian Song[1,2,3†], Yijiang Bai[1,2,3], Yalan Liu[1,2,3], Xinzhang Cai[1,2,3], Lingyun Mei[1,2,3], Lu Ma[4], Chufeng He[1,2,3*] and Yong Feng[1,4*]

[1] Department of Otorhinolaryngology, Xiangya Hospital Central South University, Changsha, China, [2] Province Key Laboratory of Otolaryngology Critical Diseases, Changsha, China, [3] Department of Geriatrics, National Clinical Research Centre for Geriatric Disorders, Xiangya Hospital, Central South University, Changsha, China, [4] Department of Otorhinolaryngology, The Affiliated Changsha Central Hospital, Hengyang Medical School, University of South China, Changsha, China

Correspondence:
Chufeng He
hechufeng2013@163.com
Yong Feng
fengyong_hn@hotmail.com

† These authors have contributed equally to this work

Waardenburg syndrome (WS) is an autosomal dominant inherited disorder that is characterized by sensorineural hearing loss and abnormal pigmentation. *SOX10* is one of its main pathogenicity genes. The generation of patient-specific induced pluripotent stem cells (iPSCs) is an efficient means to investigate the mechanisms of inherited human disease. In our work, we set up an iPSC line derived from a WS patient with *SOX10* mutation and differentiated into neural crest cells (NCCs), a key cell type involved in inner ear development. Compared with control-derived iPSCs, the *SOX10* mutant iPSCs showed significantly decreased efficiency of development and differentiation potential at the stage of NCCs. After that, we carried out high-throughput RNA-seq and evaluated the transcriptional misregulation at every stage. Transcriptome analysis of differentiated NCCs showed widespread gene expression alterations, and the differentially expressed genes (DEGs) were enriched in gene ontology terms of neuron migration, skeletal system development, and multicellular organism development, indicating that *SOX10* has a pivotal part in the differentiation of NCCs. It's worth noting that, a significant enrichment among the nominal DEGs for genes implicated in inner ear development was found, as well as several genes connected to the inner ear morphogenesis. Based on the protein-protein interaction network, we chose four candidate genes that could be regulated by *SOX10* in inner ear development, namely, *BMP2, LGR5, GBX2,* and *GATA3*. In conclusion, SOX10 deficiency in this WS subject had a significant impact on the gene expression patterns throughout NCC development in the iPSC model. The DEGs most significantly enriched in inner ear development and morphogenesis may assist in identifying the underlying basis for the inner ear malformation in subjects with WS.

Keywords: Waardenburg syndrome, SOX10, induced pluripotent stem cells (hiPSC), neural crest cells (NCCs), inner ear development, transcriptome analysis

INTRODUCTION

Waardenburg syndrome (WS) is a rare autosomal dominant inherited disorder. WS is distinguished by sensorineural hearing loss (SNHL) and pigment abnormalities, such as hypopigmentation of the skin, a white forelock, premature graying, or heterochromia iridum (Waardenburg, 1951). There are four WS subtypes categorized by the presence or lack of other clinical symptoms. Clinically, WS1 and WS2 are the most frequently noted (Dourmishev et al., 1999). The actual incidence of WS is thought to be 1/42,000, and may account for 2–5% of congenital deafness (Nayak and Isaacson, 2003). Several mutations in six genes have thus far been reported to be linked to WS, including *PAX3*, *MITF*, *SOX10*, *EDNRB*, *EDN3*, and *SNAI2* (Pingault et al., 2010). Researchers have proposed several explanations for the clinical characteristics of WS. At present, the theory of neural crest hypoplasia is the most widely noted. This theory holds that the embryonic neural crest is the source of melanocytes, frontal bone, limb muscles, and intramural ganglia, and that their dysfunction due to WS impacts different tissues and organs, leading to a series of abnormalities (Bolande, 1997; Knecht and Bronner-Fraser, 2002).

As the inner ear forms and develops, neural crest cells move from rhombomere 4 to the otocyst and begin to differentiate into glial cells of the cochleovestibular ganglion and intermediate melanocytic cells of the cochlear stria vascularis, both of which are essential cell types in the inner ear (Tachibana et al., 2003; Freter et al., 2013; Kim et al., 2013). Recently, a few studies have demonstrated that neural crest cells (NCCs) also participate in the development of the inner ear neurosensory components, which are thought to be lineages derived from the otocyst. However, the contributions of NCCs to the neurosensory components of the inner ear are not completely understood (Freyer et al., 2011; Mao et al., 2014; Karpinski et al., 2016).

SOX10 is a key transcription factor during the development of the neural crest. In addition, SOX10 has a pivotal part in maintaining the pluripotency, survival, and proliferation of NCCs (Southard-Smith et al., 1998). *SOX10* mutations are primarily connected to the pathogenesis of WS2 and WS4 (Bondurand et al., 2007; Chen et al., 2010). In addition, *SOX10* mutations can induce Kallmann syndrome (KS, OMIM 308700) as well a plethora of neurological symptoms in the neural crest (PCWH), such as outer peripheral demyelinating neuropathy, central myelination disorder, WS, and Hirschsprung's disease (HD) (Pingault et al., 2000, 2013; Inoue et al., 2004). Previous studies have demonstrated that WS subjects with *SOX10* mutations more frequently exhibit different degrees of inner ear deformities. Nevertheless, additional research is needed to elucidate the target genes and pathways regulated by SOX10 in inner ear development (Breuskin et al., 2009; Elmaleh-Bergès et al., 2013).

Human-induced pluripotent stem cell (iPSC) technology is a new tool for researching human developmental disorders. Genotype-specific molecular and cellular phenotypes that occur throughout differentiation can be modeled by these cells. By reprogramming somatic cells obtained from subjects into a state resembling embryonic stem cells and then differentiating them into disease-relevant cell types, researchers can use iPSC technology to produce an almost unlimited source of human tissues with the genetic mutations found at the genesis of the disease. This technology is a powerful tool that can be used to derive patient-specific cells for human disease modeling. In addition, iPSC technology is promising for personalized cell therapies (Takahashi et al., 2007; Tang et al., 2020; Zhang et al., 2020a). It is currently thought that a global disturbance of transcriptional regulation due to SOX10 deficiency, which is still not fully understood, may be one cause of the aberrant phenotypes found in WS patients (Huang et al., 2021). Because SOX10 functions as a DNA-binding protein, the likelihood that SOX10 may directly modulate transcription in the nucleus is high. In WS patients with SOX10 mutations, no microarray-based gene expression profiling data were generated. RNA-seq analysis is urgently needed to fully reveal the transcriptional perturbation induced by SOX10 deficiency.

In the present study, we provide details about a Chinese patient with WS2, and noted a *de novo* heterozygous mutation in *SOX10*. Patient-derived fibroblasts were gathered to produce iPSCs, and we then differentiated these iPSCs into NCCs *in vitro*, and contrasted their differentiation potential with iPSCs derived from a normal healthy patient to examine disorders linked to this syndrome. Further, we completed transcriptomics analysis of the differentiating cells throughout the *in vitro* differentiation process to examine the underlying genetic basis of WS. The genes that we characterized as relevant for NCC differentiation and development will assist in the discovery of new therapies for WS. In this work, we generated a research model and offer insights for additional studies on the mechanism(s) governing WS.

MATERIALS AND METHODS

Ethics Statement

The Xiangya Ethics Committee approved the protocol for this study, and signed informed consent was provided by every donor before sample collection. The laboratory research on the derivation and use of human iPSC lines was approved by the Ethics Committee of Xiangya Hospital Central South University (XHCSU) in accordance with local regulations, and all of the animal experiments were conducted based on XHCSU ethical guidelines.

Clinical Evaluation

The proband was recruited from the Otology Clinic at XHCSU. Other family members were included, along with 100 controls comprised of unselected, unrelated, and sex-matched healthy individuals. Comprehensive clinical history, audiologic, neurologic, ophthalmologic, and dermatologic examinations were conducted on proband and all family members. The audiologic and neurologic examinations consisted of otoscopy, pure-tone audiometry (PTA), immittance, distortion product otoacoustic emission (DPOAE), and auditory brain-stem response (ABR) tests. Another auditory steady-state response (ASSR) test was conducted for those patients who did not do well with the PTA test because of their young age (II-1 and II-2). Special attention was paid to pigmentary alterations in the skin, hair, and iris—as well as additional developmental defects, such as dystopia canthorum and limb abnormalities. The degree of hearing loss was defined based on the ASSR and three frequencies: 500, 1,000, and 2,000 Hz. Hearing loss was categorized as follows: a normal hearing level (HL) at < 26 dB (decibels); mild HL, 26–40 dB; moderate HL, 41–70 dB; severe HL, 71–90 dB; and profound HL, > 90 dB.

DNA Extraction and Mutational Analysis

Genomic DNA was removed from peripheral blood samples of the subjects and healthy controls according to the standard procedure. Whole genomic DNA was isolated with a TIANamp Blood DNA Kit (Tiangen Biotech, China.) and quantified with an ultraviolet spectrophotometer Du800 (Beckman Coulter, United States). The DNA was then kept at −20°C until use. PCR and Sanger sequencing was conducted on each of the coding exons and flanking splicing sites of the WS-related genes, including *MITF*, *SOX10*, *PAX3*, *EDNRB*, *EDN3*, and *SNAI2*. The PCR products were treated with shrimp alkaline phosphatase and exonuclease-I to degrade deoxynucleotide triphosphates and unincorporated PCR primers. The purified amplicons were combined with 10 picomoles of the forward and reverse PCR primers for bidirectional sequencing on an ABI-Prism 3100 DNA sequencer via dye-termination chemistry (Applied Biosystems, United States), and the SeqMan II program (DNA-STAR, United States) was utilized to compare results. Once the mutation was determined, DNA samples from related family members and controls were then screened for the identical mutation.

Collection and Establishment of Fibroblast Cultures From Skin Tissue of a WS Patient

After obtaining written informed consent from the donor, human skin samples were collected from the proband (WS patient). The biopsy tissue was put in a sterile tube filled with phosphate-buffered saline (PBS) containing 1% penicillin/streptomycin (Invitrogen, United States), and kept at 4°C. The steps that follow were performed in a tissue culture hood under aseptic conditions and using sterile instruments.

The subcutaneous fat and capillaries were completely removed from the sample tissue, and the tissue was moved to a 50-ml Falcon tube containing 4 ml of 0.05% trypsin/EDTA (Invitrogen, United States) and incubated overnight at 4°C. The epidermis was manually extracted from the tissue, and the supernatant was discarded after adding 4 ml of freshly-prepared fibroblast culture medium [DMEM containing 10% FBS, 1% penicillin/streptomycin, 1% glutamine, and 1% non-essential amino acids (Invitrogen, United States)]. The dermal tissues were dissected into small pieces, placed in a 100-mm Petri dish, and incubated at 4°C in 5% CO_2 for 3 h to allow the tissues to adhere to the bottom of the dish. Two milliliters of fibroblast culture medium were added to cover the bottom and ensure that the pieces stay moist. The tissues were incubated at 37°C in 5% CO_2, and 3 ml of fibroblast culture medium was put in on the following day; the medium was subsequently changed every 3 day. An optical microscope was used to monitor the cultures daily. The tissues were carefully removed when dense outgrowths of fibroblasts appeared, the medium was aspirated, and fresh culture medium was added to maintain the growing fibroblasts (in passage 1). The cells were passaged with trypsin/EDTA at a ratio of 1:3 until the cells reached 80% confluency. Cells from passages 3–5 were then utilized for the induction of iPSCs.

Generation and Culture of iPSCs

The primary fibroblasts were cultured in hFib medium at 37°C in 5% CO_2. The fibroblasts (5×10^5 cells) were electroporated with 0.5 μg per vector of five episomal vectors (pCXLE-hUL, pCXLEhOCT3/4-shp53-F, pCXLE-hSK, pCXWB-EBNA1, and pCXLE-EGFP) in order to produce the iPSCs. Electroporation was conducted with the Basic Nucleofector™ Kit for Primary Mammalian Epithelial Cells (Lonza, Switzerland) and the Lonza Nucleofector™ 2b device, program X-005. Following electroporation, the cells were seeded on gelatin-coated 100-mm dishes cultured in hFib medium with the addition of 0.5 mM sodium butyrate (Sigma, United States) and 50 μg/ml VitC (Sigma, United States). The medium was emptied and refilled daily. After 8 day, the cells were moved to Matrigel (Corning)-coated six-well plates at a density of 5×10^4 cells/cm^2 and cultured in mTeSR medium (Stem Cell Technologies). Two days after the transfer, 10 μM Y-27632 (ROCK inhibitor) was added, and the medium was emptied and refilled on alternating days. The iPSC colonies were manually removed and cultured in mTeSR on Matrigel-coated 24-well plates after 14–21 days. Accutase (Gibco, United States) was used to passage the iPSCs every 6 d at a 1:6 split ratio using, and the iPSCs were kept at 37°C in a 5% CO_2 incubator (Thermo Fisher Scientific, United States).

Induction of Neural Crest Cells (NCCs) From iPSCs

The differentiation of iPSCs into NCCs was completed according to the standards detailed prior (Chambers et al., 2011). In short, embryoid bodies were generated in EB Medium (KO-DMEM supplemented with 20% KO-Serum Replacement, 1% GlutaMax-I, and 1% non-essential amino acids) with 500 nM LDN193189 (Stemgent, United Kingdom) and 10 μM SB431542 (Tocris Bioscience, United Kingdom) for 3 day. Culture was carried out in EB Medium supplemented with 2% N-2 (Life Technologies), 1% GlutaMax-I, 100 nM EDN3, 25 ng/ml BMP4, and 50 ng/ml stem cell factor (SCF) (R&D Systems, United States) for the next 3 day. On day 6, embryoid bodies were attached to feeder-free fibronectin-coated culture flasks in Neurobasal Medium supplemented with 2% B-27, 1% N-2, 1% GlutaMax-I, 100 nM EDN3, 25 ng/ml BMP4, and 50 ng/ml SCF. The cells that grew were fed on alternating days for maintenance and expansion until differentiation occurred (day 12). From day 2 and 12 onward, 3 μM CHIR99021 (Stemgent, United Kingdom) was added to the medium.

Quantitative Reverse Transcription-Polymerase Chain Reaction (qRT-PCR)

RNA was removed from samples using Trizol reagent (Sangon, China) following the company's directions, and 1 μg of RNA was reverse-transcribed utilizing the PrimeScript™ II 1st Strand cDNA Synthesis Kit (Takara, Japan). All of the qRT-PCR analyses were performed on a Step One plus Real-Time PCR System (ABI) with 2 × SYBR Master Mix (Yeasen, China). The relative expression levels of the target genes were calculated using the $2^{-\Delta\Delta Ct}$ method, and GAPDH was utilized as the internal control (the primers are shown in **Supplementary Table 1**). Each experiment was repeated thrice, and the average value was taken as the experimental result. The statistical significances for all of the RT-qPCR data were analyzed with unpaired Student's t-tests.

Western Blot (WB)

Cell extracts that were representative of three independent experiments were prepared from NCCs in a SOX10 mutant and a normal control, and the extracted proteins were analyzed. The antibodies used for Western blot included rabbit anti-SOX10 (Abcam, United Kingdom), mouse anti-GAPDH (Good Here, AB-M-M001) as a primary antibody, HRP-labeled Goat Anti-Rabbit IgG (Beyotime, China), and HRP-labeled Goat Anti-Mouse IgG (Beyotime, China) as a second antibody.

Alkaline Phosphatase (AP) Staining

An AP Staining Kit (Beyotime, China) was used to assess alkaline phosphatase (AP) activity following the manufacturer's protocol. The images were assessed using a Nikon 300 inverted confocal microscope.

Immunofluorescence Staining

The iPSCs were fixed in 4% paraformaldehyde for 20 min at room temperature and then permeabilized using 1% Triton X-100 (Sigma, United States) for 10 min. Following blocking with 5% bovine serum albumin (BSA) (Sangon, China) for 1 h at room temperature, the samples were incubated overnight with the primary antibodies in PBS solution with 5% BSA at 4°C. The next day, secondary antibodies were incubated at room temperature for 1 h. DAPI (Beyotime, China) was used for nuclear counterstaining, and images were observed and photographed using an Olympus confocal microscope and camera. Details about the antibodies are shown in **Supplementary Table 2**.

Teratoma Assay

The iPSCs (1×10^7 cells) were gathered and injected subcutaneously into the dorsal flanks of 8-week-old male nude mice (Charles River, China). Approximately 8–10 weeks after injection, teratomas had formed. They were then dissected and fixed in 4% paraformaldehyde, and then embedded in paraffin. Tissue sections were stained using hematoxylin and eosin.

RNA Sequencing

Two stages of triple replicates (three independent inducing from one source of iPSC) from two samples were obtained (iPSCs and induced neural crest cells (iNCCs) from the normal control and the SOX10 mutant) for extracting total RNA for further analysis. Total RNA was extracted and RNA integrity was evaluated using the RNA Nano 6000 Assay Kit of the Bioanalyzer 2100 system (Agilent Technologies, United States). One microgram of RNA per sample was utilized for cDNA library preparation with the NEBNext® Ultra™ RNA Library Prep Kit from Illumina® and processed according to the manufacturer's directions. The library quality was evaluated with the Agilent Bioanalyzer 2100 system. The library preparations were sequenced on an Illumina Novaseq platform, and 150 bp paired-end reads were generated. After being checked for quality control, sequencing reads were mapped to the reference genome with Hisat2 v2.0.5 (Kim et al., 2015), and the raw data were deposited into the GEO database (No. GSE176101).

Bioinformatic Analysis of RNA-Seq

The raw reads were cleaned by removing reads that had adapters, reads that contained poly-N, and reads of low quality. The resulting clean reads were aligned to the reference genome using Hisat2 v2.0.5, and FeatureCounts v1.5.0-p3 (Liao et al., 2014) was used to quantify the read numbers mapped to every gene and calculate the per kilobase of exon per million fragments mapped (FPKM) to every gene. The differentially expressed genes (DEGs) were analyzed with the DESeq2 method using the online tool NetworkAnalyst 3.0[1] (Zhou et al., 2019). DEGs had an adjusted P-value < 0.05 and | log2 (fold-change) | > 1. Gene ontology (GO) and Kyoto Encyclopedia of Genes and Genomes (KEGG) pathway-enrichment analyses of all of the DEGs were conducted with the online tool DAVID v6.8 (Huang da et al., 2009). GO terms and KEGG pathway terms with an adjusted P-value of < 0.05 were considered to be significantly enriched. The protein-protein interaction (PPI) was analyzed using STRING v11.0[2] (Szklarczyk et al., 2019), with the SOX10 gene and DEGs uploaded onto STRING with the minimal interaction score set to > 0.4. Cytoscape 3.6.1 software was used to construct the PPI network.

Statistical Analyses

Data are reported as the mean ± standard deviation (SD) of independent experiments. Statistical analyses were conducted using the Wilcoxon signed-rank test or a one-way analysis of variance (ANOVA) with Prism Graphic software. $P < 0.05$ was considered to be statistically significant.

RESULTS

Clinical Findings

The proband was 9 years of age and showed brilliant blue bilateral irides, patchy depigmented areas on his forehead, and a white forelock since birth (**Figure 1A**). The proband was unresponsive to external audio stimuli and unable to speak. Ear injury, otitis media, and contact with ototoxic drugs were

---

[1] http://www.networkanalyst.ca
[2] https://string-db.org/

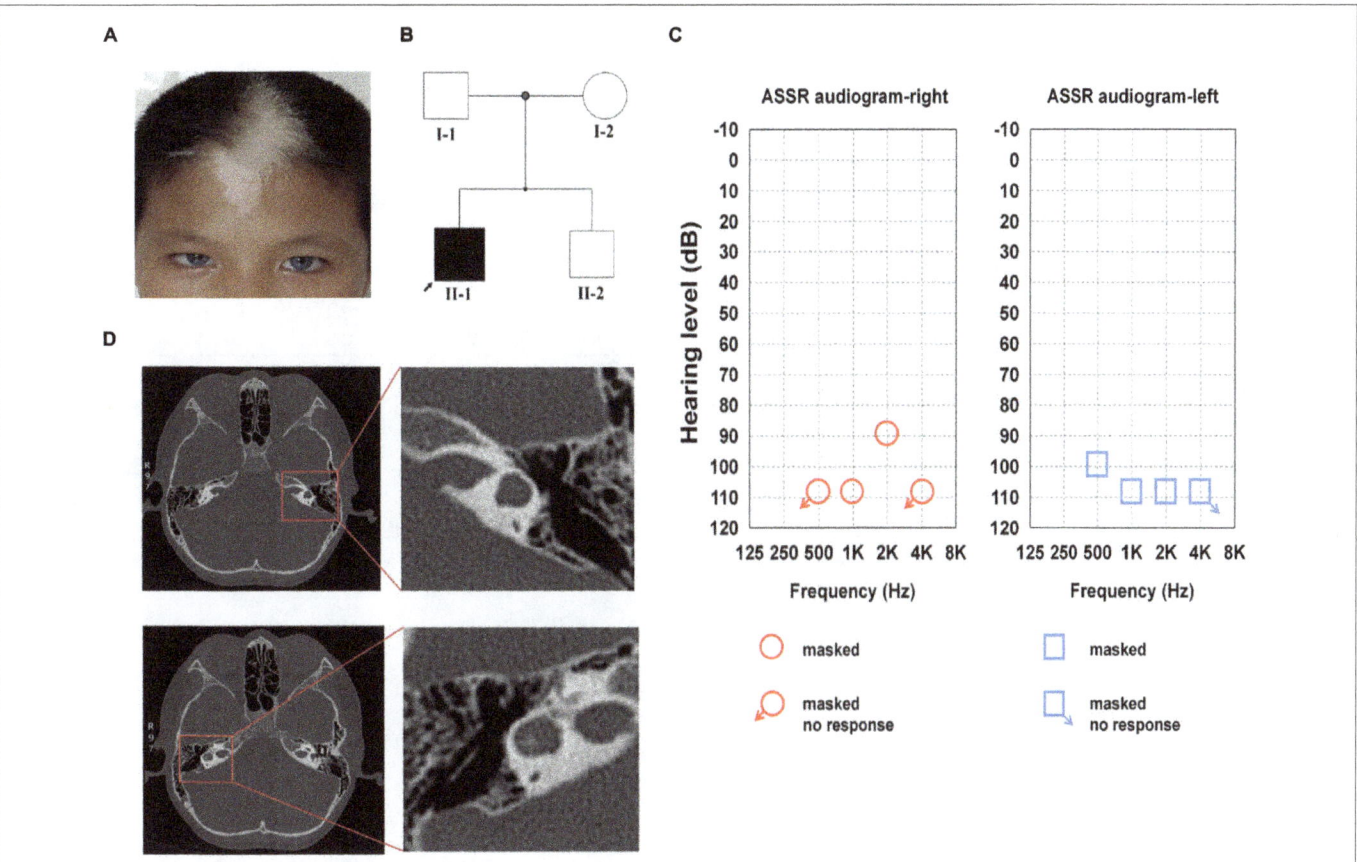

FIGURE 1 | Family history and clinical features of the proband. **(A)** The proband showed bilateral brilliant blue irides, patchy depigmented areas on forehead and white forelock. **(B)** The pedigree indicates that only Family II-1 had the WS-associated phenotypes, which are marked in black. **(C)** ASSR of the left ear: 100, 110, and 110 dB at 0.5, 1, and 2 kHz, respectively, the other frequencies showed no response. ASSR of the right ear: 110 and 90 dB at 1 and 2 kHz, respectively, the other frequencies showed no response. **(D)** Enlarged vestibule and semicircular canal abnormalities on both sides are shown on high-resolution axial CT in the red square.

not detected. Skin depigmentation was noted, eyesight and intelligence were normal, there was no dystopia cantorum (the W index < 1.95), and no digestive system or skeletal muscle abnormalities were observed. His parents and brother had no pigmentary abnormalities in their skin, hair, or eyes, and they showed no other WS-associated phenotype (**Figure 1B**).

The audiologic examination of the proband revealed profound bilateral sensorineural HL: there were no bilateral otoacoustic emissions and all of the bilateral ABR thresholds were over 105 dB nHL (the thresholds for ASSR for both ears are shown in detail in **Figure 1C**). Temporal bone CT scans revealed an enlarged vestibule on either side, left horizontal semicircular canals fused with the vestibule, and right horizontal semicircular canals enlarged and shortened; there were no obvious abnormalities in the shape and size of the bilateral cochleae (**Figure 1D**). The proband was diagnosed with WS2 based on the WS diagnostic criteria (Liu et al., 1995).

Identification of Mutations and Pathogenicity Analysis

Following screening for all of the WS-related and congenital hearing loss disease-causing genes, the proband was found to carry a heterozygous mutation of guanine (G) to adenine (A) in position 336 (c.336G > A) of the third exon of *SOX10*. This led to a substitution of the 112th codon (p.Met112Ile). Based on the standards and the guidelines of the American College of Medical Genetics and Genomics (ACMG), this variant is considered pathogenic and was initially identified by Chaoui et al. (2011). Mutations were not found in 100 unrelated healthy control subjects. The proband's parents and brother had normal phenotypes and carried no corresponding mutations as determined by Sanger sequencing, demonstrating that the mutations occurred *de novo* (**Figures 2A,B**). No further mutations connected to WS were determined in the proband. Intriguingly, the Met112 residues in SOX10 are highly conserved across various vertebrate species (**Figure 2C**), indicating the functional importance of this amino acid (Scheithauer et al., 1988).

iPSCs Derived From an Idiopathic WS Patient With a *SOX10* Mutation Were Generated and Characterized

To better understand the pathogenic mechanism subserving WS, we established an iPSC line from dermal fibroblasts from the

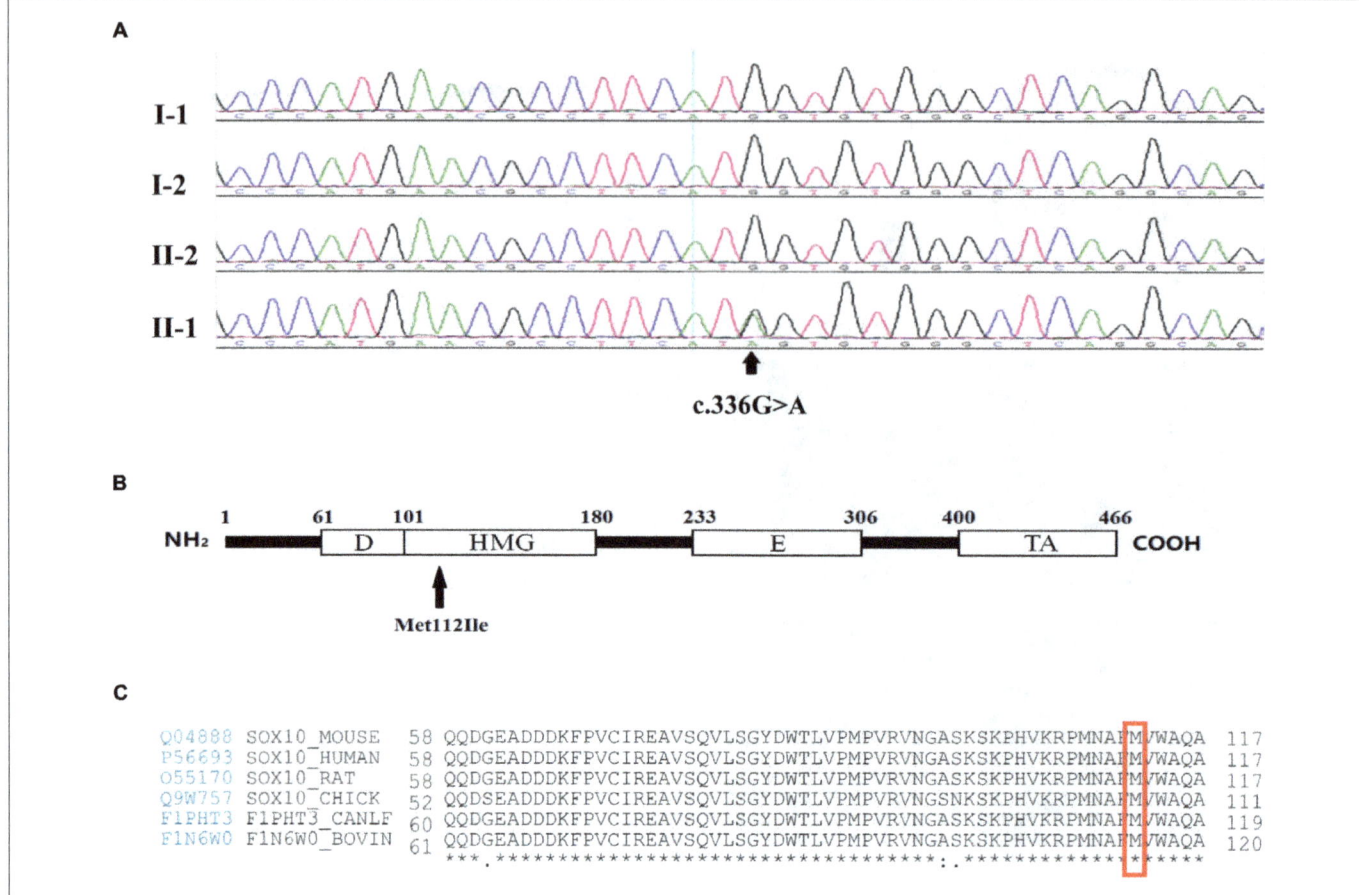

FIGURE 2 | Mutation analysis and amino acid coding diagram. **(A)** DNA sequencing profile revealed that the *SOX10* mutation c.336G > A (p.Met112Ile) was found in the proband (II-1) and not in his father (I-1), mother (I-2), or brother (II-2). The arrow indicates the area of the base substitution. **(B)** Schematic diagram of the *SOX10* gene. The black arrow indicates the mutation site. D, Dimerization domain; HMG, high mobility group domain; E, Conserved domain of SOX8/9/10; TA transactivation domain. **(C)** Protein sequence alignment of vertebrate *SOX10*; note the highly conserved Met112 residues across various species. * represents the same amino acid at the same site among different species.

proband with the *SOX10* mutation using previously described methods. We also established one normal control iPSC line from an unrelated healthy individual.

Both the *SOX10* mutant and normal control iPSC lines exhibited a typical pluripotent stem cell-like morphology and grew as compact colonies with clearly defined borders and edges. The cells had large nuclei, prominent nucleoli, and a high nuclear-to-cytoplasmic ratio (**Figure 3A**). We confirmed that the *SOX10* mutant and normal control iPSC lines expressed endogenous pluripotent genes to a high degree as measured by qPCR (**Figure 3B**). In addition, immunocytochemistry was conducted to investigate the expression of stem cell markers at the protein level. These cells were found to be positive for nuclear (OCT3/4, NANOG, and SOX2) and surface (SSEA4 and TRA1-60) markers of pluripotency, in addition to staining for AP (**Figures 3A,C**). We then examined the differentiation potential of these iPSC lines. Both lines had the ability to differentiate into the three germ layers (ectoderm, mesoderm, and endoderm) in the teratoma assay (**Figure 3F**); these iPSC lines presented a normal karyotype (**Figure 3D**). These findings indicated that the reprogramming of the fibroblasts caused no alterations in the chromosomal or genetic markers. Furthermore, genotyping confirmed the expected compound heterozygous *SOX10* mutation (c.336G > A) in the iPSC line from the WS2 patient (**Figure 3E**).

SOX10 Deficiency Results in Altered Gene Expression Patterns in iPSCs

To investigate differential gene expression in this WS patient's iPSCs resulting from *SOX10* mutation, we implemented RNA-Seq analysis of the iPSCs from a normal control. Triplicate RNA samples were isolated from the patient-derived iPSCs and an unrelated control cell line cultured under normal conditions. They were then analyzed using RNA-Seq, and differential gene-expression analysis was performed with DESeq2. A total of 405 genes were found to be differentially expressed between the patient and the pooled control iPSC line based on the differential expression criteria (adjusted P-value < 0.05 and | log2 (fold-change) | > 1). A heatmap using the FPKM value of the

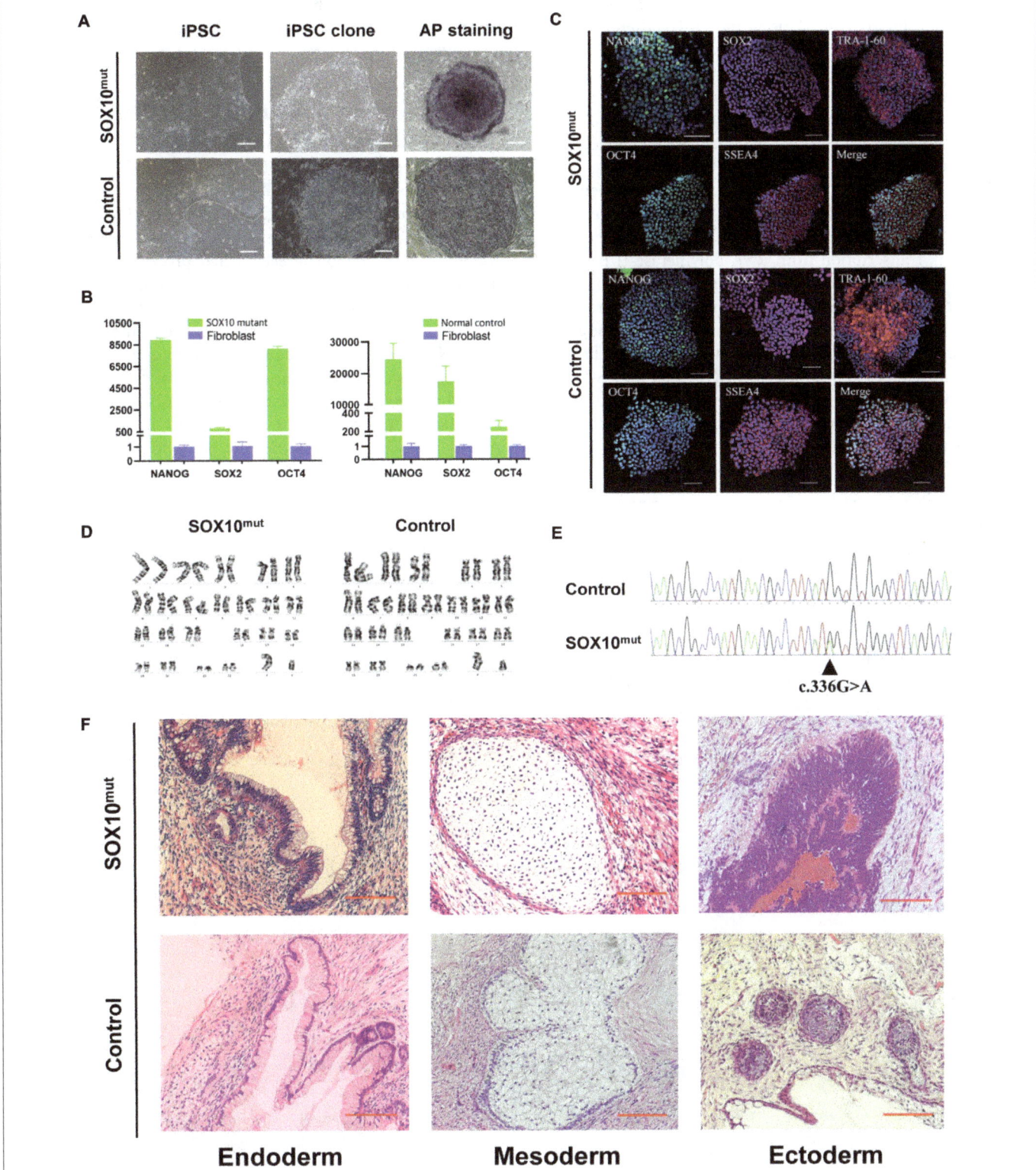

FIGURE 3 | Induction and characterization of *SOX10* mutant and normal control iPSCs. **(A)** The *SOX10* mutant and normal control iPSC clones with typical embryonic stem cell-like and positive alkaline phosphatase staining. Bar, 100 μM. **(B)** qPCR analysis of pluripotency markers in both iPSC lines showed significantly upregulated expression of OCT4, SOX2 and NANOG, in contrast to fibroblasts. **(C)** Immunofluorescence staining in both iPSC lines showed expression of pluripotency markers OCT4, NANOG, TRA-1-60, SOX2, and SSEA-4. Bar, 100 μM. **(D)** Karyotyping analysis showed normal chromosomal structure and numbers in both iPSC lines. **(E)** Sanger sequencing confirmed the mutation in *SOX10* in iPSC lines. **(F)** H&E stainings of teratomas generated from subcutaneous injection of both iPSC lines in NOD/SCID mice. Tumor sections represent differentiated structures as noted. Bar, 100 μM.

DEGs was generated and row normalization was executed using scale function (**Figure 4A**). Among the DEGs, there were 144 genes (35.6%) that displayed significantly augmented expression in the SOX10 mutant iPSCs, while 261 genes (64.4%) showed significantly diminished expression (**Figures 4B,C**).

To investigate whether the DEGs of the *SOX10* mutant iPSCs were enriched in specific functionally related gene groups and signaling pathways, we utilized Gene Ontology (GO) and KEGG (Kyoto Encyclopedia of Genes and Genomes) pathway-enrichment analyses. The significantly enriched GO terms included terms connected to DNA-templated transcription, transcription from RNA polymerase II promoter, multicellular organism development, and negative regulation of angiogenesis (**Figure 5**). Interestingly, GO enrichment for biological process identified inner ear morphogenesis enriched in the DEGs, and these related genes are listed in **Table 1**. Additionally, no DEGs of *SOX10* mutant iPSCs were significantly enriched in the KEGG pathways. Altogether, SOX10 deficiency led to subtle transcriptional perturbation with respect to the affected genes and their mRNA levels, and the *SOX10* mutant iPSCs had the ability to undergo morphologic differentiation in a manner similar to those derived from the control iPSCs.

Differentiation of Mutated *SOX10* Patient-Derived iPSCs to NCCs

Following the investigation of the impacted of lowered *SOX10* expression on WS patient-derived iPSCs at the pluripotent stage, we narrowed our study to examine differentiating the iPSCs to iNCCs as a more relevant, disorder-specific cell type. We followed a previously established protocol to differentiate patient-derived and WT iPSCs into neural crest cells (this protocol is described in the "Materials and Methods" sections of these publications, and results showed that activation of the WNT pathway induced neural border genes and neural crest markers that mimicked normal neural crest development) (Chambers et al., 2011; **Figure 6A**). Our findings indicated an apparent minor delay in neural crest induction in *SOX10* mutant iPSCs. In addition, despite being initially plated at the

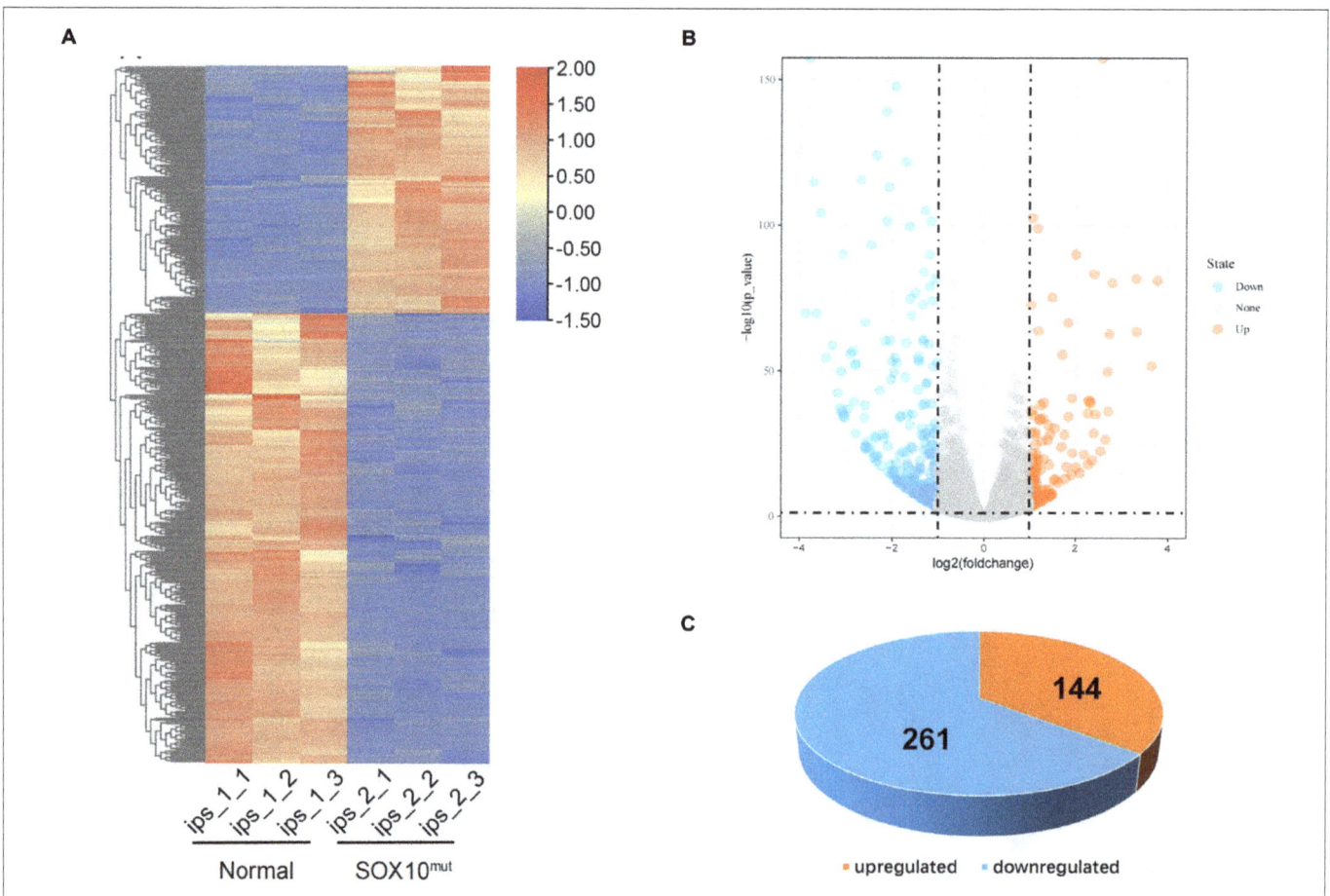

FIGURE 4 | Differentially expressed genes in *SOX10* mutant iPSCs. **(A)** The heatmap showed hierarchical clustering analysis of DEGs in *SOX10* mutant iPSCs. The FPKM values of DEGs were normalized by scale function and compared between the *SOX10* mutant iPSCs and normal control. Red and blue indicate genes with high and low expression levels, respectively. **(B)** Volcano plot showing the expression change of each gene and their significance. Red dots represent the expression of genes in *SOX10* mutant iPSCs significantly up-regulated compared to normal control. Blue dots represent the expression of genes in *SOX10* mutant iPSCs significantly down-regulated compared to normal control. **(C)** Of the DEGs, 144 genes were up-regulated and 261 genes were down-regulated.

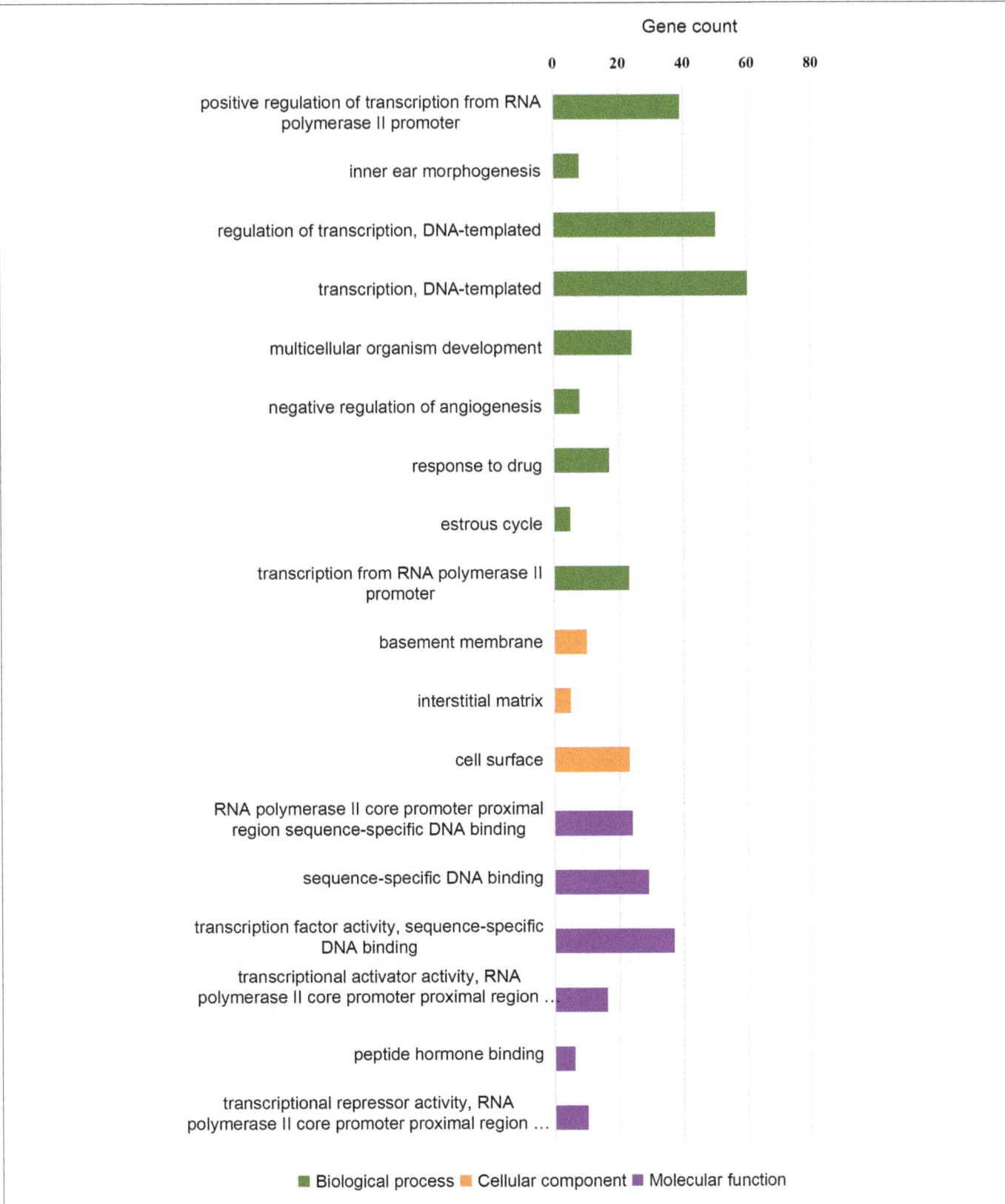

FIGURE 5 | GO enrichment analysis of differentially expressed genes in *SOX10* mutant iPSCs. A total of 18 GO terms were significantly enriched. Nine terms were significantly enriched based on biological process, three terms were significantly enriched based on cellular components, and six terms were significantly enriched based on molecular function.

TABLE 1 | Differentially expressed genes in patient iPSC enriched in inner ear morphogenesis.

No.	Gene symbol	Gene description	Log 2 fold change	Adjusted P-value
1	TBX1	T-box transcription factor 1	−3.8729	2.118E-70
2	GBX2	Gastrulation brain homeobox 2	−3.6959	1.398E-115
3	NTN1	Netrin 1	−1.8225	1.016E-34
4	PAX8	Paired box 8	−1.2506	4.331E-06
5	GATA3	GATA binding protein 3	1.1878	1.627E-05
6	SPRY2	Sprouty RTK signaling antagonist 2	−1.0997	2.516E-52
7	HMX2	H6 family homeobox 2	1.0354	2.367E-04
8	CHD7	Chromodomain helicase DNA binding protein 7	1.178	9.746E-100

identical density, less cells were noted in the mutant cultures during 7 d of culture. By day 12, the majority of the areas of the cultures had achieved confluency; in contrast, the patient-derived NCCs were denser (**Figure 6B**). Immunofluorescence analysis demonstrated that the neural crest (NC) differentiation markers SOX10, SOX9, PAX3, HNK-1, and P75 were expressed in both iNCC cell lines (**Figure 6C**). We then compared the expression of NC-related genes (SOX9, PAX3, HNK-1, P75, TWIST1, and TFAP2A including SOX10) on day 12 of the differentiation process between both types of iNCCs. Under NC induction, the iNCCs derived from SOX10 mutant iPSCs initiated significant down-regulation of the NC-related genes at the mRNA level except SOX9, compare with control (**Figure 6D**). Collectively, these observations indicated that SOX10 haploinsufficiency—through the development of NCCs-affected the proliferation and differentiation of NCCs, and reduced their overall pluripotent potential.

Global Changes in Gene Expression in the WS Patient-Derived iNCCs With the SOX10 Mutation

RNA-Seq analysis was completed in triplicate for iNCCs from the SOX10 mutant and normal control lines to evaluate cellular differentiation at the gene-expression level between the iNCC lines, and differential gene expression was determined. The methods used for data analysis and sample pooling were the same as the analysis conducted for the iPSCs in order to enable a direct comparison. The heatmap created with the FPKM value for global gene expression indicated that most of the gene-expression patterns differed between the SOX10 mutant iNCCs and controls (**Figure 7A**). DESeq2 identified a total of 1805 DEGs (P-value < 0.05 and $|\log2 \text{(fold-change)}| > 1$), among which 899 genes were downregulated in SOX10 mutant iNCCs while 906 genes were upregulated in patient iNCCs (**Figures 7B,C**). The number of DEGs was four times higher in the former relative to the iPSCs, indicating that the SOX10 mutation had a much stronger impact on the transcriptome in differentiated cells, which corresponded with the tissue-restricted phenotype.

GO and KEGG pathway-enrichment analyses were performed on all the DEGs to determine whether specific subsets of genes were differentially expressed in the patient iNCCs. In total, 78 GO terms were significantly enriched. Of them, 47 GO terms were significantly enriched to biological process (BP), 19 GO terms were significantly enriched to cellular component (CC), and 12 GO terms were significantly enriched to molecular function (MF) (the top 10 most enriched GO terms for BP, CC, and MF are revealed in **Figure 8A**). The top 10 most enriched GO terms for BP included multicellular organism development, neuron migration, regulation of transcription from RNA polymerase II promoter, ureteric bud development, skeletal system development, chemical synaptic transmission, and axon guidance. These results indicated that subsets of genes involved in tissues and cell types, including peripheral neurons and glial cells, melanocytes, secretory cells, and cranial skeletal and connective cells, were overrepresented in the DEGs, suggesting that they had strong links to defects in NCC biology and the development of multiple NC-derived systems. GO enrichment for BP also determined enriched functional networks pertaining to inner ear morphogenesis and inner ear development (the related DEGs in these two GO terms are revealed in **Tables 2, 3**). KEGG pathway analysis identified 17 terms as significantly enriched, and the top-10 KEGG terms included WNT signaling pathway, signaling pathways regulating pluripotency of stem cells, basal cell carcinoma, dopaminergic synapse, pathways in cancer, cholinergic synapse, axon guidance, morphine addiction, neuroactive ligand-receptor interaction, and glutamatergic synapse (**Figure 8B**).

In order to identify the candidate target gene regulated by SOX10 throughout inner ear development, we examined the genes pertinent to inner ear development in the GO database (GO terms were inner ear development and inner ear morphogenesis) and proteins that interacted with SOX10 in the STRING database. Fifty-nine proteins interacted directly with SOX10 (**Figure 9**). The gene lists were combined with the DEGs to acquire the target genes connected to inner ear development and morphogenesis. Considering the association between decreased RNA expression and possible SOX10-binding sites allowed us to reduce the list of candidate genes to four: BMP2, LGR5, GBX2, and GATA3. The potential SOX10-binding sites in the candidate genes were predicted using the online JASPAR database (**Table 4** shows the predicted binding site details).

DISCUSSION

WS, the most common disorder resulting in syndromic hearing loss (SHL) in the Chinese population, is a genetic disorder with locus heterogeneity and variable expression of clinical characteristics (Zhang et al., 2012; Li et al., 2019). The

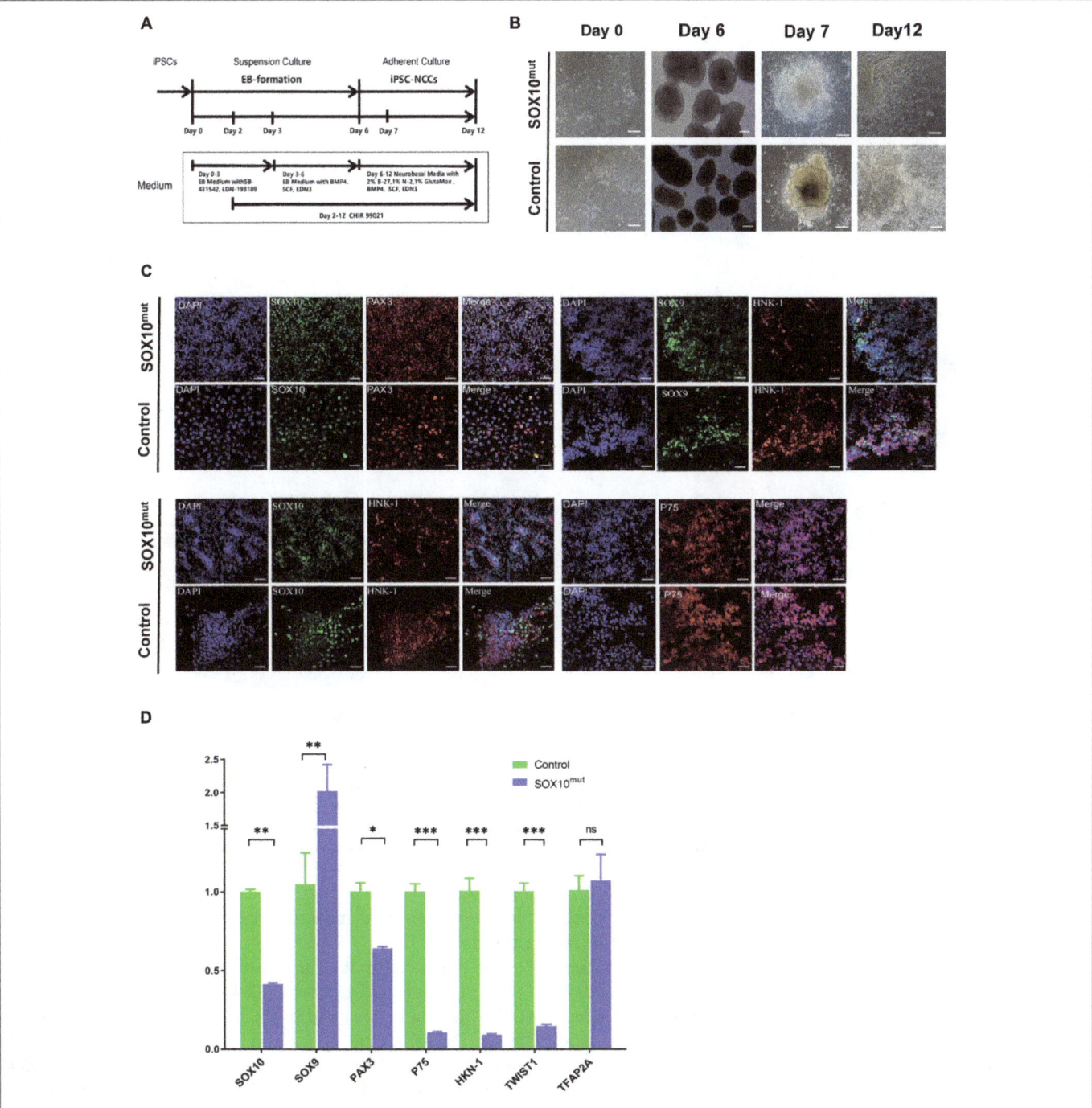

FIGURE 6 | Generation and characterization of SOX10 mutant iPSC-derived NCCs. (A) Schematic of the NCC differentiation protocol timeline. EB Medium: KO-DMEM supplemented with 20% KSR, 1% GlutaMax-I, 1%NEAA. (B) Comparison of the cell images of the SOX10 mutant and control iPSC-derived NCC at Days 0, 6, 7, and 12 following differentiation. Bar, 100 μM. (C) Immunofluorescence staining shows expression of NCC markers SOX10, PAX3, SOX9, HNK-1, and P75. Bar, 50 μM. (D) RT-qPCR for evaluating expression of NCC markers. (*represents $p < 0.05$, ** represents $p < 0.01$, *** represent $p < 0.001$ and ns represents no significant).

mechanisms underlying phenotypic variability in WS are still not fully understood (Bondurand et al., 2007; Pingault et al., 2010). SNHL is defined as a pure tone threshold shift of over 25dB, affecting more than 466 million people worldwide. SNHL includes degenerative changes of cochlear hair cells (He et al., 2017, 2021; Liu W. et al., 2019; Zhou et al., 2020; Cheng et al., 2021; Fu et al., 2021), cochlear supporting cells (Lu et al., 2017; Cheng et al., 2019; Tan et al., 2019; Zhang S. et al., 2019; Zhang et al., 2020a; Zhang Y. et al., 2020; Chen et al., 2021), and spiral ganglion neurons (Guo et al., 2016, 2020, 2021; Yan et al., 2018; Liu et al., 2021). Sound is collected and conducted by external and middle ear, then transformed into the electric

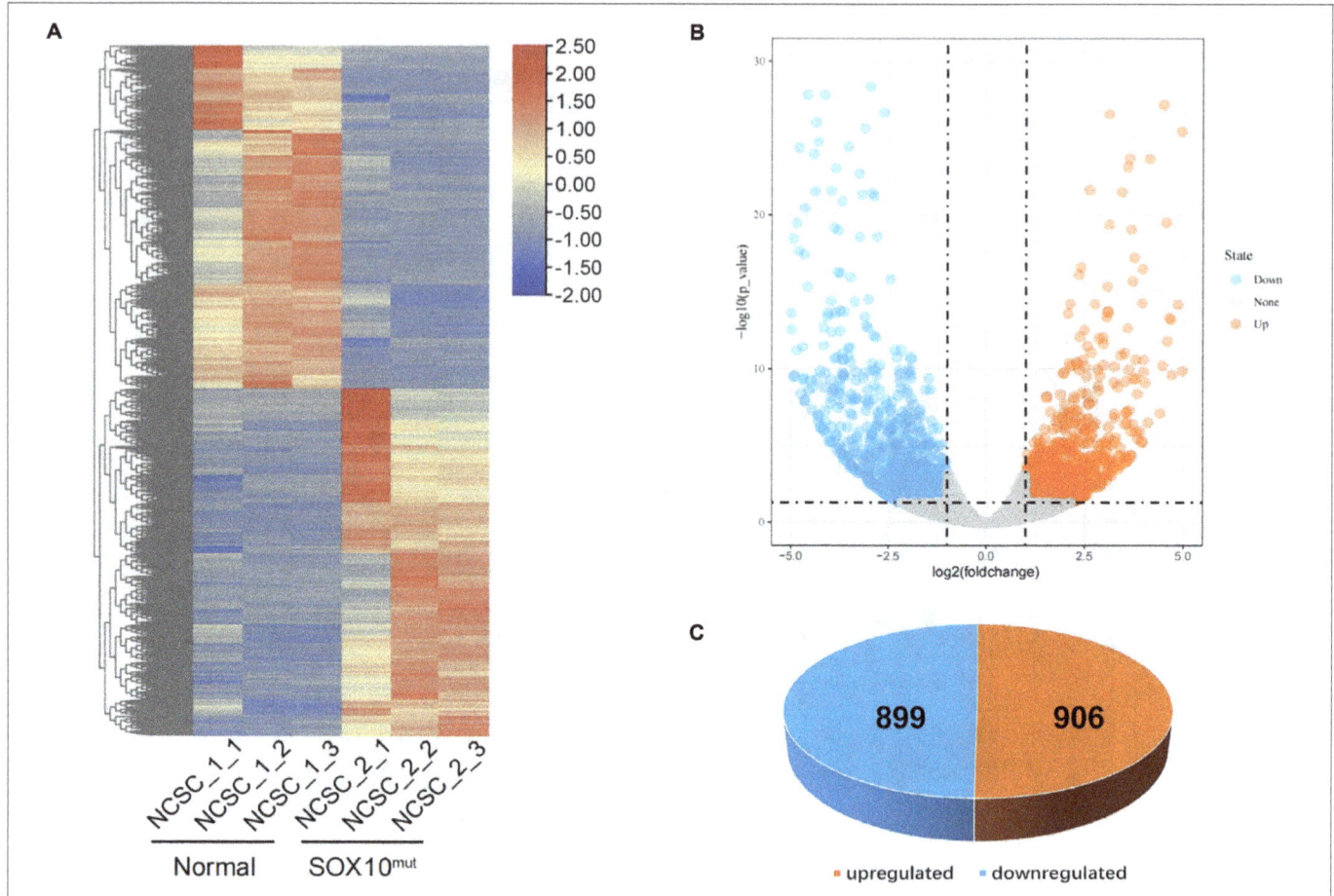

FIGURE 7 | Differentially expressed genes in *SOX10* mutant iNCCs. **(A)** The heatmap showed hierarchical clustering analysis of DEGs in *SOX10* mutant iNCCs. The FPKM values of DEGs were normalized by scale function and compared between the *SOX10* mutant iNCCs and normal control. Red and blue indicate genes with high and low expression levels, respectively. **(B)** Volcano plot showing the expression change of each gene and their significance. Red dots represent the expression of genes in *SOX10* mutant iNCCs significantly upregulated compared to normal control. Blue dots represent the expression of genes in *SOX10* mutant iNCCs significantly downregulated compared to normal control. **(C)** A total of 906 genes were up-regulated and 899 genes were down-regulated among the DEGs.

signals by cochlear hair cells (Wang et al., 2017; Liu Y. et al., 2019; Qi et al., 2019, 2020; Zhang Y. et al., 2020); while spiral ganglion neurons is function as the neural auditory transduction cells (Sun et al., 2016; Guo et al., 2019, 2021; Liu W. et al., 2019; Zhao et al., 2019). The cochlear hair cells are sensitive to aging, acoustic trauma, ototoxic drugs, and environmental or genetic influences (O'Donnell et al., 1988; Zhu et al., 2018; Fang et al., 2019; Jiang et al., 2020; Qian et al., 2020; Lv et al., 2021; Zhang et al., 2021). Previous studies have shown that oxidative stress and cell apoptosis play important roles in hair cell loss (Sun et al., 2014; Yu et al., 2017; Li et al., 2018; Gao et al., 2019; Zhang Y. et al., 2019; Zhang et al., 2020b; Zhong et al., 2020).

SOX10 is a key transcription factor related to the migration and differentiation of NCCs. Mutations in SOX10 result in abnormal pigment distribution and deafness, and are the primary cause of WS (Bondurand and Sham, 2013). SOX10 belongs to the *SOX* family, which features a high-mobility group (HMG) DNA-binding domain. The HMG domain (amino acids 102–181) identifies and binds to the promoter sequence of a target gene and induces conformational modifications in DNA throughout transcriptional regulation (Harris et al., 2010; Schock and LaBonne, 2020).

The non-sense mutation identified in the present study was found in amino acid 112, which is located in the HMG domain (DNA-binding region) and in the predicted nuclear localization signals (NLSs), resulting in a substitution of the guanine in position number 336 (Südbeck and Scherer, 1997). This *SOX10* mutant was first identified by Chaoui et al. (2011) in three independent families, and resulted from two different variations at the nucleotide level: c.336G > A and c.336G > C). The probands were associated with WS2 or PCW/PCWH based on the observed variety of phenotypes. Functional analysis revealed that the p.Met112Ile appeared to possess an increased monomer-binding capacity, leading to reduced binding of the *SOX10* mutant and reduced transactivation capacity toward the target promoter (Chaoui et al., 2011). Nevertheless, the phenotypic differences observed raise the potential for the individual genetic background being influential, which is not uncommon in neurocristopathies (Amiel et al., 2008). Since SOX10 gene is not endogenous expressed at the iPSCs stage, we collected cells at the

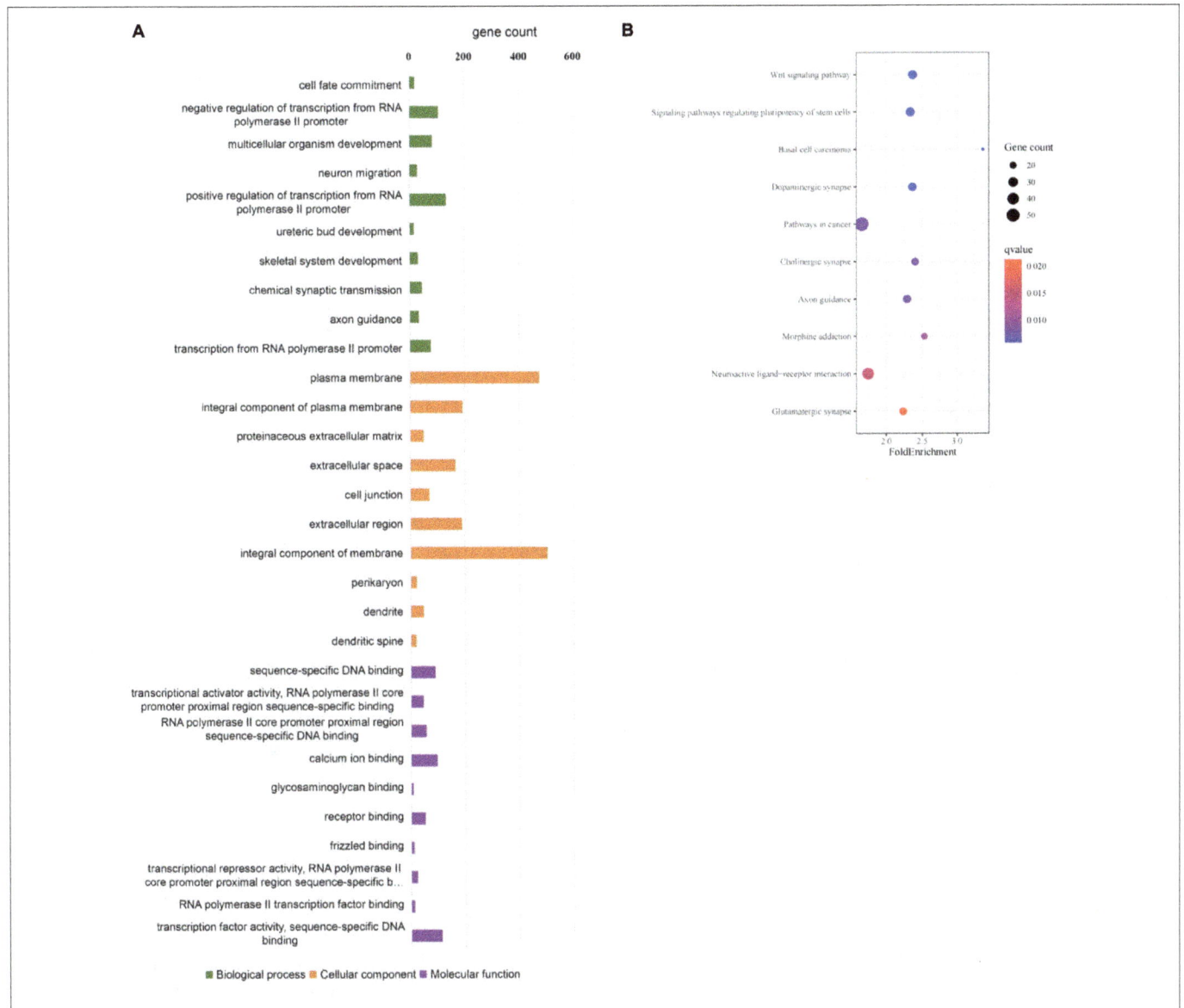

FIGURE 8 | GO enrichment analysis of differentially expressed genes in *SOX10* mutant iNCCs. **(A)** Top 10 most enriched GO terms for biological processes, cellular components, and molecular function. **(B)** Top 10 most enriched KEGG pathway terms are listed.

12th day of iNCC stage to perform qPCR and WB experiments to analyze the influence of SOX10 mutation (**Supplementary Figure 1**). The results suggest this mutation caused the decrease of its RNA and protein expression levels in the patient-derived iNCCs, thus it was speculated that it might cause functional changes through insufficient haploid dose.

To the best of our knowledge, this is the first work to document a disease model of iPSCs derived from a patient with WS. There are currently several established SOX10 animal-disease models that entail multiple species (Tachibana et al., 2003; Dutton et al., 2009; Hao et al., 2018). However, there are still many differences between the phenotypes of animal models and those of humans due to the disparities in genetic background, timeline of organ development, and underlying regulatory mechanisms between the species; it is therefore still difficult to accurately recapitulate human abnormalities such as WS in animals. Because iPSCs can differentiate into a vast array of cell types, the present system provides a powerful method to elucidate the disease mechanisms and explore potential therapeutic interventions so as to improve the well-being of patients (Chen et al., 2019; Zhang et al., 2020a).

In the current work, we generated a human cell model for WS with iPSCs harboring a *SOX10* mutation, and differentiated these iPSCs into NCCs as a specific and disease-relevant system that could be used to investigate WS *in vitro*. WS patient-derived fibroblasts were reprogrammed into *SOX10*-mutant iPSCs based on the Yamanaka method (Takahashi and Yamanaka, 2006). The *SOX10*-mutant iPSCs generated in this study could then be further cultured with relatively high efficiency and showed pluripotential characteristics, including pluripotency marker

TABLE 2 | Differentially expressed genes in patient iNCCs enriched in inner ear morphogenesis.

No.	Gene symbol	Gene description	Log 2 fold change	Adjusted P-value
1	GATA3	GATA binding protein 3	−2.5587	1.457E-04
2	USH1G	USH1 protein network component sans	−2.4423	2.017E-02
3	TBX1	T-box transcription factor 1	−2.3788	4.440E-03
4	PRRX1	Paired related homeobox 1	−1.8414	1.492E-03
5	NTN1	Netrin 1	−1.8141	2.494E-04
6	GBX2	Gastrulation brain homeobox 2	−1.7589	1.016E-04
7	ITGA8	Integrin subunit alpha 8	−1.2744	2.697E-02
8	FGF9	Fibroblast growth factor 9	1.4407	1.599E-02
9	COL11A1	Collagen type XI alpha 1 chain	1.5271	8.154E-04
10	TFAP2A	Transcription factor AP-2 alpha	1.648	3.069E-02
11	ZIC1	Zic family member 1	2.0873	3.878E-04
12	MAFB	MAF bZIP transcription factor B	2.6142	4.558E-06
13	POU4F3	POU class 4 homeobox 3	3.2812	2.775E-06
14	NEUROG1	Neurogenin 1	3.7124	1.956E-16

TABLE 3 | Differentially expressed genes in patient iNCCs enriched in inner ear development.

No	Gene symbol	Gene_description	Log 2 fold change	Adjusted P-value
1	LGR5	Leucine rich repeat containing G protein-coupled receptor 5	−5.9869	9.649E-38
2	BMPER	BMP binding endothelial regulator	−5.0578	2.041E-21
3	SHH	Sonic hedgehog signaling molecule	−3.0073	4.947E-05
4	BMP2	Bone morphogenetic protein 2	−2.3362	6.027E-12
5	HOXA1	Homeobox A1	−2.1382	8.994E-03
6	MAF	MAF bZIP transcription factor	1.5757	2.496E-04
7	CYTL1	Cytokine like 1	1.6092	4.109E-02
8	CXCL14	C-X-C motif chemokine ligand 14	1.8429	5.919E-06
9	PLPPR4	Phospholipid phosphatase related 4	1.93	1.373E-02
10	EYA4	EYA transcriptional coactivator and phosphatase 4	1.9746	6.097E-06
11	NEUROD1	Neuronal differentiation 1	3.0814	2.239E-04
12	PHOX2B	Paired like homeobox 2B	3.3696	2.151E-04

expression and the potential for teratoma formation, suggesting that the mutation in *SOX10* did not directly affect the induction and expression of the iPSCs.

In contrast to the normal control, the idiopathic *SOX10* mutant iPSCs exhibited lowered efficiency in NCC induction *in vitro* and defects in the expression of key genes in NCC specification. Interestingly, unlike other NCC markers, the expression of SOX9 was increased in the qRT-PCR of SOX10 mutated iNCC cells compared with the normal group. The SOX transcription group consists of SOX9 and SOX10, and they have a common bipartite transactivation mechanism. In addition, they share some overlap in biological functions (Haseeb and Lefebvre, 2019). The decrease of SOX10 expression may lead to the compensatory increase of SOX9 expression. Relative to the normal control, the transcriptomic analysis of *SOX10* mutant iPSCs revealed an overrepresentation of genes in the embryologic development of the tissues principally impacted in WS, such as pigmentation and skeletal and neuronal development. We identified a total of 1,805 DEGs, of which 899 (49.8%) were down-regulated. These results suggest that SOX10 mutation have a wide range of effects on the transcriptome, and that the target genes involved in the biological process are enriched, suggesting that SOX10 mutation have an impact on the proliferation and differentiation potential of NCCs, which is also in accordance with previous studies (Mollaaghababa and Pavan, 2003; Haldin and LaBonne, 2010; Schock and LaBonne, 2020).

We noted that our analyses converged, suggesting potential mechanisms of inner ear development as the proband showed conspicuous bilateral inner ear malformations. In previous studies, researchers demonstrated that, rather than resulting from an NCC defect, inner ear malformations were directly induced by a *SOX10* mutation by causing endolymphatic collapse and other abnormalities in the organ of Corti (Elmaleh-Bergès et al., 2013; Locher et al., 2015; Hao et al., 2018). However, some other researchers have explored the exact contributions of neural crest lineages to the neurosensory components of the inner ear, offering an important basis for investigating the potential NC origins of the inner ear (Freyer et al., 2011). After examining the GO and KEGG pathway enrichment analyses for the DEGs, we determined that biological processes focused on inner ear development and morphogenesis in both iPSCs and iNCCs, suggesting that the mutation in *SOX10* may have caused the inner ear malformation in this WS patient.

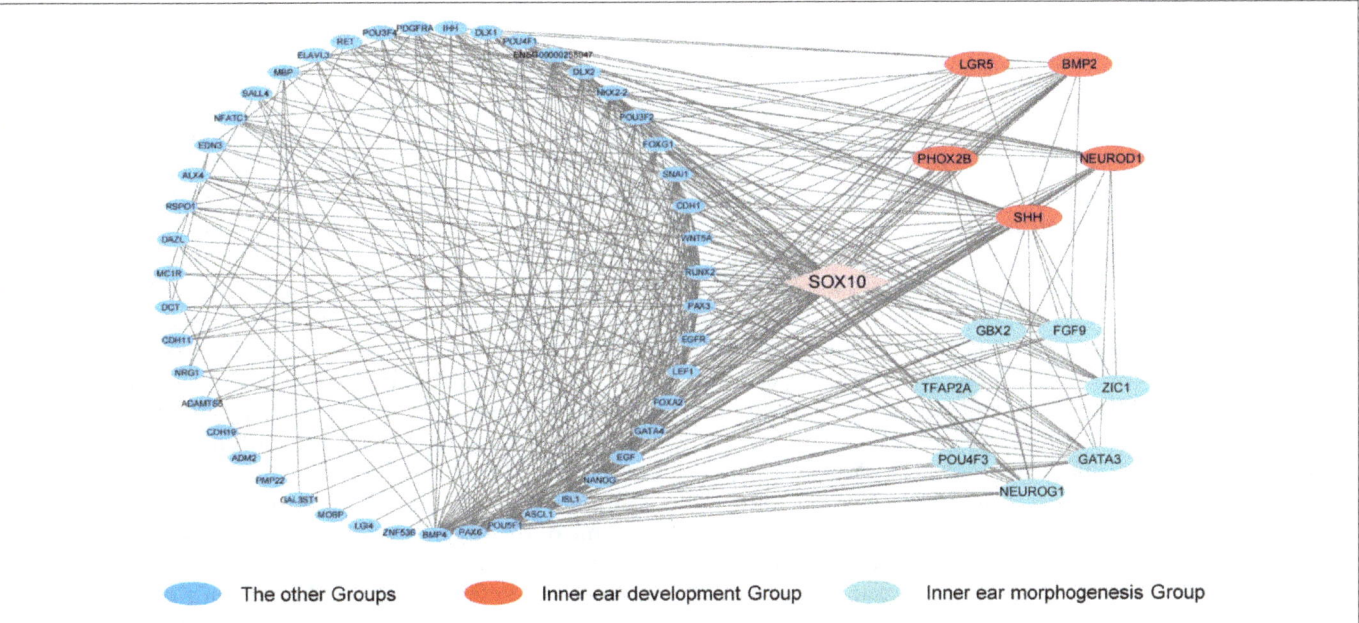

FIGURE 9 | Protein-protein interaction network of differentially expressed genes that interact with SOX10. The diamond represents SOX10. The circles indicate the proteins that interact with SOX10. Red circles represent the genes enriched in the GO term inner ear development, and cyan circles represent the genes enriched in the GO term inner ear morphogenesis. Lines represent the interaction relationship between two proteins.

TABLE 4 | The SOX10 potential binding sites predicted in the candidate genes.

Name	Score	Relative score	Start	End	Strand	Predicted sequence
BMP2	7.09699	0.91952059	395	400	+	CTGTGT
LGR5	8.90979	0.999999997	669	674	+	CTTTGT
GBX2	8.90979	0.999999997	328	333	+	CTTTGT
GATA3	7.09357	0.919368595	111	116	+	CGTTGT

While a growing body of evidence has revealed that *SOX10* mutations can cause defects of the inner ear in humans, the target genes and pathways regulated by *SOX10* that are involved in inner ear development have yet to be completely elucidated (Elmaleh-Bergès et al., 2013; Wakaoka et al., 2013; Song et al., 2016; Xu et al., 2016). We additionally performed a cluster analysis to screen the PPI network pertaining to *SOX10*, and it revealed four candidate genes that may be regulated by *SOX10* during the development of the inner ear: *BMP2, LGR5, GBX2,* and *GATA3*.

BMP2 (bone morphogenetic protein 2), a member of the transforming growth factor-beta (TGF-β) superfamily, possesses crucial functions in developmental processes, including cardiogenesis, digit apoptosis, somite formation, neuronal growth, and musculoskeletal development (Schlange et al., 2000; Benavente et al., 2012; Christen et al., 2012; Gámez et al., 2013). As mentioned in a literature review, *BMP2* plays a crucial role in the formation of three semicircular canals during inner ear development (Hwang et al., 2019). The otic-specific knockout of *Bmp2* caused the lack of all semicircular canals in a mouse model (Hwang et al., 2010). Additionally, *bmp2b* was also shown to be necessary for maintaining canal structures in zebrafish, as mutant *bmp2b* zebrafish lacked canals, which is similar to the mouse mutants. *Bmp2* is expressed in highly conserved patterns in the canals' genesis zones near the cristae, as well as in the epithelium of the developing canals (Hammond et al., 2009). Moreover, *BMP2* takes part in the regulation of NCC proliferation, migration, and differentiation—mimicking the expression patterns of the *SOX10* gene. Previous studies showed that *BMP2* is also required for enteric nervous system development. The expression of *BMP2* is significantly attenuated in Hirschsprung's disease patients—which results from defects in NCCs colonizing the intestines—and leads to an absence of enteric ganglia in the colon (Huang et al., 2019). In addition, *BMP2* selectively targets and stimulates tyrosinase (TYR) gene expression and melanogenesis in differentiated melanocytes. It has been reported that *BMP2* treatment of neural crest cells increases melanogenesis by encouraging the synthesis of melanin and the *BMP2* response-element localized upstream from the *TYR* transcriptional start site (Bilodeau et al., 2001). *SOX9* also encourages the expression of BMP2 by binding directly to the *BMP2* promoter, promoting its transcription (Xiao et al., 2019). Therefore, we suggest that *SOX9* and *SOX10* comprise a *SOX*-transcription group and share a bipartite transactivation mechanism that implicates the direct regulation of *BMP2* by *SOX10* (Haseeb and Lefebvre, 2019).

LGR5 (leucine-rich repeat-containing G-protein coupled receptor 5) is a target gene of the Wnt pathway and a known indicator of endogenous stem cells in rapidly proliferating organs

(Barker et al., 2007; Jaks et al., 2008). In addition, *LGR5* plays key roles in embryonic development and in the regeneration and preservation of adult stem cells (Chaoui et al., 2011). In a pattern emulating that of *SOX10*, *LGR5* is widely expressed in NCCs at early stages of embryonic development (Boddupally et al., 2016). *LGR5* is expressed in the apical poles of the sensory epithelium of the cochlear duct and vestibular end organs, and has limited expression in the hair cells of the organ of Corti during early embryonic development (Chai et al., 2011). Previous research has demonstrated that *Lgr5* + cochlear supporting cells (SCs) can regenerate hair cells (HCs) via direct differentiation and mitotic regeneration (Wang et al., 2015). Differentially expressed genes can be found between Lgr5$^+$ progenitors and *Lgr5*-SCs that may regulate the proliferation of the *Lgr5*$^+$ progenitors and the regenerative capacity of HCs (Cheng et al., 2017).

GBX2 (gastrulation brain homeobox 2) encodes a DNA-binding transcription factor that plays critical roles in embryogenesis. Several studies have concluded that *GBX2* is needed for the development of the inner ear, especially during the initial formation of the otic placode (Miyazaki et al., 2006; Steventon et al., 2012, 2016). The *Gbx2*$^{-/-}$ mouse displays several inner ear abnormalities, ranging from local malformation to a complete loss of vestibular and cochlear inner ear structures—including the absence of semicircular canals, malformed saccule, and cochlear duct (Lin et al., 2005). Several current studies have also depicted pivotal parts *GBX2* plays in the induction, migration, and patterning of NCCs by impacting multiple facets of NC development (Li et al., 2009; Chervenak et al., 2014; Roeseler et al., 2020). The loss of *GBX2* function also modulates the Slit/Robo-signaling pathway, leading to abnormal NCC migration and abnormalities that as similar to those in congenital diseases, such as DiGeorge syndrome and in craniofacial malformations (Byrd and Meyers, 2005; Calmont et al., 2009).

GATA3 belongs to the GATA family of transcription factors and is a key regulator of auditory system development (Karis et al., 2001; Appler and Goodrich, 2011). Its expression is found in virtually all auditory cell types (Rivolta and Holley, 1998; Lawoko-Kerali et al., 2002; Milo et al., 2009). In early inner ear development from thembryonic otic placode, *GATA3* regulates the signaling of prosensory genes in a dynamic fashion and at the same time, it directs the differentiation of cochlear neurosensory cells (Duncan and Fritzsch, 2013; Moriguchi et al., 2018). Further studies have provided evidence that *GATA3* is also crucial for the coordinated maturation of sensory hair cells and their innervation (Bardhan et al., 2019). In humans, the expression of *GATA3* is localized to the cochlear duct and the spiral ganglion between weeks 8 and 12 of gestation (Roccio et al., 2018); the loss of GATA3 in inner hair cells leads to hearing loss and accounts for some of the deafness connected to hypoparathyroidism and renal anomaly (HDR) syndrome (Van Esch et al., 2000; Martins et al., 2018). Researchers have also demonstrated that *GATA3* plays critical roles in neural crest cell development and neuronal differentiation in some cranial neural crest derivatives (George et al., 1994; Lieuw et al., 1997; Lakshmanan et al., 1999).

In conclusion, in this work, we created a WS human iPSC model with a *SOX10* mutation, and allowed the differentiation of iPSC into NCCs. Relative to normal controls, the WS patient-specific iPSCs had a poor response to NCC induction *in vitro* and a compromised differentiation potential in regard to the NCCs' fate. Transcriptional perturbation in NCC differentiation in this model was revealed through the intensive analysis of high-throughput RNA-seq results. In addition, we identified numerous candidate genes that are highly likely

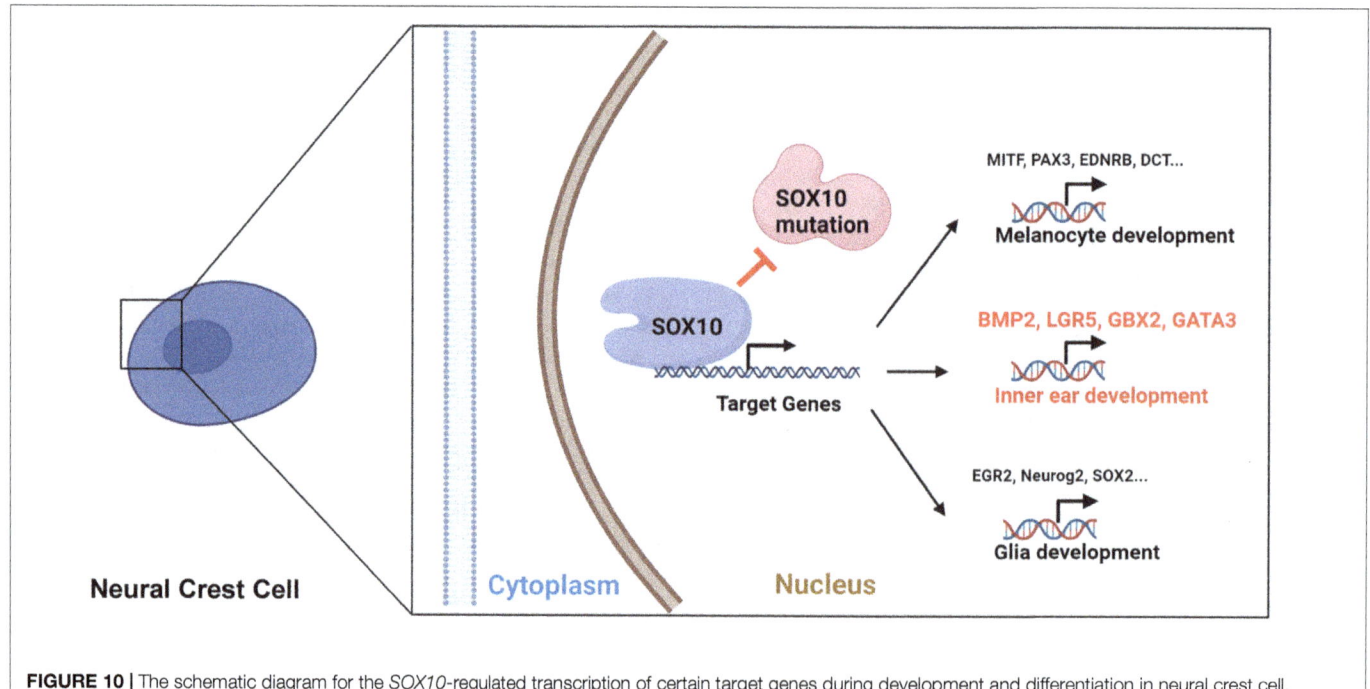

FIGURE 10 | The schematic diagram for the *SOX10*-regulated transcription of certain target genes during development and differentiation in neural crest cell.

to be related to inner ear malformation in WS patients with a *SOX10* mutation (**Figure 10**). Because the molecular mechanisms underlying the effect of *SOX10* on inner ear development have not been fully elucidated, our research offers a rich context for investigating the molecular etiology of WS in regard to inner ear malformations. Nevertheless, additional research is necessary in order to verify the part that the determined target genes and their pathways have in triggering inner ear malformations.

ETHICS STATEMENT

The studies involving human participants were reviewed and approved by the Ethics Committee of Xiangya Hospital Central South University. Written informed consent to participate in this study was provided by the participants' legal guardian/next of kin. The animal study was reviewed and approved by The Ethics Committee of Xiangya Hospital Central South University. Written informed consent was obtained from the individual(s) for the publication of any potentially identifiable images or data included in this article.

AUTHOR CONTRIBUTIONS

JS, CH, and YF conceived and designed the study. JW performed the most of the experiments. YB and LM analyzed the related data. YL contributed to the generation of iPSC lines. XC, CH, and LYM were responsible for the patient recruitment and obtaining consent for all of the patients, and clinical sample collection. JW and JS wrote the manuscript. CH and YF supervised the study. All authors approved the final version.

ACKNOWLEDGMENTS

We are truly grateful for the tissue and blood samples donated by the patient and his families and contributions to this study. We also thank LetPub (www.letpub.com) for its linguistic assistance during the preparation of this manuscript.

REFERENCES

Amiel, J., Sproat-Emison, E., Garcia-Barcelo, M., Lantieri, F., Burzynski, G., Borrego, S., et al. (2008). Hirschsprung disease, associated syndromes and genetics: a review. *J. Med. Genet.* 45, 1–14. doi: 10.1136/jmg.2007.053959

Appler, J. M., and Goodrich, L. V. (2011). Connecting the ear to the brain: Molecular mechanisms of auditory circuit assembly. *Prog. Neurobiol.* 93, 488–508. doi: 10.1016/j.pneurobio.2011.01.004

Bardhan, T., Jeng, J. Y., Waldmann, M., Ceriani, F., Johnson, S. L., Olt, J., et al. (2019). Gata3 is required for the functional maturation of inner hair cells and their innervation in the mouse cochlea. *J. Physiol.* 597, 3389–3406. doi: 10.1113/jp277997

Barker, N., van Es, J. H., Kuipers, J., Kujala, P., van den Born, M., Cozijnsen, M., et al. (2007). Identification of stem cells in small intestine and colon by marker gene Lgr5. *Nature* 449, 1003–1007. doi: 10.1038/nature06196

Benavente, F., Pinto, C., Parada, M., Henríquez, J. P., and Osses, N. (2012). Bone morphogenetic protein 2 inhibits neurite outgrowth of motor neuron-like NSC-34 cells and up-regulates its type II receptor. *J. Neurochem.* 122, 594–604. doi: 10.1111/j.1471-4159.2012.07795.x

Bilodeau, M. L., Greulich, J. D., Hullinger, R. L., Bertolotto, C., Ballotti, R., and Andrisani, O. M. (2001). BMP-2 stimulates tyrosinase gene expression and melanogenesis in differentiated melanocytes. *Pigment Cell Res.* 14, 328–336. doi: 10.1034/j.1600-0749.2001.140504.x

Boddupally, K., Wang, G., Chen, Y., and Kobielak, A. (2016). Lgr5 marks neural crest derived multipotent oral stromal stem cells. *Stem Cells* 34, 720–731. doi: 10.1002/stem.2314

Bolande, R. P. (1997). Neurocristopathy: its growth and development in 20 years. *Pediatr Pathol Lab Med* 17, 1–25.

Bondurand, N., Dastot-Le Moal, F., Stanchina, L., Collot, N., Baral, V., Marlin, S., et al. (2007). Deletions at the SOX10 gene locus cause Waardenburg syndrome types 2 and 4. *Am. J. Hum. Genet.* 81, 1169–1185. doi: 10.1086/522090

Bondurand, N., and Sham, M. H. (2013). The role of SOX10 during enteric nervous system development. *Dev. Biol.* 382, 330–343. doi: 10.1016/j.ydbio.2013.04.024

Breuskin, I., Bodson, M., Thelen, N., Thiry, M., Borgs, L., Nguyen, L., et al. (2009). Sox10 promotes the survival of cochlear progenitors during the establishment of the organ of Corti. *Dev. Biol.* 335, 327–339. doi: 10.1016/j.ydbio.2009.09.007

Byrd, N. A., and Meyers, E. N. (2005). Loss of Gbx2 results in neural crest cell patterning and pharyngeal arch artery defects in the mouse embryo. *Dev. Biol.* 284, 233–245. doi: 10.1016/j.ydbio.2005.05.023

Calmont, A., Ivins, S., Van Bueren, K. L., Papangeli, I., Kyriakopoulou, V., Andrews, W. D., et al. (2009). Tbx1 controls cardiac neural crest cell migration during arch artery development by regulating Gbx2 expression in the pharyngeal ectoderm. *Development* 136, 3173–3183. doi: 10.1242/dev.028902

Chai, R., Xia, A., Wang, T., Jan, T. A., Hayashi, T., Bermingham-McDonogh, O., et al. (2011). Dynamic expression of Lgr5, a Wnt target gene, in the developing and mature mouse cochlea. *J. Assoc. Res. Otolaryngol.* 12, 455–469. doi: 10.1007/s10162-011-0267-2

Chambers, S. M., Mica, Y., Studer, L., and Tomishima, M. J. (2011). Converting human pluripotent stem cells to neural tissue and neurons to model neurodegeneration. *Methods Mol. Biol.* 793, 87–97. doi: 10.1007/978-1-61779-328-8_6

Chaoui, A., Watanabe, Y., Touraine, R., Baral, V., Goossens, M., Pingault, V., et al. (2011). Identification and functional analysis of SOX10 missense mutations in different subtypes of Waardenburg syndrome. *Hum. Mutat.* 32, 1436–1449. doi: 10.1002/humu.21583

Chen, H., Jiang, L., Xie, Z., Mei, L., He, C., Hu, Z., et al. (2010). Novel mutations of PAX3, MITF, and SOX10 genes in Chinese patients with type I or type II Waardenburg syndrome. *Biochem. Biophys. Res. Commun.* 397, 70–74. doi: 10.1016/j.bbrc.2010.05.066

Chen, Y., Gu, Y., Li, Y., Li, G. L., Chai, R., Li, W., et al. (2021). Generation of mature and functional hair cells by co-expression of Gfi1, Pou4f3, and Atoh1 in the postnatal mouse cochlea. *Cell Rep.* 35:109016. doi: 10.1016/j.celrep.2021.109016

Chen, Y., Zhang, S., Chai, R., and Li, H. (2019). Hair cell regeneration. *Adv. Exp. Med. Biol.* 1130, 1–16. doi: 10.1007/978-981-13-6123-4_1

Cheng, C., Guo, L., Lu, L., Xu, X., Zhang, S., Gao, J., et al. (2017). Characterization of the transcriptomes of Lgr5+ hair cell progenitors and Lgr5- supporting cells in the Mouse Cochlea. *Front. Mol. Neurosci.* 10:122. doi: 10.3389/fnmol.2017.00122

Cheng, C., Hou, Y., Zhang, Z., Wang, Y., Lu, L., Zhang, L., et al. (2021). Disruption of the autism-related gene Pak1 causes stereocilia disorganization, hair cell loss, and deafness in mice. *J. Genet. Genom.* doi: 10.1016/j.jgg.2021.03.010 [Online ahead of print].

Cheng, C., Wang, Y., Guo, L., Lu, X., Zhu, W., Muhammad, W., et al. (2019). Age-related transcriptome changes in Sox2+ supporting cells in the mouse cochlea. *Stem Cell Res. Ther.* 10:365. doi: 10.1186/s13287-019-1437-0

Chervenak, A. P., Bank, L. M., Thomsen, N., Glanville-Jones, H. C., Jonathan, S., Millen, K. J., et al. (2014). The role of Zic genes in inner ear development in the mouse: exploring mutant mouse phenotypes. *Dev. Dyn.* 243, 1487–1498. doi: 10.1002/dvdy.24186

Christen, B., Rodrigues, A. M., Monasterio, M. B., Roig, C. F., and Izpisua Belmonte, J. C. (2012). Transient downregulation of Bmp signalling induces extra limbs in vertebrates. *Development* 139, 2557–2565. doi: 10.1242/dev.078774

Dourmishev, A. L., Dourmishev, L. A., Schwartz, R. A., and Janniger, C. K. (1999). Waardenburg syndrome. *Int. J. Dermatol.* 38, 656–663. doi: 10.1046/j.1365-4362.1999.00750.x

Duncan, J. S., and Fritzsch, B. (2013). Continued expression of GATA3 is necessary for cochlear neurosensory development. *PLoS One* 8:e62046. doi: 10.1371/journal.pone.0062046

Dutton, K., Abbas, L., Spencer, J., Brannon, C., Mowbray, C., Nikaido, M., et al. (2009). A zebrafish model for Waardenburg syndrome type IV reveals diverse roles for Sox10 in the otic vesicle. *Dis. Model Mech.* 2, 68–83. doi: 10.1242/dmm.001164

Elmaleh-Bergès, M., Baumann, C., Noël-Pétroff, N., Sekkal, A., Couloigner, V., Devriendt, K., et al. (2013). Spectrum of temporal bone abnormalities in patients with Waardenburg syndrome and SOX10 mutations. *AJNR Am. J. Neuroradiol.* 34, 1257–1263. doi: 10.3174/ajnr.A3367

Fang, Q., Zhang, Y., Da, P., Shao, B., Pan, H., He, Z., et al. (2019). Deletion of Limk1 and Limk2 in mice does not alter cochlear development or auditory function. *Sci. Rep.* 9:3357. doi: 10.1038/s41598-019-39769-z

Freter, S., Fleenor, S. J., Freter, R., Liu, K. J., and Begbie, J. (2013). Cranial neural crest cells form corridors prefiguring sensory neuroblast migration. *Development* 140, 3595–3600. doi: 10.1242/dev.091033

Freyer, L., Aggarwal, V., and Morrow, B. E. (2011). Dual embryonic origin of the mammalian otic vesicle forming the inner ear. *Development* 138, 5403–5414. doi: 10.1242/dev.069849

Fu, X., An, Y., Wang, H., Li, P., Lin, J., Yuan, J., et al. (2021). Deficiency of Klc2 induces low-frequency sensorineural hearing loss in C57BL/6 J mice and human. *Mol. Neurobiol.* doi: 10.1007/s12035-021-02422-w [Online ahead of print].

Gámez, B., Rodriguez-Carballo, E., and Ventura, F. (2013). BMP signaling in telencephalic neural cell specification and maturation. *Front. Cell Neurosci.* 7:87. doi: 10.3389/fncel.2013.00087

Gao, S., Cheng, C., Wang, M., Jiang, P., Zhang, L., Wang, Y., et al. (2019). Blebbistatin Inhibits neomycin-induced apoptosis in hair cell-like HEI-OC-1 cells and in cochlear hair cells. *Front. Cell Neurosci.* 13:590. doi: 10.3389/fncel.2019.00590

George, K. M., Leonard, M. W., Roth, M. E., Lieuw, K. H., Kioussis, D., Grosveld, F., et al. (1994). Embryonic expression and cloning of the murine GATA-3 gene. *Development* 120, 2673–2686.

Guo, R., Li, J., Chen, C., Xiao, M., Liao, M., Hu, Y., et al. (2021). Biomimetic 3D bacterial cellulose-graphene foam hybrid scaffold regulates neural stem cell proliferation and differentiation. *Colloids Surf. B. Biointerf.* 200, 111590. doi: 10.1016/j.colsurfb.2021.111590

Guo, R., Ma, X., Liao, M., Liu, Y., Hu, Y., Qian, X., et al. (2019). Development and application of cochlear implant-based electric-acoustic stimulation of spiral ganglion neurons. *ACS Biomater. Sci. Eng.* 5, 6735–6741. doi: 10.1021/acsbiomaterials.9b01263

Guo, R., Xiao, M., Zhao, W., Zhou, S., Hu, Y., Liao, M., et al. (2020). 2D Ti(3)C(2)T(x)MXene couples electrical stimulation to promote proliferation and neural differentiation of neural stem cells. *Acta Biomater.* doi: 10.1016/j.actbio.2020.12.035 [Online ahead of print].

Guo, R., Zhang, S., Xiao, M., Qian, F., He, Z., Li, D., et al. (2016). Accelerating bioelectric functional development of neural stem cells by graphene coupling: Implications for neural interfacing with conductive materials. *Biomaterials* 106, 193–204. doi: 10.1016/j.biomaterials.2016.08.019

Haldin, C. E., and LaBonne, C. (2010). SoxE factors as multifunctional neural crest regulatory factors. *Int. J. Biochem. Cell Biol.* 42, 441–444. doi: 10.1016/j.biocel.2009.11.014

Hammond, K. L., Loynes, H. E., Mowbray, C., Runke, G., Hammerschmidt, M., Mullins, M. C., et al. (2009). A late role for bmp2b in the morphogenesis of semicircular canal ducts in the zebrafish inner ear. *PLoS One* 4:e4368. doi: 10.1371/journal.pone.0004368

Hao, Q. Q., Li, L., Chen, W., Jiang, Q. Q., Ji, F., Sun, W., et al. (2018). Key genes and pathways associated with inner ear malformation in SOX10? (p.R109W) mutation pigs. *Front. Mol. Neurosci.* 11:181. doi: 10.3389/fnmol.2018.00181

Harris, M. L., Baxter, L. L., Loftus, S. K., and Pavan, W. J. (2010). Sox proteins in melanocyte development and melanoma. *Pigment Cell Melanoma Res.* 23, 496–513. doi: 10.1111/j.1755-148X.2010.00711.x

Haseeb, A., and Lefebvre, V. (2019). The SOXE transcription factors-SOX8, SOX9 and SOX10-share a bi-partite transactivation mechanism. *Nucleic Acids Res.* 47, 6917–6931. doi: 10.1093/nar/gkz523

He, Z., Guo, L., Shu, Y., Fang, Q., Zhou, H., Liu, Y., et al. (2017). Autophagy protects auditory hair cells against neomycin-induced damage. *Autophagy* 13, 1884–1904. doi: 10.1080/15548627.2017.1359449

He, Z. H., Li, M., Fang, Q. J., Liao, F. L., Zou, S. Y., Wu, X., et al. (2021). FOXG1 promotes aging inner ear hair cell survival through activation of the autophagy pathway. *Autophagy* 1–22. doi: 10.1080/15548627.2021.1916194 [Online ahead of print].

Huang, S., Song, J., He, C., Cai, X., Yuan, K., Mei, L., et al. (2021). Genetic insights, disease mechanisms, and biological therapeutics for Waardenburg syndrome. *Gene Ther.* doi: 10.1038/s41434-021-00240-2 [Online ahead of print].

Huang, S., Wang, Y., Luo, L., Li, X., Jin, X., Li, S., et al. (2019). BMP2 is related to hirschsprung's disease and required for enteric nervous system development. *Front. Cell Neurosci.* 13:523. doi: 10.3389/fncel.2019.00523

Huang da, W., Sherman, B. T., and Lempicki, R. A. (2009). Systematic and integrative analysis of large gene lists using DAVID bioinformatics resources. *Nat. Protoc.* 4, 44–57. doi: 10.1038/nprot.2008.211

Hwang, C. H., Guo, D., Harris, M. A., Howard, O., Mishina, Y., Gan, L., et al. (2010). Role of bone morphogenetic proteins on cochlear hair cell formation: analyses of Noggin and Bmp2 mutant mice. *Dev. Dyn.* 239, 505–513. doi: 10.1002/dvdy.22200

Hwang, C. H., Keller, J., Renner, C., Ohta, S., and Wu, D. K. (2019). Genetic interactions support an inhibitory relationship between bone morphogenetic protein 2 and netrin 1 during semicircular canal formation. *Development* 146, dev174748. doi: 10.1242/dev.174748

Inoue, K., Khajavi, M., Ohyama, T., Hirabayashi, S., Wilson, J., Reggin, J. D., et al. (2004). Molecular mechanism for distinct neurological phenotypes conveyed by allelic truncating mutations. *Nat. Genet.* 36, 361–369. doi: 10.1038/ng1322

Jaks, V., Barker, N., Kasper, M., van Es, J. H., Snippert, H. J., Clevers, H., et al. (2008). Lgr5 marks cycling, yet long-lived, hair follicle stem cells. *Nat. Genet.* 40, 1291–1299. doi: 10.1038/ng.239

Jiang, P., Zhang, S., Cheng, C., Gao, S., Tang, M., Lu, L., et al. (2020). The Roles of Exosomes in Visual and Auditory Systems. *Front. Bioeng. Biotechnol.* 8:525. doi: 10.3389/fbioe.2020.00525

Karis, A., Pata, I., van Doorninck, J. H., Grosveld, F., de Zeeuw, C. I., de Caprona, D., et al. (2001). Transcription factor GATA-3 alters pathway selection of olivocochlear neurons and affects morphogenesis of the ear. *J. Comp. Neurol.* 429, 615–630. doi: 10.1002/1096-9861(20010122)429:4<615::aid-cne8>3.0.co;2-f

Karpinski, B. A., Bryan, C. A., Paronett, E. M., Baker, J. L., Fernandez, A., Horvath, A., et al. (2016). A cellular and molecular mosaic establishes growth and differentiation states for cranial sensory neurons. *Dev. Biol.* 415, 228–241. doi: 10.1016/j.ydbio.2016.03.015

Kim, D., Langmead, B., and Salzberg, S. L. (2015). HISAT: a fast spliced aligner with low memory requirements. *Nat. Methods* 12, 357–360. doi: 10.1038/nmeth.3317

Kim, H. J., Gratton, M. A., Lee, J. H., Perez Flores, M. C., Wang, W., Doyle, K. J., et al. (2013). Precise toxigenic ablation of intermediate cells abolishes the "battery" of the cochlear duct. *J. Neurosci.* 33, 14601–14606. doi: 10.1523/jneurosci.2147-13.2013

Knecht, A. K., and Bronner-Fraser, M. (2002). Induction of the neural crest: a multigene process. *Nat. Rev. Genet.* 3, 453–461. doi: 10.1038/nrg819

Lakshmanan, G., Lieuw, K. H., Lim, K. C., Gu, Y., Grosveld, F., Engel, J. D., et al. (1999). Localization of distant urogenital system-, central nervous system-, and endocardium-specific transcriptional regulatory elements in the GATA-3 locus. *Mol. Cell Biol.* 19, 1558–1568. doi: 10.1128/mcb.19.2.1558

Lawoko-Kerali, G., Rivolta, M., and Holley, M. (2002). Expression of the transcription factors GATA3 and Pax2 during development of the mammalian inner ear. *J. Comp. Neurol.* 442, 378–391. doi: 10.1002/cne.10088

Li, A., You, D., Li, W., Cui, Y., He, Y., Li, W., et al. (2018). Novel compounds protect auditory hair cells against gentamycin-induced apoptosis by maintaining the expression level of H3K4me2. *Drug Deliv.* 25, 1033–1043. doi: 10.1080/10717544.2018.1461277

Li, B., Kuriyama, S., Moreno, M., and Mayor, R. (2009). The posteriorizing gene Gbx2 is a direct target of Wnt signalling and the earliest factor in neural crest induction. *Development* 136, 3267–3278. doi: 10.1242/dev.036954

Li, W., Mei, L., Chen, H., Cai, X., Liu, Y., Men, M., et al. (2019). New genotypes and phenotypes in patients with 3 subtypes of waardenburg syndrome identified by diagnostic next-generation sequencing. *Neural. Plast* 2019:7143458. doi: 10.1155/2019/7143458

Liao, Y., Smyth, G. K., and Shi, W. (2014). featureCounts: an efficient general purpose program for assigning sequence reads to genomic features. *Bioinformatics* 30, 923–930. doi: 10.1093/bioinformatics/btt656

Lieuw, K. H., Li, G., Zhou, Y., Grosveld, F., and Engel, J. D. (1997). Temporal and spatial control of murine GATA-3 transcription by promoter-proximal regulatory elements. *Dev. Biol.* 188, 1–16. doi: 10.1006/dbio.1997.8575

Lin, Z., Cantos, R., Patente, M., and Wu, D. K. (2005). Gbx2 is required for the morphogenesis of the mouse inner ear: a downstream candidate of hindbrain signaling. *Development* 132, 2309–2318. doi: 10.1242/dev.01804

Liu, W., Xu, L., Wang, X., Zhang, D., Sun, G., Wang, M., et al. (2021). PRDX1 activates autophagy via the PTEN-AKT signaling pathway to protect against cisplatin-induced spiral ganglion neuron damage. *Autophagy* 1–23. doi: 10.1080/15548627.2021.1905466 [Online ahead of print].

Liu, W., Xu, X., Fan, Z., Sun, G., Han, Y., Zhang, D., et al. (2019). Wnt signaling activates TP53-induced glycolysis and apoptosis regulator and protects against cisplatin-induced spiral ganglion neuron damage in the mouse cochlea. *Antioxid Redox Signal.* 30, 1389–1410. doi: 10.1089/ars.2017.7288

Liu, X. Z., Newton, V. E., and Read, A. P. (1995). Waardenburg syndrome type II: phenotypic findings and diagnostic criteria. *Am. J. Med. Genet.* 55, 95–100. doi: 10.1002/ajmg.1320550123

Liu, Y., Qi, J., Chen, X., Tang, M., Chu, C., Zhu, W., et al. (2019). Critical role of spectrin in hearing development and deafness. *Sci. Adv.* 5:eaav7803. doi: 10.1126/sciadv.aav7803

Locher, H., de Groot, J. C., van Iperen, L., Huisman, M. A., Frijns, J. H., and Chuva de Sousa Lopes, S. M. (2015). Development of the stria vascularis and potassium regulation in the human fetal cochlea: insights into hereditary sensorineural hearing loss. *Dev. Neurobiol.* 75, 1219–1240. doi: 10.1002/dneu.22279

Lu, X., Sun, S., Qi, J., Li, W., Liu, L., Zhang, Y., et al. (2017). Bmi1 regulates the proliferation of cochlear supporting cells via the canonical wnt signaling pathway. *Mol. Neurobiol.* 54, 1326–1339. doi: 10.1007/s12035-016-9686-8

Lv, J., Fu, X., Li, Y., Hong, G., Li, P., Lin, J., et al. (2021). Deletion of Kcnj16 in mice does not alter auditory function. *Front. Cell Dev. Biol.* 9:630361. doi: 10.3389/fcell.2021.630361

Mao, Y., Reiprich, S., Wegner, M., and Fritzsch, B. (2014). Targeted deletion of Sox10 by Wnt1-cre defects neuronal migration and projection in the mouse inner ear. *PLoS One* 9:e94580. doi: 10.1371/journal.pone.0094580

Martins, F. T. A., Ramos, B. D., and Sartorato, E. L. (2018). A rare case of deafness and renal abnormalities in HDR syndrome caused by a de novo mutation in the GATA3 gene. *Genet. Mol. Biol.* 41, 794–798. doi: 10.1590/1678-4685-gmb-2017-0194

Milo, M., Cacciabue-Rivolta, D., Kneebone, A., Van Doorninck, H., Johnson, C., Lawoko-Kerali, G., et al. (2009). Genomic analysis of the function of the transcription factor gata3 during development of the mammalian inner ear. *PLoS One* 4:e7144. doi: 10.1371/journal.pone.0007144

Miyazaki, H., Kobayashi, T., Nakamura, H., and Funahashi, J. (2006). Role of Gbx2 and Otx2 in the formation of cochlear ganglion and endolymphatic duct. *Dev. Growth Differ.* 48, 429–438. doi: 10.1111/j.1440-169X.2006.00879.x

Mollaaghababa, R., and Pavan, W. J. (2003). The importance of having your SOX on: role of SOX10 in the development of neural crest-derived melanocytes and glia. *Oncogene* 22, 3024–3034. doi: 10.1038/sj.onc.1206442

Moriguchi, T., Hoshino, T., Rao, A., Yu, L., Takai, J., Uemura, S., et al. (2018). A gata3 3' Distal otic vesicle enhancer directs inner ear-specific gata3 expression. *Mol. Cell Biol.* 38:e00302-18. doi: 10.1128/mcb.00302-18

Nayak, C. S., and Isaacson, G. (2003). Worldwide distribution of Waardenburg syndrome. *Ann. Otol. Rhinol. Laryngol.* 112(9 Pt. 1), 817–820. doi: 10.1177/000348940311200913

O'Donnell, L., Owens, D., McGee, C., Devery, R., Hession, P., Collins, P., et al. (1988). Effects of catecholamines on serum lipoproteins of normally fed and cholesterol-fed rabbits. *Metabolism* 37, 910–915. doi: 10.1016/0026-0495(88)90145-x

Pingault, V., Bodereau, V., Baral, V., Marcos, S., Watanabe, Y., Chaoui, A., et al. (2013). Loss-of-function mutations in SOX10 cause Kallmann syndrome with deafness. *Am. J. Hum. Genet.* 92, 707–724. doi: 10.1016/j.ajhg.2013.03.024

Pingault, V., Ente, D., Dastot-Le Moal, F., Goossens, M., Marlin, S., and Bondurand, N. (2010). Review and update of mutations causing Waardenburg syndrome. *Hum. Mutat.* 31, 391–406. doi: 10.1002/humu.21211

Pingault, V., Guiochon-Mantel, A., Bondurand, N., Faure, C., Lacroix, C., Lyonnet, S., et al. (2000). Peripheral neuropathy with hypomyelination, chronic intestinal pseudo-obstruction and deafness: a developmental "neural crest syndrome" related to a SOX10 mutation. *Ann. Neurol.* 48, 671–676.

Qi, J., Liu, Y., Chu, C., Chen, X., Zhu, W., Shu, Y., et al. (2019). A cytoskeleton structure revealed by super-resolution fluorescence imaging in inner ear hair cells. *Cell Discov.* 5:12. doi: 10.1038/s41421-018-0076-4

Qi, J., Zhang, L., Tan, F., Liu, Y., Chu, C., Zhu, W., et al. (2020). Espin distribution as revealed by super-resolution microscopy of stereocilia. *Am. J. Transl. Res.* 12, 130–141.

Qian, F., Wang, X., Yin, Z., Xie, G., Yuan, H., Liu, D., et al. (2020). The slc4a2b gene is required for hair cell development in zebrafish. *Aging* 12, 18804–18821. doi: 10.18632/aging.103840

Rivolta, M. N., and Holley, M. C. (1998). GATA3 is downregulated during hair cell differentiation in the mouse cochlea. *J. Neurocytol.* 27, 637–647. doi: 10.1023/a:1006951813063

Roccio, M., Perny, M., Ealy, M., Widmer, H. R., Heller, S., and Senn, P. (2018). Molecular characterization and prospective isolation of human fetal cochlear hair cell progenitors. *Nat. Commun.* 9:4027. doi: 10.1038/s41467-018-06334-7

Roeseler, D. A., Strader, L., Anderson, M. J., and Waters, S. T. (2020). Gbx2 is required for the migration and survival of a subpopulation of trigeminal cranial neural crest cells. *J. Dev. Biol.* 8:33. doi: 10.3390/jdb8040033

Scheithauer, W., Moyer, M. P., Clark, G. M., and Von Hoff, D. D. (1988). Application of a new preclinical drug screening system for cancer of the large bowel. *Cancer Chemother. Pharmacol.* 21, 31–34. doi: 10.1007/bf00262734

Schlange, T., Andrée, B., Arnold, H. H., and Brand, T. (2000). BMP2 is required for early heart development during a distinct time period. *Mech. Dev.* 91, 259–270. doi: 10.1016/s0925-4773(99)00311-1

Schock, E. N., and LaBonne, C. (2020). Sorting sox: diverse roles for sox transcription factors during neural crest and craniofacial development. *Front. Physiol.* 11:606889. doi: 10.3389/fphys.2020.606889

Song, J., Feng, Y., Acke, F. R., Coucke, P., Vleminckx, K., and Dhooge, I. J. (2016). Hearing loss in Waardenburg syndrome: a systematic review. *Clin. Genet.* 89, 416–425. doi: 10.1111/cge.12631

Southard-Smith, E. M., Kos, L., and Pavan, W. J. (1998). Sox10 mutation disrupts neural crest development in Dom Hirschsprung mouse model. *Nat. Genet.* 18, 60–64. doi: 10.1038/ng0198-60

Steventon, B., Mayor, R., and Streit, A. (2012). Mutual repression between Gbx2 and Otx2 in sensory placodes reveals a general mechanism for ectodermal patterning. *Dev. Biol.* 367, 55–65. doi: 10.1016/j.ydbio.2012.04.025

Steventon, B., Mayor, R., and Streit, A. (2016). Directional cell movements downstream of Gbx2 and Otx2 control the assembly of sensory placodes. *Biol. Open* 5, 1620–1624. doi: 10.1242/bio.020966

Südbeck, P., and Scherer, G. (1997). Two independent nuclear localization signals are present in the DNA-binding high-mobility group domains of SRY and SOX9. *J. Biol. Chem.* 272, 27848–27852. doi: 10.1074/jbc.272.44.27848

Sun, G., Liu, W., Fan, Z., Zhang, D., Han, Y., Xu, L., et al. (2016). The three-dimensional culture system with matrigel and neurotrophic factors preserves the structure and function of spiral ganglion neuron in vitro. *Neural. Plast.* 2016:4280407. doi: 10.1155/2016/4280407

Sun, S., Sun, M., Zhang, Y., Cheng, C., Waqas, M., Yu, H., et al. (2014). In vivo overexpression of X-linked inhibitor of apoptosis protein protects against neomycin-induced hair cell loss in the apical turn of the cochlea during the ototoxic-sensitive period. *Front. Cell Neurosci.* 8:248. doi: 10.3389/fncel.2014.00248

Szklarczyk, D., Gable, A. L., Lyon, D., Junge, A., Wyder, S., Huerta-Cepas, J., et al. (2019). STRING v11: protein-protein association networks with increased coverage, supporting functional discovery in genome-wide experimental datasets. *Nucleic Acids Res.* 47, D607–D613. doi: 10.1093/nar/gky1131

Tachibana, M., Kobayashi, Y., and Matsushima, Y. (2003). Mouse models for four types of Waardenburg syndrome. *Pigment Cell Res.* 16, 448–454. doi: 10.1034/j.1600-0749.2003.00066.x

Takahashi, K., Tanabe, K., Ohnuki, M., Narita, M., Ichisaka, T., Tomoda, K., et al. (2007). Induction of pluripotent stem cells from adult human fibroblasts by defined factors. *Cell* 131, 861–872. doi: 10.1016/j.cell.2007.11.019

Takahashi, K., and Yamanaka, S. (2006). Induction of pluripotent stem cells from mouse embryonic and adult fibroblast cultures by defined factors. *Cell* 126, 663–676. doi: 10.1016/j.cell.2006.07.024

Tan, F., Chu, C., Qi, J., Li, W., You, D., Li, K., et al. (2019). AAV-ie enables safe and efficient gene transfer to inner ear cells. *Nat. Commun.* 10:3733. doi: 10.1038/s41467-019-11687-8

Tang, P. C., Hashino, E., and Nelson, R. F. (2020). Progress in modeling and targeting inner ear disorders with pluripotent stem cells. *Stem Cell Rep.* 14, 996–1008. doi: 10.1016/j.stemcr.2020.04.008

Van Esch, H., Groenen, P., Nesbit, M. A., Schuffenhauer, S., Lichtner, P., Vanderlinden, G., et al. (2000). GATA3 haplo-insufficiency causes human HDR syndrome. *Nature* 406, 419–422. doi: 10.1038/35019088

Waardenburg, P. J. (1951). A new syndrome combining developmental anomalies of the eyelids, eyebrows and nose root with pigmentary defects of the iris and head hair and with congenital deafness. *Am. J. Hum. Genet.* 3, 195–253.

Wakaoka, T., Motohashi, T., Hayashi, H., Kuze, B., Aoki, M., Mizuta, K., et al. (2013). Tracing Sox10-expressing cells elucidates the dynamic development of the mouse inner ear. *Hear. Res.* 302, 17–25. doi: 10.1016/j.heares.2013.05.003

Wang, T., Chai, R., Kim, G. S., Pham, N., Jansson, L., Nguyen, D. H., et al. (2015). Lgr5+ cells regenerate hair cells via proliferation and direct transdifferentiation in damaged neonatal mouse utricle. *Nat. Commun.* 6:6613. doi: 10.1038/ncomms7613

Wang, Y., Li, J., Yao, X., Li, W., Du, H., Tang, M., et al. (2017). Loss of CIB2 causes profound hearing loss and abolishes mechanoelectrical transduction in mice. *Front. Mol. Neurosci.* 10:401. doi: 10.3389/fnmol.2017.00401

Xiao, B., Zhang, W., Kuang, Z., Lu, J., Li, W., Deng, C., et al. (2019). SOX9 promotes nasopharyngeal carcinoma cell proliferation, migration and invasion through BMP2 and mTOR signaling. *Gene* 715:144017. doi: 10.1016/j.gene.2019.144017

Xu, G. Y., Hao, Q. Q., Zhong, L. L., Ren, W., Yan, Y., Liu, R. Y., et al. (2016). [SOX10 mutation is relevant to inner ear malformation in patients with Waardenburg syndrome]. *Zhonghua Er Bi Yan Hou Tou Jing Wai Ke Za Zhi* 51, 832–837. doi: 10.3760/cma.j.issn.1673-0860.2016.11.006

Yan, W., Liu, W., Qi, J., Fang, Q., Fan, Z., Sun, G., et al. (2018). A three-dimensional culture system with matrigel promotes purified spiral ganglion neuron survival and function in vitro. *Mol. Neurobiol.* 55, 2070–2084. doi: 10.1007/s12035-017-0471-0

Yu, X., Liu, W., Fan, Z., Qian, F., Zhang, D., Han, Y., et al. (2017). c-Myb knockdown increases the neomycin-induced damage to hair-cell-like HEI-OC1 cells in vitro. *Sci. Rep.* 7:41094. doi: 10.1038/srep41094

Zhang, H., Chen, H., Luo, H., An, J., Sun, L., Mei, L., et al. (2012). Functional analysis of Waardenburg syndrome-associated PAX3 and SOX10 mutations: report of a dominant-negative SOX10 mutation in Waardenburg syndrome type II. *Hum. Genet.* 131, 491–503. doi: 10.1007/s00439-011-1098-2

Zhang, S., Dong, Y., Qiang, R., Zhang, Y., Zhang, X., Chen, Y., et al. (2021). Characterization of strip1 expression in mouse cochlear hair cells. *Front. Genet.* 12:625867. doi: 10.3389/fgene.2021.625867

Zhang, S., Liu, D., Dong, Y., Zhang, Z., Zhang, Y., Zhou, H., et al. (2019). Frizzled-9+ supporting cells are progenitors for the generation of hair cells in the postnatal mouse cochlea. *Front. Mol. Neurosci.* 12:184. doi: 10.3389/fnmol.2019.00184

Zhang, S., Qiang, R., Dong, Y., Zhang, Y., Chen, Y., Zhou, H., et al. (2020a). Hair cell regeneration from inner ear progenitors in the mammalian cochlea. *Am. J. Stem Cells* 9, 25–35.

Zhang, S., Zhang, Y., Dong, Y., Guo, L., Zhang, Z., Shao, B., et al. (2020b). Knockdown of Foxg1 in supporting cells increases the trans-differentiation of supporting cells into hair cells in the neonatal mouse cochlea. *Cell Mol. Life Sci.* 77, 1401–1419. doi: 10.1007/s00018-019-03291-2

Zhang, Y., Li, W., He, Z., Wang, Y., Shao, B., Cheng, C., et al. (2019). Pre-treatment with fasudil prevents neomycin-induced hair cell damage by reducing the accumulation of reactive oxygen species. *Front. Mol. Neurosci.* 12:264. doi: 10.3389/fnmol.2019.00264

Zhang, Y., Zhang, S., Zhang, Z., Dong, Y., Ma, X., Qiang, R., et al. (2020). Knockdown of Foxg1 in Sox9+ supporting cells increases the trans-differentiation of supporting cells into hair cells in the neonatal mouse utricle. *Aging* 12, 19834–19851. doi: 10.18632/aging.104009

Zhao, J., Tang, M., Cao, J., Ye, D., Guo, X., Xi, J., et al. (2019). Structurally tunable reduced graphene oxide substrate maintains mouse embryonic stem cell pluripotency. *Adv. Sci.* 6:1802136. doi: 10.1002/advs.201802136

Zhong, Z., Fu, X., Li, H., Chen, J., Wang, M., Gao, S., et al. (2020). Citicoline protects auditory hair cells against neomycin-induced damage. *Front. Cell. Dev. Biol.* 8:712. doi: 10.3389/fcell.2020.00712

Zhou, G., Soufan, O., Ewald, J., Hancock, R. E. W., Basu, N., and Xia, J. (2019). NetworkAnalyst 3.0: a visual analytics platform for comprehensive gene expression profiling and meta-analysis. *Nucleic Acids Res.* 47, W234–W241. doi: 10.1093/nar/gkz240

Zhou, H., Qian, X., Xu, N., Zhang, S., Zhu, G., Zhang, Y., et al. (2020). Disruption of Atg7-dependent autophagy causes electromotility disturbances, outer hair cell loss, and deafness in mice. *Cell Death Dis.* 11:913. doi: 10.1038/s41419-020-03110-8

Zhu, C., Cheng, C., Wang, Y., Muhammad, W., Liu, S., Zhu, W., et al. (2018). Loss of ARHGEF6 causes hair cell stereocilia deficits and hearing loss in mice. *Front. Mol. Neurosci.* 11:362. doi: 10.3389/fnmol.2018.00362

Tlr2/4 Double Knockout Attenuates the Degeneration of Primary Auditory Neurons: Potential Mechanisms From Transcriptomic Perspectives

Quan Wang[1,2†], Yilin Shen[1,2†], Yi Pan[1,2†], Kaili Chen[1,2], Rui Ding[1,2], Tianyuan Zou[1,2], Andi Zhang[1,2], Dongye Guo[1,2], Peilin Ji[1,2], Cui Fan[1,2], Ling Mei[2], Haixia Hu[1,2], Bin Ye[1,2]* and Mingliang Xiang[1,2]*

[1] Department of Otolaryngology and Head and Neck Surgery, Ruijin Hospital, Shanghai Jiao Tong University School of Medicine, Shanghai, China,
[2] Ear Institute, Shanghai Jiao Tong University School of Medicine, Shanghai, China

*Correspondence:
Mingliang Xiang
mingliangxiang@163.com
Bin Ye
aydyebin@126.com

†These authors have contributed equally to this work

The transcriptomic landscape of mice with primary auditory neurons degeneration (PAND) indicates key pathways in its pathogenesis, including complement cascades, immune responses, tumor necrosis factor (TNF) signaling pathway, and cytokine-cytokine receptor interaction. Toll-like receptors (TLRs) are important immune and inflammatory molecules that have been shown to disrupt the disease network of PAND. In a PAND model involving administration of kanamycin combined with furosemide to destroy cochlear hair cells, Tlr 2/4 double knockout (DKO) mice had auditory preservation advantages, which were mainly manifested at 4–16 kHz. DKO mice and wild type (WT) mice had completely damaged cochlear hair cells on the 30th day, but the density of spiral ganglion neurons (SGN) in the Rosenthal canal was significantly higher in the DKO group than in the WT group. The results of immunohistochemistry for p38 and p65 showed that the attenuation of SGN degeneration in DKO mice may not be mediated by canonical Tlr signaling pathways. The SGN transcriptome of DKO and WT mice indicated that there was an inverted gene set enrichment relationship between their different transcriptomes and the SGN degeneration transcriptome, which is consistent with the morphology results. Core module analysis suggested that DKO mice may modulate SGN degeneration by activating two clusters, and the involved molecules include EGF, STAT3, CALB2, LOX, SNAP25, CAV2, SDC4, MYL1, NCS1, PVALB, TPM4, and TMOD4.

Keywords: hearing loss, spiral ganglion neurons, degeneration, Tlr2/4, transcriptome analysis

INTRODUCTION

Sensorineural hearing loss (SNHL), the most common sensory deficit in the world, affects nearly 300 million individuals and costs 980 billion USD annually. SNHL mainly arises from the damage or death of auditory hair cells (Liu et al., 2016; Cheng et al., 2019; Gao et al., 2019; Han et al., 2020; Zhang S. et al., 2020, p. 1; Zhang Y. et al., 2020) and spiral ganglion neurons (SGN) (Guo et al., 2016, 2019, 2020; Liu W. et al., 2019; Ding et al., 2020; Liu et al., 2021; Yuan T. F. et al., 2021). These cells can be damaged by environmental insult (such as overexposure to loud sounds or exposure to aminoglycoside antibiotics or chemotherapeutics) (He et al., 2017, 2020, 2021; Qi et al., 2019; Jiang et al., 2020; Zhong et al., 2020; Zhou et al., 2020) or by genetic factors (Wang et al., 2017; Liu Y. et al., 2019; Qi et al., 2020, p. 4; Qian et al., 2020; Cheng et al., 2021; Fu et al., 2021; Zhang et al., 2021). As these mature cells lack the capacity for self-repair, the damage is permanent (Géléoc and Holt, 2014; Cheng et al., 2019; Tan et al., 2019; Zhang S. et al., 2020, p. 1; Chen et al., 2021).

Researchers have confirmed that many environmental insults immediately and directly damage hair cells, but the resulting SGN degeneration is chronic because of a lack of neurotrophic factors and peripheral stimuli (Kujawa and Liberman, 2009; Makary et al., 2011; Wu et al., 2021). The degeneration of the SGN leads to the loss and/or distortion of auditory information in the brain. Even as little as 10% of neural tissue degeneration can lead to a disproportionate change in the stimulation profile of the auditory nerve (Sriperumbudur et al., 2020). Spiral ganglion neurons would mainly have Ic subtype loss if the loss of peripheral stimulus occurs, which is similar to SGN aging (Shrestha et al., 2018). The degeneration of SGNs could induce distinct forms of plasticity in cortical excitatory and inhibitory neurons that culminate in net hyperactivity, increased neural gain, and reduce the adaptation to background noise (Resnik and Polley, 2021). On the other hand, once SGN degeneration occurs, cochlear implants will inevitably have poor performance. Histology of 12 temporal bones from 6 subjects indicated that higher residual SGNs could predict better performance after implantation in a given patient (Riss et al., 2008; Cusumano et al., 2017).

To elucidate the mechanism of SGN degeneration, a mouse model of rapid hair cell ablation with a single dose injection of kanamycin sulfate and furosemide (Taylor et al., 2008; Hu et al., 2017, p. 3; Ye et al., 2019), has frequently been used. In this SGN degeneration model, a single dose injection of kanamycin sulfate and furosemide immediately damaged hair cells but not SGNs (Gao et al., 2017). As auditory epithelia ablated, SGN, lacking neurotrophic factors and stimulus, will degenerate with increased lipofuscin area, damaged autophagic flux, and reduced density (Hu et al., 2017; Ye et al., 2019).

Tlr polymorphisms were correlated with hearing preservation in bacterial meningitis survivors (van Well et al., 2012). Koo et al. (2015) assumed that this kind of hearing preservation difference is associated with Tlr-mediated BLB permeability. Researchers have also found that Tlr4 knockout mice had better hearing function following noise trauma without affecting sensory cell viability under physiological conditions (Vethanayagam et al., 2016). De Paola et al. (2012) found that Tlr4 inhibition attenuates motor neuron degeneration both *in vitro* and *in vivo*. Tlr4 deficiency could also protect mice against ischemia and axotomy-induced retinal ganglion cells degeneration, and they assumed that better neuron preservation was associated with reduced parenchymal stress responses via the ERK, JNK, and P38 signaling pathways (Kilic et al., 2008). The innate immune response of the nerve microenvironment is involved in functional recovery during Wallerian degeneration, and Tlr2 and Tlr4 can regulate synaptic stability in the spinal cord after peripheral nerve injury (Freria et al., 2016). Researchers have found that systemic microbial TLR2 agonists could induce neuron degeneration in Alzheimer's disease mice and direct CNS delivery of a selective TLR2 antagonist blocked the neurotoxicity of systemically administered zymosan, indicating that CNS TLR2 mediates this neuron degeneration process (Lax et al., 2020). Previous studies have also demonstrated that administration of anti-TLR2 alleviated α-synuclein accumulation in neuronal, neuroinflammation, neurodegeneration, and behavioral deficits in an α-synuclein tg mouse model of PD/DLB and proposed TLR2 immunotherapy as a novel therapeutic strategy for neuron degeneration (Kim et al., 2018). These studies suggest that Tlr molecules may regulate the degeneration pathogenesis of auditory systems, especially spiral ganglion neurons.

Although SGN degeneration is characterized by increased lipofuscin area, damaged autophagic flux, and reduced density, a comprehensive understanding of the SGN degeneration transcriptome landscape is still lacking, and the role of molecules such as Tlr that may regulate the pathogenesis remain unknown. Here, we analyzed the transcriptome landscape of SGN degeneration and identified that Tlr2 and Tlr4 (Tlr2/4) might regulate the pathogenesis of degeneration. Based on these findings, we analyzed the role of Tlr2 and Tlr4 in SGN degeneration and found that genetic deletion of Tlr2/4 in combination attenuates SGN degeneration in mice without interfering with classic Tlr signaling pathways. Furthermore, we used transcriptome analysis to identify the key modules and pathways. Identification of these specific molecules and pathways could potently facilitate the protection of the auditory system.

MATERIALS AND METHODS

Animals

B6.B10ScN-Tlr4lps-del/JthJ and C.129(B6)-Tlr2^{tm1Kir}/J mice (The Jackson Laboratory, Bar Harbor, ME, United States) were used for Tlr2/4 double knockout. Only 8-week-old male mice without a history of ototoxic damage or noise exposure were used for model establishment. The animals were housed under a standard 12-h light/dark cycle and were allowed free access to water and a regular mouse diet. The cochleae of each animal were collected and assigned to different assays to reduce animal usage and maintain sufficient sample sizes. The following genotyping primers were used to examine the Tlr2 knockout allele: 5′-CTTCCTGAATTTGTCCAGTACA-3′; 5′-GGGCCAGCTCATTCCTCCCAC-3′; 5′-ACGAGCAAGATC AACAGGAGA-3′ (mutation allele 334 bp, WT allele 499 bp). The following genotyping primers were used to examine the Tlr4 knockout allele: 5′-GCAAGTTTCTATATGCATTCTC-3′; 5′-CCTCCATTTCCAATAGGTAG-3′; 5′-ATATGCATGATCAA CACCACAG-3′; 5′-TTTCCATTGCTGCCCTATAG-3′ (mutated allele 140 bp, WT allele 390 bp). The procedures were approved by the Ethics Committee of Xinhua Hospital, affiliated with Shanghai Jiao Tong University School of Medicine (Shanghai, China).

Spiral Ganglion Neurons Degeneration Model

Mice of the SGN degeneration group were subcutaneously injected with 1 g/kg kanamycin sulfate (Sigma-Aldrich, E004000), and intraperitoneally injected with 0.4 g/kg furosemide (Tianjin Pharmaceutical Group, H12020527; 10 mg/ml) after 30 min (Hu et al., 2017; Ye et al., 2019). Mice in the control group were simultaneously and intraperitoneally treated with equal doses of saline. The mice were sacrificed 7, 15, and 30 days after drug administration, and the temporal bones were removed and dissected in PBS at 4°C.

Measurement of Auditory Brainstem Response

The mice were anesthetized with a ketamine (0.1 mg/g)/xylazine (0.01 mg/g) mixture. Body temperature was maintained at 37°C with a warming blanket. An active needle electrode was placed in the midline of the vertex of the skull, a reference electrode at the mastoid areas, and a ground electrode in the low back area. The ABRs were provoked with tone bursts of 4, 8, 11, 16, 22, and 32 kHz, generated by a D/A converter (RP2.1; TDT) and relayed to an attenuator (PA5; TDT), an amplifier (SA1; TDT), and a magnetic speaker (MF1; TDT). Mouse auditory brainstem responses were filtered (100–3,000 Hz), amplified, and averaged using TDT hardware and software. Responses were recorded from 90 dB SPL to 10 dB below the threshold level in 5 dB descending steps. The ABR threshold was defined as the lowest intensity that reliably elicited a detectable response. The average ABR threshold shifts between wild-type and DKO mice were compared using two-way ANOVA with the two factors group × frequency. If significant group effects were identified, the Welch two-sample t-test was used to evaluate each frequency between the two groups.

Histopathological Analysis

The excised cochlea was immersed in 4% paraformaldehyde in phosphate-buffered saline solution for 12 h and decalcified in 10% EDTA for 5 days. Specimens were sliced into 4 μm sections, mounted onto silane-coated slides, stained, and observed under a light microscope. The evaluation of cochlear histology included the apical, middle, and basal regions in the Rosenthal canal and the organ of Corti. Every fifth modiolar section for a certain cochlea (four in total) was subjected to histopathological assessment. The same animals were used for the IHC staining. Primary antibodies against the following antigens were used: Caspase 3 (Abcam, ab44976), p65 (Abcam, ab32536), and p38 (Abcam, ab170099). For immunofluorescence staining, frozen sections were blocked with 10% donkey serum (Jackson, 017-000-121) and 0.5% Triton X-100 (Sigma-Aldrich, 9002-93-1) and then incubated with rabbit anti- Caspase 3 (Abcam, ab44976; 1:400) or p65 (Abcam, ab32536; 1:500) overnight at 4°C. After the sections were washed 3 times with PBS, donkey anti-rabbit Alexa Fluor 594 (Jackson, 711-585-152; 1: 500) were used to incubate samples at 37°C in the dark for 30 min. Finally, the sections were stained with DAPI (Beyotime, C1002; 1:2,000) for 5 min. For immunohistochemical staining, paraffin sections were heated at 67°C for 2 h and then deparaffinized in deparaffinized in xylene and rehydrated in alcohol. After the sections were washed 3 times with 0.1 M PBS, they were incubated with 3.0% H2O2 for 30 min at room temperature. The sections were then incubated with the primary p38 (Abcam, ab170099; 1:200) antibody overnight at 4°C. The secondary horseradish peroxidase-labeled goat anti-rabbit IgG antibody (Beyotime, A0208, 1:500) was added for 1 h, and finally, the sections were stained with 3,3N-diaminobenzidine (Beyotime, P0203). Unless otherwise stated, middle cochlear tissues (11–16 kHz region) were used for analyses.

High Throughput Sequencing

Total RNA from Cochlear modiolus tissues was extracted using the QIAGEN RNA Extraction Kit (Cat. No.74104). Agarose gels (1.5%) were used to detect RNA degradation and contamination. Illumina Hiseq 2,500 and Hiseq 4,000 were used to characterize the transcriptome landscape of SGN following the manufacturer's recommendations. The following procedures were performed using Hisat2 (version 2.1.0) to align the clean reads with the reference genome of mice (Kim et al., 2015) and StringTie (version 1.3.3b) to evaluate gene expression (Pertea et al., 2015).

Functional Annotation

Gene set enrichment analysis (GSEA) (Subramanian et al., 2005; Yu et al., 2012) was used to extract biological insight from RNA-seq data. GSEA aims to determine whether members of gene set S tend to occur in the extremes (top or bottom) of a given list from RNA-seq results. The enrichment score (ES) indicates the degree of a set S overrepresentation at the extremes of the gene ranked list L. ES was calculated as follows:

$$P_h(S, j) = \sum_{g_j \in S} \frac{|r_j|^w}{\sum_{g_j \in S} |r_j|^w} \quad (1)$$

$$P_m(S, j) = \sum_{g_j \in S} \frac{1}{(N-N_h)} \quad (2)$$

$$ES = max(|P_h - P_m|) \quad (3)$$

P-value was calculated by estimating the statistical significance of the ES by empirical phenotype-based permutation test procedures.

Terms used for functional annotation include Gene Ontology (Ashburner et al., 2000) and Kyoto Encyclopedia of Genes and Genomes (KEGG) (Kanehisa and Goto, 2000). Functional annotation of GO, including biological processes, cellular components, and molecular functions, and KEGG is a common omnibus to systematically interpret gene functions, facilitating an intensive understanding of genomic information and higher-order functional information.

Protein-Protein Interaction and Module Analysis

The construction of PPI networks imported the Search Tool for the Retrieval of Interacting Genes database (STRING)

(Szklarczyk et al., 2021), and was analyzed using Cytoscape (version 3.6.1) software (Shannon et al., 2003). STRING (version 11.0) covers 2,000 million interactions of 24.6 million proteins from 5,090 organisms. When fed with differentially expressed genes, STRING was able to identify the most significantly interactive associations, in which a criterion of a combined score > 0.4, was set as the significance level. Cytoscape plugin molecular complex detection (MCODE) can illustrate the core modules in the PPI network. The false degree cut-off, node score cut-off, haircut, false K-core, and maximum depth from seed were set at 2, 0.2, true, 2, and 100, respectively (Wang et al., 2018, 2020; Yan et al., 2019).

Statistical Analysis

Computations and data visualization were performed using R 4.0.2. Distribution of the data was assumed to be normal, but this was not formally tested. No statistical methods were used predetermine sample sizes, but our sample sizes are like those reported in our previous publications (Hu et al., 2017; Ye et al., 2019). Statistical differences in auditory physiology, SGN counts were analyzed using two-way ANOVA, followed by Welch t-test. All statistical analysis results were expressed as the mean ± standard error of the mean (SEM). Statistical significance was defined as $P < 0.05$.

RESULTS

Spiral Ganglion Neurons Degeneration Established by Cochlear Sensory Epithelial Ablation

SGN degeneration was successfully induced by the destruction of cochlear hair cells, which is consistent with the results of previous studies (Hu et al., 2017; Ye et al., 2019). Apoptotic activities in hair cells were significantly upregulated within the following 7 days, whereas no change was seen in SGNs (**Figure 1A**). The structure of the organ of Corti was almost completely collapsed and destroyed, and nearly no sensory epithelial cells remained in the middle turn on the 30th day after kanamycin and furosemide injection, while almost only a continuous layer of flattened cubic epithelial cells remained on the basilar membrane (**Figure 2B**). A time-series evaluation of SGN density was conducted on the 7th, 15th, and 30th day after kanamycin and furosemide injection (**Figure 1B**, auditory physiology data in **Supplementary Figure 1** and **Supplementary Table 1**). On the 30th day after kanamycin and furosemide injection, SGN density has significantly decreased in the apical, middle, and basal region of the cochlea (Welch two sample t-test, apical: $t = 8.4$, $P = 0.00009$; middle: $t = 7.53$, $P = 0.0005$; basal: $t = 10.33$, $P = 0.00003$). Thus, this time point was used to decipher the transcriptome changes during SGN degeneration.

Transcriptome Landscape of Spiral Ganglion Neurons Degeneration

We identified 674 upregulated and 390 downregulated genes in a background of 34147 non-significant genes during SGN degeneration (**Supplementary Table 1**). Among them, 972 differentially expressed genes (DEGs) had clear autosome positions, and chromosomes 1–19 had 60, 73, 52, 60, 76, 63, 60, 52, 58, 29, 65, 35, 30, 44, 52, 53, 42, 29, and 39 DEGs, of which the most significant ones were Atf3, Prrg4, Gatad2b, Sdr16c5, Ocm, Gm5737, Cep41, Car7, Mmp13, Tspan8, Ccl7, Serpina3n, Bmp6, Clu, Mal2, Gap43, Tnfrsf12a, Lox, and Ptar1 (**Figure 3A**). Among the differentially expressed genes, there were 76 genes encoding transcription factors (**Figure 3B**), of which the 10 most significant were Atf3, Stat3, Chgb, Irf6, Scrt1, Hipk2, Zfp871, Rxrg, Lmx1a, and Setbp1.

Gene set enrichment analysis (GSEA) showed that the top30 significantly enriched KEGG pathways included 20 upregulated pathways (**Figure 4A**), including complement and coagulation cascades, ubiquinone and other terpenoidquinone biosynthesis, linoleic acid metabolism, non-homologous end-joining, basal transcription factors, butanoate metabolism, inflammatory mediator regulation of TRP channels, phenylalanine metabolism, Hippo signaling pathway, endometrial cancer, EGFR tyrosine kinase inhibitor resistance, ErbB signaling pathway, cytokine-cytokine receptor interaction, hepatitis C, arachidonic acid metabolism, neuroactive ligand-receptor interaction, retinol metabolism, JAK-STAT signaling pathway, coronavirus disease (COVID-19), and TNF signaling pathway. The other 10 downregulated KEGG pathways (**Figure 4A**) were ribosome biogenesis, ribosome, oxidative phosphorylation, collecting duct acid secretion, glycosaminoglycan degradation, glycolysis/gluconeogenesis, regulation of lipolysis in adipocytes, DNA replication, cGMP-PKG signaling pathway, and mTOR signaling pathway. Autophagy and mTOR signaling pathways have been validated to regulate SGN degeneration in our previous work (Ye et al., 2019), which is consistent with the transcriptome results.

GO analysis showed that the dysregulated functions included positive regulation of peptidyl-serine phosphorylation of STAT protein, type I interferon receptor binding, T cell activation involved in immune response, B cell proliferation, natural killer cell activation involved in the immune response, membrane disruption, negative regulation of B cell apoptosis, and embryonic brain development (**Figure 4B**). The analysis of PPI interactions indicated six key modules (**Table 1**), and 10 molecules were the most significant, including COMP, COL1A1, STAT3, HAPLN1, HBEGF, CCL2, MMP13, SMAD4, CXCL1, and CTSK. We noticed that these enriched activities of immune responses, TNF signaling pathway, and cytokine-cytokine receptor interaction could be regulated by Tlr molecules (Peek et al., 2020). At the same time, Tlr2 and Tlr4 disrupted the SGN degeneration signaling network (**Figure 3C**). Based on these results, we hypothesized that Tlr might contribute to the regulation of SGN degeneration.

Tlr2/4 Double Knockout Mice Has Auditory Advantage in Spiral Ganglion Neurons Degeneration

Given that Tlr may play an important role in SGN degeneration, we established Tlr2 and Tlr4 knockout mice. We detected the

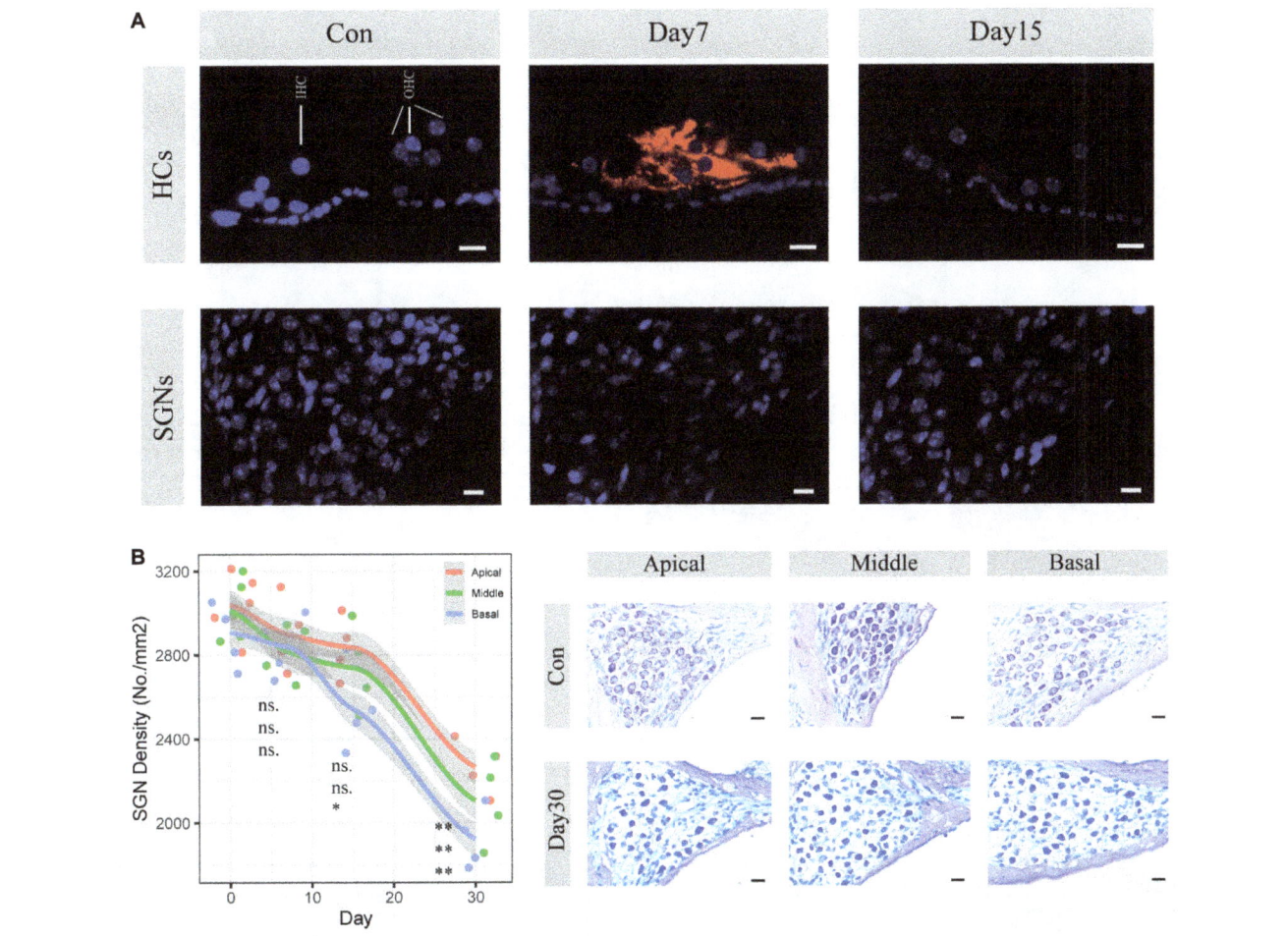

FIGURE 1 | SGN degeneration established by cochlear sensory epithelial ablation. **(A)** Representative images of CASP3 IF staining in hair cells and spiral ganglion areas. Hair cell apoptotic activities were significantly upregulated within 7 days but disappeared 15 days after injection of kanamycin and furosemide. There are no apoptosis activities seen in the SGN areas during the period. HCs: hair cells; SGNs: spiral ganglion neurons. Red: caspase3; Blue: DAPI. Scale bar: 10 μm. **(B)** SGN density evaluation 7, 15, and 30 days after the injection of kanamycin and furosemide. On the 30th day, SGN density significantly decreased at the apical, middle, and basal turn of the cochlea (apical: $N = 9$, $t = 8.14$, $P < 0.01$, middle: $N = 9$, $t = 7.53$, $P < 0.01$; basal: $N = 9$, $t = 10.33$, $P < 0.01$). Statistical significance of other time points was also denoted with the order of apical, middle and basal, respectively (ns: not significant; *$P < 0.05$; **$P < 0.01$.). Gray area indicated the standard error range calculated by loess method. Right panel shows the representative images of SGN before and 30 days after the injection of kanamycin and furosemide. Scale bar: 10 μm.

hearing threshold of Tlr2/4 DKO mice and wild-type littermates before and 30 days after SGN degeneration. The Tlr DKO group of mice treated with normal saline (NS) and the wild type (WT) mice maintained normal hearing thresholds (**Figure 2A**), and there was no significant difference in the hearing thresholds of the two groups of mice ($P = 0.748$, $F = 0.105$, two-way ANOVA). The Tlr DKO mice of the SGN degeneration group exhibited hearing threshold advantages ($P = 0.00446$, $F = 8.700$, two-way ANOVA) on the 30th day after kanamycin and furosemide injection, and the hearing preservation advantage was mainly manifested in 4–16 kHz (4 kHz, $t = -3.16$, $P = 0.012$; 8 kHz, $t = -3.12$, $P = 0.0012$; 11 kHz, $t = -2.51$, $P = 0.041$, 16 kHz, $t = -3.77$, $P = 0.0059$; 22 kHz, $t = -1.44$, $P = 0.19$, 32 kHz, $t = -0.22$, $P = 0.83$; $N = 17$, Welch Two Sample t-test) (**Figure 2A** and **Supplementary Table 1**).

We also observed morphological changes in the Organ of Corti and spiral ganglion neurons. The Tlr2/4 DKO mice and their wild-type littermates treated with normal saline (NS) maintained relatively intact inner and outer hair cells, while the Tlr DKO mice and their wild-type littermates under the SGN degeneration model lost most inner and outer hair cells, and the tunnel of Corti collapsed (**Figure 2B**).

The Tlr DKO mice and their wild-type littermates treated with NS maintained a relatively normal density, with no significant difference in neuron density ($P = 0.675$, $t = 0.43$, $N = 24$, Welch Two Sample t-test). SGN density significantly decreased in Tlr DKO mice and wild-type mice under the SGN degeneration model (**Figure 2C**), but the SGN density was significantly higher in the DKO group mice ($P < 0.001$, $t = 11.71$, $N = 32$, Welch Two Sample t-test) (**Figure 2D**). These results suggest that the hearing preservation advantage of Tlr2/4 DKO mice mainly relies on the protection of spiral ganglion neurons.

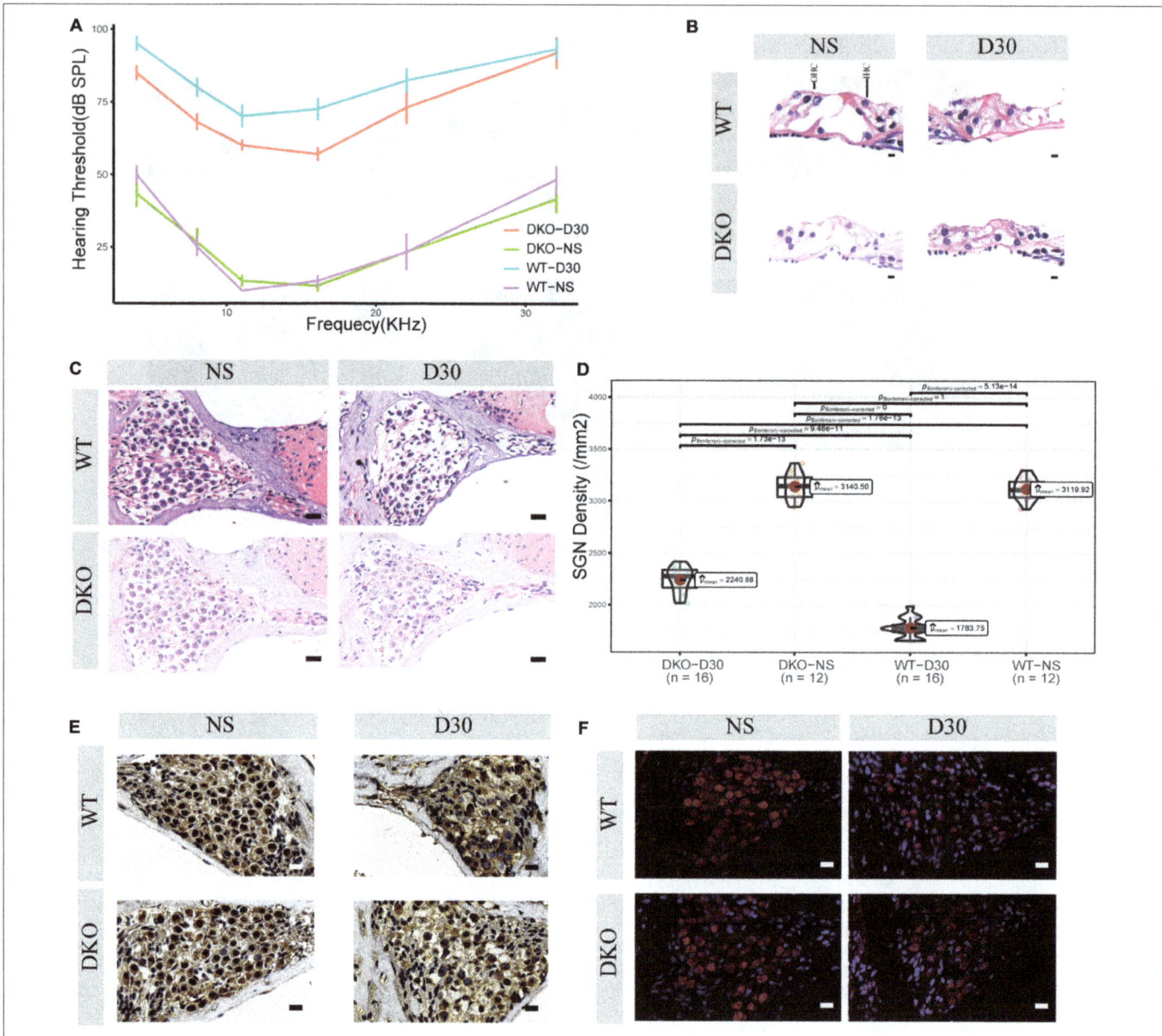

FIGURE 2 | Physiological and morphological changes in Tlr2/4 DKO mice and WT littermates. **(A)** The hearing threshold of auditory brainstem response of WT and DKO mice in the SGN degeneration model. Mice maintained normal hearing threshold in the normal saline treated group ($N = 8$, $P = 0.7148$, $F = 0.105$, two-way ANOVA). On the 30th day after kanamycin and furosemide injection, DKO mice exhibited a hearing preservation advantage compared with WT mice ($N = 13$, $P = 0.00446$, $F = 8.700$, two-way ANOVA). **(B)** Hair cell loss of WT and DKO mice. Saline treated mice had normal hair cells. On the 30th day of kanamycin and furosemide injection, both DKO and WT mice lost all hair cells and the tunnel of Corti had collapsed. Scale bar: 10 μm. **(C)** SGN loss of DKO and WT mice. Mice maintained a normal SGN count in normal saline treated group ($N = 24$, $P = 0.675$, $t = 0.43$, Welch Two Sample t-test). On the 30th day of kanamycin and furosemide injection, DKO mice have higher SGN density compared with WT mice Scale bar: 10 μm. **(D)** Statistics of panel C. On the 30th day of kanamycin and furosemide injection, DKO mice have higher SGN density compared with WT mice ($N = 32$, $P < 0.001$, $t = 11.471$ Welch Two Sample t-test). **(E)** Representative IHC image of p38 expression of SGN in WT and DKO mice. Scale Bar: Scale bar: 10 μm. **(F)** Representative IHC image of p65 expression of SGN in WT and DKO mice. Scale Bar: Scale bar: 10 μm.

Inverted Gene Set Enrichment of Double Knockout Mice During Spiral Ganglion Neurons Degeneration

The p38-mediated MAPK and p65-mediated NF-κB signaling pathways are canonical signaling pathways of Tlr molecules (Li et al., 2010). We used immunohistochemistry to detect the expression of these genes in SGNs. SGN p38 expression was found in both DKO and WT mice, mainly in the cytoplasm and nuclei. There was no significant difference in p38 expression between the two groups on the 30th day of degeneration induction (**Figure 2E**, neuron density evaluation

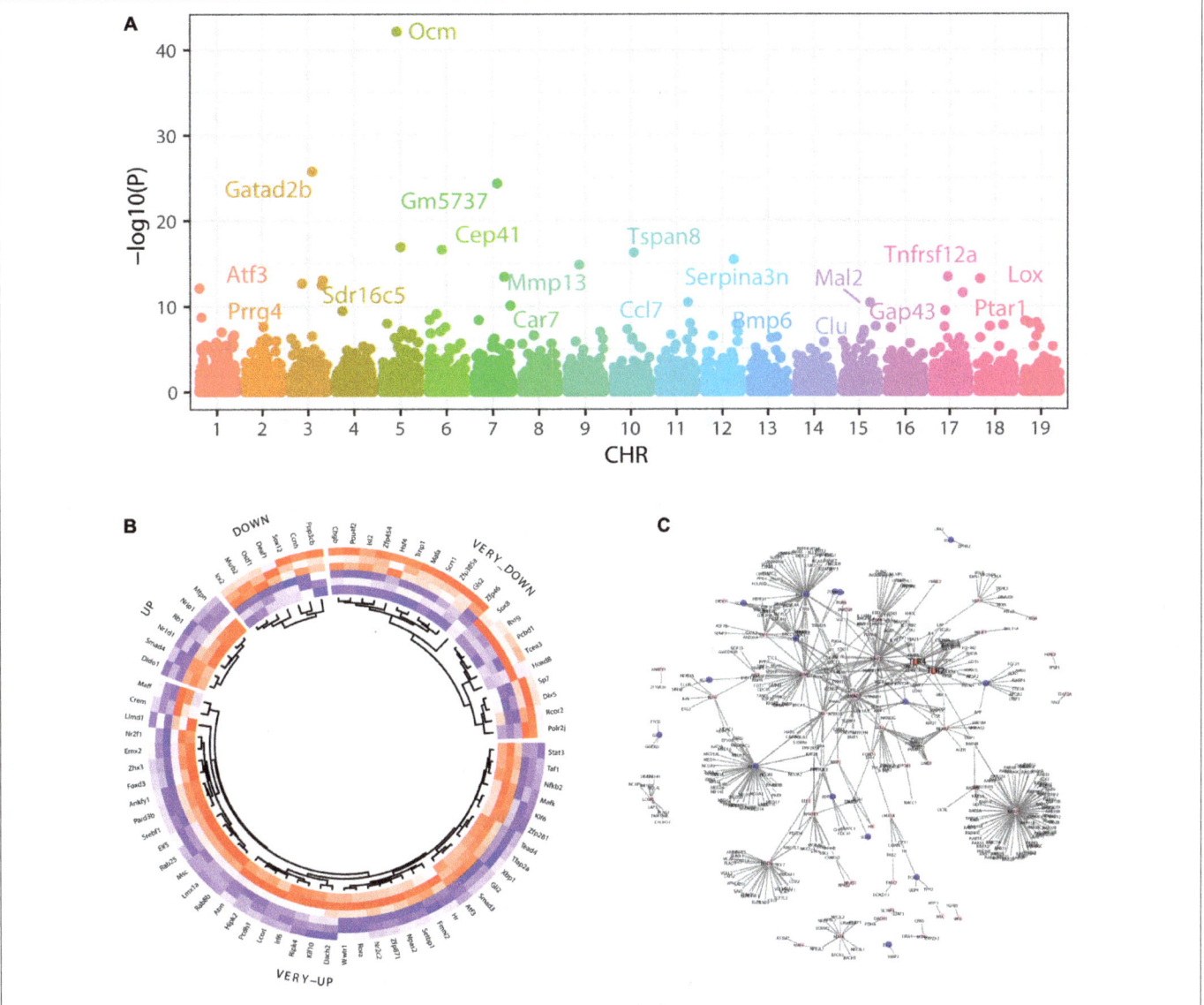

FIGURE 3 | Differentially expressed genes during SGN degeneration. **(A)** Manhattan plot of all genes, including the DEGs. The abscissa indicates the chromosomes, and the ordinate represents the p-values of those genes. The most significant gene of each chromosome is labeled. **(B)** Heatmap of the top upregulated and downregulated genes. Blue indicates relatively lower expression, and red indicates relatively higher expression. **(C)** The disturbance of Tlr2/4 on the SGN degeneration network. Blue indicates transcription factors with relatively downregulated expression, and pink indicates relatively upregulated expression. DEGs: differentially expressed genes.

in **Supplementary Figure 2**). The SGNs of DKO and WT mice express p65 (RelA), which is mainly located in the cytoplasm and nuclei. P65 expression decreased 30 days after SGN degeneration, but no significant differences in expression were identified between the two groups (**Figure 2F**, neuron density evaluation in **Supplementary Figure 2**).

Transcriptomic analysis was performed on the modiolus of DKO and WT mice on the 30th day after kanamycin and furosemide administration. We identified 1029 upregulated genes and 833 downregulated genes with the criteria of $P < 0.01$, and $|\log_2$ fold change$| > 0.2$) (**Figure 5A**; **Supplementary Table 1**). Among them, 1,747 had a clear autosomal location and there were 136, 133, 86, 103, 125, 107, 126, 82, 96, 80, 149, 70, 65, 78, 76, 56, 75, 39, 65 on chromosome 1–19, respectively. The most strongly differentially expressed genes on autosomal chromosomes were identified, including Sned1, Ttn, Gbp2, Tlr4, Jchain, Clec7a, Itgax, Nlrc5, Mmp3, Dcn, Gh, Serpina3n, Sfrp4, Dnah12, Glycam1, Parp14, C4b, Iigp1, and Ifit3 (**Figure 5B**). **Figure 5C** shows the differentially expressed transcription factors.

In general, Tlr2/4 DKO mice showed downregulated biological activities during SGN degeneration compared to WT mice. The top 30 enriched KEGG pathways included 1 upregulated and 29 downregulated pathways (**Figure 6A**). Oxidative phosphorylation was downregulated during SGN degeneration, but upregulated in DKO mice compared with

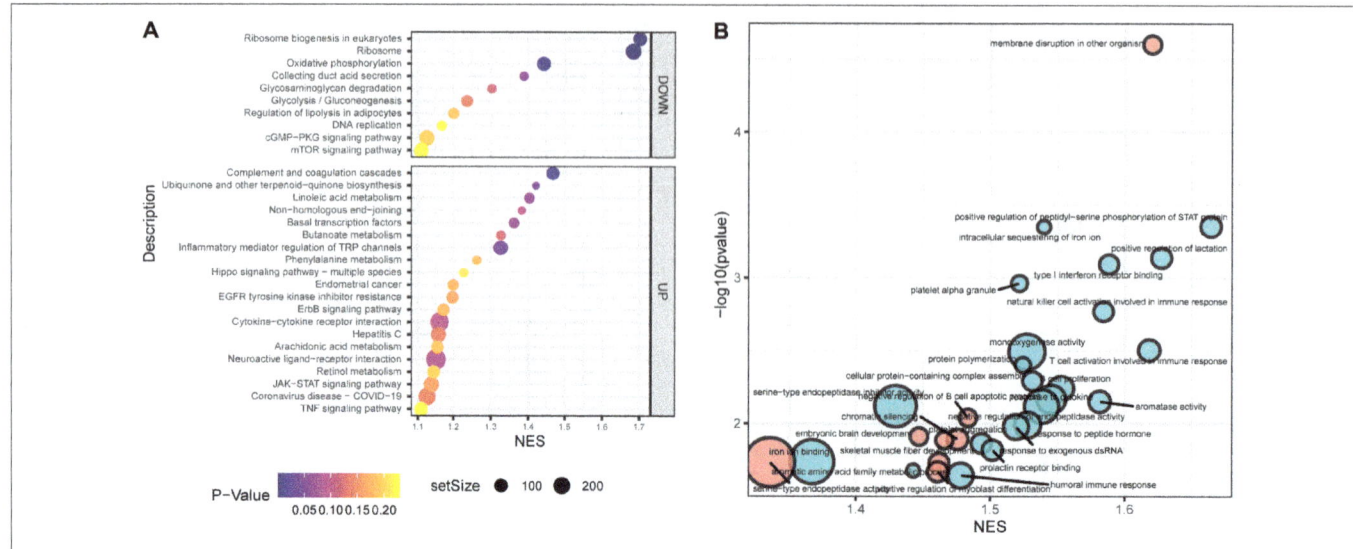

FIGURE 4 | Functional annotation of SGN degeneration. **(A)** KEGG pathway enrichment analysis of SGN degeneration. The abscissa represents the enrichment scores, and the ordinate suggests the KEGG terms. **(B)** GO enrichment analysis of SGN degeneration. The abscissa represents the enrichment scores, and the ordinate shows the –lg (p-value). Red: downregulated terms; Blue: upregulated terms.

TABLE 1 | Key modules of SGN degeneration in WT mice.

Modules	Scores	No.	Edges/Interactions	Gene name
1	4.222	10	27	COMP, COL1A1, STAT3, HAPLN1, HBEGF, CCL2, MMP13, SMAD4, CXCL1, CTSK
2	4	7	14	SNAP25, SYN2, NGFR, CALB2, GAP43, NEFH, SYP
3	3.667	7	12	LOX, ITPKB, CDH1, SMAD3, EGF, CTGF, TIMP2
4	3.2	6	10	MMP9, COL4A1, SDC4, CCL12, CCL7, VCL
5	3	3	4	SDR16C5, PLAG1, LCORL
6	2.8	6	10	CALM3, TMOD4, TPM4, CALM2, TCAP, PNCK

WT mice, which is called inverted gene set enrichment. The top 10 KEGG terms with inverted gene set enrichments included arachidonic acid metabolism, complement and coagulation cascades, coronavirus disease—COVID-19, cytokine-cytokine receptor interaction, hepatitis C, inflammatory mediator regulation of TRP channels, JAK-STAT signaling pathway, neuroactive ligand-receptor interaction, TNF signaling pathway, and oxidative phosphorylation (**Figure 6B**).

Similarly, the top 30 enriched GO terms included one upregulated and 29 downregulated activities (**Figure 6C**). The top 10 KEGG terms with inverted gene set enrichments included iron ion binding, monooxygenase activity, negative regulation of endopeptidase activity, platelet aggregation, positive regulation of myoblast differentiation, protein polymerization, response to cytokines, response to peptide hormones, serine-type endopeptidase activity, and serine-type endopeptidase inhibitor activity (**Figure 6D**).

Suspectable Core Modules That Attenuate Spiral Ganglion Neurons Degeneration in Double Knockout Mice

In order to detect whether DKO mice had consistent morphology across the entire signaling network, i.e., whether there is an inverted gene set enrichment relationship with the primary auditory neurons degeneration (PAND)-specific gene set, we analyzed the different genes in the PAND-specific gene set. We found that there was an inverted GSEA relationship between the PAND process and the PAND-specific gene set in DKO mice, and the PAND-associated DEGs were relatively reverse regulated in the progression of PAND in DKO mice (NES = –1.84, $P < 0.001$).

We further analyzed the attenuation of SGN degeneration in DKO mice from the perspective of the entire signaling network (**Supplementary Figure 3**). We found that 130 of the 661 genes specifically upregulated during the degeneration of SGN in WT mice were downregulated mice during the degeneration of spiral neurons in DKO mice, and 380 genes were specifically downregulated during the degeneration of SGN in WT mice; 116 genes were downregulated during the degeneration of spiral neurons in DKO mice.

Protein interaction analysis of the proteins encoded by these genes showed that DKO mice had a specific anti-degenerative signal network compared to WT mice. The disease module analysis showed that there were two key modules (**Table 2**). The score of the first module was 3.667, including seven genes, namely *EGF, STAT3, CALB2, LOX, SNAP25, CAV2*, and *SDC4*. The score of the second module was 3.5, which included five genes: *MYL1, NCS1, PVALB, TPM4,* and *TMOD4. In addition, EGF, STAT3,*

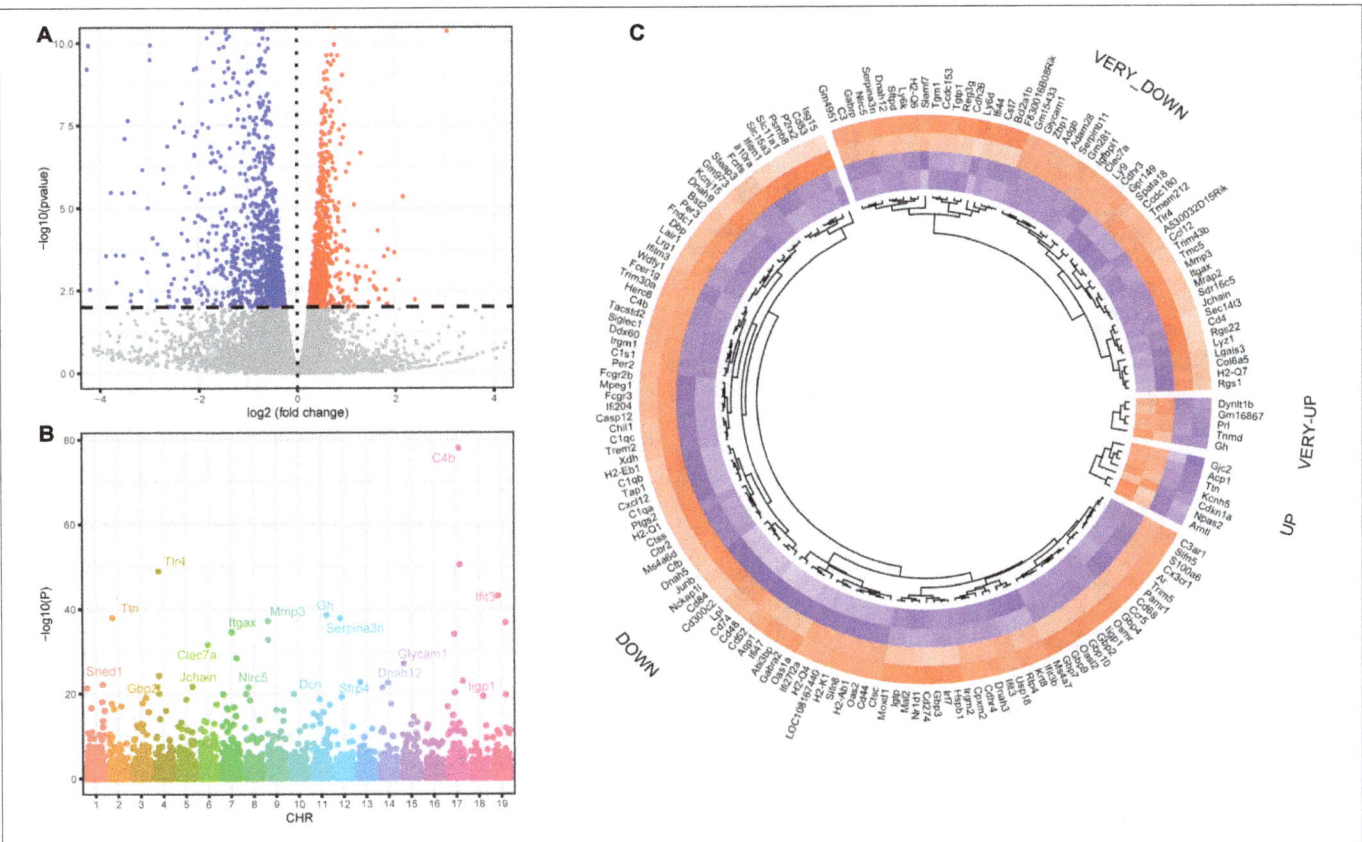

FIGURE 5 | Differentially expressed genes of DKO VS. WT SGN transcriptome on the 30th day. **(A)** Volcano plot of all detected genes including the DEGs. Red dots indicate upregulated genes and blue dots indicate downregulated genes. **(B)** Manhattan plot of all genes including the DEGs. The abscissa indicates the chromosomes, and the ordinate represents the *p*-values of those genes. The most significant gene of each chromosome is labeled. **(C)** Heatmap of the top upregulated and downregulated transcription factors. If the log$_2$ fold change is higher than 2, the category is labeled with VERY. Blue indicates relatively lower expression, and red indicates relatively higher expression.

CALB2, SNAP25, SDC4, TPM4, and *TMOD4* are key molecules involved in SGN degeneration. CALB2 is a specific marker of the SGN Ia and Ib subtypes in mice (Shrestha et al., 2018), PVALB is a neuron-specific marker (Petitpré et al., 2018), and the interaction of these molecules may contribute to the attenuation of SGN degeneration in DKO mice.

DISCUSSION

Studies have shown that primary and secondary SGN degeneration may account for half of the SGN degeneration (Makary et al., 2011; Waqas et al., 2017; Guo et al., 2021). Morphological studies of the human cochlea show that with the growth of age, even if there is no loss of inner and outer hair cells, SGN will be lost at a rate of about 100 cells per year. This rate can increase to approximately 185 cells per year when there is simultaneous loss of inner and outer hair cells (Makary et al., 2011). Unlike auditory hair cells, which are easily damaged by noise and ototoxic drugs such as aminoglycosides and cisplatin, spiral ganglion neurons are relatively robust. In a study of animal models and human temporal bone, histopathological analysis of acquired sensorineural hearing loss showed that severe degeneration of cochlear spiral neurons is often accompanied by a significant loss of hair cells (Miller et al., 1997; McFadden et al., 2004). The degeneration of SGNs seems to be related to the loss of inner hair cells, because 95% of spiral neurons only have synaptic connections with inner hair cells. However, the causal relationship based on histopathological correlation is often frustrated (Zilberstein et al., 2012), which may be because the loss of inner hair cells is usually accompanied by the loss or complete destruction of the organ of Corti after cochlear injury, and both hair cells and supporting cells contribute to the support of SGN in the cochlea (Sugawara et al., 2005). Temporal bone studies from 54 to 89 years of age without ear diseases suggest that the number of hair cells is almost normal, but the pattern of axonal degeneration of the cochlear nerve may be an important form of human presbycusis (Viana et al., 2015).

Transcriptome analysis of age-related cochlear degeneration indicated that no immune or inflammatory activity was enriched (**Supplementary Figure 4**). Therefore, the present study utilized the secondary SGN degeneration model of a single dose injection of kanamycin and furosemide, and the SGN degeneration model is suitable for the study of Tlr regulation during SGN degeneration. In the present SGN degeneration model, almost all outer hair cells were destroyed within 7 days after the injection of

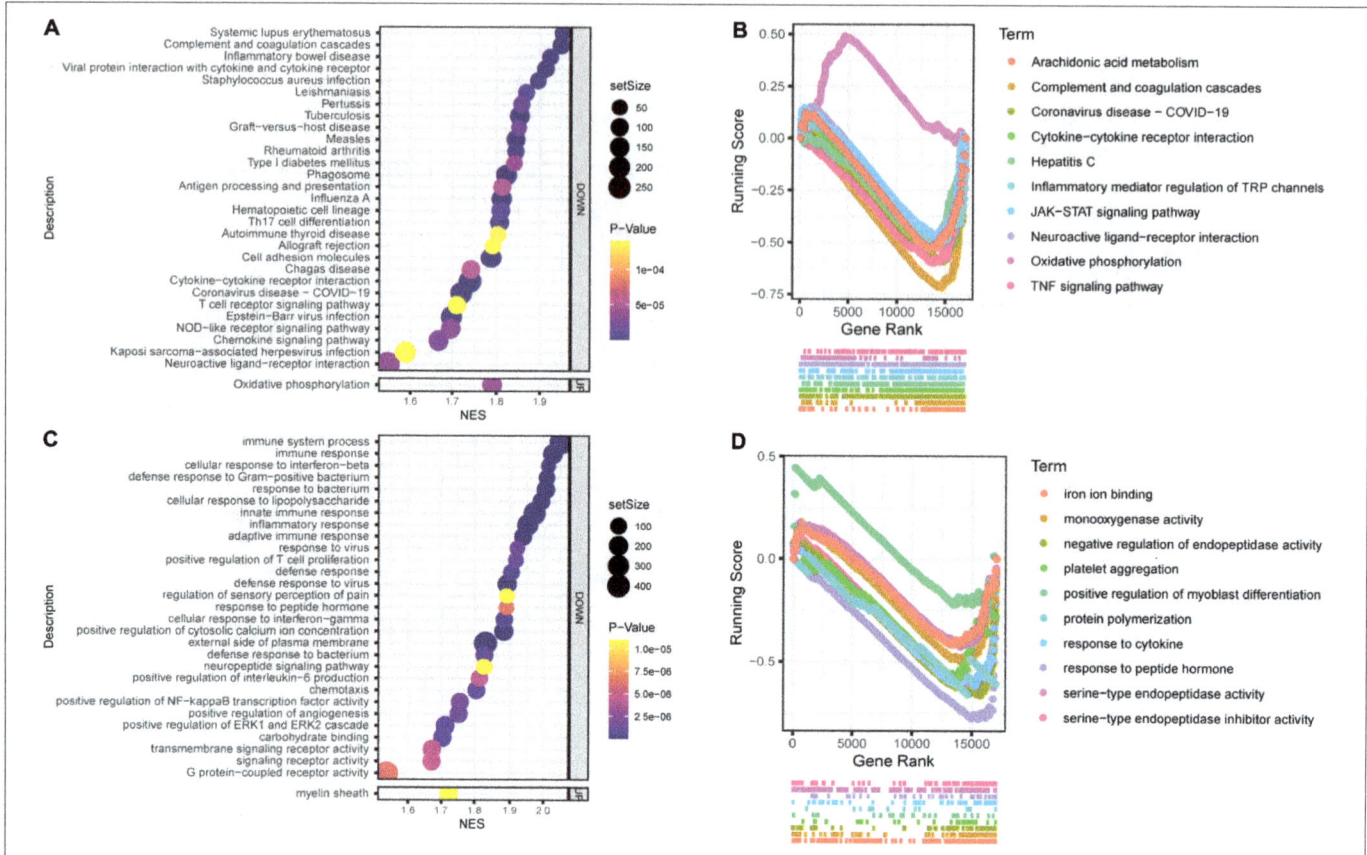

FIGURE 6 | Functional annotation of DKO VS. WT SGN transcriptome on the 30th day. **(A)** KEGG pathway enrichment analysis. The abscissa represents the enrichment scores, and the ordinate suggests KEGG terms. **(B)** The running score visualization of the top 10 enriched KEGG terms which are also involved in the SGN degeneration process. **(C)** GO enrichment analysis of SGN degeneration. The abscissa represents the enrichment scores, and the ordinate suggests KEGG terms. **(D)** The running score visualization of the top 10 enriched KEGG terms which are also involved in SGN degeneration process.

TABLE 2 | Key modules of the attenuation of SGN degeneration in DKO mice.

Modules	Score	No.	Edges/interactions	Gene name
1	3.667	7	12	*EGF, STAT3, CALB2, LOX, SNAP25, CAV2, SDC4*
2	3.5	5	9	*MYL1, NCS1, PVALB, TPM4, TMOD4*

kanamycin and furosemide. Inner hair cells seemed more robust and about 15% inner hair cells were preserved 30 days after the treatment. In other words, <5% hair cells (including OHCs and IHCs) remain alive on the 30 day (Hu et al., 2017; Ye et al., 2019). These results were also in consistent with the study of Taylor (Taylor et al., 2008).

Another important question is when this transcriptome changes happen in DKO mice. We consider that the key points might be the opposite regulated direction of DKO mice compared with a normal SGN degeneration transcriptome change. In other words, the overlapping and opposite terms would be highlighted that might play key role in the alleviation of SGN degeneration in DKO mice whenever it happened. But we should acknowledge that it is preferred if these changes occurred after the degeneration induction, otherwise a systematic influence and specific delivery of these molecules should be considered. Tlr-regulated innate immune signaling regulates neuron-glia interactions (McLaughlin et al., 2019). McLaughlin et al. demonstrated that glia non-canonical Toll-like receptor signaling could be non-autonomously activated by neuronal apoptosis, priming their capacity to engulf apoptotic neurons and regulate the maintenance of a healthy brain (Kashio and Miura, 2019). Glia continuously surveys neuronal health during development, providing trophic support to healthy neurons, while rapidly engulfing dying ones. With neuronal health being surveyed, glia could provide trophic support to healthy neurons and rapidly engulf dying neurons. Glia necessitates a foolproof mechanism to unambiguously identify those neurons to support vs. engulf. To ensure specificity, glia is proposed to interact with dying neurons via a series of carefully choreographed steps. Dying neurons and glia communicate via toll-receptor-regulated innate immune signaling, while neuronal apoptosis drives the processing and activation of the Toll-6 ligand and activates the dSARM-mediated Toll-6 transcriptional pathway, which controls the expression of the Draper engulfment receptor. Pathway loss drives early onset neurodegeneration, underscoring its functional importance.

Zhang et al. (2019) demonstrated that in the cochleae (lateral wall and spiral ganglion neurons), TLR-4 and the downstream signaling molecule MyD88 were significantly upregulated 3 d after noise exposure. It has also been reported that Tlr4 knockout mice could inhibit the expression of major histocompatibility complex class II and participate in the antigen-presenting function of macrophages after acoustic trauma (Vethanayagam et al., 2016). Their results suggested that Tlr4 regulates multiple aspects of the immune response in the cochlea and contributes to cochlear pathogenesis after acoustic injury. According to the single-cell transcriptome of Shrestha et al. (2018) and our IHC results (data not shown), SGN may rarely be Tlr2/4 positive. Tlr2/4 double knockout may attenuate SGN degeneration by disturbing the local microenvironment of circular macrophage cells or Schwann cells and detecting Tlr downstream in SGN fails to signify the attenuation of SGN degeneration.

We identified some relatively novel molecules that may play an essential role in attenuating SGN degeneration in Tlr2/4 DKO mice. Researchers have found that the interaction between Tlr and these molecules may regulate the pathogenesis of many diseases. For example, myofibroblast Tlr signaling promotes colitis-associated carcinogenesis by mediating macrophage M2 polarization and STAT3 activation via intracellular communication (Yuan Q. et al., 2021, p. 88). Hsu et al. (2010) found that the differentially regulated expression of Tlr-associated epidermal growth factor influences mucosal healing.

DFNA44, an autosomal dominant deafness, is tightly associated with the effector of EGF-mediated cell signaling (Modamio-Hoybjor et al., 2007). Rats administered oral epigallocatechin-3-gallate demonstrated reduced cisplatin-induced hearing loss, experienced reduced loss of OHCs in the basal region of the cochlea and reduced oxidative stress and apoptotic markers. The preservation of STAT3 and Bcl-xL activation and increased STAT3/STAT1 ratio may contribute to protection (Borse et al., 2017). STAT3 and its activated form are specifically expressed in hair cells during cochlear development (Chen et al., 2017). CALB2 is a candidate gene for human dominant optic atrophy (Carelli et al., 2011, p. 8). Calb2 is highly expressed in the Ia and Ib subtypes of SGN (Shrestha et al., 2018; Sun et al., 2018). In noise-induced hearing loss (NIHL), noise exposure damages cochlear sensory hair cells, which lack the capacity to regenerate. Following noise insult, intense metabolic activity occurs, resulting in a free-radical imbalance in the cochlea. Oxidative stress and antioxidant enzyme alterations, including lipoxygenase (LOX) upregulation, have been linked to chronic inflammation, which contributes to hearing impairment. Inhibition of LOX showed greater efficacy in the treatment of NIHL (Rodriguez et al., 2017). LOX products may contribute to the hypersensitivity of SGN to hair cell inputs in a variety of pathological conditions (Balaban et al., 2003). Snap25 is a key marker of neuronal identity. Noda et al. (2018) used the neurogenic pioneer transcription factor Ascl1 and the auditory neuron differentiation factor NeuroD1 to reprogram spiral ganglion non-neuronal cells into induced neurons.

Their transcriptome results indicated that induced neurons maintained some key markers of neuronal identity, such as Tubb3, Map2, Prph, Snap25, and Prox1 (Noda et al., 2018). The mutation of the otoferlin C2 domain, which causes deafness in humans, impairs the ability of otoferlin to bind syntaxin, SNAP-25, and the Cav1.3 calcium channel, which may mediate regulation by otoferlin of hair cell synaptic exocytosis, which is critical to inner ear hair cell function (Ramakrishnan et al., 2009). The damaged interaction between SDC4 and GIPCs also contributes to the progression of non-syndromic hearing loss (Katoh, 2013).

CONCLUSION

In conclusion, our results suggest that the SGN degeneration of Tlr2/4 DKO mice and their wild-type littermates exhibits an inverted GSEA relationship, and DKO mice may attenuate SGN degeneration by the differential regulation of some core molecules, including EGF, STAT3, CALB2, LOX, SNAP25, CAV2, SDC4, MYL1, NCS1, PVALB, TPM4, and TMOD4.

ETHICS STATEMENT

The animal study was reviewed and approved by the Ethics Committee of Xinhua Hospital, affiliated with Shanghai Jiao Tong University School of Medicine.

AUTHOR CONTRIBUTIONS

MX and QW were responsible for the initiation and conduction, respectively. QW was responsible for writing the manuscript. QW, YS, YP, TZ, AZ, DG, CF, HH, LM, KC, and BY performed the experiments. BY and QW processed and analyzed the data. All authors contributed to the article and approved the submitted version.

SUPPLEMENTARY MATERIAL

Supplementary Figure 1 | The hearing threshold of auditory brainstem response of WT mice in the SGN degeneration model. Mice maintained normal hearing threshold in the normal saline treated group. On the 30th day after kanamycin and furosemide injection, mice exhibited a hearing deteriation compared with NS treated mice ($N = 13$, $P < 0.00001$, $F = 275.910$, two-way ANOVA).

Supplementary Figure 2 | Reconfirmation of SGN density of sections with histopathological analysis. The upper panel for p38 and the lower panel for p65.

Supplementary Figure 3 | Protein-protein interaction network constructed DKO VS. WT SGN transcriptome on the 30th day. Red: upregulated molecules. Blue: downregulated molecules.

Supplementary Figure 4 | Differentially expressed genes during whole cochlear aging. **(A)** Manhattan plot of all genes, including the DEGs. The abscissa indicates the chromosomes, and the ordinate represents the p-values of those genes. The most significant gene of each chromosome is labeled. **(B)** Heatmap of the top upregulated and downregulated genes. Blue indicates relatively lower expression, and red indicates relatively higher expression. **(C)** KEGG pathway enrichment analysis. The abscissa represents the enrichment scores, and the ordinate suggests $-\lg$ (p-value).

REFERENCES

Ashburner, M., Ball, C. A., Blake, J. A., Botstein, D., Butler, H., Cherry, J. M., et al. (2000). Gene ontology: tool for the unification of biology. The gene ontology consortium. *Nat. Genet.* 25, 25–29. doi: 10.1038/75556

Balaban, C. D., Zhou, J., and Li, H. S. (2003). Type 1 vanilloid receptor expression by mammalian inner ear ganglion cells. *Hear. Res.* 175, 165–170. doi: 10.1016/s0378-5955(02)00734-7

Borse, V., Al Aameri, R. F. H., Sheehan, K., Sheth, S., Kaur, T., Mukherjea, D., et al. (2017). Epigallocatechin-3-gallate, a prototypic chemopreventative agent for protection against cisplatin-based ototoxicity. *Cell Death Dis.* 8:e2921. doi: 10.1038/cddis.2017.314

Carelli, V., Schimpf, S., Fuhrmann, N., Valentino, M. L., Zanna, C., Iommarini, L., et al. (2011). A clinically complex form of dominant optic atrophy (OPA8) maps on chromosome 16. *Hum. Mol. Genet.* 20, 1893–1905. doi: 10.1093/hmg/ddr071

Chen, Q., Quan, Y., Wang, N., Xie, C., Ji, Z., He, H., et al. (2017). Inactivation of STAT3 signaling impairs hair cell differentiation in the developing mouse cochlea. *Stem Cell Rep.* 9, 231–246. doi: 10.1016/j.stemcr.2017.05.031

Chen, Y., Gu, Y., Li, Y., Li, G. L., Chai, R., Li, W., et al. (2021). Generation of mature and functional hair cells by co-expression of Gfi1, Pou4f3, and Atoh1 in the postnatal mouse cochlea. *Cell Rep.* 35:109016. doi: 10.1016/j.celrep.2021.109016

Cheng, C., Hou, Y., Zhang, Z., Wang, Y., Lu, L., Zhang, L., et al. (2021). Disruption of the autism-related gene Pak1 causes stereocilia disorganization, hair cell loss, and deafness in mice. *J. Genet. Genomics* 48, 324–332. doi: 10.1016/j.jgg.2021.03.010

Cheng, C., Wang, Y., Guo, L., Lu, X., Zhu, W., Muhammad, W., et al. (2019). Age-related transcriptome changes in Sox2+ supporting cells in the mouse cochlea. *Stem Cell Res. Ther.* 10:365. doi: 10.1186/s13287-019-1437-0

Cusumano, C., Friedmann, D. R., Fang, Y., Wang, B., Roland, J. T., and Waltzman, S. B. (2017). Performance plateau in prelingually and postlingually deafened adult cochlear implant recipients. *Otol. Neurotol.* 38, 334–338. doi: 10.1097/MAO.0000000000001322

De Paola, M., Mariani, A., Bigini, P., Peviani, M., Ferrara, G., Molteni, M., et al. (2012). Neuroprotective effects of toll-like receptor 4 antagonism in spinal cord cultures and in a mouse model of motor neuron degeneration. *Mol. Med.* 18, 971–981. doi: 10.2119/molmed.2012.00020

Ding, Y., Meng, W., Kong, W., He, Z., and Chai, R. (2020). The role of FoxG1 in the inner ear. *Front. Cell Dev. Biol.* 8:614954. doi: 10.3389/fcell.2020.614954

Freria, C. M., Bernardes, D., Almeida, G. L., Simões, G. F., Barbosa, G. O., and Oliveira, A. L. R. (2016). Impairment of toll-like receptors 2 and 4 leads to compensatory mechanisms after sciatic nerve axotomy. *J. Neuroinflammation* 13:118. doi: 10.1186/s12974-016-0579-6

Fu, X., An, Y., Wang, H., Li, P., Lin, J., Yuan, J., et al. (2021). Deficiency of Klc2 induces low-frequency sensorineural hearing loss in C57BL/6 J mice and human. *Mol. Neurobiol.* 58, 4376–4391. doi: 10.1007/s12035-021-02422-w

Gao, K., Ding, D., Sun, H., Roth, J., and Salvi, R. (2017). Kanamycin damages early postnatal, but not adult spiral ganglion neurons. *Neurotox. Res.* 32, 603–613. doi: 10.1007/s12640-017-9773-2

Gao, S., Cheng, C., Wang, M., Jiang, P., Zhang, L., Wang, Y., et al. (2019). Blebbistatin inhibits neomycin-induced apoptosis in hair cell-like HEI-OC-1 cells and in cochlear hair cells. *Front. Cell. Neurosci.* 13:590. doi: 10.3389/fncel.2019.00590

Géléoc, G. S. G., and Holt, J. R. (2014). Sound strategies for hearing restoration. *Science* 344:1241062. doi: 10.1126/science.1241062

Guo, R., Li, J., Chen, C., Xiao, M., Liao, M., Hu, Y., et al. (2021). Biomimetic 3D bacterial cellulose-graphene foam hybrid scaffold regulates neural stem cell proliferation and differentiation. *Colloids Surf. B Biointerfaces* 200:111590. doi: 10.1016/j.colsurfb.2021.111590

Guo, R., Ma, X., Liao, M., Liu, Y., Hu, Y., Qian, X., et al. (2019). Development and application of cochlear implant-based electric-acoustic stimulation of spiral ganglion neurons. *ACS Biomater. Sci. Eng.* 5, 6735–6741. doi: 10.1021/acsbiomaterials.9b01265

Guo, R., Xiao, M., Zhao, W., Zhou, S., Hu, Y., Liao, M., et al. (2020). 2D Ti3C2TxMXene couples electrical stimulation to promote proliferation and neural differentiation of neural stem cells. *Acta Biomater.* (in press). doi: 10.1016/j.actbio.2020.12.035

Guo, R., Zhang, S., Xiao, M., Qian, F., He, Z., Li, D., et al. (2016). Accelerating bioelectric functional development of neural stem cells by graphene coupling: implications for neural interfacing with conductive materials. *Biomaterials* 106, 193–204. doi: 10.1016/j.biomaterials.2016.08.019

Han, S., Xu, Y., Sun, J., Liu, Y., Zhao, Y., Tao, W., et al. (2020). Isolation and analysis of extracellular vesicles in a Morpho butterfly wing-integrated microvortex biochip. *Biosens. Bioelectron.* 154:112073. doi: 10.1016/j.bios.2020.112073

He, Z., Guo, L., Shu, Y., Fang, Q., Zhou, H., Liu, Y., et al. (2017). Autophagy protects auditory hair cells against neomycin-induced damage. *Autophagy* 13, 1884–1904. doi: 10.1080/15548627.2017.1359449

He, Z.-H., Li, M., Fang, Q.-J., Liao, F.-L., Zou, S.-Y., Wu, X., et al. (2021). FOXG1 promotes aging inner ear hair cell survival through activation of the autophagy pathway. *Autophagy* 318, 1–22. doi: 10.1080/15548627.2021.1916194

He, Z. H., Zou, S. Y., Li, M., Liao, F. L., Wu, X., Sun, H. Y., et al. (2020). The nuclear transcription factor FoxG1 affects the sensitivity of mimetic aging hair cells to inflammation by regulating autophagy pathways. *Redox Biol.* 28:101364. doi: 10.1016/j.redox.2019.101364

Hsu, D., Fukata, M., Hernandez, Y. G., Sotolongo, J. P., Goo, T., Maki, J., et al. (2010). Toll-like receptor 4 differentially regulates epidermal growth factor-related growth factors in response to intestinal mucosal injury. *Lab. Invest.* 90, 1295–1305. doi: 10.1038/labinvest.2010.100

Hu, H., Ye, B., Zhang, L., Wang, Q., Liu, Z., Ji, S., et al. (2017). Efr3a insufficiency attenuates the degeneration of spiral ganglion neurons after hair cell loss. *Front. Mol. Neurosci.* 10:86. doi: 10.3389/fnmol.2017.00086

Jiang, P., Zhang, S., Cheng, C., Gao, S., Tang, M., Lu, L., et al. (2020). The roles of exosomes in visual and auditory systems. *Front. Bioeng. Biotechnol.* 8:525. doi: 10.3389/fbioe.2020.00525

Kanehisa, M., and Goto, S. (2000). KEGG: kyoto encyclopedia of genes and genomes. *Nucleic Acids Res.* 28, 27–30. doi: 10.1093/nar/28.1.27

Kashio, S., and Miura, M. (2019). Tolling of a bell at a neuron's death. *Dev. Cell* 48, 427–428. doi: 10.1016/j.devcel.2019.02.009

Katoh, M. (2013). Functional proteomics, human genetics and cancer biology of GIPC family members. *Exp. Mol. Med.* 45:e26. doi: 10.1038/emm.2013.49

Kilic, U., Kilic, E., Matter, C. M., Bassetti, C. L., and Hermann, D. M. (2008). TLR-4 deficiency protects against focal cerebral ischemia and axotomy-induced neurodegeneration. *Neurobiol. Dis.* 31, 33–40. doi: 10.1016/j.nbd.2008.03.002

Kim, C., Spencer, B., Rockenstein, E., Yamakado, H., Mante, M., Adame, A., et al. (2018). Immunotherapy targeting toll-like receptor 2 alleviates neurodegeneration in models of synucleinopathy by modulating α-synuclein transmission and neuroinflammation. *Mol Neurodegener* 13:43. doi: 10.1186/s13024-018-0276-2

Kim, D., Langmead, B., and Salzberg, S. L. (2015). HISAT: a fast spliced aligner with low memory requirements. *Nat. Methods* 12, 357–360. doi: 10.1038/nmeth.3317

Koo, J. W., Quintanilla-Dieck, L., Jiang, M., Liu, J., Urdang, Z. D., Allensworth, J. J., et al. (2015). Endotoxemia-mediated inflammation potentiates aminoglycoside-induced ototoxicity. *Sci. Transl. Med.* 7:298ra118. doi: 10.1126/scitranslmed.aac5546

Kujawa, S. G., and Liberman, M. C. (2009). Adding insult to injury: cochlear nerve degeneration after "temporary" noise-induced hearing loss. *J. Neurosci.* 29, 14077–14085. doi: 10.1523/JNEUROSCI.2845-09.2009

Lax, N., Fainstein, N., Nishri, Y., Ben-Zvi, A., and Ben-Hur, T. (2020). Systemic microbial TLR2 agonists induce neurodegeneration in Alzheimer's disease mice. *J Neuroinflammation* 17:55. doi: 10.1186/s12974-020-01738-z

Li, X., Jiang, S., and Tapping, R. I. (2010). Toll-like receptor signaling in cell proliferation and survival. *Cytokine* 49, 1–9. doi: 10.1016/j.cyto.2009.08.010

Liu, L., Chen, Y., Qi, J., Zhang, Y., He, Y., Ni, W., et al. (2016). Wnt activation protects against neomycin-induced hair cell damage in the mouse cochlea. *Cell Death Dis.* 7:e2136. doi: 10.1038/cddis.2016.35

Liu, W., Xu, L., Wang, X., Zhang, D., Sun, G., Wang, M., et al. (2021). PRDX1 activates autophagy via the PTEN-AKT signaling pathway to protect against cisplatin-induced spiral ganglion neuron damage. *Autophagy* 1–23. doi: 10.1080/15548627.2021.1905466 [Epub ahead of print].

Liu, W., Xu, X., Fan, Z., Sun, G., Han, Y., Zhang, D., et al. (2019). Wnt signaling activates TP53-induced glycolysis and apoptosis regulator and protects against cisplatin-induced spiral ganglion neuron damage in the mouse cochlea. *Antioxid. Redox Signal.* 30, 1389–1410. doi: 10.1089/ars.2017.7288

Liu, Y., Qi, J., Chen, X., Tang, M., Chu, C., Zhu, W., et al. (2019). Critical role of spectrin in hearing development and deafness. *Sci. Adv.* 5:eaav7803. doi:

10.1126/sciadv.aav7803

Makary, C. A., Shin, J., Kujawa, S. G., Liberman, M. C., and Merchant, S. N. (2011). Age-related primary cochlear neuronal degeneration in human temporal bones. *J. Assoc. Res. Otolaryngol.* 12, 711–717. doi: 10.1007/s10162-011-0283-2

McFadden, S. L., Ding, D., Jiang, H., and Salvi, R. J. (2004). Time course of efferent fiber and spiral ganglion cell degeneration following complete hair cell loss in the chinchilla. *Brain Res.* 997, 40–51. doi: 10.1016/j.brainres.2003.10.031

McLaughlin, C. N., Perry-Richardson, J. J., Coutinho-Budd, J. C., and Broihier, H. T. (2019). Dying neurons utilize innate immune signaling to prime glia for phagocytosis during development. *Dev. Cell* 48, 506–522.e6. doi: 10.1016/j.devcel.2018.12.019

Miller, J. M., Chi, D. H., O'Keeffe, L. J., Kruszka, P., Raphael, Y., and Altschuler, R. A. (1997). Neurotrophins can enhance spiral ganglion cell survival after inner hair cell loss. *Int. J. Dev. Neurosci.* 15, 631–643. doi: 10.1016/s0736-5748(96)00117-7

Modamio-Hoybjor, S., Mencia, A., Goodyear, R., del Castillo, I., Richardson, G., Moreno, F., et al. (2007). A mutation in CCDC50, a gene encoding an effector of epidermal growth factor-mediated cell signaling, causes progressive hearing loss. *Am. J. Hum. Genet.* 80, 1076–1089. doi: 10.1086/518311

Noda, T., Meas, S. J., Nogami, J., Amemiya, Y., Uchi, R., Ohkawa, Y., et al. (2018). Direct reprogramming of spiral ganglion non-neuronal cells into neurons: toward ameliorating sensorineural hearing loss by gene therapy. *Front. Cell Dev. Biol.* 6:16. doi: 10.3389/fcell.2018.00016

Peek, V., Neumann, E., Inoue, T., Koenig, S., Pflieger, F. J., Gerstberger, R., et al. (2020). Age-dependent changes of adipokine and cytokine secretion from rat adipose tissue by endogenous and exogenous toll-like receptor agonists. *Front. Immunol.* 11:1800. doi: 10.3389/fimmu.2020.01800

Pertea, M., Pertea, G. M., Antonescu, C. M., Chang, T. C., Mendell, J. T., and Salzberg, S. L. (2015). StringTie enables improved reconstruction of a transcriptome from RNA-seq reads. *Nat. Biotechnol.* 33, 290–295. doi: 10.1038/nbt.3122

Petitpré, C., Wu, H., Sharma, A., Tokarska, A., Fontanet, P., Wang, Y., et al. (2018). Neuronal heterogeneity and stereotyped connectivity in the auditory afferent system. *Nat. Commun.* 9:3691. doi: 10.1038/s41467-018-06033-3

Qi, J., Liu, Y., Chu, C., Chen, X., Zhu, W., Shu, Y., et al. (2019). A cytoskeleton structure revealed by super-resolution fluorescence imaging in inner ear hair cells. *Cell Discov.* 5:12. doi: 10.1038/s41421-018-0076-4

Qi, J., Zhang, L., Tan, F., Liu, Y., Chu, C., Zhu, W., et al. (2020). Espin distribution as revealed by super-resolution microscopy of stereocilia. *Am. J. Transl. Res.* 12, 130–141.

Qian, F., Wang, X., Yin, Z., Xie, G., Yuan, H., Liu, D., et al. (2020). The slc4a2b gene is required for hair cell development in zebrafish. *Aging (Albany, NY)* 12, 18804–18821. doi: 10.18632/aging.103840

Ramakrishnan, N. A., Drescher, M. J., and Drescher, D. G. (2009). Direct interaction of otoferlin with syntaxin 1A, SNAP-25, and the L-type voltage-gated calcium channel Cav1.3. *J. Biol. Chem.* 284, 1364–1372. doi: 10.1074/jbc.M803605200

Resnik, J., and Polley, D. B. (2021). Cochlear neural degeneration disrupts hearing in background noise by increasing auditory cortex internal noise. *Neuron* 109, 984–996.e4. doi: 10.1016/j.neuron.2021.01.015

Riss, D., Arnoldner, C., Baumgartner, W. D., Kaider, A., and Hamzavi, J. S. (2008). A new fine structure speech coding strategy: speech perception at a reduced number of channels. *Otol. Neurotol.* 29, 784–788. doi: 10.1097/MAO.0b013e31817fe00f

Rodriguez, I., Hong, B. N., Nam, Y. H., Kim, E. Y., Park, G. H., Ji, M. G., et al. (2017). Bioconversion of *Scutellaria baicalensis* extract can increase recovery of auditory function in a mouse model of noise-induced hearing loss. *Biomed. Pharmacother.* 93, 1303–1309. doi: 10.1016/j.biopha.2017.07.069

Shannon, P., Markiel, A., Ozier, O., Baliga, N. S., Wang, J. T., Ramage, D., et al. (2003). Cytoscape: a software environment for integrated models of biomolecular interaction networks. *Genome Res.* 13, 2498–2504. doi: 10.1101/gr.1239303

Shrestha, B. R., Chia, C., Wu, L., Kujawa, S. G., Liberman, M. C., and Goodrich, L. V. (2018). Sensory neuron diversity in the inner ear is shaped by activity. *Cell* 174, 1229–1246.e17. doi: 10.1016/j.cell.2018.07.007

Sriperumbudur, K. K., Appali, R., Gummer, A. W., and van Rienen, U. (2020). Neural tissue degeneration in Rosenthal's canal and its impact on electrical stimulation of the auditory nerve by cochlear implants: an image-based modeling study. *Int. J. Mol. Sci.* 21:8511. doi: 10.3390/ijms21228511

Subramanian, A., Tamayo, P., Mootha, V. K., Mukherjee, S., Ebert, B. L., Gillette, M. A., et al. (2005). Gene set enrichment analysis: a knowledge-based approach for interpreting genome-wide expression profiles. *Proc. Natl Acad. Sci. U.S.A.* 102, 15545–15550. doi: 10.1073/pnas.0506580102

Sugawara, M., Corfas, G., and Liberman, M. C. (2005). Influence of supporting cells on neuronal degeneration after hair cell loss. *J. Assoc. Res. Otolaryngol.* 6, 136–147. doi: 10.1007/s10162-004-5050-1

Sun, S., Babola, T., Pregernig, G., So, K. S., Nguyen, M., Su, S.-S. M., et al. (2018). Hair cell mechanotransduction regulates spontaneous activity and spiral ganglion subtype specification in the auditory system. *Cell* 174, 1247–1263.e15. doi: 10.1016/j.cell.2018.07.008

Szklarczyk, D., Gable, A. L., Nastou, K. C., Lyon, D., Kirsch, R., Pyysalo, S., et al. (2021). The STRING database in 2021: customizable protein–protein networks, and functional characterization of user-uploaded gene/measurement sets. *Nucleic Acids Res.* 49, D605–D612. doi: 10.1093/nar/gkaa1074

Tan, F., Chu, C., Qi, J., Li, W., You, D., Li, K., et al. (2019). AAV-ie enables safe and efficient gene transfer to inner ear cells. *Nat. Commun.* 10:3733. doi: 10.1038/s41467-019-11687-8

Taylor, R. R., Nevill, G., and Forge, A. (2008). Rapid hair cell loss: a mouse model for cochlear lesions. *J. Assoc. Res. Otolaryngol.* 9, 44–64. doi: 10.1007/s10162-007-0105-8

van Well, G. T. J., Sanders, M. S., Ouburg, S., van Furth, A. M., and Morré, S. A. (2012). Polymorphisms in Toll-like receptors 2, 4, and 9 are highly associated with hearing loss in survivors of bacterial meningitis. *PLoS One* 7:e35837. doi: 10.1371/journal.pone.0035837

Vethanayagam, R. R., Yang, W., Dong, Y., and Hu, B. H. (2016). Toll-like receptor 4 modulates the cochlear immune response to acoustic injury. *Cell Death Dis.* 7:e2245. doi: 10.1038/cddis.2016.156

Viana, L. M., O'Malley, J. T., Burgess, B. J., Jones, D. D., Oliveira, C. A. C. P., Santos, F., et al. (2015). Cochlear neuropathy in human presbycusis: confocal analysis of hidden hearing loss in post-mortem tissue. *Hear. Res.* 327, 78–88. doi: 10.1016/j.heares.2015.04.014

Wang, Q., Shen, Y., Hu, H., Fan, C., Zhang, A., Ding, R., et al. (2020). Systematic transcriptome analysis of noise-induced hearing loss pathogenesis suggests inflammatory activities and multiple susceptible molecules and pathways. *Front. Genet.* 11:968. doi: 10.3389/fgene.2020.00968

Wang, Q., Shen, Y., Ye, B., Hu, H., Fan, C., Wang, T., et al. (2018). Gene expression differences between thyroid carcinoma, thyroid adenoma and normal thyroid tissue. *Oncol. Rep.* 40, 3359–3369. doi: 10.3892/or.2018.6717

Wang, Y., Li, J., Yao, X., Li, W., Du, H., Tang, M., et al. (2017). Loss of CIB2 causes profound hearing loss and abolishes mechanoelectrical transduction in mice. *Front. Mol. Neurosci.* 10:401. doi: 10.3389/fnmol.2017.00401

Waqas, M., Sun, S., Xuan, C., Fang, Q., Zhang, X., Islam, I. U., et al. (2017). Bone morphogenetic protein 4 promotes the survival and preserves the structure of flow-sorted Bhlhb5+ cochlear spiral ganglion neurons in vitro. *Sci. Rep.* 7:3506. doi: 10.1038/s41598-017-03810-w

Wu, P. Z., O'Malley, J. T., de Gruttola, V., and Liberman, M. C. (2021). Primary neural degeneration in noise-exposed human cochleas: correlations with outer hair cell loss and word-discrimination scores. *J. Neurosci.* 41, 4439–4447. doi: 10.1523/JNEUROSCI.3238-20.2021

Yan, S., Wang, Q., Huo, Z., Yang, T., Yin, X., Wang, Z., et al. (2019). Gene expression profiles between cystic and solid vestibular schwannoma indicate susceptible molecules and pathways in the cystic formation of vestibular schwannoma. *Funct. Integr. Genomics* 19, 673–684. doi: 10.1007/s10142-019-00672-5

Ye, B., Wang, Q., Hu, H., Shen, Y., Fan, C., Chen, P., et al. (2019). Restoring autophagic flux attenuates cochlear spiral ganglion neuron degeneration by promoting TFEB nuclear translocation via inhibiting MTOR. *Autophagy* 15, 998–1016. doi: 10.1080/15548627.2019.1569926

Yu, G., Wang, L. G., Han, Y., and He, Q. Y. (2012). clusterProfiler: an R package for comparing biological themes among gene clusters. *Omics* 16, 284–287. doi: 10.1089/omi.2011.0118

Yuan, Q., Gu, J., Zhang, J., Liu, S., Wang, Q., Tian, T., et al. (2021). MyD88 in myofibroblasts enhances colitis-associated tumorigenesis via promoting macrophage M2 polarization. *Cell Rep.* 34:108724. doi: 10.1016/j.celrep.2021.108724

Yuan, T. F., Dong, Y., Zhang, L., Qi, J., Yao, C., Wang, Y., et al. (2021). Neuromodulation-based stem cell therapy in brain repair: recent advances and future perspectives. *Neurosci. Bull.* 37, 735–745. doi: 10.1007/s12264-021-00667-y

Zhang, G., Zheng, H., Pyykko, I., and Zou, J. (2019). The TLR-4/NF-κB signaling pathway activation in cochlear inflammation of rats with noise-induced hearing loss. *Hear. Res.* 379, 59–68. doi: 10.1016/j.heares.2019.04.012

Zhang, S., Dong, Y., Qiang, R., Zhang, Y., Zhang, X., Chen, Y., et al. (2021). Characterization of Strip1 expression in mouse cochlear hair cells. *Front. Genet.* 12:625867. doi: 10.3389/fgene.2021.625867

Zhang, S., Zhang, Y., Dong, Y., Guo, L., Zhang, Z., Shao, B., et al. (2020). Knockdown of Foxg1 in supporting cells increases the trans-differentiation of supporting cells into hair cells in the neonatal mouse cochlea. *Cell. Mol. Life Sci.* 77, 1401–1419. doi: 10.1007/s00018-019-03291-2

Zhang, Y., Zhang, S., Zhang, Z., Dong, Y., Ma, X., Qiang, R., et al. (2020). Knockdown of Foxg1 in Sox9+ supporting cells increases the trans-differentiation of supporting cells into hair cells in the neonatal mouse utricle. *Aging (Albany, NY)* 12, 19834–19851. doi: 10.18632/aging.104009

Zhong, Z., Fu, X., Li, H., Chen, J., Wang, M., Gao, S., et al. (2020). Citicoline protects auditory hair cells against neomycin-induced damage. *Front. Cell Dev. Biol.* 8:712. doi: 10.3389/fcell.2020.00712

Zhou, H., Qian, X., Xu, N., Zhang, S., Zhu, G., Zhang, Y., et al. (2020). Disruption of Atg7-dependent autophagy causes electromotility disturbances, outer hair cell loss, and deafness in mice. *Cell Death Dis.* 11:913. doi: 10.1038/s41419-020-03110-8

Zilberstein, Y., Liberman, M. C., and Corfas, G. (2012). Inner hair cells are not required for survival of spiral ganglion neurons in the adult cochlea. *J. Neurosci.* 32, 405–410. doi: 10.1523/JNEUROSCI.4678-11.2012

Hearing Loss in Neurological Disorders

Siyu Li[1,2†], Cheng Cheng[1,2†], Ling Lu[1,2†], Xiaofeng Ma[1†], Xiaoli Zhang[1,2†], Ao Li[1,2], Jie Chen[1,2]*, Xiaoyun Qian[1,2]* and Xia Gao[1,2]*

[1] Department of Otolaryngology Head and Neck Surgery, Affiliated Drum Tower Hospital of Nanjing University Medical School, Jiangsu Provincial Key Medical Discipline (Laboratory), Nanjing, China, [2] Research Institute of Otolaryngology, Nanjing, China

*Correspondence:
Jie Chen
njjiechen@163.com
Xiaoyun Qian
qxy522@163.com
Xia Gao
xiagaogao@hotmail.com

†These authors have contributed equally to this work

Sensorineural hearing loss (SNHL) affects approximately 466 million people worldwide, which is projected to reach 900 million by 2050. Its histological characteristics are lesions in cochlear hair cells, supporting cells, and auditory nerve endings. Neurological disorders cover a wide range of diseases affecting the nervous system, including Alzheimer's disease (AD), Parkinson's disease (PD), Huntington's disease (HD), autism spectrum disorder (ASD), etc. Many studies have revealed that neurological disorders manifest with hearing loss, in addition to typical nervous symptoms. The prevalence, manifestations, and neuropathological mechanisms underlying vary among different diseases. In this review, we discuss the relevant literature, from clinical trials to research mice models, to provide an overview of auditory dysfunctions in the most common neurological disorders, particularly those associated with hearing loss, and to explain their underlying pathological and molecular mechanisms.

Keywords: hearing loss, neurodegenerative diseases, autism spectrum disorder, pathological mechanisms, molecular mechanisms

INTRODUCTION

Hearing loss is defined by an average pure-tone threshold detection exceeding 20 dB, affecting approximately 466 million people worldwide. According to the value of pure tone thresholds, it can be classified as mild (20–35 dB), moderate (35–50 dB), moderately severe (50–65 dB), severe (65–80 dB), profound (80–95 dB), and total ($\geq$95 dB) hearing loss. Lesions in the cochlea, auditory nerve, and central auditory pathway induce sensorineural hearing loss (SNHL); nearly a third of the population over the age of 65 is suffering from it[1]. Histological characteristics of age-related hearing loss include degenerative pathology in cochlear hair cells, supporting cells, and auditory nerve endings, resulting in irreversible damage to the sensory epithelium of the cochlea (He et al., 2020; Keithley, 2020; Wu et al., 2020b). Sound is collected and conducted by the external and middle ear, then transformed into electrical signals by cochlear mechanosensory cells: the inner and outer hair cells (OHCs) (Dallos, 1986). OHCs function to enhance sound frequency selectivity

---
[1] https://www.who.int

and mechanical amplification, and inner hair cells (IHCs) are responsible for subsequent sound detection and transmission. Hair cells are sensitive to aging, acoustic trauma, ototoxic drugs (Fu et al., 2021b), and environmental or genetic influences (Wang et al., 2017; Qian et al., 2020; Fu et al., 2021a; Lv et al., 2021). As damages to either type of hair cells can result in permanent SNHL, many studies have focused on biological treatments for hearing restoration, including gene therapy, hair cell regeneration, etc. (Liu et al., 2016; Li et al., 2018b; Chen et al., 2021; He et al., 2021). These electrical signals are then transduced to the auditory cortex by spiral ganglion neurons (SGNs). SGNs are located in the Rosenthal's canal of the cochlea and work as the primary sensory neurons to connect the peripheral and central auditory systems, which are susceptible to aging and ototoxic drugs. Hence, preventing the degeneration of SGNs carries critical implications for improving the restoration of hearing (Appler and Goodrich, 2011; Coate and Kelley, 2013; Sun et al., 2016; Liu et al., 2019, 2021; Guo et al., 2021). The pulses ascend into the cochlear nuclei, superior olivary complex, and inferior colliculus for the perception of time and intensity, then target toward the medial geniculate body, and finally, the auditory information is integrated into and further processed by the auditory cortex (Grothe et al., 2010; Profant et al., 2015; Wu et al., 2015). The ascending and reversed descending pathways (originating from the cerebral cortex to the cochlea) form the complete auditory circuitry. Pathology in any portion of the auditory circuitry will lead to auditory dysfunctions, including hearing impairments and central auditory processing disorder, which can be addressed through pure tone audiometry (PTA) and speech tests (such as speech discrimination and speech-in-noise tests). The effects of hearing loss are widespread and profound, resulting in social isolation, psychological illness. And hearing loss is reported to be closely associated with cognitive decline and dementia independently in the elderly population (Lin et al., 2011a, 2013; Jafari et al., 2019).

Neurological disorders include a broad range of diseases that affect the nervous system, of which neurodegenerative diseases and neurodevelopmental disorders have been widely discussed. In the elderly, neurodegenerative diseases are common causes of morbidity and cognitive impairment (Kritsilis et al., 2018; Hou et al., 2019). The progression of these diseases is characterized by the diffusion of protein aggregates, which correlates with clinical severity (Ross and Poirier, 2004; Herrero and Morelli, 2017; Davis et al., 2018). Autism spectrum disorder (ASD) is a neurodevelopmental disorder characterized by social isolation, stereotypical behaviors, and interests. Genetic and environmental risk factors jointly account for phenotypic variations in ASD (Johnson et al., 2007; Lai et al., 2014a). Recent studies have reported that patients suffering from these neurological disorders are accompanied by hearing impairments and other auditory dysfunctions, especially in Alzheimer's disease (AD), Parkinson's disease (PD), Huntington's disease (HD), and ASD. Meanwhile, many mechanisms may account for the complex interplay, including neuropathological changes in the central and peripheral auditory system, social isolation caused by hearing decline, or other potential molecular mechanisms (Fortunato et al., 2016; Shen et al., 2018). It remains unclear whether auditory dysfunction is intrinsic or secondary to these diseases. Here, we discuss the relevant clinical literature to review the most common neurological disorders, particularly those associated with hearing loss, and explain their underlying pathological and molecular mechanisms.

ALZHEIMER'S DISEASE

Alzheimer's disease is a progressive neurodegenerative disorder and the most common form of dementia. One in 10 people aged over 65 years is affected by AD, and the incidence increases with age (Soria Lopez et al., 2019; Alzheimer's Association, 2020). Late-onset AD (LOAD) is the onset of AD later than 65 years of age, accounting for approximately 94% of all cases. Symptomatic AD exhibits insidious impairments in learning and memory at the initial stage, and then progresses toward impairments in cognition and executive function at the later stage (Long and Holtzman, 2019). AD patients are usually present with deficient perceptual and semantic processing of sounds (Perez et al., 2009; Benarroch, 2010; Ruan et al., 2012; Attems et al., 2014; Albers et al., 2015; van Wijngaarden et al., 2017). Since the 1980s, the association between hearing impairments and AD has been discussed. Evidence has shown that cognitive impairment is often accompanied by hearing loss, and in turn, hearing loss increases the incidence of cognitive decline and AD (Gallacher et al., 2012; Hung et al., 2015; Panza et al., 2015; Fortunato et al., 2016; Ford et al., 2018). Ford et al. (2018) estimated that midlife hearing loss might account for 9.1% of dementia cases globally. Lin et al. (2011a) demonstrated that for every 10 dB increase above the pure tone threshold of 25 dB, the risk of dementia increased by approximately 20%, with risk ratios for mild, moderate, and severe hearing loss of 1.89, 3.00, and 4.94, respectively. Taljaard et al. (2016) conducted a meta-analysis illustrating that hearing impairments coexisted with more inferior cognitive ability in older individuals, and receiving hearing interventions improved cognitive outcomes.

Neuropathological changes in the auditory system of AD have been widely explored, and typical AD pathological changes have been observed in auditory pathways (Uhlmann et al., 1986). Extracellular amyloid-β (Aβ) peptide aggregation and intracellular neurofibrillary tangles (NFTs) are the neuropathological hallmarks of AD (**Figure 1**; Long and Holtzman, 2019). In the amyloidogenic pathway, amyloid precursor proteins (APP) are membrane proteins that are sequentially cleaved by β-secretase and γ-secretase, resulting in the release of extracellular amyloid-β peptides, where they clump together to form deposits (Aβ plaques) and initiate a cascade of pathogenic processes and neurodegeneration. Tau protein plays a critical role in the development of neurons, and its hyperphosphorylation leads to the production of NFTs. Aβ peptides and NFTs coalesce to induce cellular dysfunctions (inflammation, oxidative stress, etc.), synaptic loss, and neurodegeneration (Guo et al., 2017; Makin, 2018). Genetically, AD is classified into familial (FAD) and sporadic cases. FAD accounts for 5% of AD cases and has an autosomal dominant

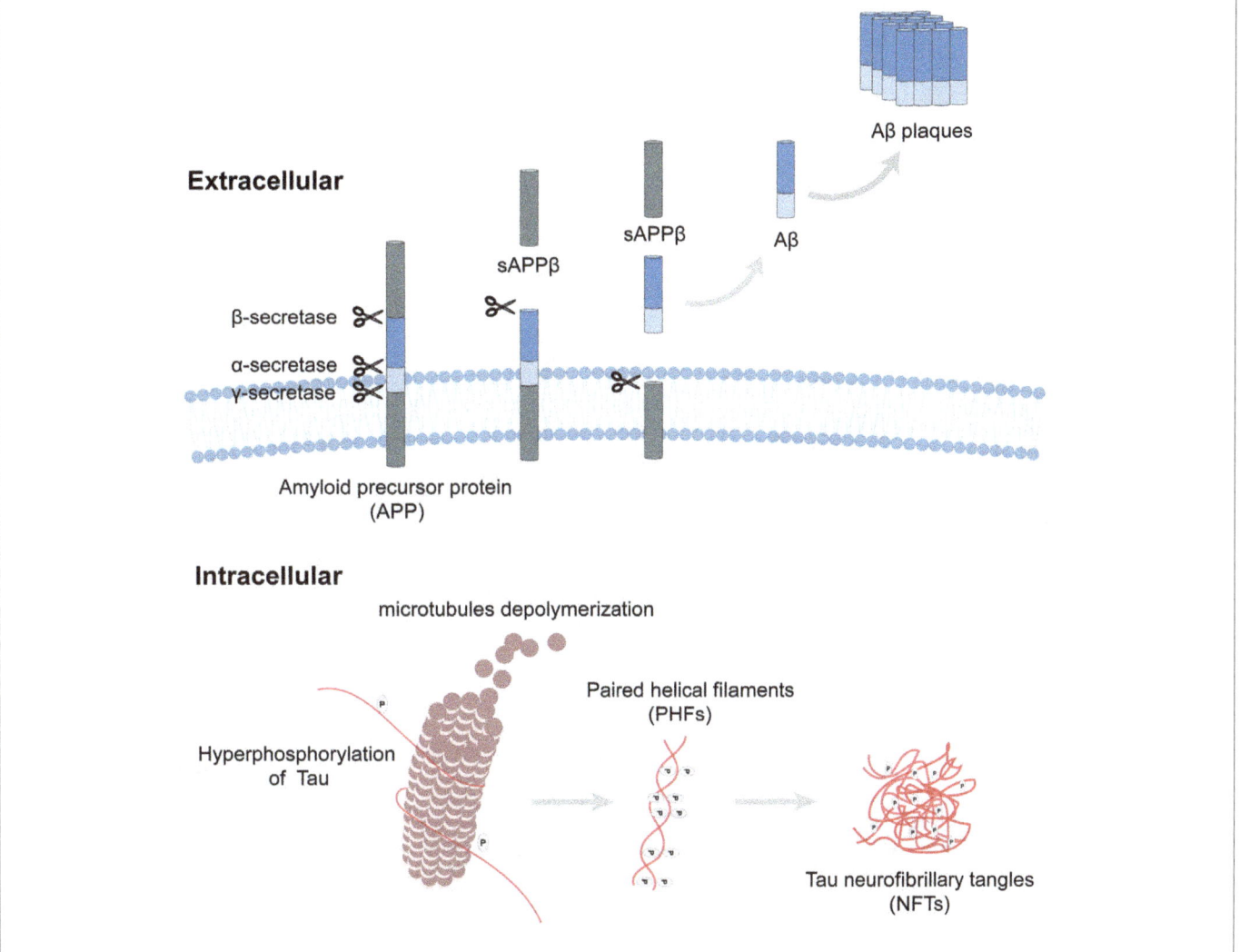

FIGURE 1 | Amyloid plaque formation extracellular and tau pathology intracellular. Amyloid precursor protein (APP) is a transmembrane protein that can be cleaved by three kinds of secretases. In the process of amyloid plaque formation, APP is cleaved by β-secretase and γ-secretase sequentially, then amyloid-β peptides release to extracellular and clump together to form deposits (Aβ plaques). Tau plays a critical role in microtubule assembly and stabilization, hyperphosphorylation of tau leads to microtubules depolymerization, and paired helical filaments (PHF) aggregate to form tau neurofibrillary tangles (NFTs).

inheritance pattern. Mutations in *APP*, *PSEN1* (Presenilin 1), and *PSEN2* (Presenilin 2) are responsible for the occurrence of FAD, and it was reported that mutations in these genes alter APP processing, induce Aβ formation, and then initiate tau pathology. In contrast, more than 90% of AD patients appear sporadically, which usually presents with late-onset AD (Piaceri et al., 2013). The only confirmed risk gene for sporadic AD is apolipoprotein E (APOE), which encodes an amino acid lipoprotein that can bind to amyloid precursor proteins. The Epsilon4 allele in APOE is strongly associated with an increased risk of AD in either homozygous or heterozygous states. Over 60% of sporadic cases are unrelated to APOE, suggesting that the interplay of genetic and environmental elements contributes to the occurrence of sporadic AD (Verghese et al., 2011). Similar neuropathology is also observed in sporadic AD without such mutations, indicating that Aβ plaques may be the driving force behind tau pathology, but not the sole one (van der Kant et al., 2020).

In the early stage of AD, brain atrophy occurs in the central auditory cortex and related functional nuclei; senile plaques (SPs) and NFTs are extensively distributed throughout relay stations in the ascending auditory pathway (Sinha et al., 1993; Parvizi et al., 2001; Rub et al., 2016). Many AD mouse models have been used to explore hearing dysfunction and their underlying mechanisms (summarized in **Table 1**). Studies have shown that AD mouse models initially exhibit high-frequency hearing loss and finally progress to the entire frequency. 5xFAD and APP/PS1 mice are mainly characterized by β-amyloid plaque deposition and show elevated auditory brainstem response (ABR) thresholds. 5xFAD mice co-express gene mutations in five FAD and can generate Aβ deposits rapidly (Oakley et al., 2006). In 5xFAD mice, amyloid depositions were observed at 2 months of age, while cochlear histopathology revealed a large amount of apical and basal hair cell loss at 13 months of age (O'Leary et al., 2017). The onset of auditory dysfunctions in APP/PS1

TABLE 1 | List of AD, HD, ASD mice models that have been used for auditory function and anatomy study.

	Mice lines	Mutations	Neuropathological abnormalities/manifestations	Auditory dysfunction	Auditory circuit anatomy	Reporter and year of publication
AD	3xTg-AD	APP PSEN1 Tau	• Neuroinflammation: 6-month-old • Aβ deposits: Initiate at 6-month-old Apparent at 12-month-old • Tau pathology: 12-month-old • Synaptic dysfunction	• ABR: thresholds increased at 9-month-old • DPOAE: normal	• SGNs loss: at 9–12 months	Wang and Wu, 2015
	5xFAD	APP K670N/M671L (Swedish) + I716V (Florida) + V717I (London) PS1 M146L + L286V	• Aβ deposition: Onset at 2-month-old Apparent at 4-month-old • Neurodegeneration and cognitive deficits: 4–5 months	• ASR: thresholds elevated at 3–4 months • ABR: thresholds increased at 8–32 kHz at 13–14 months	• HC loss: Apical and basal IHCs And OHCs at 15–16 months	O'Leary et al., 2017
	APP/PS1	APP PSEN1	• Aβ deposition: 6–7 months	• ABR: 1) High frequency increased at 2–3 months; 2) Whole frequency increased at 3–4 months; 3) Wave IV and V reduction at 3-month-old • DPOAE 16 and 20 kHz increased at 3-month-old • CM: normal	/	Liu et al., 2021
HD	Hdh(CAG)^{150}	Huntingtin knock-in	• mHtt aggregation: at 10–14 months	• ABR: thresholds at 4 and 8 kHz increased at 15-month-old	• Spiral ganglion/the organ of Corti: 1) mHtt aggregation; 2) Reduced CKB expression; 3) At 15–20 months	Lin et al., 2011b
	R6/2	Huntingtin (around 150 CAG repeats)	• mHtt aggregation: 5–6 weeks of age	• ABR: thresholds increased at 2–3 months • DPOAE: thresholds increased at 2–3 months	• Reduced prestin level: at 3-month-old • HC loss: at 3-month-old • SGNs loss: at 3-month-old	Wang and Wu, 2015
ASD	16p11.2 deletion ±	16p11.2 deletion	• Low body weight • Perinatal mortality • Spontaneous locomotor activity • Sporadic motor stereotypies	• No ASR at any decibel level • No ABR to wide frequencies: Between 8 and 100 kHz;	/	Yang et al., 2015
	Cntnap2$^{-/-}$	Cntnap2 knockout	• Reduced social interaction • Hyperactivity • Repetitive behaviors • Reduced ultrasonic vocalization output	• Auditory-processing dissociation: 1) Impairs Silent Gap Detection 2) Enhanced Tone Discrimination	• Medial Geniculate Nucleus: 1) Reduced neuron numbers 2) Smaller neurons	Truong et al., 2015
	Adnp±	truncated Adnp	• Irregular tooth eruption • Short stature • Social and vocal impediments • Motor delays • Learning and memory deficits	• ABR: Increased thresholds; Prolonged latency; at 2.5-month-old	• Normal hair-cell morphology at P0 • Expression of autism and auditory related proteins 1) Auditory cortex: Decreased ChAT in male Adnp± Decreased PVALB in male Adnp± 2) Cerebellum: Increased GAD67 in female Adnp± Decreased VGLUT2, CX32, and ChAT in female Adnp±	Hacohen-Kleiman et al., 2019

ABR, auditory brainstem responses; ADNP, activity-dependent neuroprotective protein; APP, amyloid precursor proteins; ASR, auditory startle response; CKB, brain-type creatine kinase; CNTNAP2, contactin-associated protein-like 2; DPOAE, distortion product otoacoustic emission; HC, hair cell; IHC, inner hair cell; mHtt, mutant Huntingtin; OHC, Outer Hair Cell; PSEN1, Presenilin 1; SGNs, Spiral Ganglion Neurons.
"/" means that information on the item is not available in the relevant research.

mice preceded before neuropathological changes, suggesting that acoustic measurements might be a non-invasive indicator for AD detection (Liu et al., 2020). 3xTg-AD mice express 3 AD-related transgenes, and its neuropathology developments are similar to FAD patients, characterized by Aβ deposition, tau pathology, and neuroinflammation. In 3xTg-AD mice, a reduction of SGN's relative densities was observed at 9–12 months of age. A transgenic mouse model with overexpression of Aβ peptides in hair cells was established by Omata et al. (2016) and high-frequency hearing impairments were found at 4 months of age. Aligned with the electrophysiological assessment, basal hair cell loss was observed. They further established another model overexpressing tau pathology but found no significant hearing dysfunctions. Nevertheless, double transgenic mice showed an advanced and exaggerated hearing impairments, suggesting that Aβ deposition was a fundamental pathological etiology for hearing defects exhibited by AD and that tau pathology enhanced the dysfunction (Omata et al., 2016). Many previous studies have shown that both oxidative stress and apoptosis play essential roles in the death of hair cells (Yu et al., 2017; Li et al., 2018a), whether hair cell loss observed in the researches can be attributed to Aβ-induced oxidative stress and cell apoptosis need further study.

Clinical literature suggests that midlife hearing loss is independently correlated with accelerated progression of sporadic AD and incident dementia. The degree of hearing loss was positively associated with an increased risk of dementia. AD-related neuropathology was found in the central auditory pathway but was not clinically identified in the peripheral auditory pathway. Although multiple clinical studies have been designed to determine the relationship between hearing loss and AD, there are still some flaws in the experimental design. Most of the important information has been neglected, including the extent of hearing loss, measurements of auditory processing, differences between sexes, and auditory condition in different AD classifications, resulting in restricted access to information to determine the relationship between auditory dysfunction and AD. Mouse model studies further illustrated that hearing loss is associated with AD development. In the APP/PS1 mouse model, the shifts of ABR and distortion product otoacoustic emission (DPOAE) preceded the neuropathy observed in the brain. Loss of hair cells and SGNs was observed in AD mouse models, which was likely induced by the spread of AD-related neuropathology (Aβ deposition and tau pathology) in the cochlea. However, the three AD-related mouse models were all designed with mutations in FAD genes, which could not completely mimic the pathogenesis of sporadic AD. The central auditory pathway has not yet been studied in these mouse models. High-frequency hearing loss has been observed in patients with AD and incident dementia. Moreover, both the central and peripheral auditory pathways are affected by AD-related neuropathology, but the concrete cochlear pathology is still debated. The results vary among studies due to different mouse models, sampling times, and hearing measurements. Hence, for a comprehensive understanding of AD-related hearing loss, standard observation criteria should be established in further studies.

HUNTINGTON'S DISEASE

Huntington's disease is an autosomal-dominantly inherited disorder with a mean prevalence of 2.71 per 100,000 individuals worldwide (Pringsheim et al., 2012). HD manifests with midlife cognitive impairment, motor incoordination, and psychiatric symptoms (Martin and Gusella, 1986; Walker, 2007). Late-stage HD patients often present with auditory sensory, processing, and memory problems other than typical dysfunctions. Studies have illustrated that hearing impairment is involved in and is closely correlated with motor deficits in HD (Josiassen et al., 1984; Lin et al., 2011b). Lin et al. (2011b) recruited 19 HD patients and assessed hearing impairments using PTA and ABR. The PTA thresholds showed that an average increase of 15 dB was detected in high frequencies of HD patients, and no significant differences were observed in latency and inter-peak intervals of ABRs, indicating that hearing impairments in HD were more associated with the peripheral auditory pathway than retrocochlear lesions (Lin et al., 2011b). In contrast, other researchers found that HD patients displayed normal sound sensation, but with a significant decrease in speech understanding and sound source lateralization, suggesting that HD-associated neuropathology affects the central auditory system (cortical and subcortical parts) (Beste et al., 2008; Saft et al., 2008; Profant et al., 2017). Wetter et al. (2005) revealed that HD patients had delayed auditory event-related potentials (ERPs), which were also found in individuals at risk for HD. These findings showed HD-related dysfunction during sound processing (Homberg et al., 1986; Josiassen et al., 1988; Wetter et al., 2005).

The pathophysiological mechanisms underlying HD-related auditory dysfunction are poorly understood; nonetheless, recent studies in transgenic mouse models provide new insight into these mechanisms (Walker, 2007). Aggregated mutant huntingtin (mHtt) is the most classic cellular pathological characteristic of HD; extra amplificated CAG repeats in exon 1 of *huntingtin* lead to polyglutamine (polyQ) extension at the N-terminal of Htt protein, and mutant Htt accumulates to cause neuronal loss (**Figure 2**; Macdonald et al., 1993; Mangiarini et al., 1996; Ha and Fung, 2012). Neuronal loss preferentially affects the cortico-striatal circuits, which leads to characteristic chorea, and as HD progresses, mHtt spreads to peripheral tissues, including the inner ear (Vonsattel and DiFiglia, 1998; Cepeda et al., 2007; Snowden, 2017). Mouse models were also used to illustrate auditory dysfunction and pathology in HD (summarized in **Table 1**). R6/2-HD mice express mHtt and present with HD-related phenotypes at 5–6 weeks of age. Lin et al. (2011b) found that R6/2-HD mice exhibited approximately 10 dB elevation of ABR thresholds at 2 months of age before the presentation of motor deficits. After 3 weeks, the motor defects became apparent, and a 30 dB threshold shift for click stimuli and a 15 dB threshold shift for tone bursts at all frequencies were also observed. In addition, they found no difference in ABR latency and peak intervals between R6/2-HD mice and wild type mice (Lin et al., 2011b). As described in Wang's research, R6/2-HD mice exhibited increased distortion product otoacoustic emission and ABR thresholds at 2–3 months of age. Furthermore, the relative expression of prestin was reduced in OHCs, which was

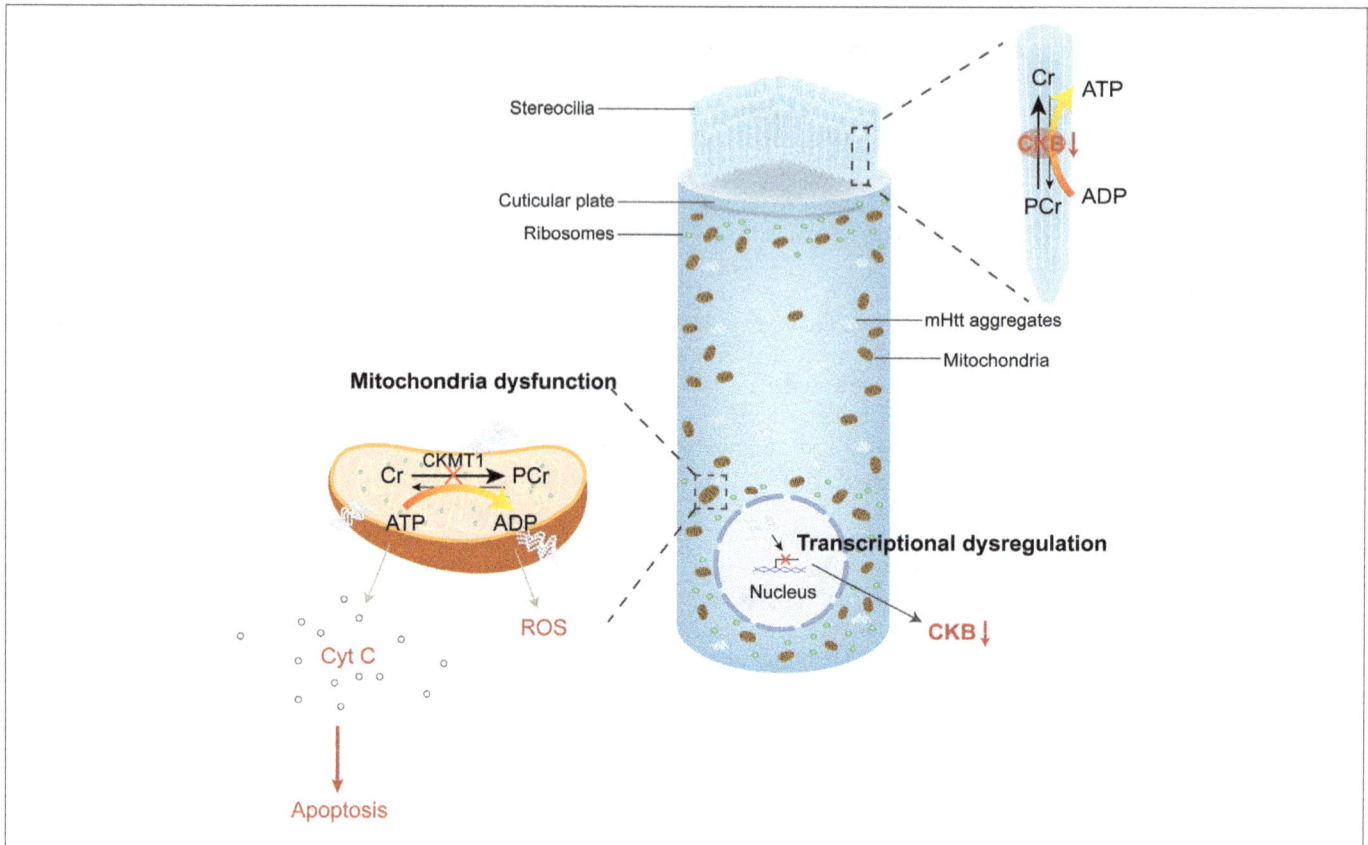

FIGURE 2 | mHtt aggregates induced toxicity and dysregulated PCr-CK system in hair cells. The PCr-CK system plays a critical role in providing ATP in hair bundles of hair cells, mitochondrial creatine kinase (CKMT1) phosphorylates creatine (Cr) to phosphocreatine (PCr). In the stereocilia, brain-type creatine kinase (CKB) regenerates ATP from PCr. Expression of mHtt in hair cells impairs the function of mitochondria, releases cytochrome C and reactive oxygen species (ROS) to the cytoplasm. On the other hand, mHtt aggregates lead to protein sequestration (including many transcriptional factors), then induce transcriptional dysregulation, which reduces the expression of CKB (creatine kinase).

reported to be responsible for dysfunction in hearing sensitivity and frequency selectivity. Cochlear SGN reduction and hair cell loss (especially OHCs) were observed histologically after that (Wang and Wu, 2015), suggesting that mHtt pathology in the central and peripheral auditory system contributed to the presence of hearing impairments in HD. Hdh(CAG)^{150} mice are knock-in mice that carry 150 CAG repeats on the Htt locus, of which mHtt aggregation in the nervous system and HD-related characteristics initiate at approximately 10 months of age. In Hdh(CAG)^{150} mice, thresholds measured by click and tone bursts ABR analysis at 15 months of age revealed that approximately 20 dB thresholds were increased for click and tone bursts at frequencies of 4 and 8 kHz. No differences were observed at frequencies of 16 and 32 kHz because wild type mice developed presbycusis at 15 months of age (Lin et al., 2011b). Moreover, aggregated mHtt and continuing loss of brain-type creatine kinase (CKB), which was previously reported to decline in HD patients, were both obtained in the organ of Corti and the spiral ganglion in both mouse models (Perluigi et al., 2005; Sorolla et al., 2008; Kim et al., 2010; Lin et al., 2011b). Aggregation of mHtt is thought to affect many transcriptional factors and induce mitochondrial dysfunction, which directly leads to the release of cytochrome C and oxidative stress (Kim and Kim, 2014). CKB, a cytosolic enzyme, can regenerate ATP by reversibly transferring high-energy phosphate from phosphocreatine (PCr) to ADP (Jacobus and Lehninger, 1973; Wallimann et al., 1992; Wyss and Kaddurah-Daouk, 2000). CKB also localizes in cochlear hair cells and ligaments and is critical for hearing function (Spicer and Schulte, 1992; Spicer et al., 1997). CKB-knockout mice presented with high-tone hearing loss that can be restored by dietary creatine supplements (Shin et al., 2007; Lin et al., 2011c). These studies suggest that CKB dysregulation may be associated with HD-related auditory dysfunction, synergistic with mHtt (**Figure 2**).

Auditory dysfunction appears to be authentic for HD. Clinical studies have shown that hearing impairments and auditory processing dysfunction are present in HD patients. Delayed ERPs are suggested to be a potential predictor of HD. While there is no consensus that auditory sense, processing, or discrimination is uniparted or jointly present in HD, more research objectives, detailed acoustic measurements, and specified auditory items should be included. Hearing impairment is solid in HD mouse models, and hearing loss precedes the occurrence of motor defects and worsens with the progression of HD in R6/2-HD mice. The loss of hair cells and SGNs was also observed. Hdh(CAG)^{150} mice exhibited significant low-frequency hearing impairment compared to wild type mice, which was accompanied by presbycusis-related high-frequency hearing loss, suggesting that hearing impairments in HD patients was not merely related to the auditory pathway degeneration caused by natural aging and clarifying that hearing loss was authentic to HD, while the cochlear anatomy has not been assessed in Hdh(CAG)^{150} mice. Moreover, pathological studies of the central auditory pathway, including cochlear nuclei, superior olivary complex, and auditory cortex, should be performed to determine auditory-related lesions and guide auditory-related tests carried out for HD patients and high-risk groups.

PARKINSON'S DISEASE

Parkinson's disease is a neurodegenerative disorder characterized by static tremor, bradykinesia, rigidity, and postural instability, affecting 1–2 per 1,000 individuals (Dorsey et al., 2007; Ascherio and Schwarzschild, 2016). Before the onset of typical motor symptoms, patients with PD often manifest with cognitive impairment, olfactory dysfunction, fatigue, etc. (Postuma et al., 2012; Khoo et al., 2013). Recently, hearing impairment has been considered as another non-motor feature in PD patients. Studies have shown that the incidence of developing PD in the hearing loss group was 1.77 higher than in the control group (Lai et al., 2014b), and high-frequency hearing impairment was observed in PD patients without self-perceiving (Yylmaz et al., 2009; Santos-Garcia et al., 2010; Shetty et al., 2019), which is positively related to PD duration and worsens as it progresses (Scarpa et al., 2020). PTA results showed an average elevation of 10 dB in 4 and 8 kHz in PD patients, and significantly increased latencies in wave V and interpeak were obtained (Yylmaz et al., 2009). PTA performed among the relatively younger (age < 55 years old) population of PD showed that thresholds were elevated at high frequency and low to mid frequencies. This ratio was even higher for low-mid-frequency hearing loss. Concurrently, the brain stem auditory-evoked potentials were comparable to the control group, indicating that hearing loss in PD was independent of aging and that the underlying mechanism appeared to be peripheral according to the study (Shetty et al., 2019). Vitale et al. (2013) calculated the proportion of different degrees of hearing loss in 75 patients with PD and found that 89% of them had mild to moderate hearing loss, and 11% had severe hearing loss. In addition, they revealed that the prevalence of PD with hearing impairments was higher in the male elderly (Vitale et al., 2013). Whole frequencies of distortion product otoacoustic emission thresholds in PD patients also increased. It can be alleviated by dopaminergic treatment (Georgiev et al., 2015; Pisani et al., 2015), which uncovered an undermined dopamine-dependent cochlear dysfunction undermined. Sisto et al. (2020) found that the ipsilateral cochlear dysfunction developed in parallel with asymmetric motor impairment. The abilities of speech discrimination and sound lateralization were also markedly reduced in PD patients (Lewald et al., 2004; Vitale et al., 2016; Folmer et al., 2017), and abnormal auditory evoked potentials were suggested as a measurement of PD duration and severity (Yylmaz et al., 2009; Jafari et al., 2020).

The association between hearing dysfunction and PD suggests a common neuropathological background. Lewy pathology and dopaminergic neuronal degeneration are two primary neuropathological features of PD that spread as PD progresses (Dickson et al., 2009; Dickson, 2012; Kordower et al., 2013). Other protein aggregations, such as Aβ plaques and NFTs, are also present in the nervous system of PD patients (Kalia and Lang, 2015). Lewy pathology consists of insoluble misfolded α-synuclein that can be found in certain regions of the central and peripheral nervous system in PD (Wakabayashi et al., 1989; Spillantini et al., 1997; Beach et al., 2010; Del Tredici et al., 2010; Goedert et al., 2013). In the inner ear, α-synuclein is located predominantly in the efferent neuronal system, especially in the OHC, and contributes to the physiological maintenance of auditory function. Hence, Lewy pathology in the auditory system has been speculated to be associated with PD-related auditory disorders (Akil et al., 2008; Park et al., 2011). On the other hand, common neurotransmitters between the auditory system and basal ganglia were indicated by the curative effect of dopaminergic therapy on auditory responses (Rey et al., 1996; Erro et al., 2015; Georgiev et al., 2015; Pisani et al., 2015). Furthermore, dopamine and glutamate mediate the synaptic interplay oppositely in the basal ganglia. In the auditory system, dopamine also counteracts the excitotoxic effects caused by glutamate to modulate auditory processing and neural plasticity. Since glutamate overdose can induce excitotoxic damage to primary auditory neurons, it was speculated that excessive glutamate caused by the degeneration of dopaminergic neurons might account for PD-related auditory dysfunction (Lendvai et al., 2011). Other common underlying mechanisms, including mitochondrial dysfunction, reduced neurotransmitter levels, perturbed protein homeostasis, and oxidative stress, have also been discussed in previous studies (Simon and Johns, 1999; Raza et al., 2019).

There have been no reports on auditory dysfunction and auditory anatomy in PD mouse model. Although manipulation of specific genes reported in familial PD, including transgenic overexpression for α-synuclein and leucine-rich repeat kinase 2 and knockout models for Parkin, DJ-1, phosphatase, and tensin homolog-induced novel kinase 1, made it possible to establish many mouse models, none of them recapitulate key clinical and neuropathological features of PD entirely, especially in the absence of neurodegeneration of dopaminergic neurons (Dawson et al., 2010). While the objective is to gain insight into the molecular mechanisms underlying auditory dysfunction and PD, studies of auditory function in mouse models with specific gene mutations are still needed. PD is a global neurodegenerative disorder that affects the central and peripheral nervous system, and extensive literature indicated a broad range of auditory dysfunctions from the peripheral auditory system to cortical areas in PD (Pekkonen et al., 1995; Kofler et al., 2001; Putzki et al., 2008; Bronnick et al., 2010; Pisani et al., 2015; Potter-Nerger et al., 2015; Seidel et al., 2015; Liu et al., 2017; Shalash et al., 2017; Guducu et al., 2019), asymptomatic hearing impairments appeared to be a newly non-motor manifestation of both early and late-onset PD, and it can be speculated that the natural aging process combined with PD-related neurodegenerative changes coalesce to induce that. Moreover, the central auditory dysfunctions, including abnormal speech discrimination and sound lateralization, cannot be ignored. The literature suggests hearing measurement as a non-invasive potential biomarker and indicator of disease severity for PD, widespread alpha-synuclein neuropathology, and loss of dopaminergic neurons were suspected of interfering with such auditory dysfunction, and PD mouse models should be applied for precise assessment of hearing function and pathological mechanism exploration.

AUTISM SPECTRUM DISORDER

Autism spectrum disorder is a neurodevelopmental disorder characterized by social isolation, stereotypical behaviors, and interests, with a prevalence of approximately 1% worldwide and has a strong male predominance (Johnson et al., 2007; Lai et al., 2014a). Sense dysfunction, including the feeling of touch, smell, taste, vision, and hearing, is another feature of ASD. The pathogenesis of ASD is not entirely understood, but comorbidities and maternal exposures in placental life may act as risk factors (Arndt et al., 2005). Researchers have suggested that genetic polymorphisms and environmental factors jointly contribute to the phenotypic variation in ASD (Bailey et al., 1995; Veenstra-VanderWeele et al., 2004; Lopez-Rangel and Lewis, 2006). Cerebellar and brainstem hypoplasia was observed in patients with ASD (Courchesne et al., 1988; Hashimoto et al., 1992, 1995), and multiregional neuropathy defects have been identified, including a reduced number of Purkinje cells in the cerebellum, delayed neuron maturation of the forebrain, abnormal development of the frontal and temporal lobes, and sporadic malformation in the brainstem and neocortex (Hardan et al., 2004; Pickett and London, 2005; Lainhart, 2006; Wegiel et al., 2010, 2014; Hampson and Blatt, 2015). These structural abnormalities lead to typical behavioral manifestations and sense dysfunctions in ASD.

Currently, most previous studies identified increased rates of audiological dysfunctions in ASD, including hearing impairments, hyperacusis, difficulty in sound discrimination with background noise and speech sounds encoding (Tomchek and Dunn, 2007; Russo et al., 2009; Stiegler and Davis, 2010). A higher incidence of hearing loss (from unilateral to bilateral) and hyperacusis was demonstrated in the ASD population (Rosenhall et al., 1999; Demopoulos and Lewine, 2016; Do et al., 2017). Fitzpatrick et al. (2014) found that approximately 29.4% of children with ASD had profound hearing loss and that those children with hearing loss benefited from the use of hearing aids. In addition, hearing dysfunction was attributed to ASD-related neuronal degeneration of the auditory pathway (Smith et al., 2019). In contrast, Szymanski et al. (2012) found a high prevalence of ASD among children with hearing loss, supporting that peripheral auditory dysfunction may be associate with functional impairment in ASD (Demopoulos and Lewine, 2016). Previous studies have provided an abundance of evidence supporting both abnormal structure and function in the auditory brainstem of ASD, but there remains a battery of literature showing that the peripheral auditory manifestations of children with ASD were comparable to controls (Gravel et al., 2006; Tharpe et al., 2006). Beers et al. (2014) reviewed 22 articles about peripheral hearing loss in ASD and concluded that there was no solid evidence for an increased risk of peripheral hearing loss among children with ASD. Tas et al. (2007) also evaluated the auditory function of children with ASD through transient evoked otoacoustic emission and ABR. The positive emission and normal hearing level at ABR revealed an insusceptible peripheral auditory system in patients with ASD. Nevertheless, the ABR results showed a prolonged III–V interpeak latencies (IPLs) in children with autism (Rosenhall et al., 2003; Tas et al., 2007).

Approximately 10% of ASD cases have an identifiable genetic background. Many ASD-related genetic and chromosomal disorders have been shown to present with auditory dysfunction (**Table 2**), underlying a potential common genetic etiology between ASD and auditory dysfunction. Many chromosomal disorders have been reported to manifest with auditory dysfunctions, ASD, developmental retardation, seizures, facial dysmorphism, and multisystem defects. Deletions and duplications range from specific loci to large segments and comprise a considerable number of related genes. Genes with remarkably high risk accounting for these manifestations are listed in **Table 2**. Most of them are involved in neuron and synaptic development (Smith et al., 2002; Sinajon et al., 2015; Yang et al., 2015; Lahbib et al., 2019; Wu et al., 2020a), among which only two genes are known to be auditory-related: *ELMOD3* and *FGF2*. *ELMOD3* is involved in autosomal recessive non-syndromic deafness disability (Lahbib et al., 2019), and *FGF2* plays a role in the proliferation and survival of auditory neuroblasts (Wu et al., 2020a). Three monogenic disorders were reported to present with auditory dysfunction and ASD simultaneously, including Fragile X syndrome, *MEIS2* syndrome, and *ADNP* syndrome (Rotschafer et al., 2015; Douglas et al., 2018; Hacohen-Kleiman et al., 2019), related genes all function in brain development, and *MEIS2* is responsible for the development of the inner ear in chicken (Douglas et al., 2018). Restricted information about genes and their functions is insufficient to illustrate the genetic association between auditory dysfunction and ASD. Whether these certified ASD-related genes also participate in auditory function is unclear.

ASD-related mouse models have been developed to study auditory dysfunction (**Table 1**). Chromosomal disorder mice characterized by 16p 11.2 deletions showed whole frequency increased ABR and auditory startle response (ASR) thresholds, indicating that genes located in the area were responsible for auditory dysfunctions, of which *KCTD13*, *SEZ6L2*, and *MAPK3* were considered to be highly correlated with autism (Konyukh et al., 2011; Golzio et al., 2012; Blumenthal et al., 2014; Yang et al., 2015), while their relationship with the auditory function has not been determined. Monogenic disorder mice were also studied; $Fmr1^{-/-}$, $Cntnap2^{-/-}$ and $Adnp^{\pm}$ mice presented with classical characteristics of ASD and showed impaired hearing and auditory process functions. Anatomy of auditory circuits, such as the ventral cochlear nucleus and the medial nucleus of the trapezoid body exhibited reduced neuron size and number. Altered hearing-related protein levels, including VGAT, ChAT,

TABLE 2 | List of ASD-related chromosomal and monogenic disorders that have been reported co-presented with auditory dysfunction.

	Chromosomal/ genetical abnormalities	Map position	Incidence	Manifestations	Potential related genes and function	References

Chromosomal disorder	chromosomal 13q12→q13 deletion	• deletion at the distal third of band 13q12
		• deletion at the proximal two-thirds of band 13q13
			/	• auditory processing defects
				• autism spectrum disorder
				• language deficit
					• *NBEA*:
					  1) encodes a neuron-specific multidomain protein
					  2) functions as a protein kinase anchor protein
					  3) post-Golgi neuronal membrane trafficking
					• *MAB21L1*: neural development
					• *DCAMKL1*:
					  1) encodes a brain-specific transmembrane kinase
					  2) cortical development
					• *DCX*:
					  1) encodes doublecortin, a brain-specific putative signaling protein
					  2) neuronal migration
					• *MADH9*: a member of the *SMAD* family
					  1) mediate the TGF beta signaling pathway
					  2) proliferation and differentiation of many different cell types
					  3) synaptic junction differentiation
						Smith et al., 2002

	16p11.2 deletions and duplications	heterozygous deletions and duplications of 16p11.2	1% of individuals with autism	• auditory dysfunction:
				  1) hearing loss
				  2) absence of acoustic startle responses
				• autism spectrum disorder
				• developmental delays, speech delay
				• obesity (deletion) and low body weight (duplication)
				• intellectual impairment
				• psychiatric disorders
				• seizures, syringomyelia
				• cardiac defects
				• motor hypotonia
				• immune deficiency
					• *KCTD13*:
					• encodes the polymerase delta-interacting protein 1 (PDIP1)
					• regulation of cell cycle during neurogenesis
					• *SEZ6L2*: epilepsy and language disorders
					• *MAPK3*:
					  1) a member of the MAP kinase family
					  2) cellular proliferation, differentiation, and cell cycle
					• *NRX1, NRXN3*: synaptic transmission and cell-cell interaction
					• *CHD8, EHMT1, MECP2, SOX5, TBF4, SATB2, FOXP1*: chromatin modifiers and transcription factors
					• *FMR1* and *CEP290*: intellectual disability
						Yang et al., 2015

	chromosome 8q22.2-q22.3 deletion	deletion at chromosome 8q22.2-q22.3	/	• bilateral hearing loss: hypoplastic auditory canals • autism spectrum disorder • macrocephaly • childhood seizure disorder • moderate intellectual disability • facial phenotype • congenital heart defect	• *GRHL2*: non-syndromic autosomal dominant deafness gene • *VPS13B*: the causative gene for Cohen syndrome • *SPAG1*: responsible for primary ciliary dyskinesia • *RRM2B*: encodes a small subunit of p53 mitochondrial DNA disorders and depletions • *NCALD*: neuronal signal transduction process	Sinajon et al., 2015

	chromosome 2p11.2 deletion	homozygous deletion in 2p11.2	/	• hearing impairment
				• autism spectrum disorder
				• intellectual disability
				• language delay
				• behavioral disturbances
					• *ELMOD3*: involves in autosomal recessive non-syndromic deafness-88 (DFNB88)
					• *CAPG*:
					  1) member of actin regulatory proteins
					  2) cytoskeletal rearrangements regulation
					  3) involves in Rett syndrome
					• *SH2D6*: signal transduction of receptor tyrosine kinase pathways
						Lahbib et al., 2019

(Continued)

TABLE 2 | Continued

	Chromosomal/ genetical abnormalities	Map position	Incidence	Manifestations	Potential related genes and function	References

	Chromosome 4q deletion and 7q duplication	• deletion of chromosome 4
		• microduplication of chromosome 7
			/	• unilateral hearing impairment
				• autism spectrum disorder
				• multisystem malformation:
				  1) facial dysmorphism: microcephaly
				  2) ocular malformation: ocular hypertelorism; exophthalmos
				  3) auditory malformation: low-set ears
				  4) appendicular malformation: single palmar flexion crease; overlapping toes
				  6) cardiopulmonary system: discontinued cyanosis recurrent respiratory infections patent foramen ovale tracheobronchomalacia
				  6) nervous system: persistent falcine sinus with a thin corpus callosum
					• *SPATA5*:
					  1) mitochondrial function (morphology and dynamics)
					  2) neuronal development
					  3) spermatogenesis
					• *FGF2*:
					  6) Angiogenesis
					  6) cell survival, division, differentiation, and migration
					  6) proliferation and survival of auditory neuroblast
					• limb development
					• wound healing
					• tumor growth
					• *NAA15*: encodes a component of the Nat A Nacetyl-transferase complex, which tethering the complex to the ribosome for posttranslational modification of proteins
					• *SMAD1*: development of pulmonary hypertension
					• *HHIP*: development of lung malformation
						Wu et al., 2020a

Monogenic disorder	Fragile X Syndrome	• *FMR1* gene locates in Xq27.3
		• *FMR1* gene silencing by:
		• amplification of a CGG repeat
		• methylation of the promoter region
			1 in 1250 males and 1 in 2500 females	• hearing loss:
				  1) elevated cortical responses to sound stimuli
				  2) aberrant ABRs
				• autism spectrum disorder
				• cognitive impairments
				• seizures
				• aberrant dendritic spine morphology
				• enhancement of response to sensory stimuli
					• a modulator of mRNA translation
					• regulates synaptic proteins production
						Rotschafer et al., 2015

	MEIS2(MRG1)	locates in chromosome 15q14	/	• hearing loss • autism spectrum disorder • atrial or ventricular septal defect • developmental delay • intellectual disability • short stature • cleft palate • gastrointestinal, skeletal, limb, and skin abnormalities	• encodes a homeodomain protein implicated as a transcriptional activator • cell proliferation • development of inner ear in chickens • development of heart, brain, limb • differentiation of various tissues and organs	Douglas et al., 2018
	ADNP syndrome	locates in chromosome 20	0.17% of individuals with autism	• mild hearing loss: > 10% of children • autism spectrum disorder • intellectual, motor, social, and speech delays/disabilities	• regulates ion channels genes • regulates the protein translation process • neural tube closure • associates with the cytoskeleton • synaptic plasticity • microtubule-dependent axonal transport • dendritic spine formation • brain development • mental function	Hacohen-Kleiman et al., 2019

CAPG, Capping Actin Protein, Gelsolin Like; CEP290, Centrosomal Protein 290; CHD8: Chromodomain Helicase Dna Binding Protein 8; DCAMKL1, Doublecortin Like Kinase 1; DCX, Doublecortin; EHMT1, Euchromatic Histone Lysine Methyltransferase 1; ELMOD3, Domain Containing 3; FGF2, Fibroblast Growth Factor-2; FMR1, Fmrp Translational Regulator 1; FOXP1, Forkhead Box P1; GRHL2, Grainyhead Like Transcription Factor 2; HHIP, Hedgehog Interacting Protein; KCTD13, Potassium Channel Tetramerization Domain Containing 13; MAB21L, Mab-21 Like 1; MADH9, Smad Family Member 9; MAPK3, Mitogen-Activated Protein Kinase 3; MECP2, Methyl-Cpg Binding Protein 2; NAA15, N-Alpha-Acetyltransferase 15; NBEA, Neurobeachin; NCALD, Neurocalcin Delta; NRX1, nucleoredoxin 1; NRXN3, neurexin 3; RRM2B, ribonucleotide reductase regulatory TP53 inducible subunit M2B; SATB2, SATB homeobox 2; SEZ6L2, seizure related 6 homolog like 2; SH2D6, SH2 domain containing 6; SMAD1, SMAD family member 1; SOX5, SRY-box transcription factor 5; SPAG1, sperm associated antigen 1; SPATA5, spermatogenesis associated 5; VPS13B, vacuolar protein sorting 13 homolog.
"/" means that information on the item is not available in the relevant research.

and GAD67, were observed in the auditory cortex and cerebellum (Rotschafer et al., 2015; Ruby et al., 2015; Truong et al., 2015; Hacohen-Kleiman et al., 2019), underlying a central auditory and synaptic pathology.

Increased rates of auditory dysfunction, including hearing impairments, hyperacusis, difficulties in sound discrimination, and speech sounds encoding, were detected in patients with ASD. ASD children with hearing impairments were identified later than those with normal hearing for auditory disorders and related communication delays. Although hearing impairment is an uncommon manifestation of ASD, both diseases affect communication abilities in children, and hearing impairment may contribute to the development of ASD. Comprehensive audiological assessments of confirmed and suspected ASD in children and early hearing interventions are recommended to improve social communication and reduce the aggression of ASD. ASD with chromosomal and monogenetic disorders has been shown to manifest with hearing impairments and auditory process problems, which correspond to auditory dysfunctions in ASD mouse models, and reduced neuron size and number were observed in auditory brainstem nuclei. Studies have also reviewed the genes that might be involved in chromosomal and monogenetic disorders. They concluded that most of them function in neuronal development, suggesting that defective neuropathy in the auditory pathway leads to hearing dysfunction and raises the idea that ASD-related genes may act as potential deafness genes. Hence, specific transgenic mouse models should be applied to clarify their function and influence on the auditory system. For further analysis, next-generation sequencing should be applied to identify more potential ASD-related candidate genes for deafness.

CONCLUSION AND PERSPECTIVES

In this review, we presented research on hearing loss in four common neurological disorders (AD, PD, HD, and ASD) and concluded that hearing loss was present in these four disorders. However, the related auditory lesions and underlying mechanisms vary among them.

In AD, high-frequency hearing loss was observed in both the patient and mouse models. Moreover, Aβ deposition appeared to be the initial neurological etiology. Auditory studies on AD mouse models raise the possibility that the auditory pathway is more sensitive to AD-related neuropathology and auditory dysfunction, especially hearing loss, presents before the onset of cognitive impairments. Thus, auditory measurements can provide a reference for preliminary diagnosis and early interventions for patients with AD. Hearing impairments and auditory processing dysfunction have been observed in HD patients. In R6/2-HD mice, hearing loss precedes the characterized presentations of HD, and in the SGNs of Hdh(CAG)^{150} mice, mHtt aggregation was observed. However, for a comprehensive understanding of auditory dysfunction in AD and HD, more clinical trials involving more subjects and including a variety of detailed auditory measurements should be carried out, and complete studies on auditory circuitry (from the cochlea to the auditory cortex) of mouse models should be conducted in the future.

A broad range of auditory dysfunctions, including hearing loss, abnormal speech discrimination, and sound lateralization, have been reported in PD, and asymptomatic hearing impairments appear to be a new non-motor symptom of PD patients, and hearing measurements may act as a non-invasive potential biomarker and indicator of disease severity. There are no transgenic mouse models that can completely mimic the important neuropathological features of PD, especially the neurodegeneration of dopaminergic neurons. Hence, better PD mouse models should be established, and to gain insight into the underlying molecular mechanisms, auditory studies in existing mouse models still worth exploring.

Many auditory dysfunctions, including hearing impairments, hyperacusis, difficulty in sound discrimination, and speech sound encoding, have been detected in patients with ASD. Concomitant hearing loss makes the diagnosis of ASD more challenging. As both disorders affect communication abilities in children and early hearing interventions have been reported to improve social communication and reduce aggression in ASD, comprehensive audiological assessments should be carried out in confirmed and suspected ASD in children. Moreover, approximately 10% of ASD cases have an identifiable genetic background. Clinical and transgenic mouse model studies revealed the involvement of hearing impairments, raising the possibility that associated genes may act as potential deafness genes. Hence, more potential ASD-related candidate genes should be identified, and specific transgenic mouse models should be applied to explore the function of autism-related genes in the auditory system.

Sensorineural hearing loss affects a large population of people worldwide, and the impact of hearing loss is broad and profound, including delayed language development in children, social isolation, and psychological illness. Hearing loss is not only present in neurological disorders mentioned above but can also affect the prognosis of these diseases to some extent. Hence, exploring hearing loss in neurological disorders is beneficial for understanding the pathogenesis and improving the prognosis of these diseases.

AUTHOR CONTRIBUTIONS

SL and CC wrote the manuscript. LL, XM, XZ, and AL collated the resource. JC, XQ, and XG wrote and reviewed the manuscript. All authors contributed to the article and approved the submitted version.

FUNDING

This work was supported by the National Natural Science Foundation of China (82071059, 82071044, 81970884, 81900941, 81970885, 81900944, 81870721, and 81771019), the Natural Science Foundation of Jiangsu Province (BK20190121), the Jiangsu Provincial Key Research and Development Fund (BE2018605), and the China Postdoctoral Science Foundation (2020M681555).

REFERENCES

Alzheimer's Association (2020). 2020 Alzheimer's disease facts and figures. *Alzheimers Dement.* 16, 391–460. doi: 10.1002/alz.12068

Akil, O., Weber, C. M., Park, S. N., Ninkina, N., Buchman, V., and Lustig, L. R. (2008). Localization of synucleins in the mammalian cochlea. *J. Assoc. Res. Otolaryngol.* 9, 452–463. doi: 10.1007/s10162-008-0134-y

Albers, M. W., Gilmore, G. C., Kaye, J., Murphy, C., Wingfield, A., Bennett, D. A., et al. (2015). At the interface of sensory and motor dysfunctions and Alzheimer's disease. *Alzheimers Dement.* 11, 70–98. doi: 10.1016/j.jalz.2014.04.514

Appler, J. M., and Goodrich, L. V. (2011). Connecting the ear to the brain: molecular mechanisms of auditory circuit assembly. *Prog. Neurobiol.* 93, 488–508. doi: 10.1016/j.pneurobio.2011.01.004

Arndt, T. L., Stodgell, C. J., and Rodier, P. M. (2005). The teratology of autism. *Int. J. Dev. Neurosci.* 23, 189–199. doi: 10.1016/j.ijdevneu.2004.11.001

Ascherio, A., and Schwarzschild, M. A. (2016). The epidemiology of Parkinson's disease: risk factors and prevention. *Lancet Neurol* 15, 1257–1272. doi: 10.1016/s1474-4422(16)30230-7

Attems, J., Walker, L., and Jellinger, K. A. (2014). Olfactory bulb involvement in neurodegenerative diseases. *Acta Neuropathol.* 127, 459–475. doi: 10.1007/s00401-014-1261-7

Bailey, A., Lecouteur, A., Gottesman, I., Bolton, P., Simonoff, E., Yuzda, E., et al. (1995). Autism as a strongly genetic disorder - evidence from a British twin study. *Psychol. Med.* 25, 63–77. doi: 10.1017/S0033291700028099

Beach, T. G., Adler, C. H., Sue, L. I., Vedders, L., Lue, L., White Iii, C. L., et al. (2010). Multi-organ distribution of phosphorylated alpha-synuclein histopathology in subjects with Lewy body disorders. *Acta Neuropathol.* 119, 689–702. doi: 10.1007/s00401-010-0664-3

Beers, A. N., McBoyle, M., Kakande, E., Dar Santos, R. C., and Kozak, F. K. (2014). Autism and peripheral hearing loss: a systematic review. *Int. J. Pediatr. Otorhinolaryngol.* 78, 96–101. doi: 10.1016/j.ijporl.2013.10.063

Benarroch, E. E. (2010). Olfactory system: functional organization and involvement in neurodegenerative disease. *Neurology* 75, 1104–1109. doi: 10.1212/WNL.0b013e3181f3db84

Beste, C., Saft, C., Gunturkun, O., and Falkenstein, M. (2008). Increased cognitive functioning in symptomatic Huntington's disease as revealed by behavioral and event-related potential indices of auditory sensory memory and attention. *J. Neurosci.* 28, 11695–11702. doi: 10.1523/JNEUROSCI.2659-08.2008

Blumenthal, I., Ragavendran, A., Erdin, S., Klei, L., Sugathan, A., Guide, J. R., et al. (2014). Transcriptional consequences of 16p11.2 deletion and duplication in mouse cortex and multiplex autism families. *Am. J. Hum. Genet.* 94, 870–883. doi: 10.1016/j.ajhg.2014.05.004

Bronnick, K. S., Nordby, H., Larsen, J. P., and Aarsland, D. (2010). Disturbance of automatic auditory change detection in dementia associated with Parkinson's disease: a mismatch negativity study. *Neurobiol. Aging* 31, 104–113. doi: 10.1016/j.neurobiolaging.2008.02.021

Cepeda, C., Wu, N., Andre, V. M., Cummings, D. M., and Levine, M. S. (2007). The corticostriatal pathway in Huntington's disease. *Prog. Neurobiol.* 81, 253–271. doi: 10.1016/j.pneurobio.2006.11.001

Chen, Y., Gu, Y., Li, Y., Li, G. L., Chai, R., Li, W., et al. (2021). Generation of mature and functional hair cells by co-expression of Gfi1, Pou4f3, and Atoh1 in the postnatal mouse cochlea. *Cell Rep.* 35:109016. doi: 10.1016/j.celrep.2021.109016

Coate, T. M., and Kelley, M. W. (2013). Making connections in the inner ear: recent insights into the development of spiral ganglion neurons and their connectivity with sensory hair cells. *Semin. Cell Dev. Biol.* 24, 460–469. doi: 10.1016/j.semcdb.2013.04.003

Courchesne, E., Yeungcourchesne, R., Press, G. A., Hesselink, J. R., and Jernigan, T. L. (1988). Hypoplasia of cerebellar vermal Lobule-Vi and Lobule-Vii in autism. *N. Engl. J. Med.* 318, 1349–1354. doi: 10.1056/Nejm198805263182102

Dallos, P. (1986). Neurobiology of cochlear inner and outer hair cells: intracellular recordings. *Hear. Res.* 22, 185–198. doi: 10.1016/0378-5955(86)90095-x

Davis, A. A., Leyns, C. E. G., and Holtzman, D. M. (2018). Intercellular spread of protein aggregates in neurodegenerative disease. *Annu. Rev. Cell Dev. Biol.* 34, 545–568. doi: 10.1146/annurev-cellbio-100617-062636

Dawson, T. M., Ko, H. S., and Dawson, V. L. (2010). Genetic animal models of Parkinson's disease. *Neuron* 66, 646–661. doi: 10.1016/j.neuron.2010.04.034

Del Tredici, K., Hawkes, C. H., Ghebremedhin, E., and Braak, H. (2010). Lewy pathology in the submandibular gland of individuals with incidental Lewy body disease and sporadic Parkinson's disease. *Acta Neuropathol.* 119, 703–713. doi: 10.1007/s00401-010-0665-2

Demopoulos, C., and Lewine, J. D. (2016). Audiometric profiles in autism spectrum disorders: does subclinical hearing loss impact communication? *Autism Res.* 9, 107–120. doi: 10.1002/aur.1495

Dickson, D. W. (2012). Parkinson's disease and parkinsonism: neuropathology. *Cold Spring Harb. Perspect. Med.* 2:a009258. doi: 10.1101/cshperspect.a009258

Dickson, D. W., Braak, H., Duda, J. E., Duyckaerts, C., Gasser, T., Halliday, G. M., et al. (2009). Neuropathological assessment of Parkinson's disease: refining the diagnostic criteria. *Lancet Neurol.* 8, 1150–1157. doi: 10.1016/S1474-4422(09)70238-8

Do, B., Lynch, P., Macris, E. M., Smyth, B., Stavrinakis, S., Quinn, S., et al. (2017). Systematic review and meta-analysis of the association of Autism spectrum disorder in visually or hearing impaired children. *Ophthalmic Physiol. Opt.* 37, 212–224. doi: 10.1111/opo.12350

Dorsey, E. R., Constantinescu, R., Thompson, J. P., Biglan, K. M., Holloway, R. G., Kieburtz, K., et al. (2007). Projected number of people with Parkinson disease in the most populous nations, 2005 through 2030. *Neurology* 68, 384–386. doi: 10.1212/01.wnl.0000247740.47667.03

Douglas, G., Cho, M. T., Telegrafi, A., Winter, S., Carmichael, J., Zackai, E. H., et al. (2018). De novo missense variants in MEIS2 recapitulate the microdeletion phenotype of cardiac and palate abnormalities, developmental delay, intellectual disability and dysmorphic features. *Am. J. Med. Genet. A* 176, 1845–1851. doi: 10.1002/ajmg.a.40368

Erro, R., Picillo, M., Amboni, M., Moccia, M., Vitale, C., Longo, K., et al. (2015). Nonmotor predictors for levodopa requirement in de novo patients with Parkinson's disease. *Mov. Disord.* 30, 373–378. doi: 10.1002/mds.26076

Fitzpatrick, E. M., Lambert, L., Whittingham, J., and Leblanc, E. (2014). Examination of characteristics and management of children with hearing loss and autism spectrum disorders. *Int. J. Audiol.* 53, 577–586. doi: 10.3109/14992027.2014.903338

Folmer, R. L., Vachhani, J. J., Theodoroff, S. M., Ellinger, R., and Riggins, A. (2017). Auditory processing abilities of Parkinson's disease patients. *Biomed. Res. Int.* 2017:2618587. doi: 10.1155/2017/2618587

Ford, A. H., Hankey, G. J., Yeap, B. B., Golledge, J., Flicker, L., and Almeida, O. P. (2018). Hearing loss and the risk of dementia in later life. *Maturitas* 112, 1–11. doi: 10.1016/j.maturitas.2018.03.004

Fortunato, S., Forli, F., Guglielmi, V., De Corso, E., Paludetti, G., Berrettini, S., et al. (2016). A review of new insights on the association between hearing loss and cognitive decline in ageing. *Acta Otorhinolaryngol. Ital.* 36, 155–166. doi: 10.14639/0392-100X-993

Fu, X., An, Y., Wang, H., Li, P., Lin, J., Yuan, J., et al. (2021a). Deficiency of Klc2 induces low-frequency sensorineural hearing loss in C57BL/6 J mice and human. *Mol. Neurobiol.* doi: 10.1007/s12035-021-02422-w

Fu, X., Wan, P., Li, P., Wang, J., Guo, S., Zhang, Y., et al. (2021b). Mechanism and prevention of ototoxicity induced by aminoglycosides. *Front. Cell Neurosci.* 15:692762. doi: 10.3389/fncel.2021.692762

Gallacher, J., Ilubaera, V., Ben-Shlomo, Y., Bayer, A., Fish, M., Babisch, W., et al. (2012). Auditory threshold, phonologic demand, and incident dementia. *Neurology* 79, 1583–1590. doi: 10.1212/WNL.0b013e31826e263d

Georgiev, D., Jahanshahi, M., Dreo, J., Cus, A., Pirtosek, Z., and Repovs, G. (2015). Dopaminergic medication alters auditory distractor processing in Parkinson's disease. *Acta Psychol.* 156, 45–56. doi: 10.1016/j.actpsy.2015.02.001

Goedert, M., Spillantini, M. G., Del Tredici, K., and Braak, H. (2013). 100 years of Lewy pathology. *Nat. Rev. Neurol.* 9, 13–24. doi: 10.1038/nrneurol.2012.242

Golzio, C., Willer, J., Talkowski, M. E., Oh, E. C., Taniguchi, Y., Jacquemont, S., et al. (2012). KCTD13 is a major driver of mirrored neuroanatomical phenotypes of the 16p11.2 copy number variant. *Nature* 485, 363–367. doi: 10.1038/nature11091

Gravel, J. S., Dunn, M., Lee, W. W., and Ellis, M. A. (2006). Peripheral audition of children on the autistic spectrum. *Ear Hear.* 27, 299–312. doi: 10.1097/01.aud.0000215979.65645.22

Grothe, B., Pecka, M., and McAlpine, D. (2010). Mechanisms of sound localization in mammals. *Physiol. Rev.* 90, 983–1012. doi: 10.1152/physrev.00026.2009

Guducu, C., Eskicioglu, E., Oz, D., Oniz, A., Cakmur, R., and Ozgoren, M. (2019). Auditory brain oscillatory responses in drug-naive patients with Parkinson's disease. *Neurosci. Lett.* 701, 170–174. doi: 10.1016/j.neulet.2019.02.039

Guo, R. R., Li, J., Chen, C. T., Xiao, M., Liao, M. H., Hu, Y. N., et al. (2021). Biomimetic 3D bacterial cellulose-graphene foam hybrid scaffold regulates neural stem cell proliferation and differentiation. *Colloids Surf. B-Biointerfaces* 200:111590. doi: 10.1016/j.colsurfb.2021.111590

Guo, T., Noble, W., and Hanger, D. P. (2017). Roles of tau protein in health and disease. *Acta Neuropathol.* 133, 665–704. doi: 10.1007/s00401-017-1707-9

Ha, A. D., and Fung, V. S. (2012). Huntington's disease. *Curr. Opin. Neurol.* 25, 491–498. doi: 10.1097/WCO.0b013e3283550c97

Hacohen-Kleiman, G., Yizhar-Barnea, O., Touloumi, O., Lagoudaki, R., Avraham, K. B., Grigoriadis, N., et al. (2019). Atypical auditory brainstem response and protein expression aberrations related to asd and hearing loss in the adnp haploinsufficient mouse brain. *Neurochem. Res.* 44, 1494–1507. doi: 10.1007/s11064-019-02723-6

Hampson, D. R., and Blatt, G. J. (2015). Autism spectrum disorders and neuropathology of the cerebellum. *Front. Neurosci.* 9:420. doi: 10.3339/fnins.2075.00420

Hardan, A. Y., Jou, R. J., Keshavan, M. S., Varma, R., and Minshew, N. J. (2004). Increased frontal cortical folding in autism: a preliminary MRI study. *Psychiatry Res.* 131, 263–268. doi: 10.1016/j.pscychresns.2004.06.001

Hashimoto, T., Tayama, M., Miyazaki, M., Sakurama, N., Yoshimoto, T., Murakawa, K., et al. (1992). Reduced brainstem size in children with autism. *Brain Dev.* 14, 94–97. doi: 10.1016/s0387-7604(12)80093-3

Hashimoto, T., Tayama, M., Murakawa, K., Yoshimoto, T., Miyazaki, M., Harada, M., et al. (1995). Development of the brainstem and cerebellum in autistic patients. *J. Autism Dev. Disord.* 25, 1–18. doi: 10.1007/BF02178163

He, Z. H., Li, M., Fang, Q. J., Liao, F. L., Zou, S. Y., Wu, X., et al. (2021). FOXG1 promotes aging inner ear hair cell survival through activation of the autophagy pathway. *Autophagy* 1–22. doi: 10.1080/15548627.2021.1916194

He, Z. H., Zou, S. Y., Li, M., Liao, F. L., Wu, X., Sun, H. Y., et al. (2020). The nuclear transcription factor FoxG1 affects the sensitivity of mimetic aging hair cells to inflammation by regulating autophagy pathways. *Redox Biol.* 28:101364. doi: 10.1016/j.redox.2019.101364

Herrero, M. T., and Morelli, M. (2017). Multiple mechanisms of neurodegeneration and progression. *Prog. Neurobiol.* 155:1. doi: 10.1016/j.pneurobio.2017.06.001

Homberg, V., Hefter, H., Granseyer, G., Strauss, W., Lange, H., and Hennerici, M. (1986). Event-related potentials in patients with Huntington's disease and relatives at risk in relation to detailed psychometry. *Electroencephalogr. Clin. Neurophysiol.* 63, 552–569. doi: 10.1016/0013-4694(86)90143-4

Hou, Y., Dan, X., Babbar, M., Wei, Y., Hasselbalch, S. G., Croteau, D. L., et al. (2019). Ageing as a risk factor for neurodegenerative disease. *Nat. Rev. Neurol.* 15, 565–581. doi: 10.1038/s41582-019-0244-7

Hung, S. C., Liao, K. F., Muo, C. H., Lai, S. W., Chang, C. W., and Hung, H. C. (2015). Hearing loss is associated with risk of Alzheimer's disease: a case-control study in older people. *J. Epidemiol.* 25, 517–521. doi: 10.2188/jea.JE20140147

Jacobus, W. E., and Lehninger, A. L. (1973). Creatine kinase of rat heart mitochondria. coupling of creatine phosphorylation to electron transport. *J. Biol. Chem.* 248, 4803–4810.

Jafari, Z., Kolb, B. E., and Mohajerani, M. H. (2019). Age-related hearing loss and tinnitus, dementia risk, and auditory amplification outcomes. *Ageing Res. Rev.* 56:100963. doi: 10.1016/j.arr.2019.100963

Jafari, Z., Kolb, B. E., and Mohajerani, M. H. (2020). Auditory dysfunction in Parkinson's disease. *Mov. Disord.* 35, 537–550. doi: 10.1002/mds.28000

Johnson, C. P., Myers, S. M., and American Academy of Pediatrics Council on Children With Disabilities (2007). Identification and evaluation of children with autism spectrum disorders. *Pediatrics* 120, 1183–1215. doi: 10.1542/peds.2007-2361

Josiassen, R. C., Shagass, C., Mancall, E. L., and Roemer, R. A. (1984). Auditory and visual evoked potentials in Huntington's disease. *Electroencephalogr. Clin. Neurophysiol.* 57, 113–118. doi: 10.1016/0013-4694(84)90169-x

Josiassen, R. C., Shagass, C., Roemer, R. A., and Mancall, E. (1988). A sensory evoked potential comparison of persons 'at risk' for Huntington's disease and hospitalized neurotic patients. *Int. J. Psychophysiol.* 6, 281–289. doi: 10.1016/0167-8760(88)90015-3

Kalia, L. V., and Lang, A. E. (2015). Parkinson's disease. *Lancet* 386, 896–912. doi: 10.1016/s0140-6736(14)61393-3

Keithley, E. M. (2020). Pathology and mechanisms of cochlear aging. *J. Neurosci. Res.* 98, 1674–1684. doi: 10.1002/jnr.24439

Khoo, T. K., Yarnall, A. J., Duncan, G. W., Coleman, S., O'Brien, J. T., Brooks, D. J., et al. (2013). The spectrum of nonmotor symptoms in early Parkinson disease. *Neurology* 80, 276–281. doi: 10.1212/WNL.0b013e31827deb74

Kim, J., Amante, D. J., Moody, J. P., Edgerly, C. K., Bordiuk, O. L., Smith, K., et al. (2010). Reduced creatine kinase as a central and peripheral biomarker in Huntington's disease. *Biochim. Biophys. Acta Mol. Basis Dis.* 1802, 673–681. doi: 10.1016/j.bbadis.2010.05.001

Kim, S., and Kim, K. T. (2014). Therapeutic approaches for inhibition of protein aggregation in Huntington's disease. *Exp. Neurobiol.* 23, 36–44. doi: 10.5607/en.2014.23.1.36

Kofler, M., Muller, J., Wenning, G. K., Reggiani, L., Hollosi, P., Bosch, S., et al. (2001). The auditory startle reaction in parkinsonian disorders. *Mov. Disord.* 16, 62–71. doi: 10.1002/1531-8257(200101)16:1<62::aid-mds1002>3.0.co;2-v

Konyukh, M., Delorme, R., Chaste, P., Leblond, C., Lemiere, N., Nygren, G., et al. (2011). Variations of the candidate SEZ6L2 gene on Chromosome 16p11.2 in patients with autism spectrum disorders and in human populations. *PLoS One* 6:e17289. doi: 10.1371/journal.pone.0017289

Kordower, J. H., Olanow, C. W., Dodiya, H. B., Chu, Y., Beach, T. G., Adler, C. H., et al. (2013). Disease duration and the integrity of the nigrostriatal system in Parkinson's disease. *Brain* 136(Pt 8), 2419–2431. doi: 10.1093/brain/awt192

Kritsilis, M., Rizou, S. V., Koutsoudaki, P. N., Evangelou, K., Gorgoulis, V. G., and Papadopoulos, D. (2018). Ageing, cellular senescence and neurodegenerative disease. *Int. J. Mol. Sci.* 19:2937. doi: 10.3390/ijms19102937

Lahbib, S., Leblond, C. S., Hamza, M., Regnault, B., Lemee, L., Mathieu, A., et al. (2019). Homozygous 2p11.2 deletion supports the implication of ELMOD3 in hearing loss and reveals the potential association of CAPG with ASD/ID etiology. *J. Appl. Genet.* 60, 49–56. doi: 10.1007/s13353-018-0472-3

Lai, M.-C., Lombardo, M. V., and Baron-Cohen, S. (2014a). Autism. *Lancet* 383, 896–910. doi: 10.1016/s0140-6736(13)61539-1

Lai, S. W., Liao, K. F., Lin, C. L., Lin, C. C., and Sung, F. C. (2014b). Hearing loss may be a non-motor feature of Parkinson's disease in older people in Taiwan. *Eur. J. Neurol.* 21, 752–757. doi: 10.1111/ene.12378

Lainhart, J. E. (2006). Advances in autism neuroimaging research for the clinician and geneticist. *Am. J. Med. Genet. C Semin. Med. Genet.* 142C, 33–39. doi: 10.1002/ajmg.c.30080

Lendvai, B., Halmos, G. B., Polony, G., Kapocsi, J., Horvath, T., Aller, M., et al. (2011). Chemical neuroprotection in the cochlea: the modulation of dopamine release from lateral olivocochlear efferents. *Neurochem. Int.* 59, 150–158. doi: 10.1016/j.neuint.2011.05.015

Lewald, J., Schirm, S. N., and Schwarz, M. (2004). Sound lateralization in Parkinson's disease. *Brain Res. Cogn. Brain Res.* 21, 335–341. doi: 10.1016/j.cogbrainres.2004.06.008

Li, A., You, D., Li, W. Y., Cui, Y. J., He, Y. Z., Li, W., et al. (2018a). Novel compounds protect auditory hair cells against gentamycin-induced apoptosis by maintaining the expression level of H3K4me2. *Drug Deliv.* 25, 1033–1043. doi: 10.1080/10717544.2018.1461277

Li, H., Song, Y. D., He, Z. H., Chen, X. Y., Wu, X. M., Li, X. F., et al. (2018b). Meclofenamic acid reduces reactive oxygen species accumulation and apoptosis, inhibits excessive autophagy, and protects hair cell-like HEI-OC1 cells from Cisplatin-induced damage. *Front. Cell. Neurosci.* 12:139. doi: 10.3389/fncel.2018.00139

Lin, F. R., Metter, E. J., O'Brien, R. J., Resnick, S. M., Zonderman, A. B., and Ferrucci, L. (2011a). Hearing loss and incident dementia. *Arch. Neurol.* 68, 214–220. doi: 10.1001/archneurol.2010.362

Lin, F. R., Yaffe, K., Xia, J., Xue, Q. L., Harris, T. B., Purchase-Helzner, E., et al. (2013). Hearing loss and cognitive decline in older adults. *JAMA Intern. Med.* 173, 293–299. doi: 10.1001/jamainternmed.2013.1868

Lin, Y. S., Chen, C. M., Soong, B. W., Wu, Y. R., Chen, H. M., Yeh, W. Y., et al. (2011b). Dysregulated brain creatine kinase is associated with hearing impairment in mouse models of Huntington disease. *J. Clin. Invest.* 121, 1519–1523. doi: 10.1172/JCI43220

Lin, Y. S., Wang, C. H., and Chern, Y. (2011c). Besides Huntington's disease, does brain-type creatine kinase play a role in other forms of hearing impairment resulting from a common pathological cause? *Aging* 3, 657–662. doi: 10.18632/aging.100338

Liu, C., Zhang, Y., Tang, W., Wang, B., Wang, B., and He, S. (2017). Evoked potential changes in patients with Parkinson's disease. *Brain Behav.* 7:e00703. doi: 10.1002/brb3.703

Liu, L., Chen, Y., Qi, J., Zhang, Y., He, Y., Ni, W., et al. (2016). Wnt activation protects against neomycin-induced hair cell damage in the mouse cochlea. *Cell Death Dis.* 7:e2136. doi: 10.1038/cddis.2016.35

Liu, W. W., Xu, L., Wang, X., Zhang, D. G., Sun, G. Y., Wang, M., et al. (2021). PRDX1 activates autophagy via the PTEN-AKT signaling pathway to protect against cisplatin-induced spiral ganglion neuron damage. *Autophagy* 1–23. doi: 10.1080/15548627.2021.1905466

Liu, W. W., Xu, X. C., Fan, Z. M., Sun, G. Y., Han, Y. C., Zhang, D. G., et al. (2019). Wnt signaling activates TP53-induced glycolysis and apoptosis regulator and protects against cisplatin-induced spiral ganglion neuron damage in the mouse cochlea. *Antioxid. Redox Signal.* 30, 1389–1410. doi: 10.1089/ars.2017.7288

Liu, Y., Fang, S., Liu, L. M., Zhu, Y., Li, C. R., Chen, K., et al. (2020). Hearing loss is an early biomarker in APP/PS1 Alzheimer's disease mice. *Neurosci. Lett.* 717:134705. doi: 10.1016/j.neulet.2019.134705

Long, J. M., and Holtzman, D. M. (2019). Alzheimer disease: an update on pathobiology and treatment strategies. *Cell* 179, 312–339. doi: 10.1016/j.cell.2019.09.001

Lopez-Rangel, E., and Lewis, M. E. (2006). Loud and clear evidence for gene silencing by epigenetic mechanisms in autism spectrum and related neurodevelopmental disorders. *Clin. Genet.* 69, 21–22. doi: 10.1111/j.1399-0004.2006.00543a.x

Lv, J., Fu, X., Li, Y., Hong, G., Li, P., Lin, J., et al. (2021). Deletion of Kcnj16 in mice does not alter auditory function. *Front. Cell. Dev. Biol.* 9:630361. doi: 10.3389/fcell.2021.630361

Macdonald, M. E., Ambrose, C. M., Duyao, M. P., Myers, R. H., Lin, C., Srinidhi, L., et al. (1993). A novel gene containing a trinucleotide repeat that is expanded and unstable on Huntingtons-disease chromosomes. *Cell* 72, 971–983. doi: 10.1016/0092-8674(93)90585-E

Makin, S. (2018). The amyloid hypothesis on trial. *Nature* 559, S4–S7. doi: 10.1038/d41586-018-05719-4

Mangiarini, L., Sathasivam, K., Seller, M., Cozens, B., Harper, A., Hetherington, C., et al. (1996). Exon 1 of the HD gene with an expanded CAG repeat is sufficient to cause a progressive neurological phenotype in transgenic mice. *Cell* 87, 493–506. doi: 10.1016/S0092-8674(00)81369-0

Martin, J. B., and Gusella, J. F. (1986). Huntington's disease. pathogenesis and management. *N. Engl. J. Med.* 315, 1267–1276. doi: 10.1056/NEJM198611133152006

O'Leary, T. P., Shin, S., Fertan, E., Dingle, R. N., Almuklass, A., Gunn, R. K., et al. (2017). Reduced acoustic startle response and peripheral hearing loss in the 5xFAD mouse model of Alzheimer's disease. *Genes Brain Behav.* 16, 554–563. doi: 10.1111/gbb.12370

Oakley, H., Cole, S. L., Logan, S., Maus, E., Shao, P., Craft, J., et al. (2006). Intraneuronal beta-amyloid aggregates, neurodegeneration, and neuron loss in transgenic mice with five familial Alzheimer's disease mutations: potential factors in amyloid plaque formation. *J. Neurosci.* 26, 10129–10140. doi: 10.1523/JNEUROSCI.1202-06.2006

Omata, Y., Tharasegaran, S., Lim, Y. M., Yamasaki, Y., Ishigaki, Y., Tatsuno, T., et al. (2016). Expression of amyloid-beta in mouse cochlear hair cells causes an early-onset auditory defect in high-frequency sound perception. *Aging* 8, 427–439. doi: 10.18632/aging.100899

Panza, F., Solfrizzi, V., and Logroscino, G. (2015). Age-related hearing impairment-a risk factor and frailty marker for dementia and AD. *Nat. Rev. Neurol.* 11, 166–175. doi: 10.1038/nrneurol.2015.12

Park, S. N., Back, S. A., Choung, Y. H., Kim, H. L., Akil, O., Lustig, L. R., et al. (2011). alpha-Synuclein deficiency and efferent nerve degeneration in the mouse cochlea: a possible cause of early-onset presbycusis. *Neurosci. Res.* 71, 303–310. doi: 10.1016/j.neures.2011.07.1835

Parvizi, J., Van Hoesen, G. W., and Damasio, A. (2001). The selective vulnerability of brainstem nuclei to Alzheimer's disease. *Ann. Neurol.* 49, 53–66. doi: 10.1002/1531-8249(200101)49:1<53::aid-ana30>3.0.co;2-q

Pekkonen, E., Jousmaki, V., Reinikainen, K., and Partanen, J. (1995). Automatic auditory discrimination is impaired in Parkinson's disease. *Electroencephalogr. Clin. Neurophysiol.* 95, 47–52. doi: 10.1016/0013-4694(94)00304-4

Perez, S. E., Lumayag, S., Kovacs, B., Mufson, E. J., and Xu, S. (2009). Beta-amyloid deposition and functional impairment in the retina of the APPswe/PS1DeltaE9 transgenic mouse model of Alzheimer's disease. *Invest. Ophthalmol. Vis. Sci.* 50, 793–800. doi: 10.1167/iovs.08-2384

Perluigi, M., Poon, H. F., Maragos, W., Pierce, W. M., Klein, J. B., Calabrese, V., et al. (2005). Proteomic analysis of protein expression and oxidative modification in r6/2 transgenic mice: a model of Huntington disease. *Mol. Cell Proteomics* 4, 1849–1861. doi: 10.1074/mcp.M500090-MCP200

Piaceri, I., Nacmias, B., and Sorbi, S. (2013). Genetics of familial and sporadic Alzheimer's disease. *Front. Biosci.* 5:167–177. doi: 10.2741/e605

Pickett, J., and London, E. (2005). The neuropathology of autism: a review. *J. Neuropathol. Exp. Neurol.* 64, 925–935. doi: 10.1097/01.jnen.0000186921.42592.6c

Pisani, V., Sisto, R., Moleti, A., Di Mauro, R., Pisani, A., Brusa, L., et al. (2015). An investigation of hearing impairment in de-novo Parkinson's disease patients: a preliminary study. *Park. Relat. Disord.* 21, 987–991. doi: 10.1016/j.parkreldis.2015.06.007

Postuma, R. B., Aarsland, D., Barone, P., Burn, D. J., Hawkes, C. H., Oertel, W., et al. (2012). Identifying prodromal Parkinson's disease: pre-motor disorders in Parkinson's disease. *Mov. Disord.* 27, 617–626. doi: 10.1002/mds.24996

Potter-Nerger, M., Govender, S., Deuschl, G., Volkmann, J., and Colebatch, J. G. (2015). Selective changes of ocular vestibular myogenic potentials in Parkinson's disease. *Mov. Disord.* 30, 584–589. doi: 10.1002/mds.26114

Pringsheim, T., Wiltshire, K., Day, L., Dykeman, J., Steeves, T., and Jette, N. (2012). The incidence and prevalence of Huntington's disease: a systematic review and meta-analysis. *Mov. Disord.* 27, 1083–1091. doi: 10.1002/mds.25075

Profant, O., Roth, J., Bures, Z., Balogova, Z., Liskova, I., Betka, J., et al. (2017). Auditory dysfunction in patients with Huntington's disease. *Clin. Neurophysiol.* 128, 1946–1953. doi: 10.1016/j.clinph.2017.07.403

Profant, O., Tintera, J., Balogova, Z., Ibrahim, I., Jilek, M., and Syka, J. (2015). Functional changes in the human auditory cortex in ageing. *PLoS One* 10:e0116692. doi: 10.1371/journal.pone.0116692

Putzki, N., Graf, K., Stude, P., Diener, H. C., and Maschke, M. (2008). Habituation of the auditory startle response in cervical dystonia and Parkinson's disease. *Eur. Neurol.* 59, 172–178. doi: 10.1159/000114038

Qian, F. P., Wang, X., Yin, Z. H., Xie, G. C., Yuan, H. J., Liu, D., et al. (2020). The slc4a2b gene is required for hair cell development in zebrafish. *Aging* 12, 18804–18821. doi: 10.18632/aging.103840

Raza, C., Anjum, R., and Shakeel, N. U. A. (2019). Parkinson's disease: mechanisms, translational models and management strategies. *Life Sci.* 226, 77–90. doi: 10.1016/j.lfs.2019.03.057

Rey, R. D., Garretto, N. S., Bueri, J. A., Simonetti, D. D., Sanz, O. P., and Sica, R. E. (1996). The effect of levodopa on the habituation of the acoustic-palpebral reflex in Parkinson's disease. *Electromyogr. Clin. Neurophysiol.* 36, 357–360.

Rosenhall, U., Nordin, V., Brantberg, K., and Gillberg, C. (2003). Autism and auditory brain stem responses. *Ear Hear.* 24, 206–214. doi: 10.1097/01.AUD.0000069326.11466.7E

Rosenhall, U., Nordin, V., Sandstrom, M., Ahlsen, G., and Gillberg, C. (1999). Autism and hearing loss. *J. Autism Dev. Disord.* 29, 349–357. doi: 10.1023/a:1023022709710

Ross, C. A., and Poirier, M. A. (2004). Protein aggregation and neurodegenerative disease. *Nat. Med.* 10(Suppl.), S10–S17. doi: 10.1038/nm1066

Rotschafer, S. E., Marshak, S., and Cramer, K. S. (2015). Deletion of Fmr1 alters function and synaptic inputs in the auditory brainstem. *PLoS One* 10:e0117266. doi: 10.1371/journal.pone.0117266

Ruan, Y., Zheng, X. Y., Zhang, H. L., Zhu, W., and Zhu, J. (2012). Olfactory dysfunctions in neurodegenerative disorders. *J. Neurosci. Res.* 90, 1693–1700. doi: 10.1002/jnr.23054

Rub, U., Stratmann, K., Heinsen, H., Turco, D. D., Seidel, K., Dunnen, W., et al. (2016). The brainstem tau cytoskeletal pathology of Alzheimer's disease: a brief historical overview and description of its anatomical distribution pattern, evolutional features, pathogenetic and clinical relevance. *Curr. Alzheimer Res.* 13, 1178–1197. doi: 10.2174/1567205013666160606100509

Ruby, K., Falvey, K., and Kulesza, R. J. (2015). Abnormal neuronal morphology and neurochemistry in the auditory brainstem of Fmr1 knockout rats. *Neuroscience* 303, 285–298. doi: 10.1016/j.neuroscience.2015.06.061

Russo, N., Nicol, T., Trommer, B., Zecker, S., and Kraus, N. (2009). Brainstem transcription of speech is disrupted in children with autism spectrum disorders. *Dev. Sci.* 12, 557–567. doi: 10.1111/j.1467-7687.2008.00790.x

Saft, C., Schuttke, A., Beste, C., Andrich, J., Heindel, W., and Pfleiderer, B. (2008). fMRI reveals altered auditory processing in manifest and premanifest Huntington's disease. *Neuropsychologia* 46, 1279–1289. doi: 10.1016/j.neuropsychologia.2007.12.002

Santos-Garcia, D., Aneiros-Diaz, A., Macias-Arribi, M., Llaneza-Gonzalez, M. A., Abella-Corral, J., and Santos-Canelles, H. (2010). Sensory symptoms in Parkinson's disease. *Rev. Neurol.* 50(Suppl. 2), S65–S74.

Scarpa, A., Cassandro, C., Vitale, C., Ralli, M., Policastro, A., Barone, P., et al. (2020). A comparison of auditory and vestibular dysfunction in Parkinson's disease and multiple system atrophy. *Park. Relat. Disord.* 71, 51–57. doi: 10.1016/j.parkreldis.2020.01.018

Seidel, K., Mahlke, J., Siswanto, S., Kruger, R., Heinsen, H., Auburger, G., et al. (2015). The brainstem pathologies of Parkinson's disease and dementia with Lewy bodies. *Brain Pathol.* 25, 121–135. doi: 10.1111/bpa.12168

Shalash, A. S., Hassan, D. M., Elrassas, H. H., Salama, M. M., Mendez-Hernandez, E., Salas-Pacheco, J. M., et al. (2017). Auditory- and vestibular-evoked potentials correlate with motor and non-motor features of Parkinson's disease. *Front. Neurol.* 8:55. doi: 10.3389/fneur.2017.00055

Shen, Y., Ye, B., Chen, P., Wang, Q., Fan, C., Shu, Y., et al. (2018). cognitive decline, dementia, Alzheimer's disease and presbycusis: examination of the possible molecular mechanism. *Front. Neurosci.* 12:394. doi: 10.3389/fnins.2018.00394

Shetty, K., Krishnan, S., Thulaseedharan, J. V., Mohan, M., and Kishore, A. (2019). Asymptomatic hearing impairment frequently occurs in early-onset Parkinson's disease. *J. Mov. Disord.* 12, 84–90. doi: 10.14802/jmd.18048

Shin, J. B., Streijger, F., Beynon, A., Peters, T., Gadzala, L., McMillen, D., et al. (2007). Hair bundles are specialized for ATP delivery via creatine kinase. *Neuron* 53, 371–386. doi: 10.1016/j.neuron.2006.12.021

Simon, D. K., and Johns, D. R. (1999). Mitochondrial disorders: clinical and genetic features. *Annu. Rev. Med.* 50, 111–127.

Sinajon, P., Gofine, T., Ingram, J., and So, J. (2015). Microdeletion 8q22.2-q22.3 in a 40-year-old male. *Eur. J. Med. Genet.* 58, 569–572. doi: 10.1016/j.ejmg.2015.10.004

Sinha, U. K., Hollen, K. M., Rodriguez, R., and Miller, C. A. (1993). Auditory system degeneration in Alzheimer's disease. *Neurology* 43, 779–785. doi: 10.1212/wnl.43.4.779

Sisto, R., Viziano, A., Stefani, A., Moleti, A., Cerroni, R., Liguori, C., et al. (2020). Lateralization of cochlear dysfunction as a specific biomarker of Parkinson's disease. *Brain Commun.* 2:fcaa144. doi: 10.1093/braincomms/fcaa144

Smith, A., Storti, S., Lukose, R., and Kulesza, R. J. Jr. (2019). Structural and functional aberrations of the auditory brainstem in autism spectrum disorder. *J. Am. Osteopath. Assoc.* 119, 41–50. doi: 10.7556/jaoa.2019.007

Smith, M., Woodroffe, A., Smith, R., Holguin, S., Martinez, J., Filipek, P. A., et al. (2002). Molecular genetic delineation of a deletion of chromosome 13q12->q13 in a patient with autism and auditory processing deficits. *Cytogenet. Genome Res.* 98, 233–239. doi: 10.1159/000071040

Snowden, J. S. (2017). The neuropsychology of Huntington's disease. *Arch. Clin. Neuropsychol.* 32, 876–887. doi: 10.1093/arclin/acx086

Soria Lopez, J. A., Gonzalez, H. M., and Leger, G. C. (2019). Alzheimer's disease. *Handb. Clin. Neurol.* 167, 231–255. doi: 10.1016/B978-0-12-804766-8.00013-3

Sorolla, M. A., Reverter-Branchat, G., Tamarit, J., Ferrer, I., Ros, J., and Cabiscol, E. (2008). Proteomic and oxidative stress analysis in human brain samples of Huntington disease. *Free Radic. Biol. Med.* 45, 667–678. doi: 10.1016/j.freeradbiomed.2008.05.014

Spicer, S. S., Gratton, M. A., and Schulte, B. A. (1997). Expression patterns of ion transport enzymes in spiral ligament fibrocytes change in relation to strial atrophy in the aged gerbil cochlea. *Hear. Res.* 111, 93–102. doi: 10.1016/s0378-5955(97)00097-x

Spicer, S. S., and Schulte, B. A. (1992). Creatine kinase in epithelium of the inner ear. *J. Histochem. Cytochem.* 40, 185–192. doi: 10.1177/40.2.1313059

Spillantini, M. G., Schmidt, M. L., Lee, V. M., Trojanowski, J. Q., Jakes, R., and Goedert, M. (1997). Alpha-synuclein in Lewy bodies. *Nature* 388, 839–840. doi: 10.1038/42166

Stiegler, L. N., and Davis, R. (2010). Understanding sound sensitivity in individuals with autism spectrum disorders. *Focus Autism Other Dev. Disabil.* 25, 67–75. doi: 10.1177/1088357610364530

Sun, G., Liu, W., Fan, Z., Zhang, D., Han, Y., Xu, L., et al. (2016). The three-dimensional culture system with matrigel and neurotrophic factors preserves the structure and function of spiral ganglion neuron in vitro. *Neural Plast.* 2016:4280407. doi: 10.1155/2016/4280407

Szymanski, C. A., Brice, P. J., Lam, K. H., and Hotto, S. A. (2012). Deaf children with autism spectrum disorders. *J. Autism Dev. Disord.* 42, 2027–2037. doi: 10.1007/s10803-012-1452-9

Taljaard, D. S., Olaithe, M., Brennan-Jones, C. G., Eikelboom, R. H., and Bucks, R. S. (2016). The relationship between hearing impairment and cognitive function: a meta-analysis in adults. *Clin. Otolaryngol.* 41, 718–729. doi: 10.1111/coa.12607

Tas, A., Yagiz, R., Tas, M., Esme, M., Uzun, C., and Karasalihoglu, A. R. (2007). Evaluation of hearing in children with autism by using TEOAE and ABR. *Autism* 11, 73–79. doi: 10.1177/1362361307070908

Tharpe, A. M., Bess, F. H., Sladen, D. P., Schissel, H., Couch, S., and Schery, T. (2006). Auditory characteristics of children with autism. *Ear Hear.* 27, 430–441. doi: 10.1097/01.aud.0000224981.60575.d8

Tomchek, S. D., and Dunn, W. (2007). Sensory processing in children with and without autism: a comparative study using the short sensory profile. *Am. J. Occup. Ther.* 61, 190–200. doi: 10.5014/ajot.61.2.190

Truong, D. T., Rendall, A. R., Castelluccio, B. C., Eigsti, I. M., and Fitch, R. H. (2015). Auditory processing and morphological anomalies in medial geniculate nucleus of Cntnap2 mutant mice. *Behav. Neurosci.* 129, 731–743. doi: 10.1037/bne0000096

Uhlmann, R. F., Larson, E. B., and Koepsell, T. D. (1986). Hearing impairment and cognitive decline in senile dementia of the Alzheimer's type. *J. Am. Geriatr. Soc.* 34, 207–210. doi: 10.1111/j.1532-5415.1986.tb04204.x

van der Kant, R., Goldstein, L. S. B., and Ossenkoppele, R. (2020). Amyloid-beta-independent regulators of tau pathology in Alzheimer disease. *Nat. Rev. Neurosci.* 21, 21–35. doi: 10.1038/s41583-019-0240-3

van Wijngaarden, P., Hadoux, X., Alwan, M., Keel, S., and Dirani, M. (2017). Emerging ocular biomarkers of Alzheimer disease. *Clin. Exp. Ophthalmol.* 45, 54–61. doi: 10.1111/ceo.12872

Veenstra-VanderWeele, J., Christian, S. L., and Cook, E. H. (2004). Autism as a paradigmatic complex genetic disorder. *Annu. Rev. Genomics Hum. Genet.* 5, 379–405. doi: 10.1146/annurev.genom.5.061903.180050

Verghese, P. B., Castellano, J. M., and Holtzman, D. M. (2011). Apolipoprotein E in Alzheimer's disease and other neurological disorders. *Lancet Neurol.* 10, 241–252. doi: 10.1016/S1474-4422(10)70325-2

Vitale, C., Marcelli, V., Abate, T., Pianese, A., Allocca, R., Moccia, M., et al. (2016). Speech discrimination is impaired in parkinsonian patients: expanding the audiologic findings of Parkinson's disease. *Park. Relat. Disord.* 22(Suppl. 1), S138–S143. doi: 10.1016/j.parkreldis.2015.09.040

Vitale, C., Marcelli, V., Allocca, R., Santangelo, G., Riccardi, P., Erro, R., et al. (2013). Hearing impairment in Parkinson's disease: expanding the nonmotor phenotype (vol 27, pg 1530, 2012). *Mov. Disord.* 28, 410–410. doi: 10.1002/mds.25406

Vonsattel, J. P., and DiFiglia, M. (1998). Huntington disease. *J. Neuropathol. Exp. Neurol.* 57, 369–384. doi: 10.1097/00005072-199805000-00001

Wakabayashi, K., Takahashi, H., Takeda, S., Ohama, E., and Ikuta, F. (1989). Lewy bodies in the enteric nervous system in Parkinson's disease. *Arch. Histol. Cytol.* 52(Suppl.), 191–194. doi: 10.1679/aohc.52.suppl_191

Walker, F. O. (2007). Huntington's disease. *Lancet* 369, 218–228. doi: 10.1016/s0140-6736(07)60111-1

Wallimann, T., Wyss, M., Brdiczka, D., Nicolay, K., and Eppenberger, H. M. (1992). Intracellular compartmentation, structure and function of creatine kinase isoenzymes in tissues with high and fluctuating energy demands: the 'phosphocreatine circuit' for cellular energy homeostasis. *Biochem. J.* 281(Pt 1), 21–40. doi: 10.1042/bj2810021

Wang, S. E., and Wu, C. H. (2015). Physiological and histological evaluations of the cochlea between 3xTg-AD mouse model of Alzheimer's diseases and R6/2 mouse model of Huntington's diseases. *Chin. J. Physiol.* 58, 359–366. doi: 10.4077/CJP.2015.BAD334

Wang, Y., Li, J., Yao, X., Li, W., Du, H., Tang, M., et al. (2017). Loss of CIB2 causes profound hearing loss and abolishes mechanoelectrical transduction in mice. *Front. Mol. Neurosci.* 10:401. doi: 10.3389/fnmol.2017.00401

Wegiel, J., Flory, M., Kuchna, I., Nowicki, K., Ma, S. Y., Imaki, H., et al. (2014). Brain-region-specific alterations of the trajectories of neuronal volume growth throughout the lifespan in autism. *Acta Neuropathol. Commun.* 2:28. doi: 10.1186/2051-5960-2-28

Wegiel, J., Kuchna, I., Nowicki, K., Imaki, H., Wegiel, J., Marchi, E., et al. (2010). The neuropathology of autism: defects of neurogenesis and neuronal migration, and dysplastic changes. *Acta Neuropathol.* 119, 755–770. doi: 10.1007/s00401-010-0655-4

Wetter, S., Peavy, G., Jacobson, M., Hamilton, J., Salmon, D., and Murphy, C. (2005). Olfactory and auditory event-related potentials in Huntington's disease. *Neuropsychology* 19, 428–436. doi: 10.1037/0894-4105.19.4.428

Wu, C., Stefanescu, R. A., Martel, D. T., and Shore, S. E. (2015). Listening to another sense: somatosensory integration in the auditory system. *Cell Tissue Res.* 361, 233–250. doi: 10.1007/s00441-014-2074-7

Wu, M., Zheng, X., Wang, X., Zhang, G., and Kuang, J. (2020a). 4q27 deletion and 7q36.1 microduplication in a patient with multiple malformations and hearing loss: a case report. *BMC Med. Genomics* 13:31. doi: 10.1186/s12920-020-0697-y

Wu, P. Z., O'Malley, J. T., de Gruttola, V., and Liberman, M. C. (2020b). Age-related hearing loss is dominated by damage to inner ear sensory cells, not the cellular battery that powers them. *J. Neurosci.* 40, 6357–6366. doi: 10.1523/JNEUROSCI.0937-20.2020

Wyss, M., and Kaddurah-Daouk, R. (2000). Creatine and creatinine metabolism. *Physiol. Rev.* 80, 1107–1213. doi: 10.1152/physrev.2000.80.3.1107

Yang, M., Mahrt, E. J., Lewis, F., Foley, G., Portmann, T., Dolmetsch, R. E., et al. (2015). 16p11.2 deletion syndrome mice display sensory and ultrasonic vocalization deficits during social interactions. *Autism Res.* 8, 507–521. doi: 10.1002/aur.1465

Yu, X. Y., Liu, W. W., Fan, Z. M., Qian, F. P., Zhang, D. G., Han, Y. C., et al. (2017). c-Myb knockdown increases the neomycin-induced damage to hair-cell-like HEI-OC1 cells in vitro. *Sci. Rep.* 7:41094. doi: 10.1038/srep41094

Yylmaz, S., Karaly, E., Tokmak, A., Guclu, E., Kocer, A., and Ozturk, O. (2009). Auditory evaluation in Parkinsonian patients. *Eur. Arch. Otorhinolaryngol.* 266, 669–671. doi: 10.1007/s00405-009-0933-8

Promising Applications of Nanoparticles in the Treatment of Hearing Loss

Zilin Huang[1,2†], Qiang Xie[1,2†], Shuang Li[1,2†], Yuhao Zhou[1,2], Zuhong He[1,2], Kun Lin[1,2], Minlan Yang[1,2*], Peng Song[1,2*] and Xiong Chen[1,2*]

[1] Department of Otorhinolaryngology, Head and Neck Surgery, Zhongnan Hospital of Wuhan University, Wuhan, China,
[2] Sleep Medicine Center, Zhongnan Hospital of Wuhan University, Wuhan, China

*Correspondence:
Minlan Yang
milano062009@163.com
Peng Song
songpeng@znhospital.cn
Xiong Chen
zn_chenxiong@126.com

Hearing loss is one of the most common disabilities affecting both children and adults worldwide. However, traditional treatment of hearing loss has some limitations, particularly in terms of drug delivery system as well as diagnosis of ear imaging. The blood–labyrinth barrier (BLB), the barrier between the vasculature and fluids of the inner ear, restricts entry of most blood-borne compounds into inner ear tissues. Nanoparticles (NPs) have been demonstrated to have high biocompatibility, good degradation, and simple synthesis in the process of diagnosis and treatment, which are promising for medical applications in hearing loss. Although previous studies have shown that NPs have promising applications in the field of inner ear diseases, there is still a gap between biological research and clinical application. In this paper, we aim to summarize developments and challenges of NPs in diagnostics and treatment of hearing loss in recent years. This review may be useful to raise otology researchers' awareness of effect of NPs on hearing diagnosis and treatment.

Keywords: hearing loss, nanomaterials, drug delivery system, imaging, hair cells, cochlear implant

INTRODUCTION

Hearing loss is one of the most common disabilities affecting the quality of life. Nowadays, people's lifestyle has been changed with longer life expectancy, and the prevalence and the severity of hearing loss have increased (Cruickshanks et al., 2003; Isaacson, 2010). According to World Health Organization (WHO), more than 5% of the world's population suffer from disabling hearing loss that includes 34 million children (Chadha and Cieza, 2017), and it is more prevalent in the elderly ($\geq$70 years) (Zahnert, 2011). Hearing loss is divided into three categories: conductive, sensitive, and mixed hearing loss. Common causes of conductive hearing loss are earwax embolism, otitis media, cholesteatoma, and otosclerosis, among others (Zahnert, 2011). Sensorineural hearing loss (SNHL) is usually caused by sensory nerve transmission problems at or behind the cochlea, including presbycusis, inner ear infection (He et al., 2020), Meniere's disease (Wang et al., 2015), noise-induced hearing loss (Varela-Nieto et al., 2020), autoimmune hearing loss (Fan et al., 2019), genetic diseases (Zhu et al., 2018; Cheng et al., 2021; Fu et al., 2021a; Lv et al., 2021), age-related hearing loss (He et al., 2021), and ototoxic material hearing loss (Liu et al., 2016, 2021; Gao et al., 2019; Liu W. et al., 2019; Zhang Y. et al., 2019; Zhong et al., 2020; Fu et al., 2021b).

Attention to the treatment of hearing loss has varied, which is influenced by social status, education, and race. For example, nearly two-thirds of United States adults aged 70 years and older are affected by hearing loss, and only 15% of older people use hearing aids (Mamo et al., 2016). At present, the traditional treatment of hearing loss includes drug therapy, hearing aids, and cochlear implant (CI). Systemic administration and intratympanic (IT) steroid injection are much prevalent clinical therapy to restore hearing loss (Ermutlu et al., 2017; Mirian and Ovesen, 2020). Due to the special and complex anatomical structure of the inner ear, the blood–labyrinth barrier (BLB) prevents most drugs in the blood from reaching the inner ear, such as protein, carbohydrate, and other small molecules (Shi, 2016); most of the hearing loss drug treatment is ineffective (Nyberg et al., 2019). Compared to systemic administration, IT injection has been shown to keep high concentrations of steroids in the perilymph and can be used as a substitute or supplement for systemic steroid therapy (Chandrasekhar et al., 2000). However, there are also differences in round window membrane (RWM) size and permeability in IT injection, which makes it difficult to accurately determine the drug concentration for individualized treatment (Goycoolea, 2001).

Hair cells are the mechanical transduction cells in the cochlea, which detect sound through the deflection of mechanosensory stereocilia, and are the most critical cells in the inner ear (He et al., 2017, 2019; Liu Y. et al., 2019; Qi et al., 2019, 2020; Zhou et al., 2020). Once damaged, hair cells only have very limited regeneration ability in mammals, and it is difficult for the new neuron cell to proliferate in a specific site (Cheng et al., 2019; Tan et al., 2019; Zhang S. et al., 2019; Zhang et al., 2020b; Chen et al., 2021). Possibly, hair cells are so fragile that the generation of inflammation in the inner ear can affect hair cell survival, and the protection of these cells is the key to the treatment of hearing loss (Zhang et al., 2020a,c). Because of the limitations of traditional treatment of hearing loss, nanomaterials are more and more likely to appear in the treatment of inner ear diseases as a new type of small medical molecular particles (Liu et al., 2018; Han et al., 2020; Yuan et al., 2021; Zhao et al., 2021). Nanoparticles (NPs) with a diameter of 1–1,000 nm can not only promote the effective concentration time of drugs in vivo, but also carry drugs to specific parts of the cochlea (Pyykkö et al., 2016). NPs have been demonstrated to have high biocompatibility, good degradation, and simple synthesis in the process of diagnosis and treatment (Zha et al., 2016; Shang et al., 2018; Yang et al., 2018; Zhao et al., 2019). Because of this, nanomaterials and their related products have been widely used in drug delivery applications, including cancer treatment, diagnosis, molecular imaging, and other applications (Shaikh et al., 2018; Li D. et al., 2019; Guo J. et al., 2020; Yang et al., 2021). Also, it is possible for nanomaterials to be used in hearing loss with many advantages that have been found in many other diseases' treatment, such as the regeneration of neural stem cells, the induced differentiation of neurons, and the transmission of some specific active substances in inner ear cells (He et al., 2016; Jiang et al., 2020; Xia et al., 2020; Yang et al., 2020). There are various kinds of medical nanomaterials for hearing loss, such as poly(lactic-co-glycolic-acid) NPs, silica NPs, magnetic NPs, and lipid NPs (Pyykkö et al., 2016). This review aims to summarize the useful nanomaterials emerging in the diagnosis and treatment of hearing loss in recent years.

COMPARISON OF TRADITIONAL MEDICINE TREATMENT AND NANOMEDICINE IN HEARING LOSS

At present, systemic drug delivery and IT injection (**Figure 1**) are the traditional drug treatments for hearing loss caused by inner ear diseases (Li et al., 2018). Previous studies have reported that systemic administration has been successfully used in the treatment of sudden hearing loss (SHL), autoimmune inner ear disease (AIED), Meniere's disease, and other inner ear diseases by intravenous, intramuscular, or oral administration (Li and Ding, 2020; Liu et al., 2020). Although the drugs can reach the inner ear through systemic administration, the limited local blood supply and poor penetration of BLB often lead to the local drug concentration lower than the treatment criteria (Nyberg et al., 2019). In order to reach the expected therapeutic effect, large doses of drugs are needed, which often lead to serious ototoxicity. However, high dose of systemic glucocorticoids can lead to hypertension, hyperglycemia, osteoporosis, and immunosuppression, as well as long-term high-dose adrenal suppression (McCall et al., 2010; Stout et al., 2019), which is harmful to human health.

On the other hand, IT injects the drug into the middle ear space, allowing the drug to diffuse to the inner ear through the RWM, bypassing the labyrinthine artery and blood inner ear barrier, which is more efficient than systemic administration and avoids the side effects of high-dose medication (Buniel et al., 2009). Schuknecht (1957) first used IT injection as a means to deliver streptomycin into the inner ear to effectively treat the hearing loss of Meniere's disease. The drug concentration of IT injection in the inner ear fluid, perilymph, and endolymph was significantly higher than that of oral or non-injection (Jackson and Silverstein, 2002; Buniel et al., 2009). Although IT administration is highly efficient and reduces the toxic and side effects of systemic administration, the concentration of drug reaching the inner ear depends on the dose of drug contacting the RWM circular window membrane of the middle ear, and the difference of RWM permeability will lead to the change of drug retention and elimination rate (Buniel et al., 2009; Lehner et al., 2021), which eventually makes it difficult to formulate a standard for dosing regimen. As a result, it is difficult to achieve precision therapy for hearing loss with traditional medication.

Compared with IT injection of dexamethasone, the products of nanotechnology have great advantages in drug treatment of hearing loss. For example, hydrogel nanomaterials deliver poloxamer 407 loaded with micronized dexamethasone (mDex) to guinea pig round window, which provides sustained release of drugs, increases the total concentration of peripheral blood lymphocytes by about 1.6-fold, and increases the residence time

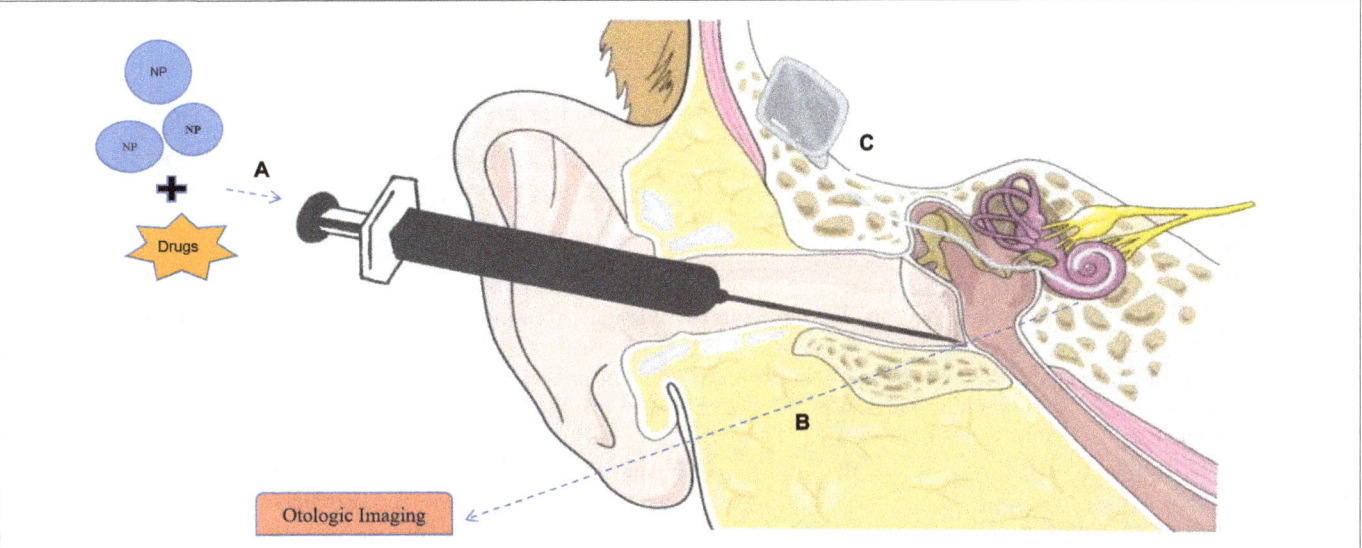

FIGURE 1 | Applications of nanomaterials in hearing loss. **(A)** Nanoparticles (NPs) can serve in drug delivery systems to the inner ear with intratympanic (IT) injection. **(B)** Nanomaterials can be used as contrast agents in otologic imaging. **(C)** Application of nanomaterial in cochlear implants (CIs). Part of the material in Figure is from https://smart.servier.com.

of drugs by about 24-fold. The initial peak concentration of dexamethasone injection before clearance from the lymphatic vessels was within 12 h, while the mDex hydrogel sustained release for 10 days (Wang et al., 2009). This study also demonstrates that mDex delivery using poloxamer 407 led to more homogenous distribution of dexamethasone along the length of the cochlea (Salt et al., 2011; Rathnam et al., 2019). In addition, some natural substances can also be transformed into NPs that promotes the growth of nerve cells or protect cells from inflammatory damage (Lambert et al., 2016), which means there will be more possibilities to find various natural NPs.

NANOMATERIALS IN OTOLOGY IMAGING

As a new medical application of nanomaterials, the nano drug delivery system not only has a wide application in drug transportation of inner ear hearing loss, but also plays a role in clinical diagnosis and treatment of inner ear hearing loss diseases because of its specific penetration, good biocompatibility, and editability (Rathnam et al., 2019). Due to the special anatomical structure of BLB and the highly complex separation of the inner ear region, it is difficult to get enough contrast agents to reach the inner ear (Kayyali et al., 2017). Therefore, conventional Computed tomography (CT) and magnetic resonance imaging (MRI) are not appropriate for the imaging of the microstructure of the cochlea. However, it is difficult for many novel contrast agents with certain biocompatibility or targeting to guarantee the sensitivity and specificity of the inner ear diseases' diagnosis (Liu et al., 2021).

Superparamagnetic nanoparticles (SPIONs) with good physical properties are characterized by nanocrystalline iron oxide (Fe_3O_4) or magnetite (γ-Fe_2O_3) nucleus, with a molecular diameter of 100–300 nm and with a certain biocompatibility (Laurent et al., 2008; Salazar-Alvarez et al., 2008). Therefore, many studies have verified its possibility as a new MRI contrast agent. Ceric ammonium nitrate oxidant stabilized γ-maghemite NPs could be detected in the inner ear using MRI after IT administration *in vivo* (Zou et al., 2017b). Besides, there are also some NPs such as superparamagnetic magnetohematite (γ-Fe_2O_3) NPs and lipid NPs that are designed to combine with traditional contrast agents to form chelates that can reflect the distribution of these contrast agents in the cochlea and form visual images (Zou et al., 2017a,b). Some metal ion NPs have great advantages in inner ear structure imaging. For example, the contrast enhancement rate of the new optical contrast agent containing nano silver clusters is more than 90%, and the ear veins can be detected much clearly (Chu et al., 2014; Ray et al., 2014). Interestingly, the nano chelate containing gold proved that the CT imaging effect of the inner ear structure was concentration gradient dependent in a certain range (Zou et al., 2015). These findings may indicate that they can be used as a potential nano template to visualize the cochlear structure in the middle ear granule in the future and to assess whether the drugs reach the designated site by positron emission tomography and MRI in the application of inner ear diagnosis and therapy.

APPLICATION OF NANOMATERIALS IN COCHLEAR IMPLANT

There are more than 324,000 CI users in the world. CI has greatly improved the quality of hearing life of patients with hearing loss. The mechanism of CI in the treatment of hearing loss is related to the connection between the CI electrode array and auditory neurons (Zhao et al., 2020). CI directly injects current into surrounding tissues through the implanted electrode array and maps the frequency of cochlea to location (Danti et al., 2020). Therefore, the emergence of nanotechnology makes significant innovation and progress of the CI electrode array. In order to reduce the damage caused by cochlear implantation, nanomaterials are applied to the corresponding electrode array to improve cochlear signal transmission and promote the growth of auditory nerve cells. Some physical stimulations as well as the influence of the cellular microenvironment are able to regulate cell migration and can direct neurite outgrowth in spiral ganglion neurons (SGNs) preferentially along a certain direction (Guo et al., 2019; Girão et al., 2020; Hu et al., 2021; Wei et al., 2021). More importantly, changes in cell culture environment can help to maintain and promote the electrophysiological properties of the SGNs, regulate the cells' polarity, promote the area of growth cones, or significantly increase the synapse density of the SGNs (Sun et al., 2016; Yan et al., 2018).

The application of nanomaterials, such as graphene and MXene, can also promote the proliferation and differentiation of neural stem cells in the inner ear, and many ultrastructures can be produced by 3D printing technology or other novel methods, so as to obtain more satisfactory biological characteristics that can be applied in hair cells (Waqas et al., 2017; Fang et al., 2019; Xia et al., 2019; Guo R. et al., 2020; Guo et al., 2021). These new technological products indicate that the application of nanomaterials in cochlea may be conducive to hearing recovery and cell regeneration (Guo et al., 2016; Li G. et al., 2019; Tang et al., 2019). Similarly, biodegradable calcium phosphate hollow nanospheres, used as CI electrode coatings and loaded with neurotrophins, attract the growth of regenerating auditory neuron dendrites through bioactive gels and finally establish direct physical contact between the auditory neurons and the CI electrodes as a result (Li et al., 2017). Carbon nanotubes (CNTs) and micro-textured nano-crystalline diamond can also enhance the transmission of inner ear electrical stimulation by increasing the contact area of the coating, which brings no additional cell damage (Burblies et al., 2016; Cai et al., 2016; Choi et al., 2019).

What is more exciting is that there are also nanomaterials in the cochlea that can be used for a longer time by spontaneous power supply. Some studies have investigated the silver NP microcoil with the micro size by aerosol jet printing. It has been demonstrated that the electromagnetic field generated by this material is not affected by cochlear environment (Sarreal and Bhatti, 2020). The eddy current generated by electromagnetic field can be used to stimulate the nearby tissues, and to improve the spatial resolution of cochlear tissues and CI function (Golestanirad et al., 2018). Some researchers have also developed electrospun piezoelectric polymer nanofibers that can transform sound waves into electrical signals through the possible synergistic effect of piezoelectric and triboelectric, which provides a basis for the development of self-powered small nano cochlea (Viola et al., 2020).

These studies may have paved the way for the development of self-powered nanofibrous implantable auditory sensors, which suggests that more and more nanomaterials may be used in the construction of cochlear materials and cochlear signal transduction technology in the future.

DISCUSSION AND OUTLOOK OF NANOMATERIALS IN THE FIELD OF HEARING LOSS

Nanomaterials and related technology products may not only provide diagnosis and treatment strategies for specific and efficient treatment of hearing loss, but also other inner ear diseases, such as otology tumors and ear inflammation. Furthermore, we can foresee that some types of nanomaterials or nanoproducts may be routinely used in the treatment of hearing loss and other inner ear diseases in the future (Li et al., 2017). Among the applications of nanomaterials in the diagnosis and treatment of hearing loss, researchers pay more attention to the biodegradability of nanomaterials and the ototoxicity *in vivo*. These substances act on the cells or tissues of the inner ear, which may also have ototoxicity, thus affecting the biological activity of hair cells and the activity of auditory neurons. Although some studies have found that NPs may have ototoxicity *in vivo*, there is no clear report on the ototoxicity of nanomaterials to humans (Murugadoss et al., 2021).

Previous studies have reported that positively charged NPs can enter the inner ear more easily through RWM, as drug carriers for inner ear diseases or CI materials, but they will produce certain ototoxicity in the process of biodegradation with cell membrane damage, production of reactive oxygen species, hair cell apoptosis, etc. (Yoon et al., 2015; Zhou et al., 2015). The time required for NPs to enter the body is longer than traditional drugs, but the possible effects of long-term residues of these NPs in animals are still unclear (Wang et al., 2009; Ray et al., 2014; Lehner et al., 2021). Therefore, future studies may need to determine whether the components of NPs will accumulate in the inner ear and the effects of these substances on hair cells.

Moreover, the cost of developing and manufacturing NPs for clinical application in the field of inner ear diseases is significantly higher than traditional treatments (Mokoena et al., 2019). Many patients with hearing loss may choose low-cost and convenient IT injection for treatment. Based on the current development of manufacturing technology, the manufacturing difficulty and cost of NPs are greatly overcome by printing technology, and it makes it easier for researchers to edit and manufacture NPs (Zhang et al., 2020d). In the future, we may choose to reduce the manufacturing cost of NPs through 3D printing, reduce the corresponding treatment costs, and try to produce NPs with more functions that are more convenient to be preserved or used. It is difficult to perfectly match the bioactivity of current nanomaterials to the conditions that are required for hair cell growth and proliferation in the inner ear, but it is possible that we may design nanomedicines that can precisely promote the differentiation of stem cells into auditory synesthesia cells, such as inner ear stem cells, mesenchymal stem cells, and pluripotent stem cells. In other words, if these novel nanomaterials can carry certain stem cells into the inner ear that promote stem cell differentiation into hair cells at specific structural locations, it will be a great advance in the treatment of hearing loss with significant hearing recovery.

CONCLUSION

The application of nanomaterials in the diagnosis and treatment of hearing loss diseases is novel and promising. In the future, ideal nanomaterials should be more universal, able to load more therapeutic drugs with various functions, such as preventing rapid degradation, retaining targeting effects, and prolonging the action time in the inner ear. This kind of materials should not only have better efficacy in various diseases of inner ear hearing loss, but also have stronger ear permeability, and ensure no impact or side effects on the human body. Many studies have attempted to deliver drugs, genes, and growth factors to the inner ear *in vivo* with nanomaterials, and promising results have also been reported. However, we do not know the specific effect of nanomaterials applied in human inner ear. There is still a big gap between basic research and clinical application of nanomaterials, so it is necessary to study the safety and effectiveness of nanomaterials. With the emergence of new biomaterials and the realization of a deeper understanding of inner ear physiology, nanomaterials will have a clearer understanding of the diagnosis and treatment of hearing loss.

AUTHOR CONTRIBUTIONS

ZLH, SL, and QX wrote the first draft of the manuscript. YZ and ZHH polished the language. KL searched the literatures. XC, PS, and MLY conceived the idea and revised the manuscript. All authors read and approved the final manuscript.

ACKNOWLEDGMENTS

We thank members of their laboratory for their research work.

REFERENCES

Buniel, M. C., Geelan-Hansen, K., Weber, P. C., and Tuohy, V. K. (2009). Immunosuppressive therapy for autoimmune inner ear disease. *Immunotherapy* 1, 425–434. doi: 10.2217/imt.09.12

Burblies, N., Schulze, J., Schwarz, H. C., Kranz, K., Motz, D., Vogt, C., et al. (2016). Coatings of different carbon nanotubes on platinum electrodes for neuronal devices: preparation, cytocompatibility and interaction with spiral ganglion cells. *PLoS One* 11:e0158571. doi: 10.1371/journal.pone.0158571

Cai, Y., Edin, F., Jin, Z., Alexsson, A., Gudjonsson, O., Liu, W., et al. (2016). Strategy towards independent electrical stimulation from cochlear implants: guided auditory neuron growth on topographically modified nanocrystalline diamond. *Acta Biomater.* 31, 211–220. doi: 10.1016/j.actbio.2015.11.021

Chadha, S., and Cieza, A. (2017). Promoting global action on hearing loss: world hearing day. *Internat. J. Audiol.* 56, 145–147. doi: 10.1080/14992027.2017.1291264

Chandrasekhar, S. S., Rubinstein, R. Y., Kwartler, J. A., Gatz, M., Connelly, P. E., Huang, E., et al. (2000). Dexamethasone pharmacokinetics in the inner ear: comparison of route of administration and use of facilitating agents. *Otolaryngol. Head Neck Surg.* 122, 521–528. doi: 10.1067/mhn.2000.102578

Chen, Y., Gu, Y., Li, Y., Li, G. L., Chai, R., Li, W., et al. (2021). Generation of mature and functional hair cells by co-expression of Gfi1, Pou4f3, and Atoh1 in the postnatal mouse cochlea. *Cell Rep.* 35:109016. doi: 10.1016/j.celrep.2021.109016

Cheng, C., Hou, Y., Zhang, Z., Wang, Y., Lu, L., Zhang, L., et al. (2021). Disruption of the autism-related gene Pak1 causes stereocilia disorganization, hair cell loss, and deafness in mice. *J. Genet. Genom.* 48, 324–332. doi: 10.1016/j.jgg.2021.03.010

Cheng, C., Wang, Y., Guo, L., Lu, X., Zhu, W., Muhammad, W., et al. (2019). Age-related transcriptome changes in Sox2+ supporting cells in the mouse cochlea. *Stem Cell Res. Ther.* 10:365. doi: 10.1186/s13287-019-1437-0

Choi, G. J., Gwon, T. M., Kim, D. H., Park, J., Kim, S. M., Oh, S. H., et al. (2019). CNT bundle-based thin intracochlear electrode array. *Biomed. Microdev.* 21:27. doi: 10.1007/s10544-019-0384-y

Chu, L., Wang, S., Li, K., Xi, W., Zhao, X., and Qian, J. (2014). Biocompatible near-infrared fluorescent nanoparticles for macro and microscopic in vivo functional bioimaging. *Biomed. Opt. Expr.* 5, 4076–4088. doi: 10.1364/boe.5.004076

Cruickshanks, K. J., Tweed, T. S., Wiley, T. L., Klein, B. E., Klein, R., Chappell, R., et al. (2003). The 5-year incidence and progression of hearing loss: the epidemiology of hearing loss study. *Archiv. Otolaryngol. Head Neck Surg.* 129, 1041–1046. doi: 10.1001/archotol.129.10.1041

Danti, S., Azimi, B., Candito, M., Fusco, A., Sorayani Bafqi, M. S., Ricci, C., et al. (2020). Lithium niobate nanoparticles as biofunctional interface material for inner ear devices. *Biointerphases* 15:031004. doi: 10.1116/6.0000067

Ermutlu, G., Süslü, N., Yılmaz, T., and Saraç, S. (2017). Sudden hearing loss: an effectivity comparison of intratympanic and systemic steroid treatments. *Eur. Archiv. Otorhinolaryngol.* 274, 3585–3591. doi: 10.1007/s00405-017-4691-8

Fan, K. Q., Li, Y. Y., Wang, H. L., Mao, X. T., Guo, J. X., Wang, F., et al. (2019). Stress-induced metabolic disorder in peripheral CD4(+) T cells leads to anxiety-like behavior. *Cell* 179, 864–879.e19. doi: 10.1016/j.cell.2019.10.001

Fang, Q., Zhang, Y., Chen, X., Li, H., Cheng, L., Zhu, W., et al. (2019). Three-dimensional graphene enhances neural stem cell proliferation through metabolic regulation. *Front. Bioeng. Biotechnol.* 7:436. doi: 10.3389/fbioe.2019.00436

Fu, X., An, Y., Wang, H., Li, P., Lin, J., Yuan, J., et al. (2021a). Deficiency of Klc2 induces low-frequency sensorineural hearing loss in C57BL/6 J mice and human. *Mol. Neurobiol.* doi: 10.1007/s12035-021-02422-w [Epub ahead of print].

Fu, X., Wan, P., Li, P., Wang, J., Guo, S., Zhang, Y., et al. (2021b). Mechanism and prevention of ototoxicity induced by aminoglycosides. *Front. Cell. Neurosci.* 15:692762. doi: 10.3389/fncel.2021.692762

Gao, S., Cheng, C., Wang, M., Jiang, P., Zhang, L., Wang, Y., et al. (2019). Blebbistatin inhibits neomycin-induced apoptosis in hair cell-like HEI-OC-1 cells and in cochlear hair cells. *Front. Cell. Neurosci.* 13:590. doi: 10.3389/fncel.2019.00590

Girão, A. F., Sousa, J., Domínguez-Bajo, A., González-Mayorga, A., Bdikin, I., Pujades-Otero, E., et al. (2020). 3D reduced graphene oxide scaffolds with a combinatorial fibrous-porous architecture for neural tissue engineering. *ACS Appl. Mater. Interf.* 12, 38962–38975. doi: 10.1021/acsami.0c10599

Golestanirad, L., Gale, J. T., Manzoor, N. F., Park, H. J., Glait, L., Haer, F., et al. (2018). Solenoidal micromagnetic stimulation enables activation of axons with specific orientation. *Front. Physiol.* 9:724. doi: 10.3389/fphys.2018.00724

Goycoolea, M. V. (2001). Clinical aspects of round window membrane permeability under normal and pathological conditions. *Acta Otolaryngol.* 121, 437–447. doi: 10.1080/000164801300366552

Guo, J., Yu, Y., Sun, L., Zhang, Z., Zhao, Y., Chai, R., et al. (2020). Bio-inspired multicomponent carbon nanotube microfibers from microfluidics for supercapacitor. *Chem. Eng. J.* 397:125517. doi: 10.1016/j.cej.2020.125517 [Epub ahead of print].

Guo, R., Li, J., Chen, C., Xiao, M., Liao, M., Hu, Y., et al. (2021). Biomimetic 3D bacterial cellulose-graphene foam hybrid scaffold regulates neural stem cell proliferation and differentiation. *Coll. Surf. B Biointerf.* 200:111590. doi: 10.1016/j.colsurfb.2021.111590

Guo, R., Ma, X., Liao, M., Liu, Y., Hu, Y., Qian, X., et al. (2019). Development and application of cochlear implant-based electric-acoustic stimulation of spiral ganglion neurons. *ACS Biomater. Sci. Eng.* 5, 6735–6741. doi: 10.1021/acsbiomaterials.9b01265

Guo, R., Xiao, M., Zhao, W., Zhou, S., Hu, Y., Liao, M., et al. (2020). 2D Ti(3)C(2)T(x)MXene couples electrical stimulation to promote proliferation and neural differentiation of neural stem cells. *Acta Biomater.* doi: 10.1016/j.actbio.2020.12.035

Guo, R., Zhang, S., Xiao, M., Qian, F., He, Z., Li, D., et al. (2016). Accelerating bioelectric functional development of neural stem cells by graphene coupling: implications for neural interfacing with conductive materials. *Biomaterials* 106, 193–204. doi: 10.1016/j.biomaterials.2016.08.019

Han, S., Xu, Y., Sun, J., Liu, Y., Zhao, Y., Tao, W., et al. (2020). Isolation and analysis of extracellular vesicles in a Morpho butterfly wing-integrated microvortex biochip. *Biosens. Bioelectron.* 154:112073. doi: 10.1016/j.bios.2020.112073

He, Z. H., Li, M., Fang, Q. J., Liao, F. L., Zou, S. Y., Wu, X., et al. (2021). FOXG1 promotes aging inner ear hair cell survival through activation of the autophagy pathway. *Autophagy* 17, 1–22. doi: 10.1080/15548627.2021.1916194

He, Z. H., Zou, S. Y., Li, M., Liao, F. L., Wu, X., Sun, H. Y., et al. (2020). The nuclear transcription factor FoxG1 affects the sensitivity of mimetic aging hair cells to inflammation by regulating autophagy pathways. *Redox Biol.* 28:101364. doi: 10.1016/j.redox.2019.101364

He, Z., Fang, Q., Li, H., Shao, B., Zhang, Y., Zhang, Y., et al. (2019). The role of FOXG1 in the postnatal development and survival of mouse cochlear hair cells. *Neuropharmacology* 144, 43–57. doi: 10.1016/j.neuropharm.2018.10.021

He, Z., Guo, L., Shu, Y., Fang, Q., Zhou, H., Liu, Y., et al. (2017). Autophagy protects auditory hair cells against neomycin-induced damage. *Autophagy* 13, 1884–1904. doi: 10.1080/15548627.2017.1359449

He, Z., Zhang, S., Song, Q., Li, W., Liu, D., Li, H., et al. (2016). The structural development of primary cultured hippocampal neurons on a graphene substrate. *Colloids Surf. B Biointerf.* 146, 442–451. doi: 10.1016/j.colsurfb.2016.06.045

Hu, Y., Li, D., Wei, H., Zhou, S., Chen, W., Yan, X., et al. (2021). Neurite extension and orientation of spiral ganglion neurons can be directed by superparamagnetic iron oxide nanoparticles in a magnetic field. *Intern. J. Nanomed.* 16, 4515–4526. doi: 10.2147/ijn.S313673

Isaacson, B. (2010). Hearing loss. *Med. Clin. North Am.* 94, 973–988. doi: 10.1016/j.mcna.2010.05.003

Jackson, L. E., and Silverstein, H. (2002). Chemical perfusion of the inner ear. *Otolaryngol. Clin. North Am.* 35, 639–653. doi: 10.1016/s0030-6665(02)00023-3

Jiang, P., Zhang, S., Cheng, C., Gao, S., Tang, M., Lu, L., et al. (2020). The roles of exosomes in visual and auditory systems. *Front. Bioeng. Biotechnol.* 8:525. doi: 10.3389/fbioe.2020.00525

Kayyali, M. N., Brake, L., Ramsey, A. J., Wright, A. C., O'Malley, B. W., and Li, D. D. (2017). A novel nano-approach for targeted inner ear imaging. *J. Nanomed. Nanotechnol.* 8:456. doi: 10.4172/2157-7439.1000456

Lambert, P. R., Carey, J., Mikulec, A. A., and LeBel, C. (2016). Intratympanic sustained-exposure dexamethasone thermosensitive gel for symptoms of ménière's disease: randomized Phase 2b safety and efficacy trial. *Otol. Neurotol.* 37, 1669–1676. doi: 10.1097/mao.0000000000001227

Laurent, S., Forge, D., Port, M., Roch, A., Robic, C., Vander Elst, L., et al. (2008). Magnetic iron oxide nanoparticles: synthesis, stabilization, vectorization, physicochemical characterizations, and biological applications. *Chem. Rev.* 108, 2064–2110. doi: 10.1021/cr068445e

Lehner, E., Liebau, A., Syrowatka, F., Knolle, W., Plontke, S. K., and Mäder, K. (2021). Novel biodegradable round window disks for inner ear delivery of dexamethasone. *Intern. J. Pharm.* 594:120180. doi: 10.1016/j.ijpharm.2020.120180

Li, A., You, D., Li, W., Cui, Y., He, Y., Li, W., et al. (2018). Novel compounds protect auditory hair cells against gentamycin-induced apoptosis by maintaining the expression level of H3K4me2. *Drug Deliv.* 25, 1033–1043. doi: 10.1080/10717544.2018.1461277

Li, D., Yan, X., Hu, Y., Liu, Y., Guo, R., Liao, M., et al. (2019). Two-photon image tracking of neural stem cells via iridium complexes encapsulated in polymeric nanospheres. *ACS Biomater. Sci. Eng.* 5, 1561–1568. doi: 10.1021/acsbiomaterials.8b01231

Li, G., Chen, K., You, D., Xia, M., Li, W., Fan, S., et al. (2019). Laminin-coated electrospun regenerated silk fibroin mats promote neural progenitor cell proliferation, differentiation, and survival in vitro. *Front. Bioeng. Biotechnol.* 7:190. doi: 10.3389/fbioe.2019.00190

Li, H., Edin, F., Hayashi, H., Gudjonsson, O., Danckwardt-Lillieström, N., Engqvist, H., et al. (2017). Guided growth of auditory neurons: bioactive particles towards gapless neural - electrode interface. *Biomaterials* 122, 1–9. doi: 10.1016/j.biomaterials.2016.12.020

Li, J., and Ding, L. (2020). Effectiveness of steroid treatment for sudden sensorineural hearing loss: a meta-analysis of randomized controlled trials. *Ann. pharmacother.* 54, 949–957. doi: 10.1177/1060028020908067

Liu, L., Chen, Y., Qi, J., Zhang, Y., He, Y., Ni, W., et al. (2016). Wnt activation protects against neomycin-induced hair cell damage in the mouse cochlea. *Cell Death Dis.* 7:e2136. doi: 10.1038/cddis.2016.35

Liu, W., Xu, L., Wang, X., Zhang, D., Sun, G., Wang, M., et al. (2021). PRDX1 activates autophagy via the PTEN-AKT signaling pathway to protect against cisplatin-induced spiral ganglion neuron damage. *Autophagy* 17, 1–23. doi: 10.1080/15548627.2021.1905466

Liu, W., Xu, X., Fan, Z., Sun, G., Han, Y., Zhang, D., et al. (2019). Wnt signaling activates TP53-induced glycolysis and apoptosis regulator and protects against cisplatin-induced spiral ganglion neuron damage in the mouse cochlea. *Antioxid. Redox Signal.* 30, 1389–1410. doi: 10.1089/ars.2017.7288

Liu, Y., Chen, Q., and Xu, Y. (2020). Research progress in refractory sudden hearing loss: steroid therapy. *J. Intern. Med. Res.* 48:300060519889426. doi: 10.1177/0300060519889426

Liu, Y., Qi, J., Chen, X., Tang, M., Chu, C., Zhu, W., et al. (2019). Critical role of spectrin in hearing development and deafness. *Sci. Adv.* 5:eaav7803. doi: 10.1126/sciadv.aav7803

Liu, Z., Tang, M., Zhao, J., Chai, R., and Kang, J. (2018). Looking into the future: toward advanced 3D biomaterials for stem-cell-based regenerative medicine. *Adv. Mater.* 30:e1705388. doi: 10.1002/adma.201705388

Lv, J., Fu, X., Li, Y., Hong, G., Li, P., Lin, J., et al. (2021). Deletion of Kcnj16 in mice does not alter auditory function. *Front. Cell Dev. Biol.* 9:630361. doi: 10.3389/fcell.2021.630361

Mamo, S. K., Nieman, C. L., and Lin, F. R. (2016). Prevalence of untreated hearing loss by income among older adults in the United States. *J. Health Care Poor Under.* 27, 1812–1818. doi: 10.1353/hpu.2016.0164

McCall, A. A., Swan, E. E., Borenstein, J. T., Sewell, W. F., Kujawa, S. G., and McKenna, M. J. (2010). Drug delivery for treatment of inner ear disease: current state of knowledge. *Ear Hear.* 31, 156–165. doi: 10.1097/AUD.0b013e3181c351f2

Mirian, C., and Ovesen, T. (2020). Intratympanic vs systemic corticosteroids in first-line treatment of idiopathic sudden sensorineural hearing loss: a systematic review and meta-analysis. *JAMA Otolaryngol. Head Neck Surg.* 146, 421–428. doi: 10.1001/jamaoto.2020.0047

Mokoena, D. R., George, B. P., and Abrahamse, H. (2019). Enhancing breast cancer treatment using a combination of cannabidiol and gold nanoparticles for photodynamic therapy. *Intern. J. Mol. Sci.* 20:4771. doi: 10.3390/ijms20194771

Murugadoss, S., Vinković Vrček, I., Pem, B., Jagiello, K., Judzinska, B., Sosnowska, A., et al. (2021). A strategy towards the generation of testable adverse outcome pathways for nanomaterials. *Altex* doi: 10.14573/altex.2102191 [Epub ahead of print].

Nyberg, S., Abbott, N. J., Shi, X., Steyger, P. S., and Dabdoub, A. (2019). Delivery of therapeutics to the inner ear: the challenge of the blood-labyrinth barrier. *Sci. Transl. Med.* 11:eaao0935. doi: 10.1126/scitranslmed.aao0935

Pyykkö, I., Zou, J., Schrott-Fischer, A., Glueckert, R., and Kinnunen, P. (2016). An overview of nanoparticle based delivery for treatment of inner ear disorders. *Methods Mol. Biol.* 1427, 363–415. doi: 10.1007/978-1-4939-3615-1_21

Qi, J., Liu, Y., Chu, C., Chen, X., Zhu, W., Shu, Y., et al. (2019). A cytoskeleton structure revealed by super-resolution fluorescence imaging in inner ear hair cells. *Cell Discov.* 5:12. doi: 10.1038/s41421-018-0076-4

Qi, J., Zhang, L., Tan, F., Liu, Y., Chu, C., Zhu, W., et al. (2020). Espin distribution as revealed by super-resolution microscopy of stereocilia. *Am. J. Transl. Res.* 12, 130–141.

Rathnam, C., Chueng, S. D., Ying, Y. M., Lee, K. B., and Kwan, K. (2019). Developments in bio-inspired nanomaterials for therapeutic delivery to treat hearing loss. *Front. Cell. Neurosci.* 13:493. doi: 10.3389/fncel.2019.00493

Ray, A., Mukundan, A., Xie, Z., Karamchand, L., Wang, X., and Kopelman, R. (2014). Highly stable polymer coated nano-clustered silver plates: a multimodal optical contrast agent for biomedical imaging. *Nanotechnology* 25:445104. doi: 10.1088/0957-4484/25/44/445104

Salazar-Alvarez, G., Qin, J., Sepelák, V., Bergmann, I., Vasilakaki, M., Trohidou, K. N., et al. (2008). Cubic versus spherical magnetic nanoparticles: the role of surface anisotropy. *J. Am. Chem. Soc.* 130, 13234–13239. doi: 10.1021/ja0768744

Salt, A. N., Hartsock, J., Plontke, S., LeBel, C., and Piu, F. (2011). Distribution of dexamethasone and preservation of inner ear function following intratympanic delivery of a gel-based formulation. *Audiol. Neurootol.* 16, 323–335. doi: 10.1159/000322504

Sarreal, R. R., and Bhatti, P. (2020). Characterization and miniaturization of silver-nanoparticle microcoil via aerosol jet printing techniques for micromagnetic cochlear stimulation. *Sensors* 20:6087. doi: 10.3390/s20216087

Schuknecht, H. F. (1957). Ablation therapy in the management of Menière's disease. *Acta Otolaryngol. Suppl.* 132, 1–42.

Shaikh, S., Rehman, F. U., Du, T., Jiang, H., Yin, L., Wang, X., et al. (2018). Real-time multimodal bioimaging of cancer cells and exosomes through biosynthesized iridium and iron nanoclusters. *ACS Appl. Mater. Interf.* 10, 26056–26063. doi: 10.1021/acsami.8b08975

Shang, L., Yu, Y., Gao, W., Wang, Y., Qu, L., Zhao, Z., et al. (2018). Bio-inspired anisotropic wettability surfaces from dynamic ferrofluid assembled templates. *Adv. Funct. Mater.* 28, 148–155.

Shi, X. (2016). Pathophysiology of the cochlear intrastrial fluid-blood barrier (review). *Hear. Res.* 338, 52–63. doi: 10.1016/j.heares.2016.01.010

Stout, A., Friedly, J., and Standaert, C. J. (2019). Systemic absorption and side effects of locally injected glucocorticoids. *J. Injury Funct. Rehabil.* 11, 409–419. doi: 10.1002/pmrj.12042

Sun, G., Liu, W., Fan, Z., Zhang, D., Han, Y., Xu, L., et al. (2016). The three-dimensional culture system with matrigel and neurotrophic factors preserves the structure and function of spiral ganglion neuron in vitro. *Neural Plastic.* 2016:4280407. doi: 10.1155/2016/4280407

Tan, F., Chu, C., Qi, J., Li, W., You, D., Li, K., et al. (2019). AAV-ie enables safe and efficient gene transfer to inner ear cells. *Nat. Commun.* 10:3733. doi: 10.1038/s41467-019-11687-8

Tang, M., Li, J., He, L., Guo, R., Yan, X., Li, D., et al. (2019). Transcriptomic profiling of neural stem cell differentiation on graphene substrates. *Colloids Surf. B Biointerf.* 182:110324. doi: 10.1016/j.colsurfb.2019.06.054

Varela-Nieto, I., Murillo-Cuesta, S., Calvino, M., Cediel, R., and Lassaletta, L. (2020). Drug development for noise-induced hearing loss. *Expert Opin. Drug Discov.* 15, 1457–1471. doi: 10.1080/17460441.2020.1806232

Viola, G., Chang, J., Maltby, T., Steckler, F., Jomaa, M., Sun, J., et al. (2020). Bioinspired multiresonant acoustic devices based on electrospun piezoelectric polymeric nanofibers. *ACS Appl. Mater. Interf.* 12, 34643–34657. doi: 10.1021/acsami.0c09238

Wang, T., Chai, R., Kim, G. S., Pham, N., Jansson, L., Nguyen, D. H., et al. (2015). Lgr5+ cells regenerate hair cells via proliferation and direct transdifferentiation in damaged neonatal mouse utricle. *Nat. Commun.* 6:6613. doi: 10.1038/ncomms7613

Wang, X., Dellamary, L., Fernandez, R., Harrop, A., Keithley, E. M., Harris, J. P., et al. (2009). Dose-dependent sustained release of dexamethasone in inner ear cochlear fluids using a novel local delivery approach. *Audiol. Neurootol.* 14, 393–401. doi: 10.1159/000241896

Waqas, M., Sun, S., Xuan, C., Fang, Q., Zhang, X., Islam, I. U., et al. (2017). Bone morphogenetic protein 4 promotes the survival and preserves the structure of flow-sorted Bhlhb5+ cochlear spiral ganglion neurons in vitro. *Sci. Rep.* 7:3506. doi: 10.1038/s41598-017-03810-w

Wei, H., Chen, Z., Hu, Y., Cao, W., Ma, X., Zhang, C., et al. (2021). Topographically conductive butterfly wing substrates for directed spiral ganglion neuron growth. *Small* 2021:e2102062. doi: 10.1002/smll.202102062

Xia, L., Shang, Y., Chen, X., Li, H., Xu, X., Liu, W., et al. (2020). Oriented neural spheroid formation and differentiation of neural stem cells guided by anisotropic inverse opals. *Front. Bioeng. Biotechnol.* 8:848. doi: 10.3389/fbioe.2020.00848

Xia, L., Zhu, W., Wang, Y., He, S., and Chai, R. (2019). Regulation of neural stem cell proliferation and differentiation by graphene-based biomaterials. *Neural Plastic.* 2019:3608386. doi: 10.1155/2019/3608386

Yan, W., Liu, W., Qi, J., Fang, Q., Fan, Z., Sun, G., et al. (2018). A three-dimensional culture system with matrigel promotes purified spiral ganglion neuron survival and function in vitro. *Mol. Neurobiol.* 55, 2070–2084. doi: 10.1007/s12035-017-0471-0

Yang, Y., Gao, B., Hu, Y., Wei, H., Zhang, C., Chai, R., et al. (2021). Ordered inverse-opal scaffold based on bionic transpiration to create a biomimetic spine. *Nanoscale* 13, 8614–8622. doi: 10.1039/d1nr00731a

Yang, Y., Zhang, Y., Chai, R., and Gu, Z. (2018). Designs of biomaterials and microenvironments for neuroengineering. *Neural Plastic.* 2018:1021969. doi: 10.1155/2018/1021969

Yang, Y., Zhang, Y., Chai, R., and Gu, Z. A. (2020). Polydopamine-functionalized carbon microfibrous scaffold accelerates the development of neural stem cells. *Front. Bioengin. Biotechnol.* 8:616. doi: 10.3389/fbioe.2020.00616

Yoon, J. Y., Yang, K. J., Kim, D. E., Lee, K. Y., Park, S. N., Kim, D. K., et al. (2015). Intratympanic delivery of oligoarginine-conjugated nanoparticles as a gene (or drug) carrier to the inner ear. *Biomaterials* 73, 243–253. doi: 10.1016/j.biomaterials.2015.09.025

Yuan, T. F., Dong, Y., Zhang, L., Qi, J., Yao, C., Wang, Y., et al. (2021). Neuromodulation-based stem cell therapy in brain repair: recent advances and future perspectives. *Neurosci. Bull.* 37, 735–745. doi: 10.1007/s12264-021-00667-y

Zahnert, T. (2011). The differential diagnosis of hearing loss. *Deutsches Arzteblatt Intern.* 108, 433–443. doi: 10.3238/arztebl.2011.0433

Zha, Y., Chai, R., Song, Q., Chen, L., Wang, X., Cheng, G., et al. (2016). Characterization and toxicological effects of three-dimensional graphene foams in rats in vivo. *J. Nanopartic. Res.* 18:122.

Zhang, S., Liu, D., Dong, Y., Zhang, Z., Zhang, Y., Zhou, H., et al. (2019). Frizzled-9+ supporting cells are progenitors for the generation of hair cells in the postnatal mouse cochlea. *Front. Mol. Neurosci.* 12:184. doi: 10.3389/fnmol.2019.00184

Zhang, Y., Li, W., He, Z., Wang, Y., Shao, B., Cheng, C., et al. (2019). Pre-treatment with fasudil prevents neomycin-induced hair cell damage by reducing the accumulation of reactive oxygen species. *Front. Mol. Neurosci.* 12:264. doi: 10.3389/fnmol.2019.00264

Zhang, S., Zhang, Y., Dong, Y., Guo, L., Zhang, Z., Shao, B., et al. (2020b). Knockdown of Foxg1 in supporting cells increases the trans-differentiation of supporting cells into hair cells in the neonatal mouse cochlea. *Cell. Mol. Life Sci.* 77, 1401–1419. doi: 10.1007/s00018-019-03291-2

Zhang, S., Qiang, R., Dong, Y., Zhang, Y., Chen, Y., Zhou, H., et al. (2020a). Hair cell regeneration from inner ear progenitors in the mammalian cochlea. *Am. J. Stem Cells* 9, 25–35.

Zhang, Y., Zhang, S., Zhang, Z., Dong, Y., Ma, X., Qiang, R., et al. (2020c). Knockdown of Foxg1 in Sox9+ supporting cells increases the trans-differentiation of supporting cells into hair cells in the neonatal mouse utricle. *Aging* 12, 19834–19851. doi: 10.18632/aging.104009

Zhang, Y. Z., Wang, Y., Jiang, Q., El-Demellawi, J. K., Kim, H., and Alshareef, H. N. (2020d). MXene printing and patterned coating for device applications. *Adv. Mater.* 32:e1908486. doi: 10.1002/adma.201908486

Zhao, C., Chen, G., Wang, H., Zhao, Y., and Chai, R. (2021). Bio-inspired intestinal scavenger from microfluidic electrospray for detoxifying lipopolysaccharide. *Bioactive Mater.* 6, 1653–1662. doi: 10.1016/j.bioactmat.2020.11.017

Zhao, E. E., Dornhoffer, J. R., Loftus, C., Nguyen, S. A., Meyer, T. A., Dubno, J. R., et al. (2020). Association of patient-related factors with adult cochlear implant speech recognition outcomes: a meta-analysis. *JAMA Otolaryngol. Head Neck Surg.* 146, 613–620. doi: 10.1001/jamaoto.2020.0662

Zhao, J., Tang, M., Cao, J., Ye, D., Guo, X., Xi, J., et al. (2019). Structurally tunable reduced graphene oxide substrate maintains mouse embryonic stem cell pluripotency. *Adv. Sci.* 6:1802136. doi: 10.1002/advs.201802136

Zhong, Z., Fu, X., Li, H., Chen, J., Wang, M., Gao, S., et al. (2020). Citicoline protects auditory hair cells against neomycin-induced damage. *Front. Cell Dev. Biol.* 8:712. doi: 10.3389/fcell.2020.00712

Zhou, H., Ma, X., Liu, Y., Dong, L., Luo, Y., Zhu, G., et al. (2015). Linear polyethylenimine-plasmid DNA nanoparticles are ototoxic to the cultured sensory epithelium of neonatal mice. *Mol. Med. Rep.* 11, 4381–4388. doi: 10.3892/mmr.2015.3306

Zhou, H., Qian, X., Xu, N., Zhang, S., Zhu, G., Zhang, Y., et al. (2020). Disruption of Atg7-dependent autophagy causes electromotility disturbances, outer hair cell loss, and deafness in mice. *Cell Death Dis.* 11:913. doi: 10.1038/s41419-020-03110-8

Zhu, C., Cheng, C., Wang, Y., Muhammad, W., Liu, S., Zhu, W., et al. (2018). Loss of ARHGEF6 causes hair cell stereocilia deficits and hearing loss in mice. *Front. Mol. Neurosci.* 11:362. doi: 10.3389/fnmol.2018.00362

Zou, J., Hannula, M., Misra, S., Feng, H., Labrador, R. H., Aula, A. S., et al. (2015). Micro CT visualization of silver nanoparticles in the middle and inner ear of rat and transportation pathway after transtympanic injection. *J. Nanobiotechnol.* 13:5. doi: 10.1186/s12951-015-0065-9

Zou, J., Ostrovsky, S., Israel, L. L., Feng, H., Kettunen, M. I., Lellouche, J. M., et al. (2017b). Efficient penetration of ceric ammonium nitrate oxidant-stabilized gamma-maghemite nanoparticles through the oval and round windows into the rat inner ear as demonstrated by MRI. *J. Biomed. Mater. Res. Part B Appl. Biomater.* 105, 1883–1891. doi: 10.1002/jbm.b.33719

Zou, J., Feng, H., Sood, R., Kinnunen, P. K. J., and Pyykko, I. (2017a). Biocompatibility of liposome nanocarriers in the rat inner ear after intratympanic administration. *Nanoscale Res. Lett.* 12:372. doi: 10.1186/s11671-017-2142-5

Single-Cell RNA Sequencing Analysis Reveals Greater Epithelial Ridge Cells Degeneration During Postnatal Development of Cochlea in Rats

Jianyong Chen[1,2,3†], Dekun Gao[1,2,3†], Junmin Chen[1,2,3†], Shule Hou[1,2,3], Baihui He[1,2,3], Yue Li[1,2,3], Shuna Li[1,2,3], Fan Zhang[1,2,3], Xiayu Sun[1,2,3], Fabio Mammano[4,5], Lianhua Sun[1,2,3]*, Jun Yang[1,2,3]* and Guiliang Zheng[1,2,3]*

[1] *Department of Otorhinolaryngology Head and Neck Surgery, Xinhua Hospital, Shanghai Jiao Tong University School of Medicine, Shanghai, China,* [2] *Shanghai Jiao Tong University School of Medicine Ear Institute, Shanghai, China,* [3] *Shanghai Key Laboratory of Translational Medicine on Ear and Nose Diseases, Shanghai, China,* [4] *Department of Physics and Astronomy "G. Galilei", University of Padova, Padua, Italy,* [5] *Department of Biomedical Sciences, Institute of Cell Biology and Neurobiology, Italian National Research Council, Monterotondo, Italy*

*Correspondence:
Lianhua Sun
sunlianhua@xinhuamed.com.cn
Jun Yang
yangjun@xinhuamed.com.cn
Guiliang Zheng
zhengguiliang@xinhuamed.com.cn

[†] *These authors have contributed equally to this work and share first authorship*

Greater epithelial ridge cells, a transient neonatal cell group in the cochlear duct, which plays a crucial role in the functional maturation of hair cell, structural development of tectorial membrane, and refinement of audio localization before hearing. Greater epithelial ridge cells are methodologically homogeneous, while whether different cell subtypes are existence in this intriguing region and the degeneration mechanism during postnatal cochlear development are poorly understood. In the present study, single-cell RNA sequencing was performed on the cochlear duct of postnatal rats at day 1 (P1) and day 7 (P7) to identify subsets of greater epithelial ridge cell and progression. Gene ontology and Kyoto Encyclopedia of Genes and Genomes pathway enrichment analysis were used to examine genes enriched biological processes in these clusters. We identified a total of 26 clusters at P1 and P7 rats and found that the cell number of five cell clusters decreased significantly, while four clusters had similar gene expression patterns and biological properties. The genes of these four cell populations were mainly enriched in Ribosome and P13K-Akt signal pathway. Among them, Rps16, Rpsa, Col4a2, Col6a2, Ctsk, and Jun are particularly interesting as their expression might contribute to the greater epithelial ridge cells degeneration. In conclusion, our study provides an important reference resource of greater epithelial ridge cells landscape and mechanism insights for further understanding greater epithelial ridge cells degeneration during postnatal rat cochlear development.

Keywords: single-cell RNA sequencing, cochlear duct, greater epithelial ridge cell, landscape, degeneration

INTRODUCTION

Mammalian hearing is dependent on the normal development of the cochlea, which includes the development of hair cells and supporting cells. The main cause of sensorineural hearing loss is damage to hair cells, which is difficult to reverse after hearing development has matured (Wagner and Shin, 2019). It has been found that hair cells in mice have a transient and limited ability to regenerate during hearing development, and further studies have revealed that this is related to the unique structural components of the inner ear (Henley et al., 1996; Chen et al., 2019).

The mammalian inner ear contains the vestibular sensory epithelium that perceives various accelerations and the auditory epithelia that perceive sound stimuli (Kelley, 2007). The auditory epithelium contains two main cell types: supporting cells and hair cells with greatly different anatomical and physiological characteristics (Scheffer et al., 2015). Hair cells continuously receive various stimuli from supporting cells and the outside world through unique receptors during their growth and development. These include the G-protein coupled P2Y receptors that activate phospholipase C (PLC) dependent production of inositor triphosphate (IP3) and release of intracellular ionized calcium (Ca^{2+}) from intracellular stores (Forsythe, 2007; Tritsch et al., 2007). In the developing cochlea, glutamate release from IHCs activates type I spiral neurons (SGNs) to generate action potentials, thereby mimicking in the pre-hearing cochlea the mechanical-electrical signal transduction effect triggered by acoustic waves transmitted via the external auditory canal (Tritsch and Bergles, 2010; Mammano and Bortolozzi, 2018; Ceriani et al., 2019), resulting in an increase in the frequency of spontaneous action potential release from IHCs and promoting the functional maturation of IHCs (Flores-Otero et al., 2007; Tritsch and Bergles, 2010; Dayaratne et al., 2014).

There are various types of supporting cells in the cochlea, and our group's previous research focused on GER cells. We found direct evidence of ATP release from supporting cells, with interactions between proteins involved in the ATP synthesis, release and action pathway in the cochlea, and the intracellular ATP-containing vesicles are lysosomes (He and Yang, 2015a). In addition, we found that not only apoptosis but also autophagy of the supporting cells occurs in GER (Yang and He, 2016; Hou et al., 2020). The GER cells are a group of broad columnar support cells located medial to the hair cells in the cochlea, and is the earliest epithelial structure to appear during cochlear development (Lim and Anniko, 1985). GER cells stimulate the production of calcium waves in the supporting cells by spontaneously releasing ATP, which excites hair cells and afferent nerve fibers, triggers the development of action potentials in auditory nerve fibers, and synchronizes the transmitters released by IHCs to encode similar frequencies, playing an important role in the development of the cochlea (Mazzarda et al., 2020). GER cells are seen in numerous mammals, including human, rat, and mouse, and undergo a series of changes in cell morphology and number during embryonic and postnatal periods (Hinojosa, 1977; Lim and Anniko, 1985), such as cell cytoplasm moving away from the cytosol, cell crumpling, gradual increase in cell gaps, gradual replacement of columnar cells by cuboidal cells, etc., eventually degenerating and leading to a mature inner sulcus region on the Corti organ structure after the animal becomes sensitive to external acoustic stimuli (Kelley, 2007; Nickel and Forge, 2008; Dayaratne et al., 2014). Eventually, the GER cells disappear while cochlear development continues, leading to a fully mature auditory function.

Transcriptome sequencing has been extensively used in previous studies of the inner ear (Liu et al., 2014; Burns et al., 2015; Cai et al., 2015; Scheffer et al., 2015; Han et al., 2018; Cheng et al., 2019; Tang et al., 2019; Li et al., 2020). However, it remains to be established whether GER cells degenerate completely during development or are partially transformed into other cell types to achieve a mature auditory function. To examine the transcriptional changes that occur during the formation of the organ of Corti, Kolla et al. (2020) performed single-cell RNA sequencing of the cochlear basilar membrane at different developmental stages and clustered them according to different gene expression patterns. Kolla's research team dissociated cochlear duct cells at four developmental time points and captured individual cells for analysis using single-cell RNAseq. They identified multiple unique cell types at each time point, including both known types, such as HCs and SCs, and previously unknown cell types, such as multiple unique cell types in Kölliker's organ. The sampling in the Kolla's team study was from E14 and E16 mice, whereas here we focussed our attention on rats at P1 and P7. However, the molecular mechanisms of how these cell clusters regulate GER cells development through changes in gene expression patterns at different times are not clear. Molecular signals released by GER cells during different periods may also shape hair cell maturation and auditory development by driving gene transcription, altering GER cell morphology, and changes in the number of GER cells, all of which are closely associated with hair cell maturation (Uziel, 1986; Legrand et al., 1988).

In the present work, we revealed the changes of GER cells profiles by single-cell RNA sequencing technology (Baslan et al., 2012; Shapiro et al., 2013; Huang et al., 2018). We also observed the change of the expression and regulation of key genes and signaling pathways enriched biological processes in these clusters during cochlear development. We identified four clusters with similar gene expression patterns and biological properties. Further investigations showed the genes of these four cell clusters were mainly enriched in Ribosome and P13K-Akt signal pathway. Among them, Rps16, Rpsa, Col4a2, Col6a2, Ctsk, and Jun are particularly interesting as their expression might contribute to degeneration of GER cells during normal development. Our present data provide a reference for the cellular landscape of the GER and suggests possible mechanism that lead to GER degeneration during normal postnatal development.

MATERIALS AND METHODS

Animals
Male and/or female Sprague-Dawley (SD) rats were purchased from Shanghai SIPPR-BK Laboratory Animals Co. Ltd. All the procedures involving rats were performed following the guidelines approved by the institutional Animal Care and Use Committee of the Shanghai Jiao Tong University School of Medicine.

In this study, the first postnatal day (P1) was the birthday, and P7 means the postnatal time points after the birthday.

Forty SD rats were randomly selected for each age group. The rats were sacrificed using an approved guillotine method. The cochlea tissue was extracted from the temporal bone, and the otic capsule was carefully transferred to a dish containing 0.01 M cold sodium phosphate-buffered saline (PBS, pH 7.35, GIBCO, Invitrogen Inc., Carlsbad, CA, United States). The stria vascularis, spiral ligament, and spiral ganglions, was gently separated by microdissection. The isolated cochlear duct was washed twice with potassium and magnesium-free PBS.

Tissue Dissociation and Preparation of Single-Cell Suspensions

The cochlear duct tissues were placed in a sterile RNase-free culture dish containing an appropriate amount of calcium-free and magnesium-free 1 × PBS on ice, the tissues were transferred into the culture dish and cut it into 0.5 mm^2 pieces, the tissues were washed with 1 × PBS, and remove as many non-purpose tissues as possible such as blood stains and fatty layers. Tissues were dissociated into single cells in dissociation solution (0.35% collagenase IV5, 2 mg/ml papain, 120 Units/ml DNase I) in 37°C water bath with shaking for 20 min at 100 rpm. Digestion was terminated with 1 × PBS containing 10% fetal bovine serum (FBS, V/V, then pipetting 5–10 times with a Pasteur pipette). The resulting cell suspension was filtered by passing through a 70–30 μm stacked cell strainer and centrifuged at 300 g for 5 min at 4°C. The cell pellet was resuspended in 100 μl 1 × PBS (0.04% BSA) and added with 1 ml 1 × red blood cell lysis buffer (MACS 130-094-183, 10×)and incubated at room temperature or on ice for 2–10 min to lyse remaining red blood cells.

After incubation, the suspension was centrifuged at 300 g for 5 min at room temperature. The suspension was resuspended in 100 μl Dead Cell Removal MicroBeads (MACS 130-090-101) and remove dead cells using Miltenyi Dead Cell Removal Kit (MACS 130-090-101). Then the suspension was resuspended in 1 × PBS(0.04% BSA) and centrifuged at 300 g for 3 min at 4°C (repeat twice). The cell pellet was resuspended in 50 μl of 1 × PBS (0.04% BSA). The overall cell viability was confirmed by trypan blue exclusion, which needed to be above 85%, single-cell suspensions were counted using a hemocytometer/Countess II Automated Cell Counter and concentration adjusted to 700–1200 cells/μ l.

Chromium 10x Genomics Library and Sequencing

Single-cell suspensions were loaded to 10x Chromium to capture 5000 single cells according to the manufacturer's instructions of the 10X Genomics Chromium Single-Cell 3′ kit (V3). The following cDNA amplification and library construction steps were performed according to the standard protocol. Libraries were sequenced on an Illumina NovaSeq 6000 sequencing system (paired-end multiplexing run, 150 bp) by LC-Bio Technology Co. Ltd. (Hangzhou, China) at a minimum depth of 20,000 reads per cell.

Bioinformatics Analysis of scRNA-Seq Data

Sequencing results were demultiplexed and converted to FASTQ format using Illumina bcl2fastq software. Sample demultiplexing, barcode processing, and single-cell 3′ gene counting by using the Cell Ranger pipeline[1] (version 3.1.0) and scRNA-seq data were aligned to Rattus norvegicus reference genome (Source: Rattus norvegicus UCSC; version: rn6). The Cell Ranger output was loaded into Seurat (version 3.1.1) to be used for dimensional reduction, clustering, and analysis of scRNA-sequencing data. Overall, 25139 cells passed the quality control threshold: all genes expressed in less than 1 cell were removed, the number of genes expressed per cell > 500 as low and <5000 as high cut-off, and UMI counts less than 500 and the percent of mitochondrial-DNA derived gene-expression < 25%.

To visualize the data, we further reduced the dimensionality of all 25139 cells using Seurat and used t-SNE to project the cells into 2D space (Satija et al., 2015), the steps include: (1) Using the Log normalize method of the "Normalization" function of the Seurat software to calculate the expression value of genes; (2) PCA (Principal component analysis) analysis was performed using the normalized expression value, Within all the PCs, the top 10 PCs were used to do clustering and t-SNE analysis; (3) To find clusters, selecting weighted Shared Nearest Neighbor (SNN) graph-based clustering method. Marker genes for each cluster were identified with the Wilcoxon rank-sum test (default parameters is "bi-mod": Likelihood-ratio test)with default parameters via the "Find All Markers" function in Seurat. This selects markers genes that are expressed in more than 10% of the cells in a cluster and average log$_2$ (Fold Change) of greater than 0.26.

Pathway Enrichment Analysis

Gene ontology (GO) enrichment analyses were performed with top GO package in R (Bioconductor) (Brionne et al., 2019) and Kyoto Encyclopedia of Genes and Genomes (KEGG) pathway enrichment analysis examining enriched processes in clusters was performed using Ingenuity Pathway Analysis (IPA) (Krämer et al., 2014). These two Functional enrichment analyses were used to identify which DEGs were significantly enriched in GO terms and/or metabolic pathways. GO is an international standard classification system for gene function. DEGs are mapped to the GO terms (biological functions) in the database. The number of genes in each term was calculated, and a hypergeometric test was performed to identify significantly enriched GO terms in the gene list out of the background of the reference gene list. GO terms and KEGG pathways with the adjusted p-value < 0.05 were considered significantly different.

Localization of Gene Expression by Fluorescence in situ Hybridization (FISH)

The Paraffin-DIG (digoxigenin)-TSA (Tyramide Signal Amplification)-ISH protocol was used to verify the localization

---
[1] https://support.10xgenomics.com/single-cell-gene-expression/software/downloads/3.1/

of gene expression. Cochleae were collected from SD rats of both sexes at postnatal day 1 (P1) and day 7 (P7) fixed in 4% paraformaldehyde overnight. The tissue was then dehydrated by gradient alcohol, paraffin, embedding, and sectioned on a cryostat at 10-μm thickness. Hybridization protocol was carried out based on the manufacturer's suggestions. After RNA ISH, sections were washed in 2 × SSC for 10 min at 37°C, with 1 × SSC two times for 5 min at 37°C, and wash in 0.5 × SSC for 10 min at room temperature. Formamide washing can be added if there are more non-specific hybrids. Blocking solution (rabbit serum) was added to the section and incubate at room temperature for 30 min, and then remove the blocking solution and add anti-digoxigenin-labeled peroxidase. Sections were incubated with secondary antibodies at 37°C for 40 min, then washed with PBS four times for 5 min each. And Nuclei were counterstained with DAPI for 15 s at room temperature. All fluorescent images were obtained on a Nikon Eclipse CI upright fluorescence microscope.

Statistical Analysis

All the statistical analyses of the cochlear cells data described in this paper were performed using Prism version 7.0 (GraphPad Software) and calculated according to the relative abundances. Experimental data are presented as the mean ± standard error of the mean. Comparisons were made by one-way analyses of variance or student's unpaired two-tailed t-tests between two different stages. P-values < 0.05 were considered statistically significant differences between these two periods.

RESULTS

scRNA-seq Identifies Multiple 26 Clusters of Cochlear Cells at P1 and P7

We performed scRNA-seq using a 10 × Genomics platform in pooled cochlear cells from 40 cochlear tissues from P1 and P7 phases. The cochlear duct cells comprise a highly diverse cellular mosaic that includes an undefined number of supporting cell (SC) types, two different types of mechanosensory hair cells (HCs), and unknown cell types in Kölliker's organ (KO).

The cochlear duct cells were isolated from the P1 and P7 cochlear duct and applied to scRNA-seq analysis (**Figure 1A**). The results obtained from Cell Ranger analyses were shown in **Supplementary Figure 1**. The estimated number of cells in the current study was 28557. Fraction reads in cells were 91.1%. Mean reads per cell were 38929 in P1 and 32218 in P7. Median genes per cell were 2151 in P1 and 2283 in P7. Total genes detected were 20866 in P1 and 20367 in P7. Reads Mapped to Genome were 96.20% in P1 and 96.30% in P7 (**Supplementary Data 1**). Following the quality control of scRNA-seq data, we retained 12826 cells in P1 and 12313 cells in P7 for the downstream analysis (**Supplementary Data 2**). After aggregated and normalized scRNA-seq data, t-distributed stochastic neighbor embedding (t-SNE) analysis (Satija et al., 2015) using Seurat R Package was performed for cell-type identification (Butler et al., 2018). The results of single-cell sequencing analysis showed that a total of 26 cell clusters were identified in P1 and P7 phases. An examination of the top five genes defining each cluster was used to assign identities to each group. **Figure 1B** showed the cell clusters in the P1 phase, and **Figure 1C** showed the cell clusters in the P7 phase. Visualization of the top five most variably expressed genes between cell clusters showed distinct transcriptional programs of the 26 clusters (**Figure 1D**).

The expression patterns of enriched genes of each cluster were analyzed. **Figure 2** shows the high expressed gene in each cell group. The darker the color, the richer the expression level of these genes in this cell's cluster. Cldn5, Loc100910270, Mt3, Plvap, Epcam, Stmn2, Rgs5, Lyz2, Ube2c, Gjb6, Gcg, Slco1a4, Cenpf, Coch, Aldh1a2 genes are highly expressed on one of the clusters, while Crym, Gpc3, Ccn3, Dbi, Col9a1, Sptssa, Pmp22 genes are co-express on several clusters (**Figure 2**). t-SEN plots of most ten abundant genes of each cell cluster were shown in **Supplementary Figures 2–28**).

scRNA-Seq Identifies Four GER Cell Clusters According to the Cells Number Dynamic Change From P1 to P7, and Gene Expression for Significant Marker Genes

Analysis of the cell numbers of each cell cluster of P1 and P7 showed that there was a significant decrease in the cell number of clusters 0, 2, 3, 4, 6, and 8, with statistically significant differences in clusters 0, 3, 6, and 8. And the cell number of clusters 1, 7, 9, and 12 increased and had statistical differences, as shown in **Supplementary Data 2** and **Figure 3**.

Great epithelial ridge cells are transient structures during cochlear development (Dayaratne et al., 2014), and a typical manifestation of this is a gradual decrease in the number of cells during auditory development. We performed genotypic analysis on these five cell clusters with significantly reduced cell numbers: clusters 0, 3, 4, 6, and 8. **Figure 4** shows the top five genes with high expression in each cell cluster (**Figure 4**). Oto and Crym were relatively highly expressed on cluster 0 (**Figure 4A**), and these two genes were also highly expressed on cluster 2 and cluster 12. On the t-SNE plot, cluster 12 and cluster 0 were closely linked in spatial position. Vcan, Edn3, and Gpc3 had similar gene expression patterns in clusters 3, 7, and 9 (**Figure 4B**). Scara3 and Aldh1a2 were relatively specifically highly expressed on cluster 4 (**Figure 4C**). More specific marker genes were present on cluster 6, including Ccn3, Irx3, Scg3, and Postn. Slc1a3 and Postn were similarly expressed on clusters 4 and 6 (**Figure 4D**). Cluster 8 lacked significant specific highly expressed genes and differed significantly from cluster 0, 3, 4, and 6 in gene expression patterns and spatial location.

The select genes with high expression in the decreased clusters of 0, 3, 4, 6, and 8 were further analyzed and the results are shown in **Figure 5**. In terms of gene expression, clusters 0, 3, 4,

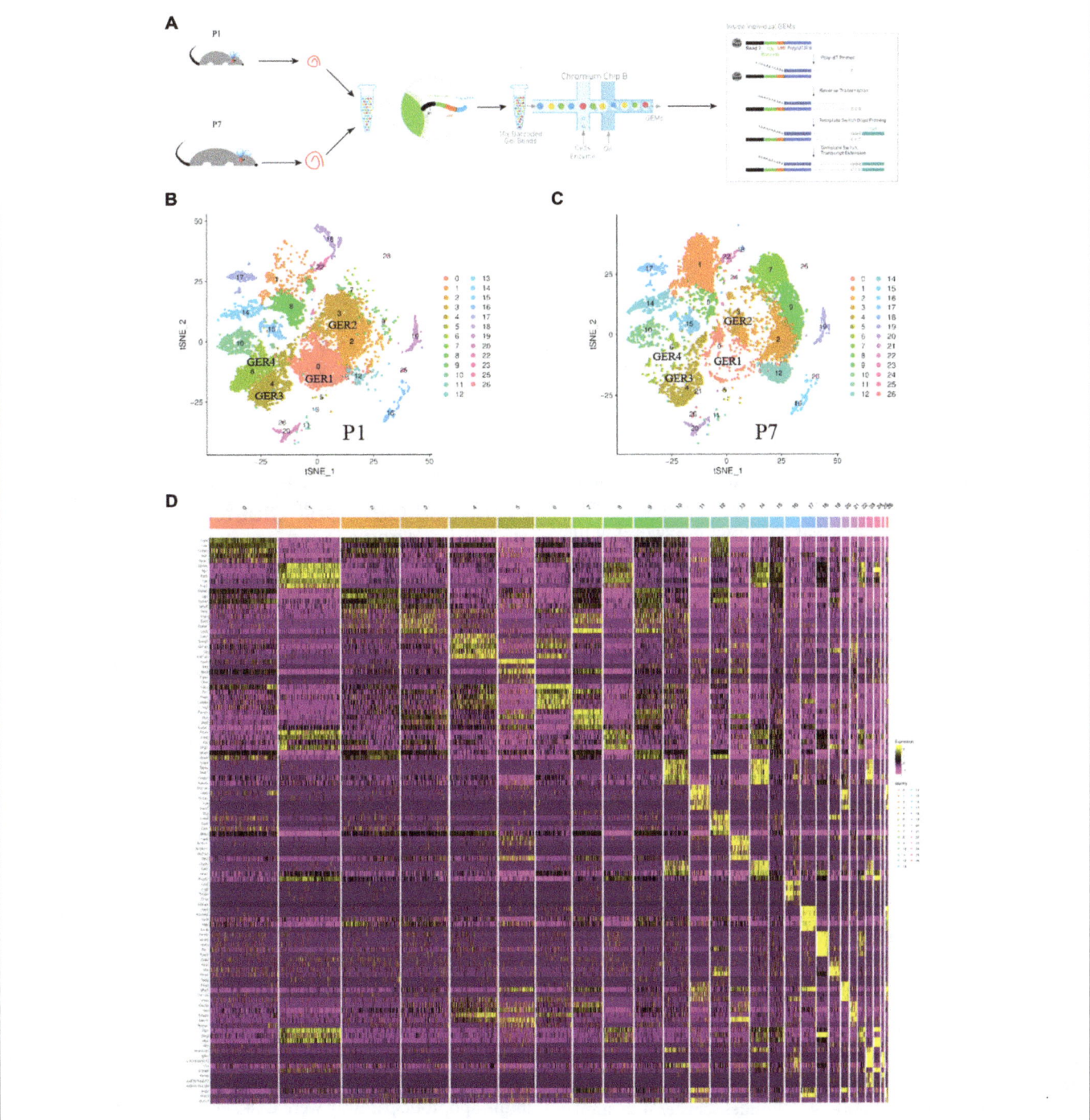

FIGURE 1 | Global expression profiling of cochlear cells by scRNA-Seq and cell clusters identification. **(A)** Scheme of cochlear duct preparation, single-cell isolation, and Chromium 10x Genomics library and scRNA-seq at P1 and P7. **(B)** t-SNE plots of cochlear cells at P1. (Left) Cell colors based on the origins (donors) are shown. **(C)** t-SNE plots of cochlear cells at P7. (Right) Cell colors based on the origins (donors) are shown. **(D)** Heat map for cochlear cell clusters. The top 5 deferentially expressed (DE) genes for the 26 identified clusters are shown. Cellular identity for each cluster is indicated by a color bar at the top of the heat map. The color ranges from blue to bright yellow indicates low to high gene expression levels, respectively.

and 6 have similar gene expression patterns. Separately, Isyna1 was more highly expressed on cluster 0; Col6a1 and Gpc3 were more highly expressed on cluster 3; Otor and Ccn3 had similar high expression levels in cluster 0, 3, 4, and 6; Clu, Scara3, and Calb2 were significantly and specifically highly expressed on cluster 4; Slc1a3 had similar expression levels on cluster 4

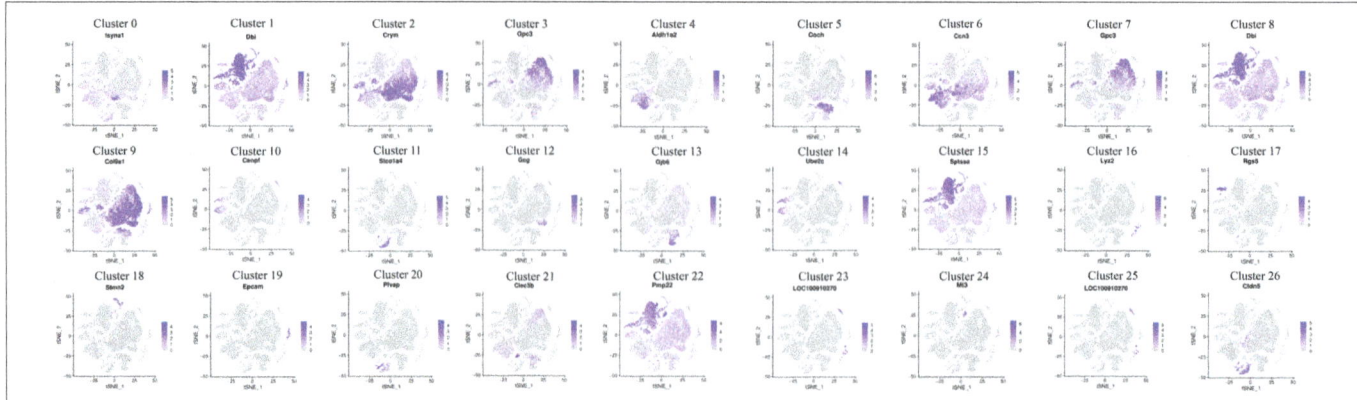

FIGURE 2 | Cochlea cells landscape revealed by scRNA-seq analysis. scRNA-seq was performed on single-cell suspensions pooled from P1 and P7 cochlea duct. All samples were analyzed using canonical correlation analysis with the Seurat R package. Cells were clustered using a graph-based shared nearest-neighbor clustering approach plotted by tSNE plot. Feature Plots of the most abundant gene in each cell cluster of cochlea cells.

and 6. In contrast to cluster 8, most of these aforementioned genes showed a lower expression on cluster 8, but the gene of Dbi was relatively highly expressed on cluster 8, suggesting that cluster 8 and the other four cell clusters are two cell types of different nature.

Gene Ontology (GO) Function Analysis Showed These Four Identified GER Cell Clusters Have Similar Expression Patterns

Gene Ontology function consists of biological processes (BP), cellular components (CC), and molecular functions (MF). We analyzed the GO functions of clusters 0, 3, 4, 6 and found the following characteristics. The gene of cluster 0 is mainly enriched in Translocation (BP), Nucleus (CC), and Structural constituent of Ribosome (MF) (**Figure 6A**). The gene of cluster 3 is mainly enriched in Negative regulation of transcription from RNA polymerase II, Biological process, Positive regulation of transcription from RNA polymerase II, Cell differentiation and translation (BP), Extracellular exosome, Extracellular space, Cytoplasm and Nucleoplasm, Cytoplasm, and Nucleus (CC) and Protein binding (MF) (**Figure 6B**). The gene of cluster 4 has similar BP and CC as cluster 3 that are mainly enriched in Translation, Cytoplasm, Extracellular exosome, and Nucleus (**Figure 6C**). Besides, cluster 4 is similar to cluster 0 in terms of MF and is enriched in Protein binding and Structural constituents of the Ribosome. Cluster 6 is similar to cluster 2 in terms of BP, mainly enriched in Translocation, Biological process, negative regulation of transcription from RNA polymerase II (**Figure 6D**). Also, in the CC, cluster 6 is mainly enriched in Cytoplasm, Nucleus, and Membrane, similar to cluster 3 and cluster 4 (**Figures 6B,C**), while enriched in Structural constituent of Ribosome, RNA-binding, and Protein binding which is similar to cluster 0 in MF, which shows that these cell clusters have similar expression patterns.

KEGG Pathway Analysis for the Identified GER Cell Clusters

The results of KEGG signaling pathway analysis for cluster 0, cluster 3, cluster 4, and cluster 6 are shown in **Figure 7**. The results showed that genes in all clusters were predominantly enriched in Ribosome signaling pathway (**Figures 7A–D**). In cluster 0, 44 genes are rich in Ribosome, and the top 5 genes are Rps16, Rps18l1, Rpsa, Rps5, Rps17 (**Supplementary Data 3**). In cluster 3, there were 13 genes enriched in Ribosome, and the top 5 genes are Rps16, Rps8, Rpl41, Rpl28, Rps12 (**Supplementary Data 4**). In cluster 4, there were 31 genes enriched in Ribosome, and the top 5 genes are Rps18l1, Rps5, Rps17, Rpl10a, Rps8 (**Supplementary Data 5**).

In cluster 6, there were 58 genes enriched in Ribosome, and the top 5 genes are Rps16, Rps19, Rps18l1, Rpsa, Rpl35 (**Supplementary Data 6**). We found that Rp16 was involved in the Ribosome signaling pathway of these three cell clusters. While in cluster 3, some genes were also clearly enriched in the P13K-Akt signal pathway, Focal adhesion, and Protein digestion and absorption. The genes enriched in the P13K-Akt signal pathway are Col4a2, Col6a2, Creb3l1, AABR07068316.1, Igf2, Col4a1, Gf1, Col6a1, Fn1, Pten, Col1a1, Spp1, and genes enriched in Protein digestion and absorption are Col5a2, Col4a2, Col6a2, Col3a1, Mme, AABR07068316.1, Col5a1, Col4a1, Col6a1, Col1a1 (**Supplementary Data 4**). In addition, we found the main genes in the apoptotic pathway were Ctsk, Fos, Ctsb, and Jun.

The Heterogeneity Analysis of These Four GER Cell Clusters

To analyze the heterogeneity of these four cell clusters, we performed a re-clustered analysis. Analysis of the top ten genes with high expression showed that the top five genes expressed on cluster 0 were Col9a1, Col2a1, Crym, Col9a2, and S100b, respectively; the top five genes expressed on cluster 3 were Dcn, Sparcl1, Col3a1, Gpc3, and Mgp, respectively. The top five expressed genes on cluster 4 were Gsn, Clu, Sat1,

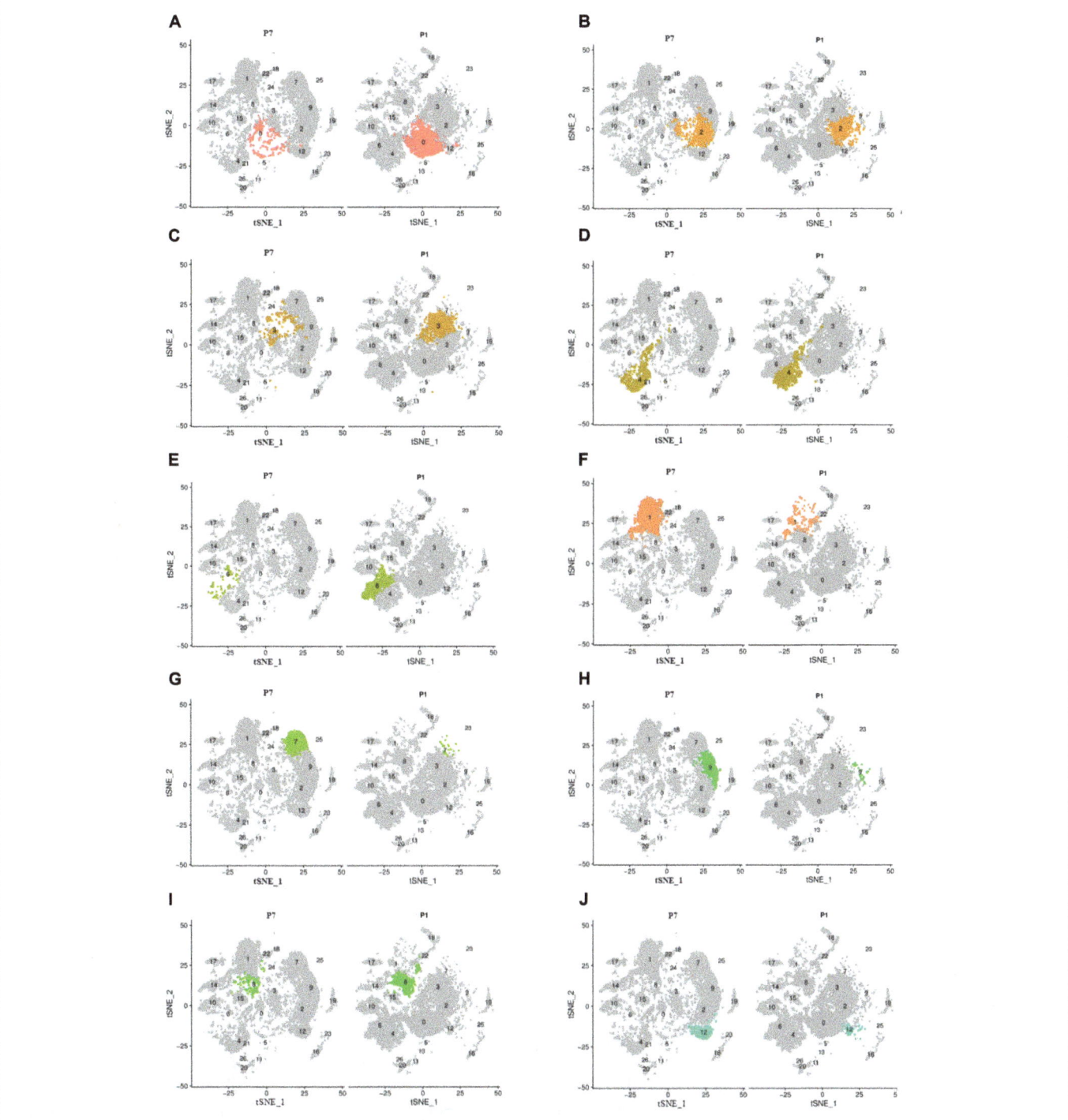

FIGURE 3 | The change of cell number of the above different cell clusters in two different periods of P1 and P7. Cells were clustered using a graph-based shared nearest-neighbor clustering approach plotted by a tSNE plot. **(A,C–E,I)** The decreased clusters of 0, 3, 4, 6, and 8. **(B,F–H,J)** The significantly increased clusters of 1, 7, 9, and 12.

Itga8, and Cavin2. The top five expressed genes on cluster 6 were Apoe, Ccn3, Postn, Ccdc80, and Nr2f1. **Figure 8** shows the top five genes highly expressed in the above four cell clusters.

The select genes of these four cell clusters were analyzed to reveal the heterogeneity, and the results are shown in **Figure 9**. In terms of gene expression, Col9a2 and S100b was more highly expressed on cluster 0 and 3; Dcn was more highly

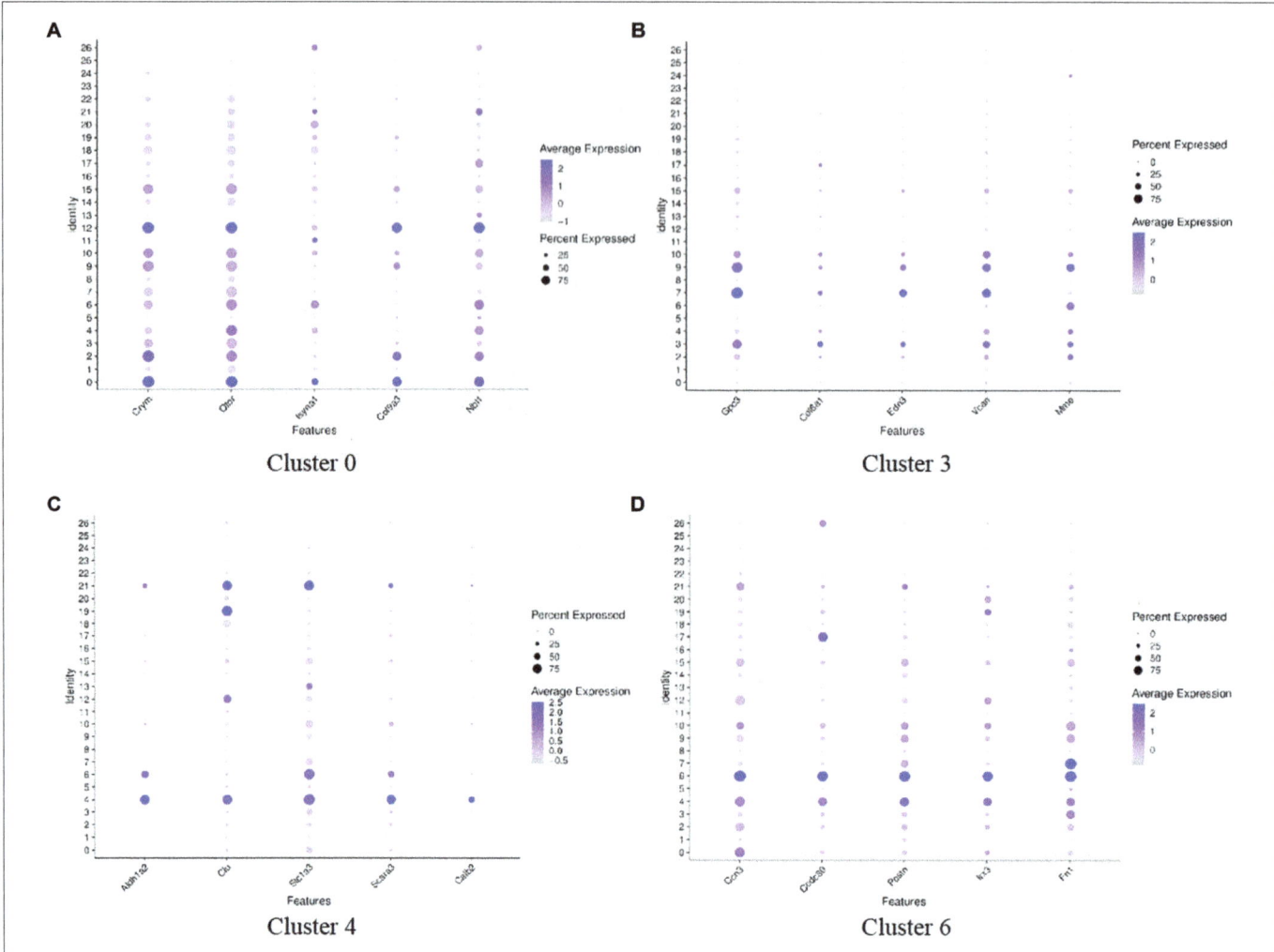

FIGURE 4 | Dot plots representing expression levels of cochlea cells. scRNA-seq was performed on single-cell suspensions pooled from the cochlea duct of SD rats including P1 and P7 stages. All samples were analyzed using Dot plot analysis with the Seurat R package. Expression levels of the top five genes on cluster 0 (A), cluster 3 (B), cluster 4 (C), cluster 6 (D) are shown. Each dot was sized to represent the proportion of cells of each type expressing the marker gene and colored to represent the mean expression of each marker gene across all cells, as shown in the key.

expressed on cluster 3; Gsn had similar high expression levels in cluster 3 and 4; Postn was highly expressed on cluster 4 and 6; Apoe had similar expression levels on this four clusters. These findings indicate that these four GER cell clusters are some heterogeneity.

The results of GO functional enrichment analysis showed that the genes in cluster 0 were mainly enriched in the extracellular space and extracellular region; the genes in cluster 3 and cluster 4 were mainly enriched in the extracellular exosome and extracellular space; the genes in cluster 6 are mainly enriched in the extracellular region and negative regulation of cell promotion. These results showed that they had similar GO functions, and the genes were mainly enriched in regulating the changes of cell spatial structure, among which cluster 3 and cluster 4 had higher homogeneity. Cluster 6 plays a major role in the negative regulation of cell proliferation (**Figure 10**).

KEGG signaling pathway analysis showed that the genes in cluster 0 were mainly enriched in protein digestion and absorption and TGF beta signaling pathway, which regulated the digestion and absorption of cell debris after apoptosis; The genes in cluster 3 are mainly enriched in the PI3K-Akt signaling pathway and pathways in cancer, which regulates cell apoptosis; The genes in Cluster 4 are mainly enriched in fluid shear stress and atherosclerosis, and hepatocellular carcinoma, which also plays a role in regulating apoptosis. The genes in cluster 6 were mainly enriched in Wnt signaling pathway, and human papillomavirus infection (**Figure 11**). According to these results, the four-cell clusters are heterogeneous.

Fluorescence *in situ* Hybridization (FISH) of GER Cell Clusters

To validate the cell-type-specific genes of clusters 0, 3, 4, and 6, we used fluorescence *in situ* hybridization (FISH) to localize

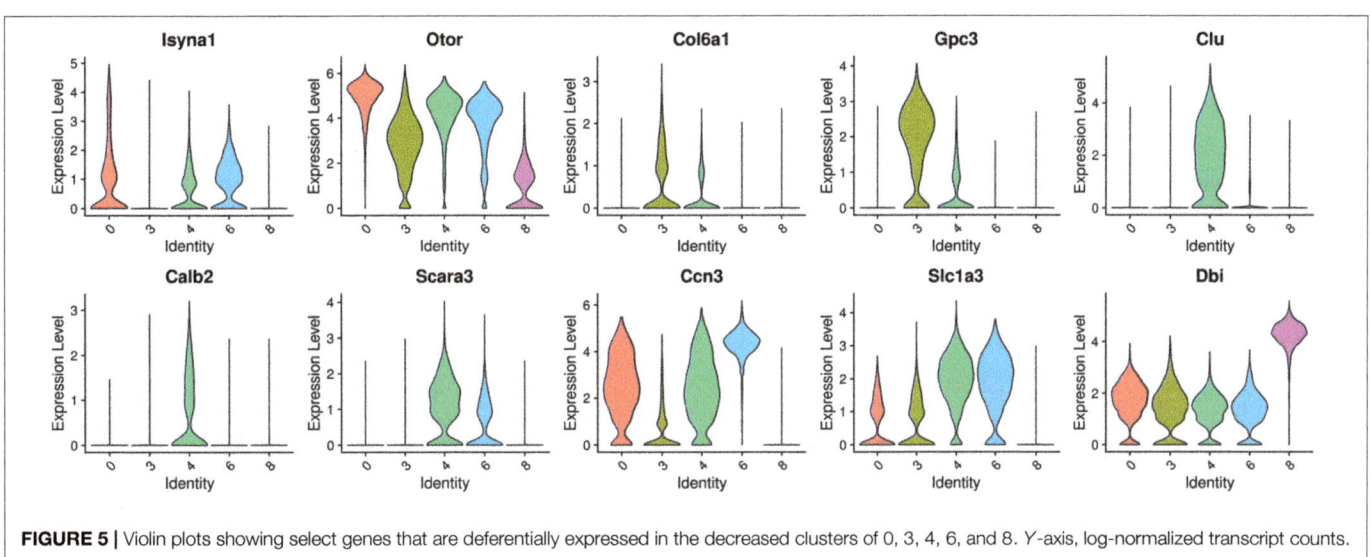

FIGURE 5 | Violin plots showing select genes that are deferentially expressed in the decreased clusters of 0, 3, 4, 6, and 8. Y-axis, log-normalized transcript counts.

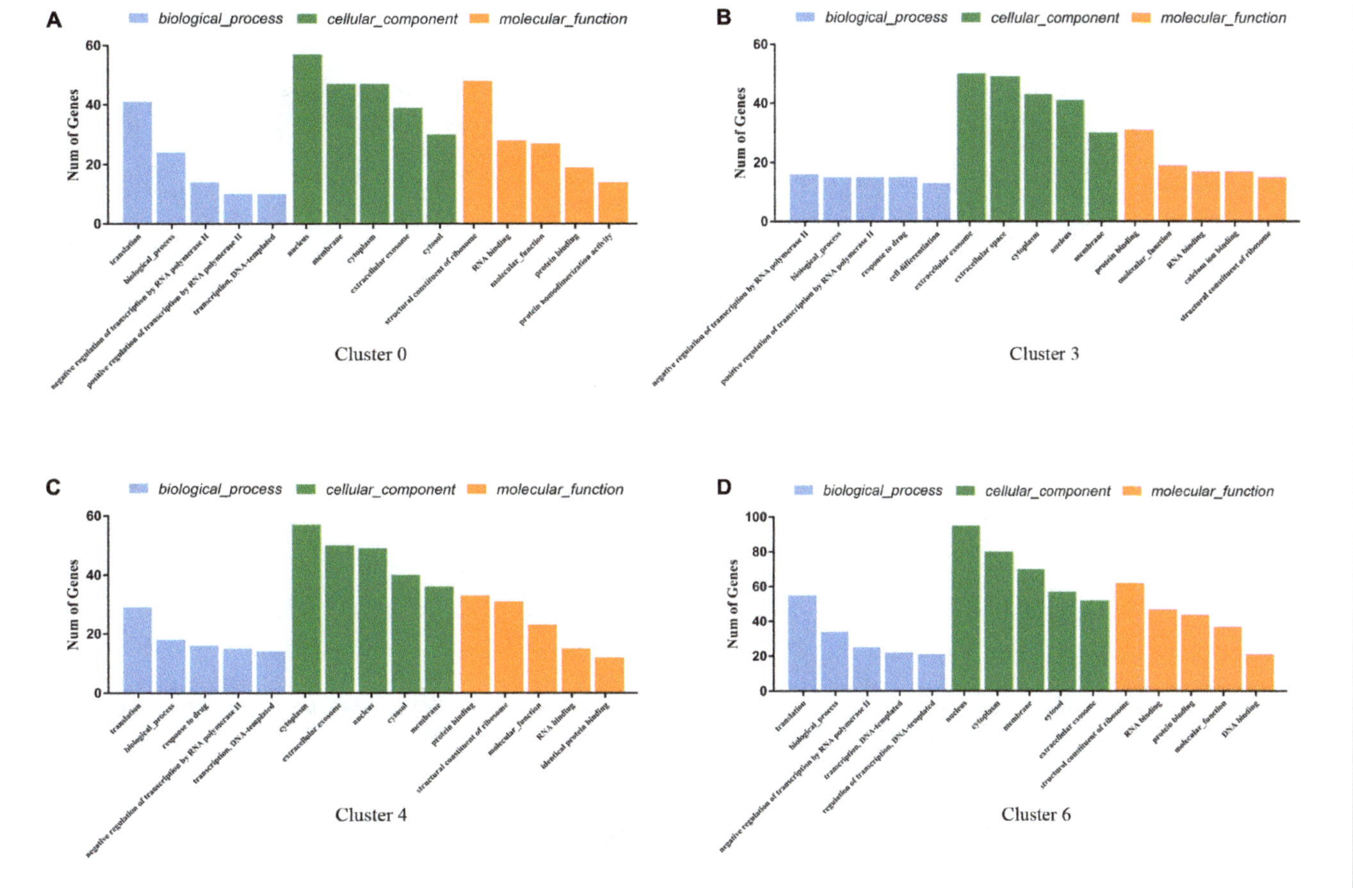

FIGURE 6 | GO enrichment analysis of genes for cluster 0 **(A)**, cluster 3 **(B)**, cluster 4 **(C)**, cluster 6 **(D)**. The Go functions include biological processes (BP, blue color), cellular components (CC, green color), and molecular functions (MF, yellow color). The horizontal coordinate-axis X is the item of go function, and the ordinate represents the genes enriched by different items.

transcripts for these four GER cells types in cross-sections from P1 to P7 cochlea (**Figure 12**). Four genes with the high expression on clusters 0, 3, 4, and 6 based on scRNA-seq results were selected for FISH: Otor, Col6a1, Scara3, and Ccn3. All four genes showed patterns of expression that were consistent with the single-cell results. Otor that was detected in all GER cell clusters, and was among the top five differentially expressed genes in cluster 0. From the FISH result, it can be seen that Otor was high and nearly

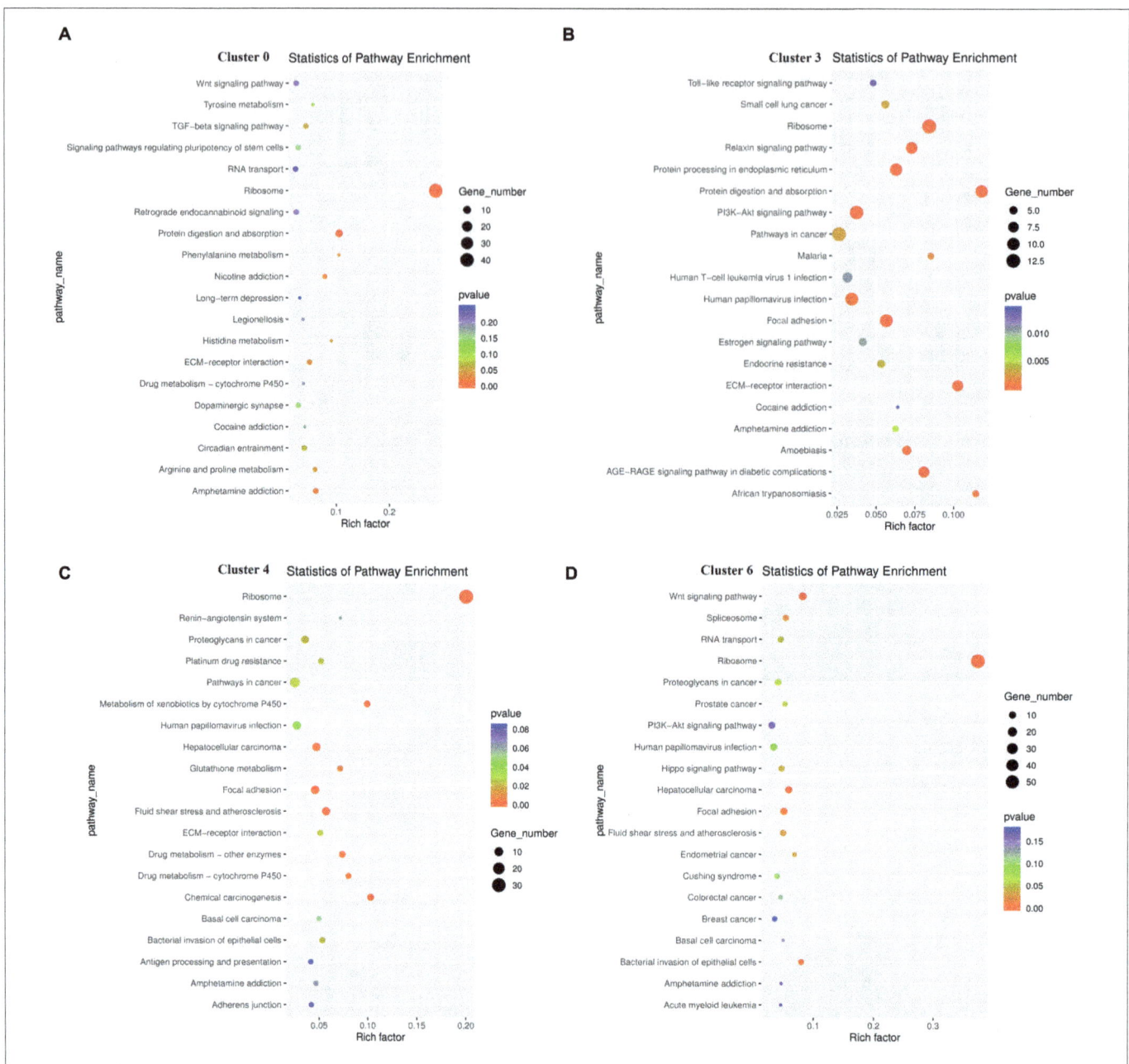

FIGURE 7 | Functional enrichment analyses using Kyoto Encyclopedia of Genes and Genomes (KEGG) pathways for cluster 0 **(A)**, cluster 3 **(B)**, cluster 4 **(C)**, cluster 6 **(D)**. The triangle size indicates the significance and corresponding significance values displayed as log10 (P-value).

restricted expressed to the whole GER cells at P1 (green color), and down-regulated expression in GER at P7 (**Figures 12A,E**). Col6a1 was significantly expressed in EGR region of the cochlea at P1, but almost disappeared at P7 (**Figures 12B,F**). Scara3 was centrally expressed in the lateral wall of the GER region of the cochlea during the P1 period but showed a significantly reduced scattered expression during the P7 period (**Figures 12C,G**). The location of Ccn3 expression in the GER region of the cochlea during P1 overlapped a lot with Otor, but the expression was also significantly reduced at P7 (**Figures 12D,H**).

DISCUSSION

As a temporary structure in the development of the cochlea, the presence of GER indicates that the cochlea is still immature (Bryant et al., 2002; Inoshita et al., 2014; Peeters et al., 2015; Mazzarda et al., 2020). GER cells undergo cellular morphological changes after birth, such as plasma membrane separation, cell shrinkage, cell gap enlargement, and columnar cells replaced by cubic cells (Uziel, 1986). At the same time, the number of cells is greatly reduced and eventually changes to a mature inner sulcus

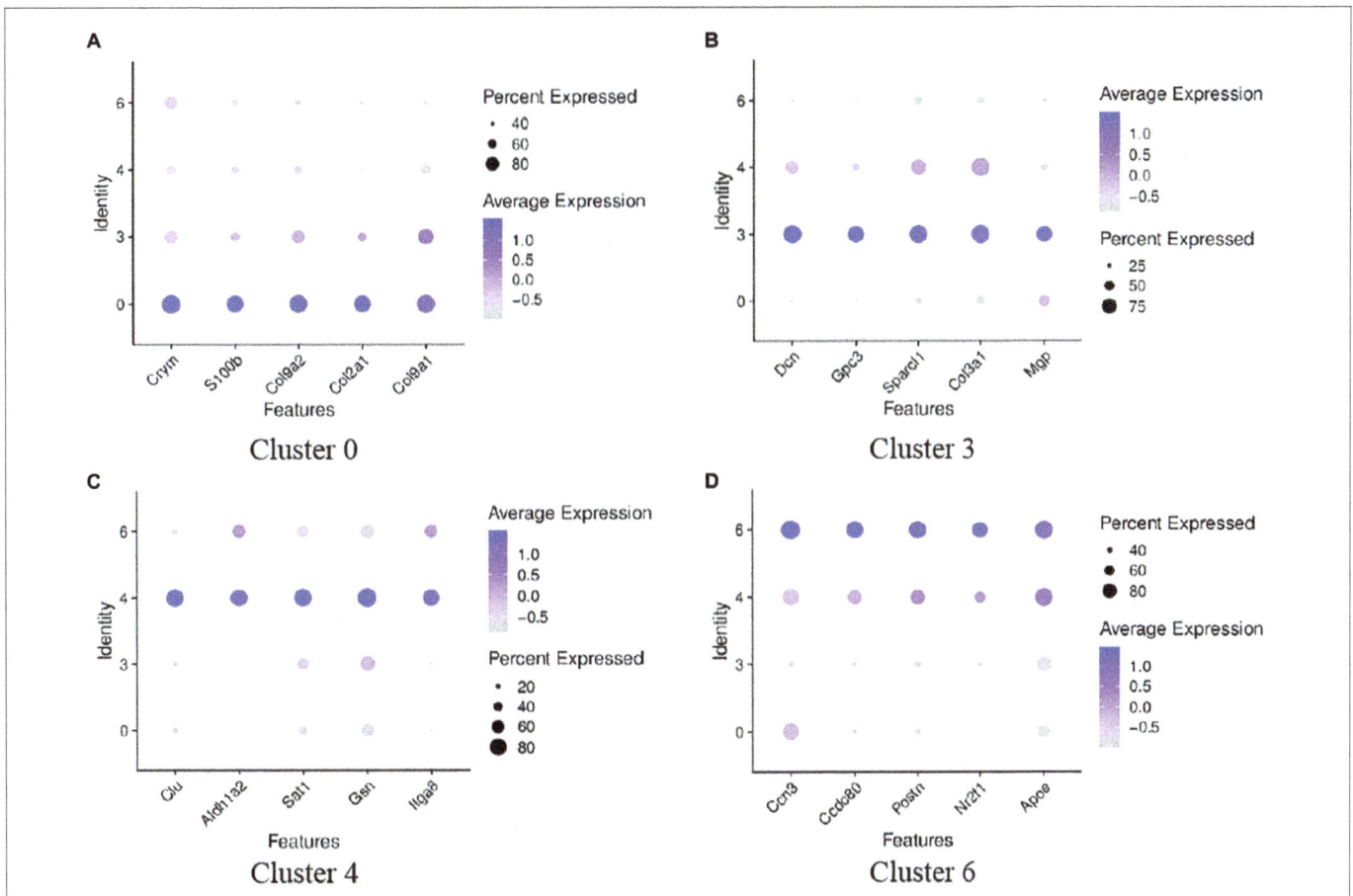

FIGURE 8 | Dot plots representing expression levels of the four GER cells. A re-clustered analysis was performed to reveal the heterogeneity of differential genes expression. Expression levels of the top five genes on cluster 0 **(A)**, cluster 3 **(B)**, cluster 4 **(C)**, cluster 6 **(D)** are shown. Each dot was sized to represent the proportion of cells of each type expressing the marker gene and colored to represent the mean expression of each marker gene across all cells, as shown in the key.

region (Hinojosa, 1977; Woods et al., 2004; Sirko et al., 2019). The present single-cell RNA sequencing results confirmed that the GER cell population decreases over time, in accord with prior work (Hinojosa, 1977; Woods et al., 2004; Sirko et al., 2019). The GER has an important role in the survival and maturation of auditory neurons, synaptic development, and refinement of auditory afferent and efferent innervation before the emergence of hearing (Chai et al., 2012; Johnson et al., 2017; Mammano and Bortolozzi, 2018; Ceriani et al., 2019). There is a high degree of morphological uniformity in a range of cell shapes in the GER region, but it is not clear whether different subtypes of cells play different regulatory roles during cochlea development (Dayaratne et al., 2014; Hayashi Y. et al., 2020). Kolla et al. (2020) classified GER cells into four different subtypes by single-cell sequencing analysis, and genes with different expression abundance on different cell subtypes. The authors named the cells as L.KO, lateral Kölliker's organ cells and M.KO, medial Kölliker's organ cells according to their expression patterns, and further divided the L.KO cells into KO1, KO2, and KO3 subtypes. Among them, KO1 cell cluster highly expresses Dcn and Rcn3; KO2 cell cluster highly expresses Cpxm2, Ctgf, Kazald1, and Tectb; KO3 cell cluster highly expresses, Gjb6, Net1, Tectb, and Tsen15; KO4 cell cluster highly expresses Calb1, Clu, Crabp1, Epyc, and Itm2a. Kubota et al. (2021) classified GER cells into S2, S3, and S4 cell subtypes based on specific gene expression. Among them, Gsn and Sparcl1 were significantly highly expressed on all three cell subtypes, Crabp1 was significantly highly expressed on the S2 cell subtype, and Scara3, Clu, and Gpc3 were highly expressed on the S2 and S3 cell subtype. From these results, three distinct GER cells groups that correlate with a specific spatial distribution of marker genes were identified, and disappeared during post-natal cochlear maturation.

In the present study, we compared cell cluster typing and numbers at P1 and P7. The results showed that the cells of clusters 0, 3, 4, 6, and 8 were significantly reduced over time. Clusters 0, 3, 4, and 6 showed high similarity in the expression patterns, GO functions, and signaling pathways. Besides, these four clusters were also closely related to each other on the tSNE plot, while cluster 8 had no spatial relationship with these clusters. Based on these results, we considered that clusters 0, 3, 4, and 6 were different subtypes of GER cells.

At the same time, we found that clusters 2, 7, 9, and 12 were highly similar to clusters 0 and 3 in terms of gene expression patterns, and the cell numbers of these four clusters showed an

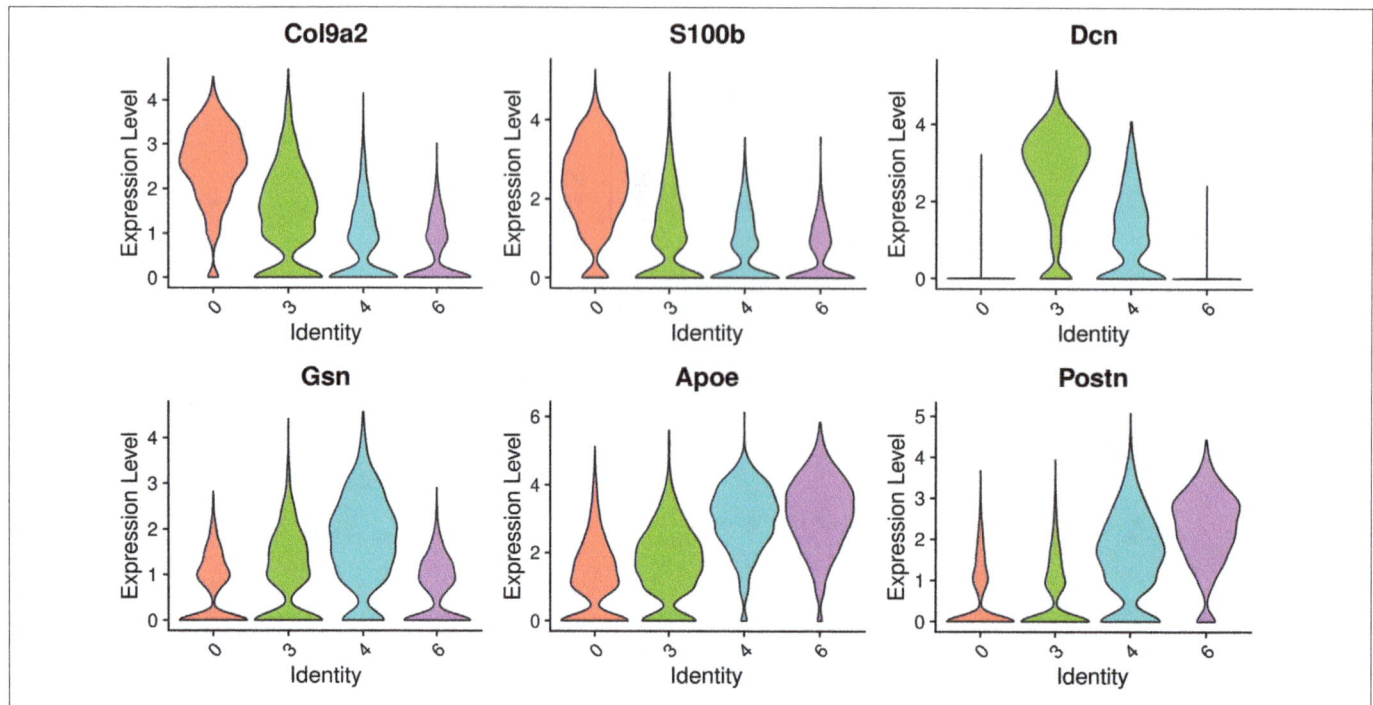

FIGURE 9 | Expression of select genes of these four GER cell clusters. Violin plots showing normalized log-transformed expression values for the select genes for cluster 0, cluster 3, cluster 4, cluster 6.

increase around P7, with a statistically significant difference in the cluster 7, 9, and 12. Vcan, Edn3 and Gpc3 had similar gene expression patterns in clusters 3, 7, and 9. Oto and Crym were closely linked in spatial locations between cluster12 and 0, and their spatial locations were close to each other. The research of Kubota et al. (2021) is consistent with this study. Kubota et al. (2021) believe that the most lateral GER group has the highest similarity with neonatal inner border and inner phalangeal cells, and thought these inner border and inner phalangeal cells have a similar organ-forming potential. However, whether these cell populations can also be considered as different subtypes of GER cells or other types of cochlear support cells that disappear after full maturation of cochlear hearing development still requires further in-depth investigation.

Although, the number of cells in clusters 0, 3, 4, and 6 decreased significantly from P1 to P7, the detailed mechanism is unclear.

Yang and He (2016) found that the morphology of GER cells in the newborn rat cochlea gradually appeared to replace the short columnar epithelium with high columnar cells from the basilar turn to the apex as they developed, and the number of cells also gradually decreased. They hypothesized that GER cells apoptosis played an important role in the development of rat cochlea. In addition, GER cells exhibited programmed apoptosis from the basilar turn to the apex turn *in vivo* experiments, but showed proliferation *in vitro* experiments (He and Yang, 2015b). The authors suggested that the initiating factors of apoptosis might come from outside of the GER cells rather than from intrinsic cellular factors. It was also found (Hou et al., 2019,

2020) that the expression levels of caspase-3, caspase-8, caspase-9, and Bcl-2 gene mRNA and protein in the basilar membrane of rat cochlea at different times after birth were significantly time-dependent. Together, those studies suggest that some GER cells undergo apoptosis while other proliferate. However, proliferating cells are outnumbered by apoptotic cells, which eventually leads to the disappearance of GER cells. Autophagy is also thought to be involved in GER cells development and both autophagy and apoptosis show a strict time dependence, with peak activity occurring at P1 or earlier in autophagic, and apoptosis occurring at P7 or later (He and Yang, 2015b; Yang and He, 2016). Autophagy and apoptosis play different roles in different stages of cochlea development (Takahashi et al., 2001; Peeters et al., 2015; Liu et al., 2017; Hayashi K. et al., 2020). Disruption of autophagy or apoptosis of supporting cells during cochlea development will result in impaired development or hearing impairment (He et al., 2017; Mammano and Bortolozzi, 2018; Zhou et al., 2020). Therefore, the dynamic balance between autophagy and apoptosis regulates the normal differentiation and development of the cochlea, but the specific regulatory mechanism is not yet clear.

The results of this scRNA sequencing showed that GER clusters have many commonalities in Go function enrichment. In terms of biological processes, the enrichment is more consistent in Translation and Negative regulation of transcription from RNA polymerase II; in terms of cellular components, the gene enrichment is more consistent in Nucleus and Cytoplasm; in terms of molecular functions, the enrichment is mainly in Protein binding and Structural constituent of Ribosome. In terms of

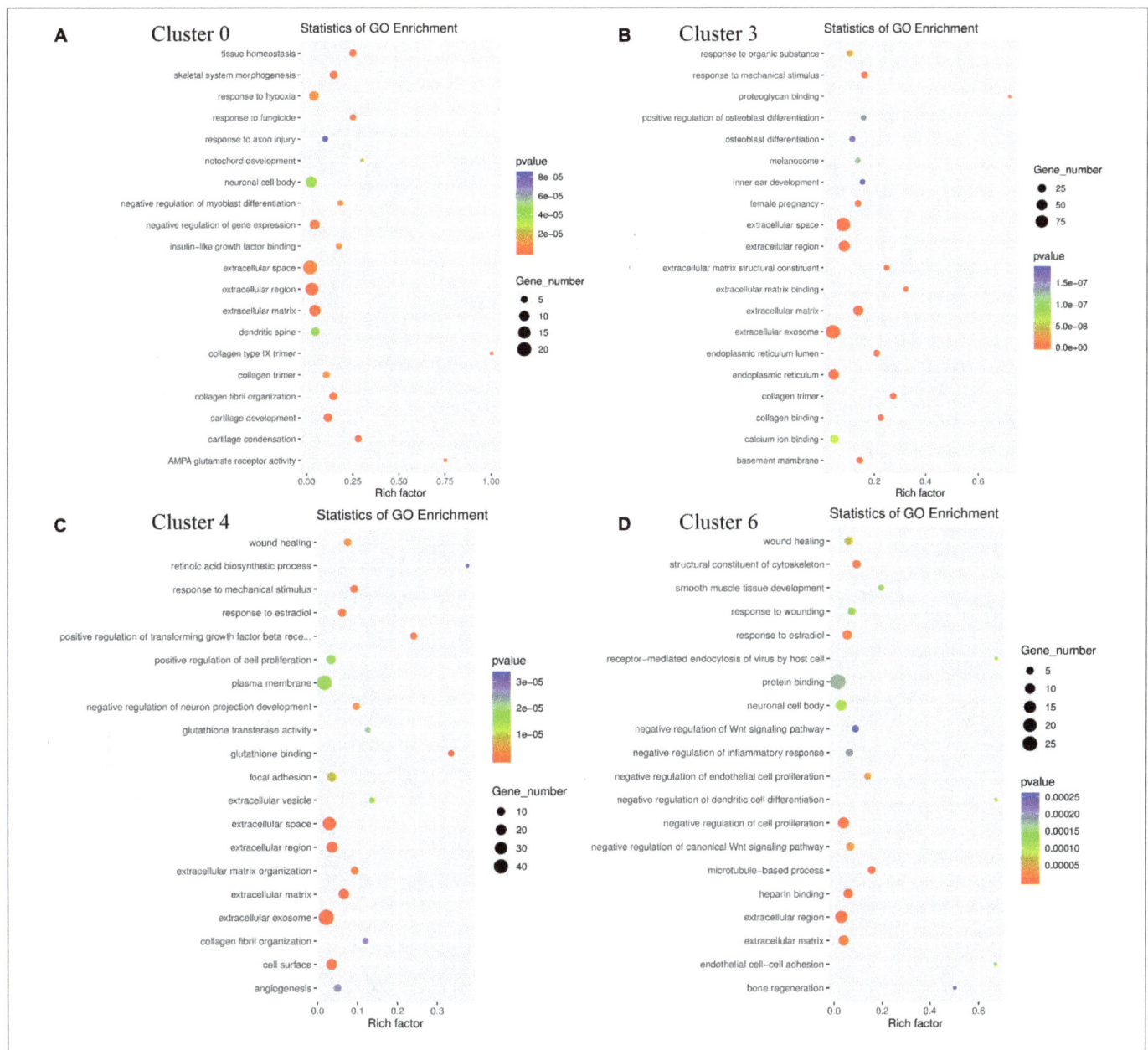

FIGURE 10 | GO enrichment analysis of genes for the heterogeneity of cluster 0 (A), cluster 3 (B), cluster 4 (C), cluster 6 (D). The triangle size indicates the significance and corresponding significance values displayed as log10 (P-value).

molecular mechanisms, transcription and translation are very active. Meanwhile, different GER cell clusters, such as clusters 3 and 4, have a large number of genes enriched in Negative regulation of transcription from RNA polymerase II, which play a negative dynamic regulatory role (Sun et al., 2015). These negatively regulated genes are mainly Nedd4, Rarb, Foxp2, Pawr, Dact1, Igf2, Egr1, H2afy2, Btg2, Calr, Foxc1, Mdfi, Rps14, Jun, Peg3, and Ets2.

At present, several genes and signaling pathways have been confirmed to play important roles in the development of the inner ear, such as the Sox2 (Yang et al., 2019), Pax2 (Patel et al., 2018), Atoh1 (Zhong et al., 2019), FGF (Yang et al., 2018) Notch (Daudet and Żak, 2020, FoxG1 (Ding et al., 2020), Shh (Bok et al., 2007), mTOR (Fu et al., 2018), and Wnt (Waqas et al., 2016) pathways. The results based on the KEGG signaling pathway showed a high degree of consistency in gene enrichment in these four GER cell clusters. Clusters 0, 4, and 6 were significantly enriched in the Ribosome signaling pathway (see **Figures 7A,C,D**); cluster 3 was enriched in PI3K-Akt and Protein digestion and absorption signaling pathway in addition to the Ribosome signaling pathway (see **Figure 7B**), which is consistent with

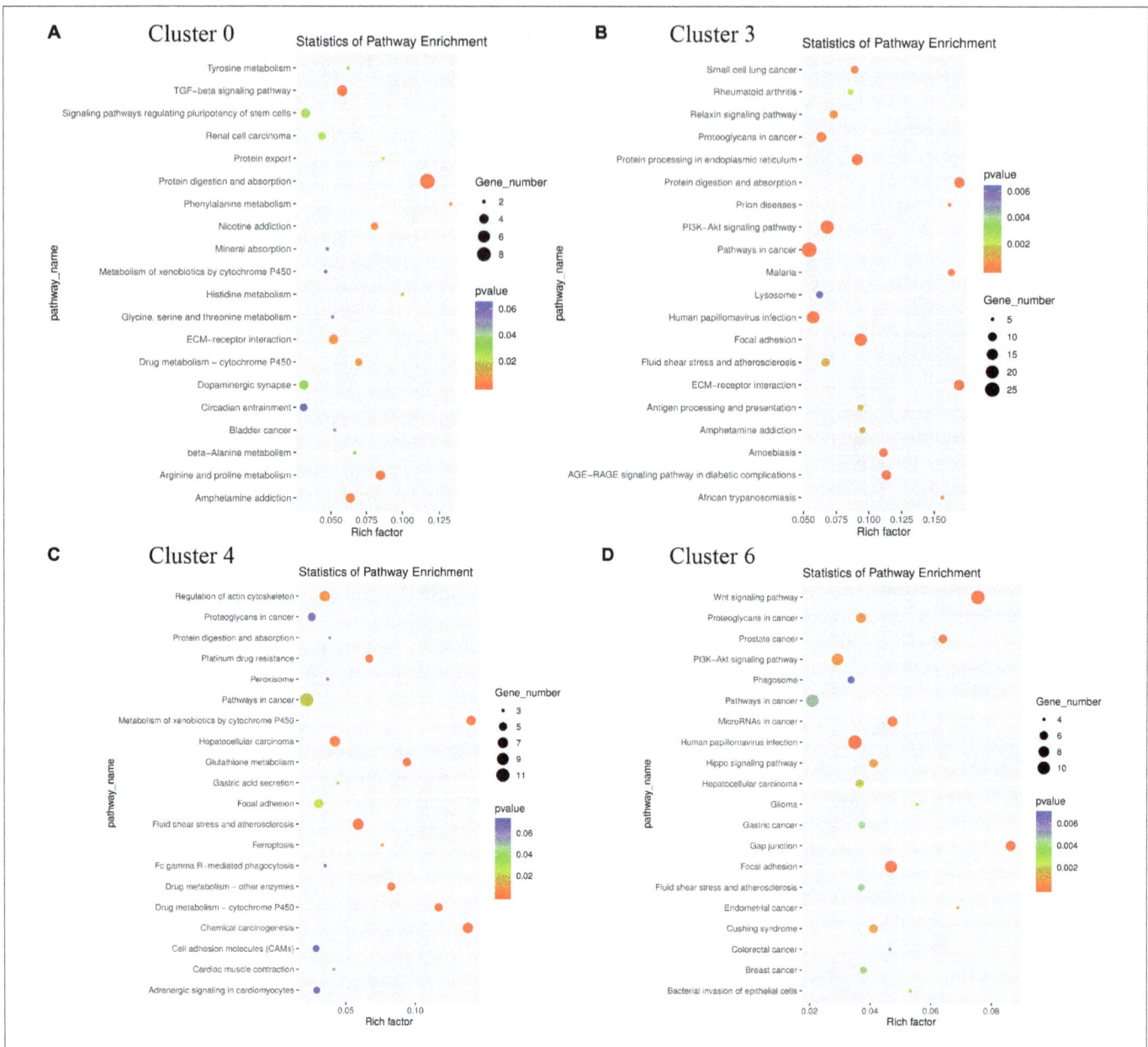

FIGURE 11 | KEGG pathways functional enrichment analyses for the heterogeneity of cluster 0 **(A)**, cluster 3 **(B)**, cluster 4 **(C)**, cluster 6 **(D)** after re-clustered. The triangle size indicates the significance and corresponding significance values displayed as log10 (*P*-value).

the Go function results. The ribosome signaling pathway is an important signaling pathway regulating development, and ribosome biosynthesis is one of the most multifaceted and energetically demanding processes in the whole of biology, involving protein assembly and maturation factors, and requiring the coordinated involvement of multiple cellular functions (Pelletier et al., 2018). Mitosis is a key process of organ development and maturation, and vigorous mitosis suggests cells are dividing and proliferating, yet the overall number of GER cells decrease during postnatal development, presumably mainly related to the negative regulatory signaling pathway of cluster 3. The PI3K-Akt signaling pathway is an important

signaling pathway that regulates cell proliferation, differentiation, apoptosis, and migration (Ediriweera et al., 2019; Jia et al., 2019). It has also been shown to regulate hair cell regeneration in cochlea developmental regeneration studies (Mullen et al., 2012; Xia et al., 2019).

Cluster 3 has a large number of genes enriched in the PI3K-Akt signaling pathway, including Col4a2, Col6a2, Creb3l1, AABR07068316.1, Igf2, Col4a1, gf1, Col6a1, Fn1, Pten, Col1a1, Spp1, which might regulate the proliferation and apoptosis of GER cells, and through Col5a2, Col4a2, Col6a2, Col3a1, Mme, AABR07068316.1, Col5a1, Col4a1, Col6a1, Col1a1 on the Protein digestion and absorption signaling pathway regulate

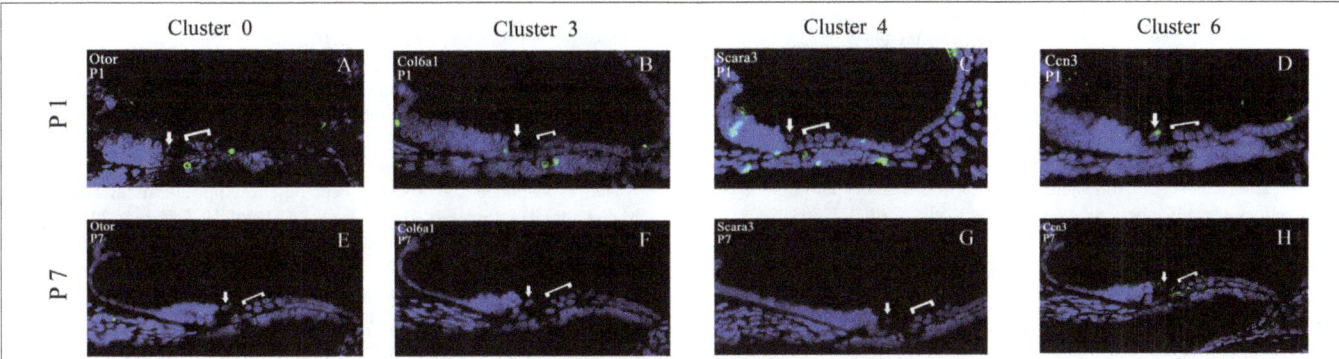

FIGURE 12 | Validation of high expression gene of GER cell clusters at P1 and P7. Otor was high and nearly restricted expressed to the whole GER cells at P1 (green color), and down-regulated expression in GER at P7 **(A,E)**. Col6a1 was significantly expressed in EGR region of the cochlea at P1, but almost disappeared at P7 **(B,F)**. Scara3 was centrally expressed in the lateral wall of the GER region of the cochlea during the P1 period, but showed a significantly reduced scattered expression during the P7 period **(C,G)**. The location of Ccn3 expression in the GER region of the cochlea during P1 overlapped a lot with Otor, but the expression was also significantly reduced at P7 **(D,H)**. For all panels, the IHC is indicated with an arrow and the three OHCs are indicated by a bracket.

these apoptotic proteins and autophagy of cellular debris, thereby directing the orderly degeneration of GER cells or possible trans-differentiation of hair cells or supporting cells. In this study, we also found that the genes enriched in the apoptotic pathway are mainly Ctsk, Fos, Ctsb, and Jun. The mechanism of these genes in regulating the degeneration of GER cells and promoting auditory development has not been reported, and the role of this signaling pathway and related genes still needs to be investigated in depth.

LIMITATION OF STUDY

The present study has the following shortcomings: (1) We did not perform localization studies of the characteristic genes expressed in these four GER subtypes; (2) Previous morphological studies showed that GER cells in rodents degenerate and disappear in 12–14 days after birth, by which time auditory function emerges. In the present study, we only studied GER cells subtypes up to P7, and found a significant decrease in the number of GER cells, but not a complete degeneration; (3) We also found that clusters 2, 7, 9, and 12 have an increased number of cells and their gene expression patterns are common to the above four subtypes of GER cells. Whether these cells are trans-differentiated hair cells, supporting cell precursor cells, or other subtypes of GER cells, and the fate transition of these cells still needs more in-depth study and exploration; (4) Although we identified several gene candidates, we did not perform mechanistic studies to determine the relationship of these genes and related signaling pathway with proliferation, apoptosis, and autophagy of GER cells.

ETHICS STATEMENT

The animal study was reviewed and approved by Animal Ethics Committee of Shanghai Jiao Tong University School of Medicine.

AUTHOR CONTRIBUTIONS

JY, FM, and GZ: study design. JiC, DG, JuC, SH, BH, and LS: acquisition of data. YL, SL, FZ, and XS: analysis and interpretation of data. JiC and DG: drafting the manuscript. JY and GZ: study supervision. All authors contributed to the article and approved the submitted version.

ACKNOWLEDGMENTS

We want to thank the National Natural Science Foundation of China to support this work and thank the staff members of the LC Sciences (Hangzhou, China) for their support and expertise.

REFERENCES

Baslan, T., Kendall, J., Rodgers, L., Cox, H., Riggs, M., Stepansky, A., et al. (2012). Genome-wide copy number analysis of single cells. *Nat. Protoc.* 7, 1024–1041. doi: 10.1038/nprot.2012.039

Bok, J., Dolson, D. K., Hill, P., Rüther, U., Epstein, D. J., and Wu, D. K. (2007). Opposing gradients of Gli repressor and activators mediate Shh signaling along the dorsoventral axis of the inner ear. *Development* 134, 1713–1722. doi: 10.1242/dev.000760

Brionne, A., Juanchich, A., and Hennequet-Antier, C. (2019). ViSEAGO: a Bioconductor package for clustering biological functions using Gene Ontology and semantic similarity. *BioData Min.* 12:16. doi: 10.1186/s13040-019-0204-1

Bryant, J., Goodyear, R. J., and Richardson, G. P. (2002). Sensory organ development in the inner ear: molecular and cellular mechanisms. *Br. Med. Bull.* 63, 39–57. doi: 10.1093/bmb/63.1.39

Burns, J. C., Kelly, M. C., Hoa, M., Morell, R. J., and Kelley, M. W. (2015). Single-cell RNA-Seq resolves cellular complexity in sensory organs from the neonatal inner ear. *Nat. Commun.* 15:8557. doi: 10.1038/ncomms9557

Butler, A., Hoffman, P., Smibert, P., Papalexi, E., and Satija, R. (2018). Integrating single-cell transcriptomic data across different conditions, technologies, and species. *Nat. Biotechnol.* 36, 411–420. doi: 10.1038/nbt.4096

Cai, T., Jen, H. I, Kang, H., Klisch, T. J., Zoghbi, H. Y., and Groves, A. K. (2015). Characterization of the transcriptome of nascent hair cells and identification of direct targets of the Atoh1 transcription factor. *J. Neurosci.* 35, 5870–5883. doi: 10.1523/JNEUROSCI.5083-14.2015

Ceriani, F., Hendry, A., Jeng, J. Y., Johnson, S. L., Stephani, F., Olt, J., et al. (2019). Coordinated calcium signalling in cochlear sensory and non-sensory cells refines afferent innervation of outer hair cells. *EMBO. J.* 38:e99839. doi: 10.15252/embj.201899839

Chai, R., Kuo, B., Wang, T., Liaw, E. J., Xia, A. P., Jan, T. A., et al. (2012). Wnt signaling induces proliferation of sensory precursors in the postnatal mouse cochlea. *Proc. Natl. Acad. Sci. U. S. A.* 109, 8167–8172. doi: 10.1073/pnas.1202774109

Chen, Y., Zhang, S., Chai, R., and Li, H. (2019). Hair Cell Regeneration. *Adv. Exp. Med. Biol.* 1130, 1–16. doi: 10.1007/978-981-13-6123-4_1

Cheng, C., Wang, Y., Guo, L., Lu, X., Zhu, W., Muhammad, W., et al. (2019). Age-related transcriptome changes in Sox2+ supporting cells in the mouse cochlea. *Stem Cell Res. Ther.* 10:365. doi: 10.1186/s13287-019-1437-0

Daudet, N., and Żak, M. (2020). Notch Signalling: the Multitask Manager of Inner Ear Development and Regeneration. *Adv. Exp. Med. Biol.* 1218, 129–157. doi: 10.1007/978-3-030-34436-8_8

Dayaratne, M. W. N., Vlajkovic, S. M., Lipski, J., and Thorne, P. R. (2014). Kölliker's organ and the development of spontaneous activity in the auditory system: implications for hearing dysfunction. *Biomed. Res. Int.* 2014:367939. doi: 10.1155/2014/367939

Ding, Y., Meng, W., Kong, W., He, Z., and Chai, R. (2020). The Role of FoxG1 in the Inner Ear. *Front. Cell Dev. Biol.* 8:614954. doi: 10.3389/fcell.2020.614954

Ediriweera, M. K., Tennekoon, K. H., and Samarakoon, S. R. (2019). Role of the PI3K/AKT/mTOR signaling pathway in ovarian cancer: biological and therapeutic significance. *Semin. Cancer Biol.* 59, 147–160. doi: 10.1016/j.semcancer.2019.05.012

Flores-Otero, J., Xue, H. Z., and Davis, R. L. (2007). Reciprocal regulation of presynaptic and postsynaptic proteins in bipolar spiral ganglion neurons by neurotrophins. *J. Neurosci.* 27, 14023–14034. doi: 10.1523/JNEUROSCI.3219-07.2007

Forsythe, I. D. (2007). Hearing: a fantasia on Kölliker's organ. *Nature* 450, 43–44. doi: 10.1038/450043a

Fu, X., Sun, X., Zhang, L., Jin, Y., Chai, R., Yang, L., et al. (2018). Tuberous sclerosis complex-mediated mTORC1 overactivation promotes age-related hearing loss. *J. Clin. Invest.* 128, 4938–4955. doi: 10.1172/JCI98058

Han, J., Wu, H., Hu, H., Yang, W., Dong, H., Liu, Y., et al. (2018). Characterization of the Transcriptome of Hair Cell Regeneration in the Neonatal Mouse Utricle. *Cell. Physiol. Biochem.* 51, 1437–1447. doi: 10.1159/000495592

Hayashi, K., Suzuki, Y., Fujimoto, C., and Kanzaki, S. (2020). Molecular Mechanisms and Biological Functions of Autophagy for Genetics of Hearing Impairment. *Genes* 11:1331. doi: 10.3390/genes11111331

Hayashi, Y., Suzuki, H., Nakajima, W., Uehara, I., Tanimura, A., Himeda, T., et al. (2020). Cochlear supporting cells function as macrophage-like cells and protect audiosensory receptor hair cells from pathogens. *Sci. Rep.* 10:6740. doi: 10.1038/s41598-020-63654-9

He, Y., and Yang, J. (2015b). The study on the proliferation and the apoptosis factors in vitro of Kölliker organ supporting cells in the cochlea of newborn rat. *Lin Chung Er Bi Yan Hou Tou Jing Wai Ke Za Zhi* 29, 152–159.

He, Y., and Yang, J. (2015a). [ATP release mechanism from the supporting cells in the Kölliker organ in vitro in the cochlea of newborn rat]. *Zhonghua Er Bi Yan Hou Tou Jing Wai Ke Za Zhi.* 50, 43–49.

He, Z., Guo, L., Shu, Y., Fang, Q., Zhou, H., Liu, Y., et al. (2017). Autophagy protects auditory hair cells against neomycin-induced damage. *Autophagy* 13, 1884–1904. doi: 10.1080/15548627.2017.1359449

Henley, C. M., Weatherly, R. A., Martin, G. K., and Lonsbury-Martin, B. (1996). Sensitive developmental periods for kanamycin ototoxic effects on distortion-product otoacoustic emissions. *Hear. Res.* 98, 93–103. doi: 10.1016/0378-5955(96)00077-9

Hinojosa, R. (1977). A note on development of Corti's organ. *Acta Otolaryngol.* 84, 238–251. doi: 10.3109/00016487709123963

Hou, S., Chen, J., and Yang, J. (2019). Autophagy precedes apoptosis during degeneration of the Kölliker's organ in the development of rat cochlea. *Eur. J. Histochem.* 63:3025. doi: 10.4081/ejh.2019.3025

Hou, S., Chen, P., Chen, J., Chen, J., Sun, L., Chen, J., et al. (2020). Distinct Expression Patterns of Apoptosis and Autophagy-Associated Proteins and Genes during Postnatal Development of Spiral Ganglion Neurons in Rat. *Neural Plast.* 2020, 1–9. doi: 10.1155/2020/9387560

Huang, X. T., Li, X., Qin, P. Z., Zhu, Y., Xu, S. N., and Chen, J. P. (2018). Technical Advances in Single-Cell RNA Sequencing and Applications in Normal and Malignant Hematopoiesis. *Front. Oncol.* 8:582. doi: 10.3389/fonc.2018.00582

Inoshita, A., Karasawa, K., Funakubo, M., Miwa, A., Ikeda, K., and Kamiya, K. (2014). Dominant negative connexin26 mutation R75W causing severe hearing loss influences normal programmed cell death in postnatal organ of Corti. *BMC Genet.* 15:1. doi: 10.1186/1471-2156-15-1

Jia, X., Wen, Z., Sun, Q., Zhao, X., Yang, H., Shi, X., et al. (2019). Apatinib suppresses the Proliferation and Apoptosis of Gastric Cancer Cells via the PI3K/Akt Signaling Pathway. *J. BUON* 24, 1985–1991.

Johnson, S. L., Ceriani, F., Houston, O., Polishchuk, R., Polishchuk, E., Crispino, G., et al. (2017). Connexin-Mediated Signaling in Nonsensory Cells Is Crucial for the Development of Sensory Inner Hair Cells in the Mouse Cochlea. *J. Neurosci.* 37, 258–268. doi: 10.1523/JNEUROSCI.2251-16.2016

Kelley, M. W. (2007). Cellular commitment and differentiation in the organ of Corti. *Int. J. Dev. Biol.* 51, 571–583. doi: 10.1387/ijdb.072388mk

Kolla, L., Kelly, M. C., Mann, Z. F., Anaya-Rocha, A., Ellis, K., Lemons, A., et al. (2020). Characterization of the development of the mouse cochlear epithelium at the single cell level. *Nat. Commun.* 11:2389. doi: 10.1038/s41467-020-16113-y

Krämer, A., Green, J., Pollard, J. J., and Tugendreich, S. (2014). Causal analysis approaches in Ingenuity Pathway Analysis. *Bioinformatics* 30, 523–530. doi: 10.1093/bioinformatics/btt703

Kubota, M., Scheibinger, M., Jan, T. A., and Heller, S. (2021). Greater epithelial ridge cells are the principal organoid-forming progenitors of the mouse cochlea. *Cell Rep.* 34:108646. doi: 10.1016/j.celrep.2020.108646

Legrand, C., Bréhier, A., Clavel, M. C., Thomasset, M., and Rabié, A. (1988). Cholecalcin (28-kDa CaBP) in the rat cochlea. Development in normal and hypothyroid animals. An immunocytochemical study. *Brain Res.* 466, 121–129. doi: 10.1016/0165-3806(88)90090-9

Li, C., Li, X., Bi, Z., Sugino, K., Wang, G., Zhu, T., et al. (2020). Comprehensive transcriptome analysis of cochlear spiral ganglion neurons at multiple ages. *Elife* 9:e50491. doi: 10.7554/eLife.50491

Lim, D. J., and Anniko, M. (1985). Developmental morphology of the mouse inner ear. A scanning electron microscopic observation. *Acta Otolaryngol. Suppl.* 422, 1–69.

Liu, H., Pecka, J. L., Zhang, Q., Soukup, G. A., Beisel, K. W., and He, D. Z. (2014). Characterization of transcriptomes of cochlear inner and outer hair cells. *J. Neurosci.* 34, 11085–11095. doi: 10.1523/JNEUROSCI.1690-14.2014

Liu, J., Cai, L. B., He, Y. Y., and Yang, J. (2017). Apoptosis pattern and alterations of expression of apoptosis-related factors of supporting cells in Kölliker's organ in vivo in early stage after birth in rats. *Eur. J. Histochem.* 61:2706. doi: 10.4081/ejh.2017.2706

Mammano, F., and Bortolozzi, M. (2018). Ca2+ signaling, apoptosis and autophagy in the developing cochlea: milestones to hearing acquisition. *Cell Calcium* 70, 117–126. doi: 10.1016/j.ceca.2017.05.006

Mazzarda, F., D'Elia, A., Massari, R., De Ninno, A., Bertani, F. R., Businaro, L., et al. (2020). Organ-on-chip model shows that ATP release through connexin hemichannels drives spontaneous Ca^{2+} signaling in non-sensory cells of the greater epithelial ridge in the developing cochlea. *Lab Chip* 20, 3011–3023. doi: 10.1039/d0lc00427h

Mullen, L. M., Pak, K. K., Chavez, E., Kondo, K., Brand, Y., and Ryan, A. F. (2012). Ras/p38 and PI3K/Akt but not Mek/Erk signaling mediate BDNF-induced neurite formation on neonatal cochlear spiral ganglion explants. *Brain Res.* 1430, 25–34. doi: 10.1016/j.brainres.2011.10.054

Nickel, R., and Forge, A. (2008). Gap junctions and connexins in the inner ear: their roles in homeostasis and deafness. *Curr. Opin. Otolaryngol. Head Neck Surg.* 16, 452–457. doi: 10.1097/MOO.0b013e32830e20b0

Patel, D., Shimomura, A., Majumdar, S., Holley, M. C., and Hashino, E. (2018). The histone demethylase LSD1 regulates inner ear progenitor differentiation through interactions with Pax2 and the NuRD repressor complex. *PLoS One* 13:e0191689. doi: 10.1371/journal.pone.0191689

Peeters, R. P., Ng, L., Ma, M., and Forrest, D. (2015). The timecourse of apoptotic cell death during postnatal remodeling of the mouse cochlea and its premature onset by triiodothyronine (T3). *Mol. Cell. Endocrinol.* 407, 1–8. doi: 10.1016/j.mce.2015.02.025

Pelletier, J., Thomas, G., and Volarević, S. (2018). Ribosome biogenesis in cancer: new players and therapeutic avenues. *Nat. Rev. Cancer* 18, 51–63. doi: 10.1038/nrc.2017.104

Satija, R., Farrell, J. A., Gennert, D., Schier, A. F., and Regev, A. (2015). Spatial reconstruction of single-cell gene expression data. *Nat. Biotechnol.* 33, 495–502. doi: 10.1038/nbt.3192

Scheffer, D. I., Shen, J., Corey, D. P., and Chen, Z. Y. (2015). Gene Expression by Mouse Inner Ear Hair Cells during Development. *J. Neurosci.* 35, 6366–6380. doi: 10.1523/JNEUROSCI.5126-14.2015

Shapiro, E., Biezuner, T., and Linnarsson, S. (2013). Single-cell sequencing-based technologies will revolutionize whole-organism science. *Nat. Rev. Genet.* 14, 618–630. doi: 10.1038/nrg3542

Sirko, P., Gale, J. E., and Ashmore, J. F. (2019). Intercellular Ca^{2+} signalling in the adult mouse cochlea. *J. Physiol.* 597, 303–317. doi: 10.1113/JP276400

Sun, J., Rockowitz, S., Chauss, D., Wang, P., Kantorow, M., Zheng, D., et al. (2015). Chromatin features, RNA polymerase II and the comparative expression of lens genes encoding crystallins, transcription factors, and autophagy mediators. *Mol. Vis.* 21, 955–973.

Takahashi, K., Kamiya, K., Urase, K., Suga, M., Takizawa, T., Mori, H., et al. (2001). Caspase-3-deficiency induces hyperplasia of supporting cells and degeneration of sensory cells resulting in the hearing loss. *Brain Res.* 894, 359–367. doi: 10.1016/s0006-8993(01)02123-0

Tang, M., Li, J., He, L., Guo, R., Yan, X., Li, D., et al. (2019). Transcriptomic profiling of neural stem cell differentiation on graphene substrates. *Colloids Surf. B. Biointerfaces* 182:110324. doi: 10.1016/j.colsurfb.2019.06.054

Tritsch, N. X., and Bergles, D. E. (2010). Developmental regulation of spontaneous activity in the Mammalian cochlea. *J. Neurosci.* 30, 1539–1550. doi: 10.1523/JNEUROSCI.3875-09.2010

Tritsch, N. X., Yi, E., Gale, J. E., Glowatzki, E., and Bergles, D. E. (2007). The origin of spontaneous activity in the developing auditory system. *Nature* 450, 50–55. doi: 10.1038/nature06233

Uziel, A. (1986). Periods of sensitivity to thyroid hormone during the development of the organ of Corti. *Acta Otolaryngol. Suppl.* 429, 23–27. doi: 10.3109/00016488609122726

Wagner, E. L., and Shin, J. B. (2019). Mechanisms of Hair Cell Damage and Repair. *Trends Neurosci.* 42, 414–424. doi: 10.1016/j.tins.2019.03.006

Waqas, M., Zhang, S., He, Z., Tang, M., and Chai, R. (2016). Role of Wnt and Notch signaling in regulating hair cell regeneration in the cochlea. *Front. Med.* 10, 237–249. doi: 10.1007/s11684-016-0464-9

Woods, C., Montcouquiol, M., and Kelley, M. W. (2004). Math1 regulates development of the sensory epithelium in the mammalian cochlea. *Nat. Neurosci.* 7, 1310–1318. doi: 10.1038/nn1349

Xia, W., Hu, J., Ma, J., Huang, J., Jing, T., Deng, L., et al. (2019). Mutations in TOP2B cause autosomal-dominant hereditary hearing loss via inhibition of the PI3K-Akt signalling pathway. *FEBS Lett.* 593, 2008–2018. doi: 10.1002/1873-3468.13482

Yang, J., and He, Y. (2016). The apoptosis of the Kölliker organ in the cochlea of newborn rat in vitro. *J. Audiol. Speech Pathol.* 24, 371–376. doi: 10.3969/j.issn.1006-7299.2016.04.012

Yang, L. M., Cheah, K. S. E., Huh, S. H., and Ornitz, D. M. (2019). Sox2 and FGF20 interact to regulate organ of Corti hair cell and supporting cell development in a spatially-graded manner. *PLoS Genet.* 15:e1008254. doi: 10.1371/journal.pgen.1008254

Yang, Z., Yao, J., and Cao, X. (2018). [Roles of the FGF signaling pathway in regulating inner ear development and hair cell regeneration]. *Yi. Chuan* 40, 515–524. doi: 10.16288/j.yczz.17-407

Zhong, C., Fu, Y., Pan, W., Yu, J., and Wang, J. (2019). Atoh1 and other related key regulators in the development of auditory sensory epithelium in the mammalian inner ear: function and interplay. *Dev. Biol.* 446, 133–141. doi: 10.1016/j.ydbio.2018.12.025

Zhou, H., Qian, X., Xu, N., Zhang, S., Zhu, G., Zhang, Y., et al. (2020). Disruption of Atg7-dependent autophagy causes electromotility disturbances, outer hair cell loss, and deafness in mice. *Cell Death Dis.* 11:913. doi: 10.1038/s41419-020-03110-8

Use of a Network-Based Method to Identify Latent Genes Associated with Hearing Loss in Children

Feng Liang[1†], Xin Fu[1†], ShiJian Ding[2] and Lin Li[3]*

[1]Anaesthesia Department, China-Japan Union Hospital, JiLin University, Changchun, China, [2]School of Life Sciences, Shanghai University, Shanghai, China, [3]Department of Otorhinolaryngology Head and Neck Surgery, China-Japan Union Hospital of Jilin University, Changchun, China

*Correspondence:
Lin Li
lilin01@jlu.edu.cn

†These authors have contributed equally to this work

Hearing loss is a total or partial inability to hear. Approximately 5% of people worldwide experience this condition. Hearing capacity is closely related to language, social, and basic emotional development; hearing loss is particularly serious in children. The pathogenesis of childhood hearing loss remains poorly understood. Here, we sought to identify new genes potentially associated with two types of hearing loss in children: congenital deafness and otitis media. We used a network-based method incorporating a random walk with restart algorithm, as well as a protein-protein interaction framework, to identify genes potentially associated with either pathogenesis. A following screening procedure was performed and 18 and 87 genes were identified, which potentially involved in the development of congenital deafness or otitis media, respectively. These findings provide novel biomarkers for clinical screening of childhood deafness; they contribute to a genetic understanding of the pathogenetic mechanisms involved.

Keywords: hearing loss, children, random walk with restart, protein-protein interaction, biomarker

INTRODUCTION

Deafness refers to a total or partial inability to hear, also known as hearing impairment or hearing loss (Olusanya et al., 2019). According to the World Health Organization, approximately 5% of people worldwide exhibit deafness or various extents of hearing impairment (Murray et al., 2019; Olusanya et al., 2019); approximately 10% of these people (34 million) are children (Murray et al., 2019). Although this number does not fully reflect the non-negligible threat imposed by hearing loss on human health, an independent report from the National Institute on Deafness and Other Communication Disorders of the United States revealed that the fight against deafness was urgent (Wass et al., 2019). In the USA, over 15% of all people currently exhibit hearing loss or have previously exhibited hearing loss (Moeller, 2000). Hearing loss is often age-associated; individuals over 60 years of age tend to have hearing impairments (Uchida et al., 2019). However, deafness or hearing loss is even more serious in children, because hearing is closely related to language-learning, social behavior, and basic emotional development (Trudeau et al., 2021). Therefore, an exploration of the pathological factors associated with childhood deafness is critical for child health and of considerable interest to researchers. The clinical pathogenesis of hearing loss in children is either congenital (Korver et al., 2017) or acquired (Pichichero, 2018). Congenital causes have been associated with genetic factors and family histories (Korver et al., 2017). X-linked hearing loss is the most typical form of congenital hearing loss, passed from mothers to their sons (O'brien et al., 2021). Genes *PRPS1*, *POU3F4*, *SMPX*, *AIFM1*, and *COL4A6* have all been associated with X-linked hearing loss (Song et al., 2012). However, otitis media and ototoxicity also trigger childhood hearing loss (Vanneste and Page, 2019). Otitis media is a complex process that involves multiple infections and specific genetic susceptibilities (Vanneste and Page, 2019). Acute otitis media (the most common form of the condition) has been associated with infections by various bacteria including *Streptococcus pneumoniae*, *Hemophilus influenzae*, *Moraxella catarrhalis*, and *Staphylococcus aureus* (Deniz et al., 2018). Additionally, acute otitis media susceptibility and recurrence have been associated with genetic factors. In 2011, researchers in Helsinki University Central Hospital reported that genetic factors contributed to childhood recurrent acute otitis media in 38.5% of affected patients and chronic otitis media in 22.1% of affected patients, highlighting the substantial contributions of genetic traits to these conditions (Hafrén et al., 2012). Furthermore, genome-wide association studies have shown that particular genes, including *FNDC1*, are associated with otitis media (Van Ingen et al., 2016), validating the essential roles of genetics in otitis media-induced hearing loss. Notably, drug ototoxicity was not significantly associated with the genetic background (Lanvers-Kaminsky et al., 2017). In summary, both congenital deafness and environmental otitis media (i.e., the two major pathogeneses of childhood hearing loss) feature strong genetic predispositions.

Although major efforts have been made to describe the pathogenesis of childhood hearing loss, the underlying mechanism remains unclear; only a few genes are known or suspected to be associated with the disease. Here, we focused on congenital hearing loss and otitis media-related hearing loss; both are associated with clear genetic predispositions. We used DisGeNet (https://www.disgenet.org/) to generate a list of genes associated with hearing loss (Piñero et al., 2017); we then employed a network-based method to identify novel latent biomarkers and genetic traits predisposing to congenital and otitis media-associated hearing loss. We used a random walk with restart (RWR) algorithm (Kohler et al., 2008; Macropol et al., 2009) by setting genes associated with otitis media or congenital deafness as the seed nodes to a STRING [19] protein-protein interaction (PPI) network to discover new candidate genes. A following screening procedure was conducted to select essential candidates. Eighteen latent congenital genes and 87 otitis media-associated genes were identified; some were associated with either pathogenesis. These may serve as novel biomarkers for clinical deafness screening in children; they will help to identify the pathogenetic mechanisms involved.

MATERIALS AND METHODS

Genes Associated with Hearing Loss in Children

We focused on genes associated with hearing loss in children. The American Speech-Language-Hearing Association (Alsarraf et al., 1998; Dhooge, 2003) defines such hearing loss in children as either acquired or associated with otitis media or congenital deafness. We downloaded the relevant genes from DisGeNet (Piñero et al., 2017) (https://www.disgenet.org/, version 7.0, accessed in April 2021). In total, 175 genes were associated with otitis media, while 72 were associated with congenital deafness and 2 were associated with acquired hearing loss; thus, we did not study acquired hearing loss. The genes associated with congenital deafness and otitis media are listed in **Supplementary Tables S1, S2**, respectively. We used a network-based method to identify novel candidate genes associated with either pathogenesis.

Network-Based Identification of Novel Genes

PPIs are widely used to explore protein or gene-related problems. Several studies have reported that compared with non-interacting proteins, interacting proteins are more likely to have similar functions (Ng et al., 2010; Hu et al., 2011; Chen et al., 2016a; Cai et al., 2017; Zhao et al., 2019; Gao et al., 2021). Such interactions can be used to identify novel genes that are associated with known disease-related genes. We used the STRING database (https://www.string-db.org/, version 10.0) (Szklarczyk et al., 2015) to construct a PPI network; we then applied the powerful, network RWR algorithm (Kohler et al., 2008; Macropol et al., 2009) to discover novel candidate genes associated with otitis media or congenital deafness. Human PPI information collected in STRING is contained in "9606.protein.links.v10.txt.gz". Each PPI features two proteins identified by their Ensembl IDs, as well as a confidence score indicating the PPI strength. Each score ranges from 1 to 999 and is derived by considering several types of PPIs. In fact, PPIs in STRING can not only indicate the interactions between proteins but also reflect functional associations of proteins. Thus, they can widely measure protein associations. We used the PPIs to build a network in which all 19,247 proteins served as nodes. Two nodes were considered adjacent if and only if they formed a PPI; thus, each edge was a PPI. We assigned a weight to each edge for indicating the strengths of the PPI, which was defined as the confidence score of the corresponding PPI. The network was termed N.

The RWR algorithm is powerful. It simulates a walker that commences at a node set and then randomly moves in the network. The start nodes are termed seed nodes. The walker delivers probabilities of seed nodes to all other nodes in the network. Given a network and k seed nodes, each seed node is assigned a probability of $1/k$; the other nodes are assigned probabilities of zero. These probabilities form a vector termed P_0. The vector is repeatedly updated as follows:

$$P_{t+1} = (1-r)A^T P_t + rP_0, \quad (1)$$

where A is the column-wise, normalized adjacency matrix of the network and r is the restarting probability, which was set to 0.8 in this study. Updating stops when P_{t+1} and P_t are sufficiently close; closeness is given by $\|P_{t+1} - P_t\|_{L_1} < 10^{-6}$. P_{t+1} is the required outcome of the algorithm. Based on this outcome, each node is assigned a probability transmitted from the seed nodes. A higher node probability is indicative of stronger associations with seed nodes.

We used the RWR program established by Li and Patra (Li and Patra, 2010). Genes associated with congenital deafness or otitis media were fed into the program, which ran on the PPI network N. Nodes with probabilities higher than 10^{-5} served as raw candidate genes for congenital deafness or otitis media.

Screening Procedure

Some raw candidate genes associated with congenital deafness or otitis media can be identified using a network-based method. However, several false-positives may be included in the results. To eliminate such genes and select only valid candidates, we used a screening procedure that featured three sequential tests.

Permutation Test

The RWR algorithm was executed on the PPI network N to discover raw candidate genes. The structure of N may influence the outcome. Some nodes are readily assigned high probabilities because of their special locations in the network. However, they may have low or no associations with congenital deafness or otitis media. Thus, there is a need to test the statistical significance of the probability that each raw candidate gene is valid. Accordingly, we randomly generated 1,000 gene sets, each of which had the same number of genes associated with congenital deafness or otitis media. For each gene set, such genes were set as the seed nodes of the RWR algorithm. Thus, each candidate gene was assigned a probability in each random gene set. When all 1,000 sets had been tested, each candidate gene had been assigned 1,000 probabilities. By comparing the probability on actual seed nodes to the probabilities on randomly generated sets, the statistical significance of each probability was revealed. We used the Z-score to evaluate significance as follows:

$$Z - score(g) = \frac{P(g) - PM(g)}{PSTD(g)}, \quad (2)$$

where g is a raw candidate gene identified by the network-based method, $P(g)$ is the probability on actual seed nodes, and $PM(g)$ and $PSTD(g)$ are the respective mean and standard deviation of the probabilities on randomly produced sets. We set the selection threshold for candidate genes to 1.96; this is a widely accepted threshold when statistical significance is essential.

Association Test

The second test directly evaluated the associations between candidate genes and congenital deafness or otitis media. For each candidate gene, such associations can be measured by associations between that gene and other genes associated with either condition. Proteins that interact in STRING always exhibit strong associations that can be quantified using confidence scores. For proteins p and q, the confidence score is denoted as $Q(p, q)$. For each candidate gene g, we computed the maximum association score (MAS) as follows:

$$MAS(g) = Max\{Q(g, g'): g'$$
is a gene associated with congenital deafness or otitis media$\}$
$$(3)$$

Genes with high MAS values are strongly associated with at least one gene linked to congenital deafness or otitis media. Thus, such genes may also be highly related to either condition. We set the threshold for selection of essential candidate genes to 900; this is the cutoff of the highest STRING confidence score.

Function Test

The last test further filtered candidate genes according to the similarities between their functional terms and the functional terms of genes associated with congenital deafness or otitis media. If the functional terms of a candidate gene are similar to the functional terms of a gene that is validly associated with either condition, that gene may also be linked to one of the conditions. We first used enrichment theory (Carmona-Saez et al., 2007; Huang et al., 2011; Huang et al., 2012; Chen et al., 2016b; Chen et al., 2019) to evaluate the associations between genes and functional terms (GO terms and KEGG pathway terms). Given one gene and one functional term, the gene set containing that gene and genes with which it interacted (in the PPI network of STRING) was constructed; another gene set containing genes annotated by the functional term was built. The associations between the gene and the functional term were calculated as the $-\log_{10}$ of the hypergeometric test p-value of the gene sets constructed above. For any gene g, its associations with all functional terms were computed and collected in a vector denoted $V(g)$. The similarity of two genes g and g' (based on their functional terms) can be evaluated by comparing their vectors as follows:

$$\Lambda(g, g') = \frac{V(g) \cdot V(g')}{\|V(g)\| \cdot \|V(g')\|} \quad (4)$$

In a manner similar to MAS calculation, for each candidate gene g, the maximum function score (MFS) was computed as follows:

$$MFS(g) = Max\{\Lambda(g, g'): g'$$
is a gene associated with congenital deafness or otitis media$\}$
$$(5)$$

Essential genes can be selected by choosing an appropriate MAS threshold.

Functional Enrichment Analyses on Identified Genes

To explore biological functions associated with identified genes, we applied gene ontology (GO) enrichment analyses using R package *topGO* (https://bioconductor.org/packages/release/bioc/html/topGO.html, v.2.42.0). The threshold of p-value was set to 0.001 for selecting enriched GO terms in three subclasses: biological processes (BP), cellular components (CC) and molecular functions (MF).

RESULTS

We sought genes associated with pediatric congenital deafness or otitis media. We used a network-based method to identify such

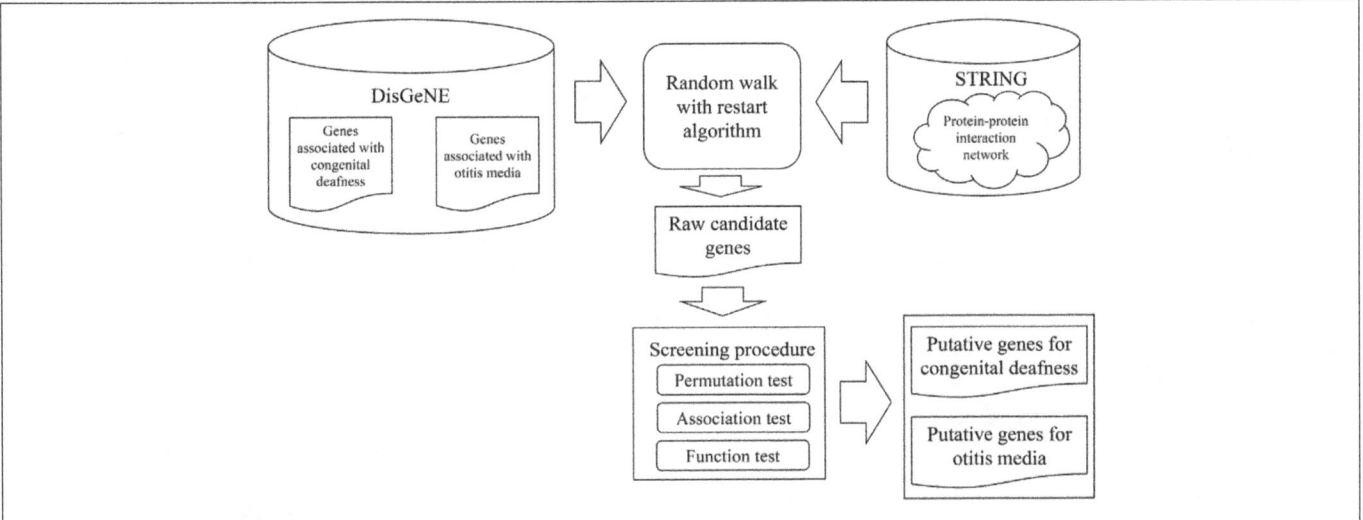

FIGURE 1 | Procedures used to identify new genes that might have roles in the development of childhood congenital deafness or otitis media-mediated hearing loss. Genes associated with either pathogenesis were retrieved from DisGeNE and the STRING protein-protein interaction networks were explored. The genes and networks were fed into a random walk with restart algorithm; we sought to discover new candidate genes. These genes were screened using three tests to select putative genes.

TABLE 1 | Numbers of candidate genes remaining after each filtration step.

Cause of childhood deafness	RWR	Permutation test	Association test	Function test
Congenital	5,426	367	117	18
Otitis media	5,631	637	502	87

genes. The entire procedure is illustrated in **Figure 1**. The numbers of genes remaining after each filtration step are listed in **Table 1**.

Congenital Deafness

Genes associated with congenital deafness were fed into the RWR algorithm, which ran on PPI network N. Each node in the network was assigned a probability. The selection threshold for raw candidate genes was set to 10^{-5}; this yielded 5,426 genes (**Supplementary Table S3**). We then engaged in screening (i.e., filtration) to identify essential genes. First, we used the permutation test to evaluate the statistical significance of probability that each raw candidate gene was essential; the Z-scores for all genes are listed in **Supplementary Table S3**. In total, 367 candidate genes were assigned Z-scores greater than 1.96. These were fed into the association test, which assigned an MAS to each gene (**Supplementary Table S3**). At a threshold of 900, 117 genes were selected; these were finally evaluated using the function test. The MFS values are listed in **Supplementary Table S3**. At an MFS threshold of 0.9, 18 genes were chosen. These "putative genes" were considered to be closely associated with congenital deafness; they are listed in **Supplementary Table S4**.

For the obtained putative genes, their associations with validated genes were investigated. We extracted all PPIs between putative and validated genes. The confidence scores of these PPIs are illustrated in a heat map, as shown in **Figure 2**. It can be observed that each putative gene had some interacting genes with confidence scores no less than 900, suggesting strong associations with validated genes. This can be further inferred that putative genes had special relationships with congenital deafness.

Otitis Media

We used the method described above to identify putative otitis media-associated genes. The RWR algorithm with genes associated with otitis media as seed nodes was performed on the PPI network N. The probabilities of all nodes were obtained. We selected nodes with probabilities over 10^{-5}; this yielded 5,631 genes (**Supplementary Table S5**). These genes were filtered as described above. The Z-scores, MAS values, and MFS values are listed in **Supplementary Table S5**. Use of thresholds of 1.96 for the Z-score, 900 for the MAS, and 0.96 for the MFS yielded 87 "putative genes" (**Supplementary Table S6**).

Likewise, the PPIs between putative and validated genes were investigated. A heat map was plotted to indicate the strength of these PPIs, as shown in **Figure 3**. Also, each putative genes had one or more interacting genes with highest confidence (confidence score ≥900). It is suggested that these putative genes may have special associations with otitis media.

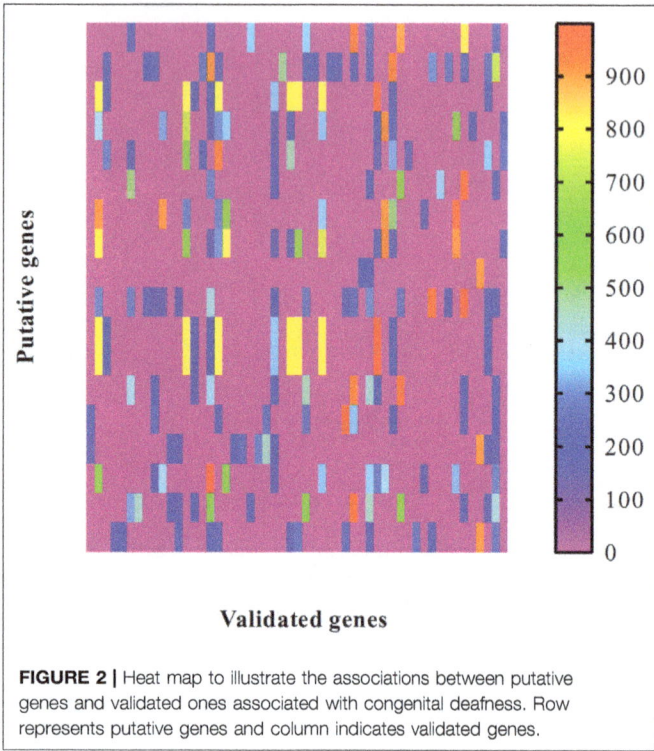

FIGURE 2 | Heat map to illustrate the associations between putative genes and validated ones associated with congenital deafness. Row represents putative genes and column indicates validated genes.

GO Enrichment Analyses on Putative Genes
GO Enrichment Analyses on Congenital Deafness Associated Putative Genes

For congenital deafness, 18 putative genes were obtained. These genes were set as gene of interest and all available genes were set as background for *topGO*. 18 enriched GO terms were obtained, which are provided in **Supplementary Table S7**. These terms and their *p*-values are also illustrated in **Figure 4**. Among these GO terms, eight were BP GO terms, six were CC GO terms and four were MF GO terms.

GO Enrichment Analyses on Otitis Media Associated Putative Genes

For 87 putative genes associated with otitis media, we did the same enrichment analysis. Results are available in **Supplementary Table S8**. We obtained 65 enriched GO terms. These GO terms and their *p*-values are shown in **Figure 5**. Of these 65 GO terms, fifty-two belonged to BP, five belonged to CC and eight belonged to MF.

DISCUSSION

We used a network-based method to identify putative genes associated with congenital deafness or otitis media. Below, we discuss some genes.

Putative Genes Associated with Congenital Deafness

We identified 18 putative genes, of which 5 were chosen for detailed analysis (**Table 2**). The first is ***PRKACB***

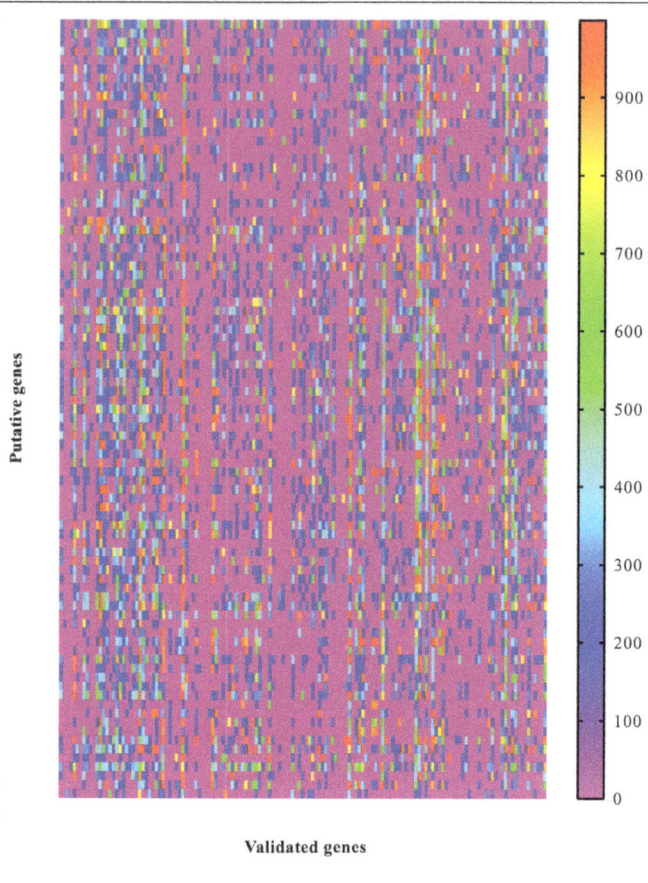

FIGURE 3 | Heat map to illustrate the associations between putative genes and validated ones associated with otitis media. Row represents putative genes and column indicates validated genes.

(ENSP00000359719), which encodes a catalytic subunit of cAMP-dependent protein kinase. The enzyme is expressed in hearing-associated organs *in utero*. In 2017, researchers from Southeast University showed that mouse *PRKACB* regulated the development of Lgr5+ hair cells (inner ear progenitor cells) (Cheng et al., 2017). Therefore, *PRKACB* is functionally associated with cochlear development; the cochlea is a sensorineural hearing organ. Cochlear impairment and abnormalities are reportedly associated with congenital hearing loss in children (O'malley et al., 1995; Korver et al., 2017; Van Wieringen et al., 2019). It is thus reasonable to expect that a regulator of cochlear development, such as *PRKACB*, would be associated with congenital pediatric deafness. We identified another putative gene with a similar biological function. ***PRKACG*** (ENSP00000366488) encodes another protein of the same complex. In 2016, researchers from the University of Bristol confirmed that the gain-of-function variant *DIAPH1* caused macrothrombocytopenia and hearing loss (Stritt et al., 2016). *PRKACG* acts downstream of *DIAPH1*, thus participating in *DIAPH1*-related biological effects. *PRKACG* may also be functionally connected to pediatric hearing loss.

The next putative gene is ***PAX2*** (ENSP00000396259), which is regarded as a key transcription factor that regulates the development of multiple systems, including the central nervous system (Ziman

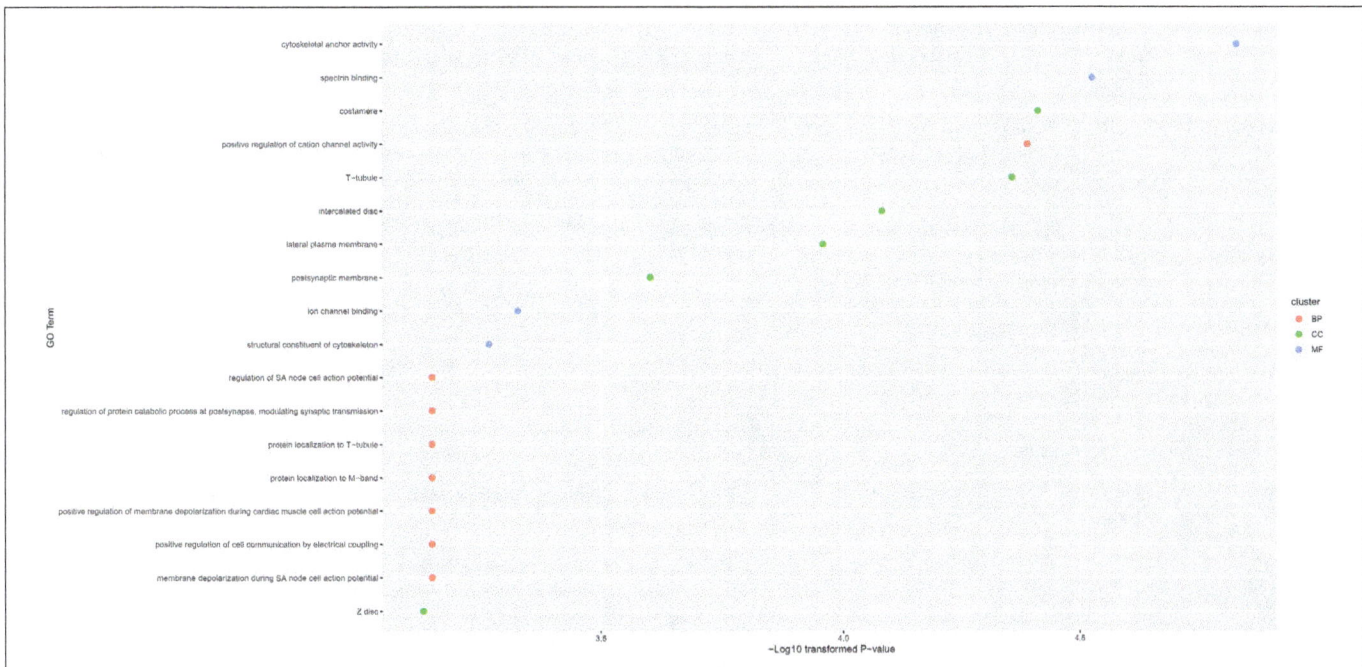

FIGURE 4 | Gene ontology (GO) enrichment results for putative genes associated with congenital deafness. GO terms with p-value less than 0.001 are selected and ranked by their p-values.

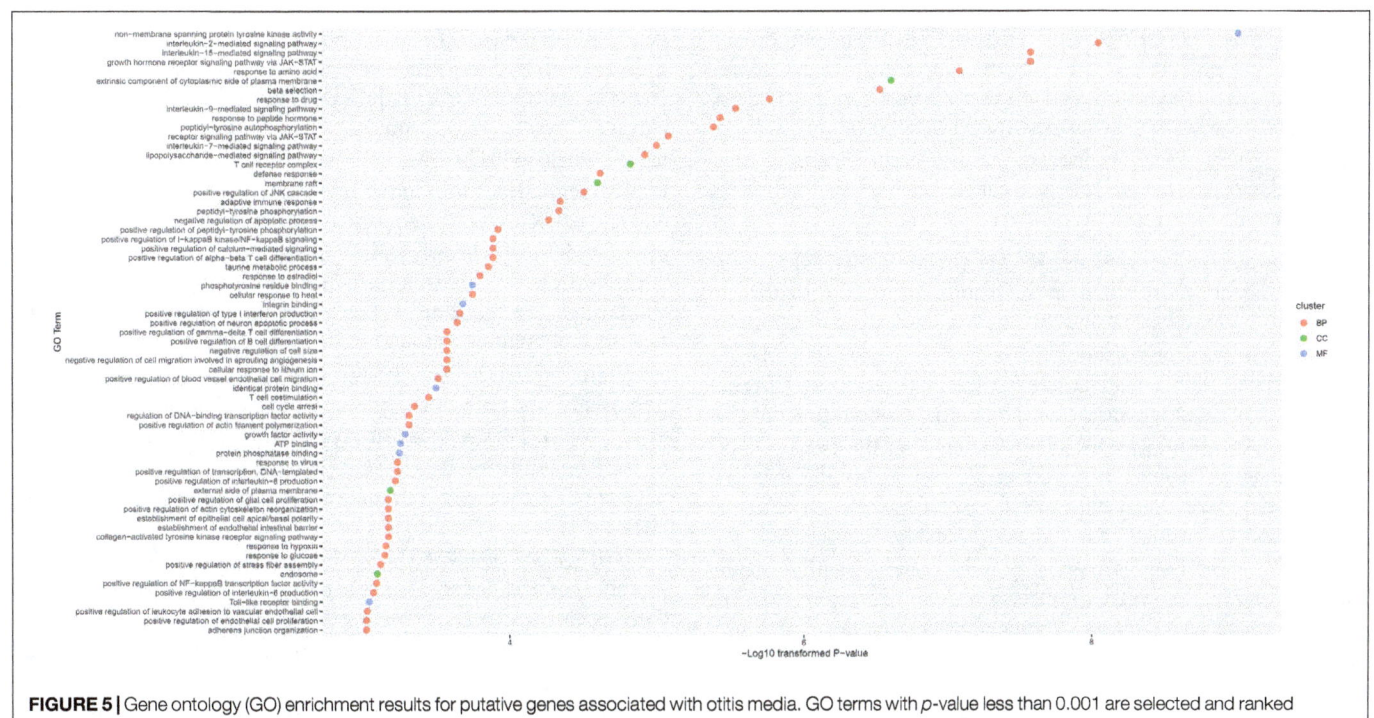

FIGURE 5 | Gene ontology (GO) enrichment results for putative genes associated with otitis media. GO terms with p-value less than 0.001 are selected and ranked by their p-values.

et al., 2001) and the eyes (Adam et al., 1993). In 2006, researchers from the McLaughlin Research Institute for Biomedical Sciences reported that *PAX2* interacted with *EYA1* to regulate the development of sensory regions in the inner ear (Zou et al., 2006). Developmental abnormalities of these regions are directly associated with congenital hearing loss (Kimura et al., 2018), implying that *PAX2* is a relevant putative gene involved in congenital pediatric deafness.

TABLE 2 | Five putative congenital deafness genes.

Ensembl ID	Gene symbol	Description	Probability	Z-score	MAS	MFS	Supporting References
ENSP00000359719	PRKACB	Protein Kinase CAMP-Activated Catalytic Subunit Beta	1.036E-04	2.2076	999	0.9884	O'malley et al. (1995), Cheng et al. (2017), Korver et al. (2017), Van Wieringen et al. (2019)
ENSP00000396259	PAX2	Paired Box 2	1.133E-04	5.0805	947	0.9877	Adam et al. (1993), Ziman et al. (2001), Zou et al. (2006), Kimura et al. (2018)
ENSP00000262848	PRKX	Protein Kinase X-Linked	1.018E-04	2.1608	987	0.9876	Song et al. (2012), Haltrich, (2019)
ENSP00000366488	PRKACG	Protein Kinase CAMP-Activated Catalytic Subunit Gamma	1.035E-04	2.1305	994	0.9862	Stritt et al. (2016)
ENSP00000378485	MATK	Megakaryocyte-Associated Tyrosine Kinase	6.746E-05	4.3589	986	0.9847	Jhun et al. (1995), Grgurevich et al. (1997), Lee et al. (2006), Costello et al. (2017)

TABLE 3 | Five putative otitis media genes.

Ensembl ID	Gene symbol	Description	Probability	Z-score	MAS	MFS	Supporting References
ENSP0000304283	RAC3	Rac Family Small GTPase 3	1.496E-04	5.0315	994	0.9984	Henrie et al. (2018)
ENSP00000365012	HCK	HCK Proto-Oncogene, Src Family Tyrosine Kinase	6.876E-05	3.8668	985	0.9959	Ernst et al. (2002) Suri et al., 2016)
ENSP00000398655	ITK	IL2 Inducible T Cell Kinase	6.657E-05	4.7676	925	0.9959	Juhn et al. (2008), Saettini et al. (2017)
ENSP00000363115	FGR	FGR Proto-Oncogene, Src Family Tyrosine Kinase	5.308E-05	2.3092	955	0.9947	Klein et al. (1988), Kim et al. (2008), Vogelnik and Matos, 2017)
ENSP00000314458	CDC42	Cell Division Cycle 42	1.377E-04	2.2400	999	0.9946	Hoppe and Swanson, (2004), Kashani et al. (2021)

PRKX (ENSP00000262848) is also associated with congenital pediatric hearing loss. A 2019 review concerning chromosomal aberrations associated with endocrine abnormalities in children confirmed that *PRKX* regulated the development of hearing (Haltrich, 2019). *PRKX* is located on the X chromosome; it is functionally connected to X-linked congenital hearing loss (Song et al., 2012).

The next putative gene is *MATK* (ENSP00000378485); this regulates signal transduction in hematopoietic cells (Grgurevich et al., 1997; Lee et al., 2006). In 2017, a clinical case report in *JAMA Otolaryngology—Head and Neck Surgery* stated that *MATK* was associated with unilateral hearing loss and otorrhea (Costello et al., 2017). Acute megakaryoblastic leukemia has been functionally connected to unilateral, congenital hearing loss; the pathogenetic backgrounds are related (Costello et al., 2017). MATK encodes megakaryocyte-associated tyrosine kinase, which is structurally similar to C-terminal Src kinase; notably, megakaryocyte-associated tyrosine kinase is associated with acute megakaryoblastic leukemia (Jhun et al., 1995). Therefore, *MATK* might be involved in the development of ear tumors that cause adaptive hearing loss.

Putative Genes Associated with Otitis Media

We identified 87 genes putatively associated with otitis media (**Supplementary Table S6**); we subjected 5 of these genes to detailed analysis (**Table 3**). The first such gene is *RAC3* (ENSP00000304283). Although there is insufficient direct evidence that *RAC3* is involved in otitis media, a clinical genomic database (ClinVar Miner) (Henrie et al., 2018) indicates that the Talkowski Laboratory of Massachusetts General Hospital has demonstrated associations of *RAC3* variants with otitis media. The next gene is **HCK** (ENSP00000365012); this member of the Src tyrosine kinase family regulates the innate immune response (Ernst et al., 2002). *HCK* was previously reported to be specifically associated with chronic otitis media and its major chronic complications in children with hearing loss (Suri et al., 2016), validating our findings. The next putative gene is *ITK* (ENSP00000398655), which encodes an IL2-and T cell-associated kinase. In 2008, the gene was reported to potentially mediate the inflammation of otitis media (Juhn et al., 2008). Furthermore, a report concerning early diagnosis of PI3Kδ syndrome in a 2-year-old girl revealed an association between *ITK* deficiency and recurrent otitis media (Saettini et al., 2017).

FGR (ENSP00000363115; also known as *SRC2*), another member of the Src tyrosine kinase family, is also associated with otitis media. This gene has roles in immune responses against pathogens in multiple organs, including ears (Kim et al., 2008). Additionally, the gene has been widely reported to participate in Epstein–Barr virus-associated malignancies (Klein et al., 1988). In 2017, Epstein–Barr virus infection was confirmed as a major etiological and pathological factor for secretory otitis media in children (Vogelnik and Matos, 2017), validating the link between *FGR* and otitis media.

CDC42 (ENSP00000314458) is an immune system-associated gene; we found that it was closely associated with otitis media. In 2021, *CDC42* deficiency was shown to be associated with recurrent pneumonia, otitis media, and bacteremia (Kashani et al., 2021). *CDC42* interacts with another effector gene, *RAC1* (Hoppe and Swanson, 2004); a homolog of *RAC1* (i.e., *RAC3*, discussed above) was shown to be associated with hearing loss, confirming that *CDC42* is linked to otitis media.

In summary, several putative genes are associated with the two types of pediatric deafness. Their identification may provide insights concerning the pathogeneses involved.

Functional Enrichment Analyses on Putative Genes

For GO functional enrichment analyses on putative genes yielded by our computational method, multiple significant GO terms were identified. The detailed analyses on the top three enriched GO terms ranking by p-values for congenital deafness and otitis media were presented below.

For congenital deafness, the first enriched GO term is cytoskeletal anchor activity (GO:0008093). According to recent publications, mutations in cytoskeletal encoding proteins have been shown to be associated with congenital deafness (Riazuddin et al., 2006), reflecting the potential associations between congenital deafness and cytoskeletal anchor activity. The second enriched term is spectrin binding (GO:0030507). In 2017, a recessive mutation on spectrin associated gene has been shown to be associated with congenital central deafness (Knierim et al., 2017), validating this result. Furthermore, costamere (GO:0043034) is the third enriched GO term (in CC) associated with congenital deafness. According to recent next-generation sequencing analyses (Schraders et al., 2011), costameres has been shown to be associated with progressive hearing impairment.

More GO terms were enriched by putative genes associated with otitis media, including non−membrane spanning protein tyrosine kinase activity (GO:0004715) and interleukin mediated signaling pathway (GO:0038100, GO0035723). Non-membrane spanning protein tyrosine kinase has been shown to be associated with specific inflammatory effects and pathogen infections (Gu et al., 2009; Rocha-Sanchez et al., 2013). Considering that otitis media is associated with infection and inflammatory effects around middle ears, it is reasonable for otitis media associated genes to enrich in inflammatory effects. As for interleukin mediated signaling pathways, middle ear inflammation has been shown to be associated with interleukin related signaling pathways, validating this result (Kerschner et al., 2006; Shi et al., 2014).

Shared Putative Genes Associated with Both Congenital Deafness and Otitis Media

By comparing the putative genes associated with congenital deafness and otitis media, only one shared gene **CDH1** (ENSG00000039068) was identified. The pathogenesis of congenital deafness and otitis media are totally different according to recent studies. Congenital deafness means the hearing loss is present at birth linking the pathogenesis to genetic factors or stimulations during pregnancy. However, as for otitis media, generally, otitis media is caused by infections and happens after birth. *CDH1* has been widely reported to be associated with hearing loss (Friedman and Avraham, 2009; Kanavy et al., 2019). Specifically, *CDH1* has been reported to be associated with congenital deafness due to the pathogenic alteration of inner ear but not middle ear (Friedman and Avraham, 2009), which has totally different pathogenic regions comparing with otitis media. As for otitis media, *CDH1* has been shown to participate in the pathogenesis of otitis media *via* regulation on the inflammatory proliferative responses against infections (Kurabi et al., 2013).Therefore, although both subtypes of hearing loss have been shown to be associated with gene *CDH1*, the contribution and regulatory role of *CDH1* on them are totally different, reflecting the complex regulatory mechanisms for childhood hearing loss.

In summary, *CHD1* is associated with two types of pediatric deafness. Its dentification may provide insights concerning the pathogeneses involved.

CONCLUSION

We used a network-based method to identify new candidate genes involved in childhood hearing loss caused by congenital deafness and otitis media. The genes included *PRKACB*, *PAX2*, *PRKX*, *PRKACG*, *MATK*, *RAC3*, *HCK*, *ITK*, *FGR*, and *CDC42*. They may be involved in the pathogenesis of childhood hearing loss.

AUTHOR CONTRIBUTIONS

LL designed the study. FL, XF and SJD performed the experiments. FL and XF analyzed the results. FL and XF wrote the manuscript. All authors contributed to the research and reviewed the manuscript.

REFERENCES

Adam, M. P., Ardinger, H. H., Pagon, R. A., Wallace, S. E., Bean, L. J. H., Mirzaa, G., et al. (1993). *GeneReviews*. Seattle (WA): University of Washington.

Alsarraf, R., Jung, C. J., Crowley, C., Perkins, J., and Gates, G. A. (1998). Otitis media Health Status Evaluation: a Pilot Study for the Investigation of Cost-Effective Outcomes of Recurrent Acute Otitis media Treatment. *Ann. Otol Rhinol Laryngol.* 107, 120–128. doi:10.1177/000348949810700207

Cai, Y.-D., Zhang, Q., Zhang, Y.-H., Chen, L., and Huang, T. (2017). Identification of Genes Associated with Breast Cancer Metastasis to Bone on a Protein-Protein Interaction Network with a Shortest Path Algorithm. *J. Proteome Res.* 16, 1027–1038. doi:10.1021/acs.jproteome.6b00950

Carmona-Saez, P., Chagoyen, M., Tirado, F., Carazo, J. M., and Pascual-Montano, A. (2007). GENECODIS: a Web-Based Tool for Finding Significant Concurrent Annotations in Gene Lists. *Genome Biol.* 8, R3. doi:10.1186/gb-2007-8-1-r3

Chen, L., Pan, X., Zhang, Y.-H., Liu, M., Huang, T., and Cai, Y.-D. (2019).

Classification of Widely and Rarely Expressed Genes with Recurrent Neural Network. *Comput. Struct. Biotechnol. J.* 17, 49–60. doi:10.1016/j.csbj.2018.12.002

Chen, L., Xing, Z., Huang, T., Shu, Y., Huang, G., and Li, H.-P. (2016a). Application of the Shortest Path Algorithm for the Discovery of Breast Cancer-Related Genes. *Cbio* 11, 51–58. doi:10.2174/1574893611666151119220024

Chen, L., Zhang, Y.-H., Zheng, M., Huang, T., and Cai, Y.-D. (2016b). Identification of Compound-Protein Interactions through the Analysis of Gene Ontology, KEGG Enrichment for Proteins and Molecular Fragments of Compounds. *Mol. Genet. Genomics* 291, 2065–2079. doi:10.1007/s00438-016-1240-x

Cheng, C., Guo, L., Lu, L., Xu, X., Zhang, S., Gao, J., et al. (2017). Characterization of the Transcriptomes of Lgr5+ Hair Cell Progenitors and Lgr5- Supporting Cells in the Mouse Cochlea. *Front. Mol. Neurosci.* 10, 122. doi:10.3389/fnmol.2017.00122

Costello, M. S., Stevens, S., and Samy, R. N. (2017). Unilateral Hearing Loss and Otorrhea. *JAMA Otolaryngol. Head Neck Surg.* 143, 727–728. doi:10.1001/jamaoto.2016.3824

Deniz, Y., Van Uum, R. T., De Hoog, M. L. A., Schilder, A. G. M., Damoiseaux, R. A. M. J., and Venekamp, R. P. (2018). Impact of Acute Otitis media Clinical Practice Guidelines on Antibiotic and Analgesic Prescriptions: a Systematic Review. *Arch. Dis. Child.* 103, 597–602. doi:10.1136/archdischild-2017-314103

Dhooge, I. J. M. (2003). Risk Factors for the Development of Otitis media. *Curr. Allergy Asthma Rep.* 3, 321–325. doi:10.1007/s11882-003-0092-8

Ernst, M., Inglese, M., Scholz, G. M., Harder, K. W., Clay, F. J., Bozinovski, S., et al. (2002). Constitutive Activation of the SRC Family Kinase Hck Results in Spontaneous Pulmonary Inflammation and an Enhanced Innate Immune Response. *J. Exp. Med.* 196, 589–604. doi:10.1084/jem.20020873

Friedman, L. M., and Avraham, K. B. (2009). MicroRNAs and Epigenetic Regulation in the Mammalian Inner Ear: Implications for Deafness. *Mamm. Genome* 20, 581–603. doi:10.1007/s00335-009-9230-5

Gao, J., Hu, B., and Chen, L. (2021). A Path-Based Method for Identification of Protein Phenotypic Annotations. *Cbio* 16, 1214–1222. doi:10.2174/1574893616666210531100035

Grgurevich, S., Linnekin, D., Musso, T., Zhang, X., Modi, W., Varesio, L., et al. (1997). The Csk-like proteins Lsk, Hyl, and Matk represent the same Csk homologous kinase (Chk) and are regulated by stem cell factor in the megakaryoblastic cell line MO7e. *Growth Factors* 14, 103–115. doi:10.3109/08977199709021514

Gu, D., Sater, A. K., Ji, H., Cho, K., Clark, M., Stratton, S. A., et al. (2009). Xenopus δ-catenin Is Essential in Early Embryogenesis and Is Functionally Linked to Cadherins and Small GTPases. *J. Cel. Sci.* 122, 4049–4061. doi:10.1242/jcs.031948

Hafrén, L., Kentala, E., Järvinen, T. M., Leinonen, E., Onkamo, P., Kere, J., et al. (2012). Genetic Background and the Risk of Otitis media. *Int. J. Pediatr. Otorhinolaryngol.* 76, 41–44. doi:10.1016/j.ijporl.2011.09.026

Haltrich, I. (2019). Chromosomal Aberrations with Endocrine Relevance (Turner Syndrome, Klinefelter Syndrome, Prader-Willi Syndrome). *Exp. Suppl.* 111, 443–473. doi:10.1007/978-3-030-25905-1_20

Henrie, A., Hemphill, S. E., Ruiz-Schultz, N., Cushman, B., Distefano, M. T., Azzariti, D., et al. (2018). ClinVar Miner: Demonstrating Utility of a Web-Based Tool for Viewing and Filtering ClinVar Data. *Hum. Mutat.* 39, 1051–1060. doi:10.1002/humu.23555

Hoppe, A. D., and Swanson, J. A. (2004). Cdc42, Rac1, and Rac2 Display Distinct Patterns of Activation during Phagocytosis. *MBoC* 15, 3509–3519. doi:10.1091/mbc.e03-11-0847

Hu, L., Huang, T., Shi, X., Lu, W.-C., Cai, Y.-D., and Chou, K.-C. (2011). Predicting Functions of Proteins in Mouse Based on Weighted Protein-Protein Interaction Network and Protein Hybrid Properties. *PloS one* 6, e14556. doi:10.1371/journal.pone.0014556

Huang, T., Chen, L., Cai, Y.-D., and Chou, K.-C. (2011). Classification and Analysis of Regulatory Pathways Using Graph Property, Biochemical and Physicochemical Property, and Functional Property. *PLoS ONE* 6, e25297. doi:10.1371/journal.pone.0025297

Huang, T., Zhang, J., Xu, Z.-P., Hu, L.-L., Chen, L., Shao, J.-L., et al. (2012). Deciphering the Effects of Gene Deletion on Yeast Longevity Using Network and Machine Learning Approaches. *Biochimie* 94, 1017–1025. doi:10.1016/j.biochi.2011.12.024

Jhun, B. H., Rivnay, B., Price, D., and Avraham, H. (1995). The MATK Tyrosine Kinase Interacts in a Specific and SH2-dependent Manner with C-Kit. *J. Biol. Chem.* 270, 9661–9666. doi:10.1074/jbc.270.16.9661

Juhn, S. K., Jung, M.-K., Hoffman, M. D., Drew, B. R., Preciado, D. A., Sausen, N. J., et al. (2008). The Role of Inflammatory Mediators in the Pathogenesis of Otitis media and Sequelae. *Clin. Exp. Otorhinolaryngol.* 1, 117–138. doi:10.3342/ceo.2008.1.3.117

Kanavy, D. M., Mcnulty, S. M., Jairath, M. K., Brnich, S. E., Bizon, C., Powell, B. C., et al. (2019). Comparative Analysis of Functional Assay Evidence Use by ClinGen Variant Curation Expert Panels. *Genome Med.* 11, 77–19. doi:10.1186/s13073-019-0683-1

Kashani, P., Marwaha, A., Feanny, S., Kim, V. H.-D., Atkinson, A. R., Leon-Ponte, M., et al. (2021). Progressive Decline of T and B Cell Numbers and Function in a Patient with CDC42 Deficiency. *Immunol. Res.* 69, 53–58. doi:10.1007/s12026-020-09168-y

Kerschner, J. E., Yang, C., Burrows, A., and Cioffi, J. A. (2006). Signaling Pathways in Interleukin-1??-Mediated Middle Ear Mucin Secretion. *The Laryngoscope* 116, 207–211. doi:10.1097/01.mlg.0000191467.63650.9e

Kim, Y.-C., Kim, S.-Y., Choi, D., Ryu, C.-M., and Park, J. M. (2008). Molecular Characterization of a Pepper C2 Domain-Containing SRC2 Protein Implicated in Resistance against Host and Non-host Pathogens and Abiotic Stresses. *Planta* 227, 1169–1179. doi:10.1007/s00425-007-0680-2

Kimura, Y., Masuda, T., and Kaga, K. (2018). Vestibular Function and Gross Motor Development in 195 Children with Congenital Hearing Loss-Assessment of Inner Ear Malformations. *Otol Neurotol* 39, 196–205. doi:10.1097/mao.0000000000001685

Klein, C., Busson, P., Tursz, T., Young, L. S., and Raab-Traub, N. (1988). Expression of Thec-Fgr Related Transcripts in Epstein-Barr Virus-Associated Malignancies. *Int. J. Cancer* 42, 29–35. doi:10.1002/ijc.2910420107

Knierim, E., Gill, E., Seifert, F., Morales-Gonzalez, S., Unudurthi, S. D., Hund, T. J., et al. (2017). A Recessive Mutation in Beta-IV-Spectrin (SPTBN4) Associates with Congenital Myopathy, Neuropathy, and central Deafness. *Hum. Genet.* 136, 903–910. doi:10.1007/s00439-017-1814-7

Köhler, S., Bauer, S., Horn, D., and Robinson, P. N. (2008). Walking the Interactome for Prioritization of Candidate Disease Genes. *Am. J. Hum. Genet.* 82, 949–958. doi:10.1016/j.ajhg.2008.02.013

Korver, A. M. H., Smith, R. J. H., Van Camp, G., Schleiss, M. R., Bitner-Glindzicz, M. A. K., Lustig, L. R., et al. (2017). Congenital Hearing Loss. *Nat. Rev. Dis. Primers* 3, 16094. doi:10.1038/nrdp.2016.94

Kurabi, A., Pak, K., Dang, X., Coimbra, R., Eliceiri, B. P., Ryan, A. F., et al. (2013). Ecrg4 Attenuates the Inflammatory Proliferative Response of Mucosal Epithelial Cells to Infection. *PloS one* 8, e61394. doi:10.1371/journal.pone.0061394

Lanvers-Kaminsky, C., Zehnhoff-Dinnesen, A. a., Parfitt, R., and Ciarimboli, G. (2017). Drug-induced Ototoxicity: Mechanisms, Pharmacogenetics, and Protective Strategies. *Clin. Pharmacol. Ther.* 101, 491–500. doi:10.1002/cpt.603

Lee, B.-C., Avraham, S., Imamoto, A., and Avraham, H. K. (2006). Identification of the Nonreceptor Tyrosine Kinase MATK/CHK as an Essential Regulator of Immune Cells Using Matk/CHK-Deficient Mice. *Blood* 108, 904–907. doi:10.1182/blood-2005-12-4885

Li, Y., and Patra, J. C. (2010). Genome-wide Inferring Gene-Phenotype Relationship by Walking on the Heterogeneous Network. *Bioinformatics* 26, 1219–1224. doi:10.1093/bioinformatics/btq108

Macropol, K., Can, T., and Singh, A. K. (2009). RRW: Repeated Random Walks on Genome-Scale Protein Networks for Local Cluster Discovery. *BMC bioinformatics* 10, 283. doi:10.1186/1471-2105-10-283

Moeller, M. P. (2000). Early Intervention and Language Development in Children Who Are Deaf and Hard of Hearing. *Pediatrics* 106, E43. doi:10.1542/peds.106.3.e43

Murray, J. J., Hall, W. C., and Snoddon, K. (2019). Education and Health of Children with Hearing Loss: the Necessity of Signed Languages. *Bull. World Health Organ.* 97, 711–716. doi:10.2471/blt.19.229427

Ng, K.-L., Ciou, J.-S., and Huang, C.-H. (2010). Prediction of Protein Functions Based on Function-Function Correlation Relations. *Comput. Biol. Med.* 40, 300–305. doi:10.1016/j.compbiomed.2010.01.001

O'brien, A., Aw, W. Y., Tee, H. Y., Naegeli, K. M., Bademci, G., Tekin, M., et al. (2021). Confirmation of COL4A6 Variants in X-Linked Nonsyndromic Hearing Loss and its Clinical Implications. *Eur. J. Hum. Genet.* doi:10.1038/s41431-021-00881-2

O'malley, B. W., Li, D., and Turner, D. S. (1995). Hearing Loss and Cochlear Abnormalities in the Congenital Hypothyroid (Hyt/hyt) Mouse. *Hearing Res.* 88, 181–189. doi:10.1016/0378-5955(95)00111-g

Olusanya, O. B., Davis, A. C., and Hoffman, H. J. (2019). Hearing Loss: Rising Prevalence and Impact. *Bull. World Health Organ.* 97, 646–646A. doi:10.2471/BLT.19.224683

Pichichero, M. E. (2018). Helping Children with Hearing Loss from Otitis media with Effusion. *The Lancet* 392, 533–534. doi:10.1016/s0140-6736(18)31862-2

Piñero, J., Bravo, A., Queralt-Rosinach, N., Gutiérrez-Sacristán, A., Deu-Pons, J., Centeno, E., et al. (2017). DisGeNET: a Comprehensive Platform Integrating Information on Human Disease-Associated Genes and Variants. *Nucleic Acids Res.* 45, D833–D839. doi:10.1093/nar/gkw943

Riazuddin, S., Khan, S. N., Ahmed, Z. M., Ghosh, M., Caution, K., Nazli, S., et al. (2006). Mutations in TRIOBP, Which Encodes a Putative Cytoskeletal-Organizing Protein, Are Associated with Nonsyndromic Recessive Deafness. *Am. J. Hum. Genet.* 78, 137–143. doi:10.1086/499164

Rocha-Sanchez, S. M., Scheetz, L. R., Siddiqi, S., Weston, M. W., Smith, L. M., Dempsey, K., et al. (2013). Lack of Rbl1/p107 Effects on Cell Proliferation and Maturation in the Inner Ear. *Jbbs* 03, 534–555. doi:10.4236/jbbs.2013.37056

Saettini, F., Pelagatti, M. A., Sala, D., Moratto, D., Giliani, S., Badolato, R., et al. (2017). Early Diagnosis of PI3Kδ Syndrome in a 2 Years Old Girl with Recurrent Otitis and Enlarged Spleen. *Immunol. Lett.* 190, 279–281. doi:10.1016/j.imlet.2017.08.021

Schraders, M., Haas, S. A., Weegerink, N. J. D., Oostrik, J., Hu, H., Hoefsloot, L. H., et al. (2011). Next-generation Sequencing Identifies Mutations of SMPX, Which Encodes the Small Muscle Protein, X-Linked, as a Cause of Progressive Hearing Impairment. *Am. J. Hum. Genet.* 88, 628–634. doi:10.1016/j.ajhg.2011.04.012

Shi, J., Li, J., Guan, H., Cai, W., Bai, X., Fang, X., et al. (2014). Anti-fibrotic Actions of Interleukin-10 against Hypertrophic Scarring by Activation of PI3K/AKT and STAT3 Signaling Pathways in Scar-Forming Fibroblasts. *PloS one* 9, e98228. doi:10.1371/journal.pone.0098228

Song, M. H., Lee, K. Y., Choi, J. Y., Bok, J., and Kim, U. K. (2012). Nonsyndromic X-Linked Hearing Loss. *Front. Biosci. (Elite Ed.* 4, 924–933. doi:10.2741/430

Stritt, S., Nurden, P., Turro, E., Greene, D., Jansen, S. B., Westbury, S. K., et al. (2016). A Gain-Of-Function Variant in DIAPH1 Causes Dominant Macrothrombocytopenia and Hearing Loss. *Blood* 127, 2903–2914. doi:10.1182/blood-2015-10-675629

Suri, D., Rawat, A., and Singh, S. (2016). X-linked Agammaglobulinemia. *Indian J. Pediatr.* 83, 331–337. doi:10.1007/s12098-015-2024-8

Szklarczyk, D., Franceschini, A., Wyder, S., Forslund, K., Heller, D., Huerta-Cepas, J., et al. (2015). STRING V10: Protein-Protein Interaction Networks, Integrated over the Tree of Life. *Nucleic Acids Res.* 43, D447–D452. doi:10.1093/nar/gku1003

Trudeau, S., Anne, S., Otteson, T., Hopkins, B., Georgopoulos, R., and Wentland, C. (2021). Diagnosis and Patterns of Hearing Loss in Children with Severe Developmental Delay. *Am. J. Otolaryngol.* 42, 102923. doi:10.1016/j.amjoto.2021.102923

Uchida, Y., Sugiura, S., Nishita, Y., Saji, N., Sone, M., and Ueda, H. (2019). Age-related Hearing Loss and Cognitive Decline - the Potential Mechanisms Linking the Two. *Auris Nasus Larynx* 46, 1–9. doi:10.1016/j.anl.2018.08.010

Van Ingen, G., Li, J., Goedegebure, A., Pandey, R., Li, Y. R., March, M. E., et al. (2016). Genome-wide Association Study for Acute Otitis media in Children Identifies FNDC1 as Disease Contributing Gene. *Nat. Commun.* 7, 12792. doi:10.1038/ncomms12792

Van Wieringen, A., Boudewyns, A., Sangen, A., Wouters, J., and Desloovere, C. (2019). Unilateral Congenital Hearing Loss in Children: Challenges and Potentials. *Hearing Res.* 372, 29–41. doi:10.1016/j.heares.2018.01.010

Vanneste, P., and Page, C. (2019). Otitis media with Effusion in Children: Pathophysiology, Diagnosis, and Treatment. A Review. *J. Otology* 14, 33–39. doi:10.1016/j.joto.2019.01.005

Vogelnik, K., and Matos, A. (2017). Facial Nerve Palsy Secondary to Epstein-Barr Virus Infection of the Middle Ear in Pediatric Population May Be More Common Than We Think. *Wien Klin Wochenschr* 129, 844–847. doi:10.1007/s00508-017-1259-y

Wass, M., Ching, T. Y. C., Cupples, L., Wang, H.-C., Lyxell, B., Martin, L., et al. (2019). Orthographic Learning in Children Who Are Deaf or Hard of Hearing. *Lshss* 50, 99–112. doi:10.1044/2018_lshss-17-0146

Zhao, R., Chen, L., Zhou, B., Guo, Z.-H., Wang, S., and Aorigele (2019). Recognizing Novel Tumor Suppressor Genes Using a Network Machine Learning Strategy. *IEEE Access* 7, 155002–155013. doi:10.1109/access.2019.2949415

Ziman, M. R., Rodger, J., Chen, P., Papadimitriou, J. M., Dunlop, S. A., and Beazley, L. D. (2001). Pax Genes in Development and Maturation of the Vertebrate Visual System: Implications for Optic Nerve Regeneration. *Histol. Histopathol* 16, 239–249. doi:10.14670/HH-16.239

Zou, D., Silvius, D., Rodrigo-Blomqvist, S., Enerbäck, S., and Xu, P.-X. (2006). Eya1 Regulates the Growth of Otic Epithelium and Interacts with Pax2 during the Development of All Sensory Areas in the Inner Ear. *Develop. Biol.* 298, 430–441. doi:10.1016/j.ydbio.2006.06.049

Stem Cell-Based Therapies in Hearing Loss

Zuhong He[1]*[†], Yanyan Ding[2][†], Yurong Mu[2][†], Xiaoxiang Xu[1], Weijia Kong[2], Renjie Chai[3,4,5,6,7]* and Xiong Chen[1]*

[1] Department of Otorhinolaryngology-Head and Neck Surgery, Zhongnan Hospital of Wuhan University, Wuhan, China, [2] Department of Otorhinolaryngology, Union Hospital, Tongji Medical College, Huazhong University of Science and Technology, Wuhan, China, [3] State Key Laboratory of Bioelectronics, Jiangsu Province High-Tech Key Laboratory for Bio-Medical Research, School of Life Sciences and Technology, Southeast University, Nanjing, China, [4] Co-Innovation Center of Neuroregeneration, Nantong University, Nantong, China, [5] Institute for Stem Cell and Regeneration, Chinese Academy of Sciences, Beijing, China, [6] Jiangsu Province High-Tech Key Laboratory for Bio-Medical Research, Southeast University, Nanjing, China, [7] Beijing Key Laboratory of Neural Regeneration and Repair, Capital Medical University, Beijing, China

*Correspondence:
Zuhong He
hezuhong@163.com
Xiong Chen
zn_chenxiong@126.com
Renjie Chai
renjiec@seu.edu.cn

[†] These authors have contributed equally to this work

In recent years, neural stem cell transplantation has received widespread attention as a new treatment method for supplementing specific cells damaged by disease, such as neurodegenerative diseases. A number of studies have proved that the transplantation of neural stem cells in multiple organs has an important therapeutic effect on activation and regeneration of cells, and restore damaged neurons. This article describes the methods for inducing the differentiation of endogenous and exogenous stem cells, the implantation operation and regulation of exogenous stem cells after implanted into the inner ear, and it elaborates the relevant signal pathways of stem cells in the inner ear, as well as the clinical application of various new materials. At present, stem cell therapy still has limitations, but the role of this technology in the treatment of hearing diseases has been widely recognized. With the development of related research, stem cell therapy will play a greater role in the treatment of diseases related to the inner ear.

Keywords: stem cell, inner ear, hair cell, spiral ganglion neurons, hearing protection

INTRODUCTION

Hearing disabilities have become one of the most common sensory disabilities in the world, but there is still no effective treatment for deafness (Wilson et al., 2017). Hearing loss can be classified as conductive hearing loss or SNHL according to the site of damage. The damage site for conductive hearing loss is mainly in the outer ear and middle ear, while the damage site for SNHL is mainly in the inner ear and auditory nerve (Weissman, 1996). At present, the treatment of SNHL mainly involves injections or oral drugs. In addition, local hormone injections, hyperbaric oxygen chamber rehabilitation, hearing aids, cochlear implantation, etc., can also be used in treatment (Chandrasekhar et al., 2019). The efficacy of treatment for patients in the acute phase is about 50%–70% (Tucci et al., 2002; Jeyakumar et al., 2006; Stachler et al., 2012). For patients who have not received effective treatment for more than 72 h after the onset of symptoms, the probability of hearing improvement will be greatly reduced. Some experts believe that the best time for initiating treatment should be within 48 h following the first aural symptoms (Ojha et al., 2020). However, even if the patient receives effective treatment in the acute phase, his hearing cannot be perfectly restored to the level before the illness (Stachler et al., 2012). Therefore, stem cell therapy may be an effective treatment for SNHL.

Inner ear hair cells and spiral ganglion neurons play a key role in the transmission of peripheral auditory signals (Nayagam et al., 2011; Moser and Starr, 2016). After exposure to the mechanical pressure of sound waves, the inner ear hair cells release neurotransmitters to the spiral ganglion cells, which then transmit signals to the auditory center. SNHL (SNHL) is caused by damage to the inner ear, auditory nerve, or central auditory pathway (Dufner-Almeida et al., 2019). The main factors that cause SNHL are damage to hair cells, damage to or loss of synapses between neurons and hair cells, and neuronal degeneration (Waqas et al., 2018). The loss of outer hair cells affects the function of the cochlear amplifier; the loss of inner hair cells or their synapses inhibits the encoding of sound signals; and the loss of spiral ganglia affects the encoding or conduction of sound signals (Moser et al., 2013). Therefore, the damage to the two kinds of inner ear nerve cells can cause permanent hearing loss (Lang, 2016). Previous studies have shown that non-mammalian vertebrates can regenerate hair cells in the cochlea and vestibular system after the hair cells are damaged to restore auditory function (Corwin and Cotanche, 1988). However, adult mammals have no regenerative ability for damaged hair cells, so hearing loss is permanent (Corwin and Cotanche, 1988; Brigande and Heller, 2009; Warchol, 2011). At present, the use of stem cells to induce differentiation to replace damaged hair cells is regarded as the most feasible treatment for regenerating hair cells. In addition, the loss of spiral ganglia, which are important to receiving incoming signals in the auditory system, is also irreversible. The loss of spiral neurons permanently damages the afferent pathways of auditory signals and causes SNHL (Shi and Edge, 2013). Therefore, implanting neural stem cells into the inner ear to regenerate spiral neurons and synaptic connections is also a potential way to restore hearing (Géléoc and Holt, 2014).

THE ROLE OF NEURAL STEM CELLS IN OTHER NEURODEGENERATIVE DISEASE TREATMENT

Neural stem cells have strong proliferation and differentiation potential and can be specifically induced to differentiate into various nerve cells, such as neurons, astrocytes, and oligodendrocytes (Vieira et al., 2018). Therefore, neural stem cells are used as a potential solution for supplementing specific cells damaged by disease, such as neurodegenerative diseases, spinal injuries, and so on. Neural stem cells can be divided into autologous neural stem cells and allogeneic neural stem cells according to their sources. According to their different stages of growth and different tissue sources, neural stem cells can be divided into embryonic stem cell-derived neural stem cells, adult neural stem cells, and non-neural tissue-derived neural stem cells (Yi and Dong, 2010; Trounson and McDonald, 2015). At present, the therapeutic mechanisms of neural stem cells are mainly divided into three types: (1) neural stem cells gather at the injury site, proliferate, and differentiate into specific cells to restore the functions of the original tissues or organs; (2) neural stem cells secrete relevant nutritional factors to promote the recovery and regeneration of damaged cells; (3) neural stem cells establish or improve synaptic connections between neuronal cells and restore nerve conduction pathways.

A number of studies have reported that cell replacement therapy (CRT) using neural stem cells has made significant progress in neurodegenerative diseases such as Parkinson's disease and Huntington's disease (Choi and Hong, 2017; Marsh and Blurton-Jones, 2017). Generating specific neurons to function by implanting neural stem cells has become the focus of current research in the treatment of Parkinson's disease. For example, newborn neurons are used to replace dopaminergic neurons in the striatum and participate in the reconstruction of the nervous system (Lindvall, 2015; Bjorklund and Parmar, 2020). Zhu et al. found that stem cells also have great potential in the treatment of amyotrophic lateral sclerosis (ALS) (Zhu and Lu, 2020). Implanted neural stem cells survive well in a damaged spinal cord. They not only replace lost motor neurons, but also act as a neuronal relay to establish connections between regenerating axons, and between their own axons and host axons so as to rebuild the body's innervation of voluntary muscles (Zhu and Lu, 2020). The main pathological feature of Alzheimer's disease (AD) is that amyloid β (Aβ) plaques accumulate in the degenerated neurons of the aging brain. Protein plaques are mainly composed of Aβ fibrils that phosphorylate tau protein and neurofibrillary tangles (NFTs). To treat AD, the implantation of neural stem cells restores damaged neurons, reduces Aβ accumulation, and ameliorates the microenvironment (Li et al., 2014; Han et al., 2020; Hayashi et al., 2020). Neural stem cell implantation also reduces brain damage in adult ischemic stroke and neonatal ischemic hypoxic encephalopathy through a variety of protective mechanisms such as immune regulation and neuroprotection. Endogenous neural stem cells can proliferate, differentiate, and repair brain damage under the stimulation of brain-derived neurotrophic factor (BDNF), NGF, EPO, etc. (Huang and Zhang, 2019). It is also reported that neural stem cell therapy is also used in the treatment of hemorrhagic encephalopathy (Gao et al., 2018), glioblastoma multiforme (Miska and Lesniak, 2015), multiple sclerosis (Xiao et al., 2018), and other diseases.

THE ROLE OF NEURAL STEM CELLS IN HEARING REGENERATION

During the embryonic development of mammals, as the expression of BMP changes, the non-neuroectoderm (NNE) at the junction of the neural tube and the ectoderm thickens, forming the pre-placodal ectoderm (PPE). Pre-placodal ectoderm forms the auditory placode at the front of the embryo. Under the induction of FGF (fibroblast growth factors) and Wnt released from the mesenchyme and neural tubes, the auditory placode is recessed and squeezed from the surface of the ectoderm to form an auditory vesicle. Then the SOX2-positive cell subset in the auditory vesicle up-regulates the pre-neural transcription factor bHLH and forms neuron precursor cells, which are separated from the auditory vesicle to form the cochlear-vestibular ganglion. The cells in the auditory vesicle form the sensory and non-sensory parts of the inner ear through proliferation, remodeling, and apoptosis

(Roccio and Edge, 2019). The cochlear precursor cells in the organ of Corti have the ability to differentiate into neurospheres after birth (Zhai et al., 2005; Wang et al., 2006). Among these cells, Lgr5, Lgr6, Abcg2, EPCAM, and CD271 positive cells can proliferate and then differentiate into hair cells and supporting cells under the positive regulation of EGF (epidermal growth factor), IGF (insulin-like growth factor-1), bFGF (basic fibroblast growth factor), Wnt, Shh, and the negative regulation of p27Kip1. Atoh1, Shh, and the Notch pathways play an important regulatory role in the differentiation of precursor cells into hair cells. Nestin and Sox2-positive neural stem cells derived from spiral ganglia proliferate and differentiate into neurons and astrocytes under the control of EGF, IGF, bFGF, LIF (leukemia inhibitory factor), and other pathways (Xia et al., 2019). In this process, BDNF, *GDNF (glial cell-derived neurotrophic factor), NT-3 (neurotrophic factor-3), RA (valproic acid), FA (ferulic acid)* and other factors play an important regulatory role (Xia et al., 2019).

In recent years, many scientists around the world have explored the application of neural stem cell therapy in the inner ear and have achieved many inspiring results. The main direction is to induce the regeneration of auditory hair cells and spiral ganglion cells to replace damaged cells and attempt to treat SNHL (Matsui et al., 2005; Nacher-Soler et al., 2019; Liu et al., 2020). Neural stem cells in the inner ear can differentiate into auditory neurons, hair cells, and supporting cells. Therefore, after the inner ear is damaged by noise, neural stem cells can make up for the damaged cells, meanwhile reduce the apoptosis of spiral ganglion cells (Xu et al., 2016). Iguchi et al. found that the effectiveness of cochlear implantation (CI) relies on residual spiral ganglion cells, and neural stem cells can differentiate into glial cells and neuronal cells after CI. GDNF and BDNF can nourish spiral ganglion cells to enhance hearing improvement after CI (Iguchi et al., 2003). The application of stem cell therapy in the inner ear mainly includes two aspects: stimulating the proliferation and differentiation of endogenous stem cells in the inner ear and implanting exogenous stem cells (**Figure 1**).

Application of Endogenous Stem Cells in Hearing Regeneration

Studies have reported that there are inner ear stem cells in the cochlea and vestibule, which are distributed in the greater epithelial ridge (GER), lesser epithelial ridge (LER), organ of Corti, vestibular sensory epithelium, and semicircular canals (Liu et al., 2014). The inner ear stem cells in the mouse cochlea can be isolated in the first week after birth, while the stem cells in the vestibule can be isolated even 4 months after birth (Oshima et al., 2007; Kanzaki et al., 2020). Inner ear stem cells are regulated by a variety of transcription factors and can differentiate into sensory precursor cells, neural precursor cells, and non-sensory cells (Kiernan et al., 2005; Raft et al., 2007). Genes such as *Jagged1* (Daudet and Lewis, 2005), *Notch1* (Liu et al., 2012), *Sox2* (Neves et al., 2007), *BMP-4* (Cole et al., 2000), *FGF* (Schimmang, 2007), *IGF-1* (Aburto et al., 2012), *Atoh1, Jagged2,* and *Delta1* (Morrison et al., 1999) play important regulatory roles in the differentiation and development of inner ear stem cells into hair cells. In addition, *Brn3c* (Xiang et al., 1997), *Espin* (Zheng et al., 2000), and *Myosin VI, VIIA,* and *XV* (Steel and Kros, 2001; Udovichenko et al., 2002) are important for the survival of hair cells, and *TGF-α* promotes the transdifferentiation of supporting cells into hair cells (Liu et al., 2014). Neural stem cells in the inner ear also have the potential to replace damaged cells, and these neural stem cells may be derived from residual spiral ganglion cells (Oshima et al., 2007, 2009). Previous audiology-related studies have found that the number of remaining spiral ganglion neurons has an effect on speech recognition after CI (Seyyedi et al., 2014).

The research on the differentiation of inner ear precursor cells (such as stem cells or supporting cells) into hair cells was first carried out in non-mammalians. Researchers found that after the inner ear hair cells of non-mammals such as birds, fish, and amphibians are damaged, the supporting cells directly or indirectly transdifferentiate into hair cells (Bodson et al., 2010; Wang et al., 2015; Kanzaki, 2018). There are two ways to regenerate hair cells from inner ear supporting cells: re-entering the cell cycle, and transdifferentiation (Chen et al., 2019). In addition, Lagarde et al. found that when the organ of Corti in newborn mice is not fully mature, two types of supporting cells, inner border cells and inner finger cells, can be effectively replenished after loss, thereby maintaining normal hearing in mice (Mellado Lagarde et al., 2014). Cox et al. found that when the cochlear hair cells of newborn mice are lost, supporting cells can regenerate hair cells through mitosis and transdifferentiation, although most of the regenerated hair cells are gradually lost with an extension of development time (Cox et al., 2014). These prove that when the cochlea of newborn mice is damaged, it can activate its ability to regenerate hair cells. It is known that the current technical methods for inducing the regeneration of supporting cells into hair cells mainly include gene editing and drug treatment (Géléoc and Holt, 2014). In 2005, Izumikawa et al. used adenoviral vectors to transfect the *Atoh1* gene into the inner ear for the first time. *Atoh1* can achieve partial hearing recovery and improvement after deafness by encoding HLH transcription factors and the key factors related to hair cell development (Izumikawa et al., 2005). Akil et al. used adeno-associated virus type 1 (AAV1) to deliver the *VGLUT3* gene to the inner ears of *VGLUT3* knockout mice and found that the morphology of the ribbon synapses between the inner hair cells was restored. Within 2 weeks, the examined result of mouse auditory brainstem response (ABR) threshold returned to normal level, and the startle reflex was partially relieved (Akil et al., 2012). At present, the application of genetic engineering in the treatment of deafness still has many limitations. For example, the research of Masahiko Izumikawa et al. failed to restore hearing in all experimental animals (Izumikawa et al., 2005). The *VGLUT3* mutation studied by Akil et al. is also not common in humans, so it does not have broad representative significance (Akil et al., 2012). However, the value and potential of therapy through the gene introduction of viral vectors have been reflected in many studies. In addition, other gene therapy methods such as the introduction of siRNA, knockout of dominant genes, systemic injection of antisense oligonucleotides, and plasmid introduction into intrauterine embryos also show good therapeutic effects and can be used as

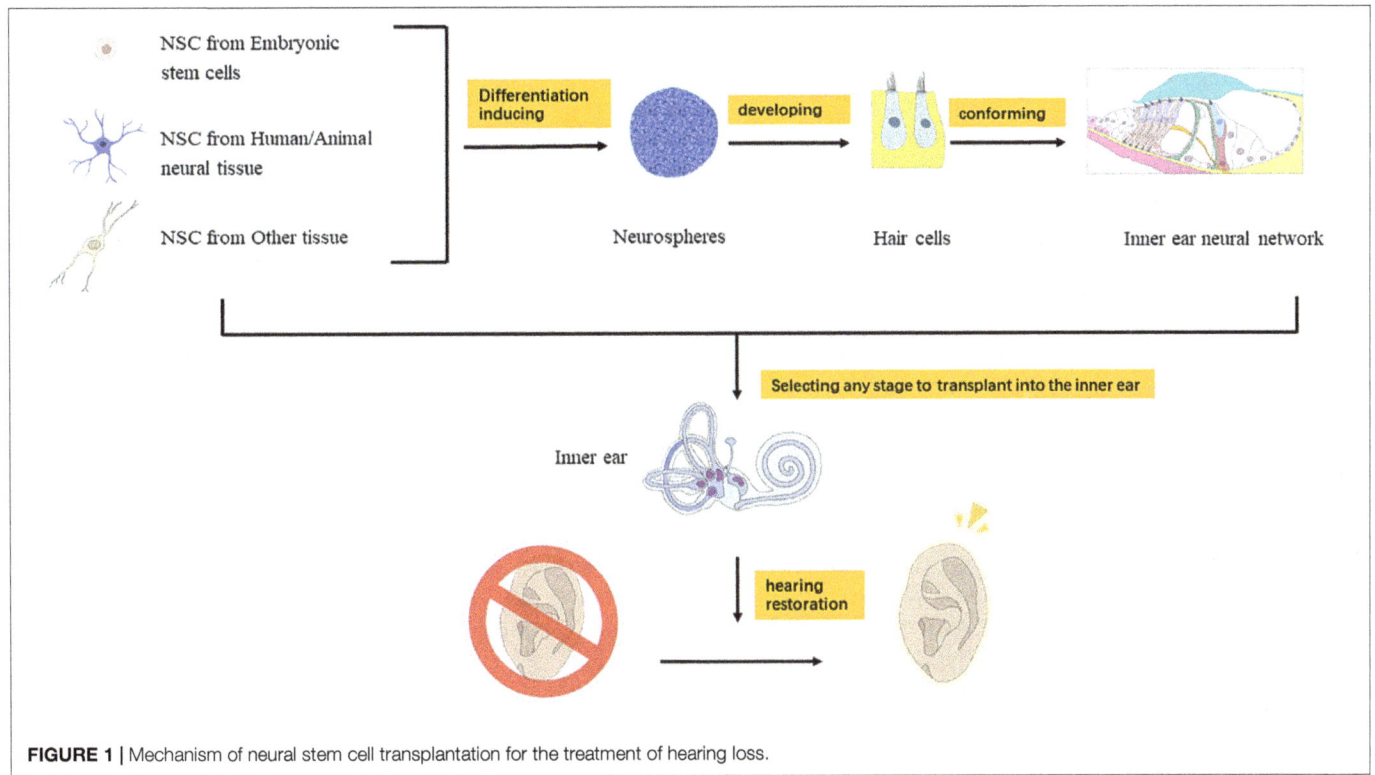

FIGURE 1 | Mechanism of neural stem cell transplantation for the treatment of hearing loss.

potential therapeutic methods (Muller and Barr-Gillespie, 2015). It has been confirmed that some genes in the signaling pathways related to the regeneration of inner ear hair cells play important regulatory roles, such as *Atoh1* (Bermingham et al., 1999; Chonko et al., 2013), *p27Kip1* (Chai et al., 2011), *pRb* (Sage et al., 2006), *Foxg1* (Ding et al., 2020), *Wnt* (Bengoa-Vergniory and Kypta, 2015), *Notch* (Kiernan, 2013), *Hedgehog* (Zhao et al., 2006), *Ephrin*, *Six1*, *Pou4f3*, and *Gfi1* (Menendez et al., 2020; Zhang et al., 2020a). White et al. found that down-regulating the expression of the cell cycle inhibitor *P27Kip1* enabled some of the supporting cells in the inner ear to re-enter the cell cycle and generate hair cells (White et al., 2006). Mizutari et al. injected γ-secretase inhibitors locally in mice with noise-induced hearing loss to inhibit the expression of Notch and increase the level of Atoh1. They found that the transdifferentiation of supporting cells into hair cells occurred in the inner ears of mice, resulting in an increase in the number of hair cells (Mizutari et al., 2013). Menendez et al. combined the four transcription factors Six1, Atoh1, Pou4f3, and Gfi1 to convert mouse embryonic fibroblasts, adult mouse tail fibroblasts and postnatal mouse supporting cells into induced hair cell-like cells (Menendez et al., 2020). Foxg1 can affect the proliferation of inner ear neural progenitor cells by regulating the expression of genes related to the cell cycle and Notch signaling pathway. Zhang et al. found that knockout *Foxg1* can promote the transdifferentiation of supporting cells to hair cells (Zhang et al., 2020b). Sage et al. found that pRb plays an important role in the maturation and survival of auditory hair cells. When the expression of pRb is deleted, the vestibular hair cells and supporting cells of postnatal mice still divide and proliferate (Sage et al., 2006).

Although the hair cells regenerated in this way cannot fully restore the number of cells before the injury, and the hearing improvement is limited (only about 10 dB), this study confirmed the feasibility of regenerating hair cells through the regulation of the cell cycle by drugs, and also promoted the application of more cell cycle regulators in the future (Mizutari et al., 2013; Géléoc and Holt, 2014; Kanzaki et al., 2020).

Recent studies have shown that microRNA is also a potential gene therapy tool. It not only affects the development of the cochlea and hair cells, but also regulates the proliferation and differentiation of inner ear stem cells, which is very important for the regeneration of inner ear hair cells (Wu et al., 2020). Jiang et al. found that regulating the expression of miR-124 in inner ear neural stem cells in spiral ganglia can change the expression of tropomyosin receptor kinase B (TrkB) and cell division cycle 42 (Cdc42), and it promotes the neuronal differentiation and neurite outgrowth of inner ear neural stem cells (Jiang et al., 2016). At present, many studies have tried to use the regulatory role of microRNA in cell proliferation and differentiation to repair and regenerate inner ear hair cells, thereby treating hearing loss (Chen et al., 2018; Zhou et al., 2018).

Application of Exogenous Stem Cells in Hearing Regeneration

Due to the limited number of existing stem cells in the inner ear, and because the mechanism of inner ear cell renewal is still unclear, many researchers have tried to repair inner ear cells by implanting neural stem cells (Waqas et al., 2020). Clarke et al. found that neural stem cells have the potential to differentiate into functional auditory neurons (Clarke et al., 2000). The reported sources of neural stem cells implanted in the inner ear include dorsal root ganglion cells, neural precursor cells, the stem cells or precursor cells isolated from the inner ear, immortalized auditory neuroblasts, embryonic stem cells and their derived neural stem cells, and bone marrow stromal cells treated with Shh and retinoic acid (Lang et al., 2008). Michael et al. developed an organoid culture system *in vitro* based on the *in vivo* embryonic development system (Perny et al., 2017). They first activated BMP and inhibited TGF-β to induce mouse embryonic stem cells (mESCs) to generate non-neuroectoderm, while avoiding the induction of mesoderm, and then inhibited BMP and activated FGF2 to further induce the generation of pre-placodal ectode (PPE) and otic placode. Spiral ganglia were stratified and differentiated in a serum-free 2D Matrigel matrix. The tissues were treated with BDNF and NT-3 for 15 days *in vitro*, and were finally differentiated into mature spiral ganglia with a clear morphology and normal function (Perny et al., 2017). Karl R. Koehler et al. used the quickly aggregated serum-free embryonic body method (SFEBq) to culture mouse embryonic neural stem cells, and regulated the expression of BMP, TGF-β, and FGF at different time points, so that the cell population formed non-neuroectoderm, PPE, and otic placode epithelial cells. The signal pathways related to the differentiation of the inner ear sensory epithelial cells were then are activated, such as the Wnt, Notch, Hippo, Shh, and MAPK pathways (Bengoa-Vergniory and Kypta, 2015; Ouyang et al., 2020; Susanto et al., 2020), resulting in a large number of hair cells with special function and structure that could sense mechanical pressure (Koehler et al., 2013; Jiao et al., 2017; Xia et al., 2019). In addition, nerve growth factor (NGF) plays an important role in the survival and differentiation of neural stem cells. A medium containing NGF has a large number of neural stem cells with high differentiation potential (Han et al., 2017).

METHOD AND FUNCTION EVALUATION OF NEURAL STEM CELL IMPLANTATION IN THE INNER EAR

Implanting stem cells into the inner ear can select proper pathway from perilymph, endolymph, cochlear axis, auditory nerve, cochlear lateral wall, and so on (Zhu et al., 2018). The perilymph path includes round window and external semicircular canal injection, and the endolymph path is through membranous cochlear duct injection (Liu et al., 2016). Zhang et al. cultivated neural stem cells for a period of time, and then injected them into the cochlea through the cochlear sidewall, allowing them to migrate to the area of the cochlea axis where the spiral ganglia were distributed (Zhang et al., 2013). This method is effective, precise, and incurs a minimal level of trauma. Due to the special structure of the cochlea, invasive cochlear surgery may cause severe hearing loss (Bogaerts et al., 2008). Therefore, when neural stem cells are implanted, different methods should be selected according to the treatment conditions and treatment purposes (**Figure 1**).

It is necessary to test the function of neural stem cells after implantation from the perspective of histology and function. Histological detection indicators mainly include the differentiation of neural stem cells, the neurotrophic factors secreted by neural stem cells, and the formation of neural networks such as the extension of axons and the establishment of synaptic connections between neurons. Functional detection indicators mainly include the improvement in the hearing level of the implanted object, whether symptoms such as tinnitus are alleviated, and whether the effect of hearing devices such as cochlear implants has been enhanced. To determine whether neural stem cells are successfully differentiated into target cells after implantation in the inner ear, detection is mainly based on morphology, protein expression, and genetic markers. For example, detection may be based on detecting specific expression genes (*MYO7A*, *BRN3A*, and *ATHO1*), auditory receptors, mechanical energy to electrical energy conversion, and hair cell electrophysiological activity to determine whether the newly generated hair cells after stem cell implantation have the characteristics of normal hair cells (Ottersen et al., 1998; Gale et al., 2001; Griesinger et al., 2002; Prosser et al., 2008; Beurg et al., 2009). The BrdU detection of cell proliferation, microscopic detection of morphology, and detection of synaptic protein expression, as well as electrophysiological detection and other methods can determine whether the implanted newly generated cells have successfully differentiated into spiral ganglion cells (Li et al., 2016).

APPLICATION OF NEW MATERIALS RELATED TO NEURAL STEM CELLS IN THE TREATMENT OF AUDITORY DISEASES

In recent years, many researchers have developed more new technologies and materials in the process of using neural stem cells to treat auditory diseases, and these technologies have promoted the clinical application of neural stem cells (**Figure 2**). As a material with excellent stability, biocompatibility, conductivity, ductility, elasticity, and mechanical strength, graphene is often used in tissue engineering research. When graphene was used as a nanocomposite carrier or scaffold material for neural stem cells, researchers found that graphene materials could promote the proliferation and differentiation of neural stem cells and the directional growth of neuronal axons, and ultimately formed biologically functional tissue (Shin et al., 2016; Yang et al., 2018; Han et al., 2019). When neural stem cells were cultured on a graphene substrate, the cell membrane potential parameters did not change, but when neural stem cells proliferated and differentiated, the resting potential of the cells increased negatively, and the amplitude of the action potential increased. In addition, the differentiation of neural stem cells accelerated, and the expression of synaptic proteins and synaptic activity increased, which showed that graphene could accelerate the development and maturation of neural stem cells (Guo et al., 2016). In addition to graphene, artificial photonic crystal materials also promote the growth of neural stem cells due to their special topological properties and electrical signal

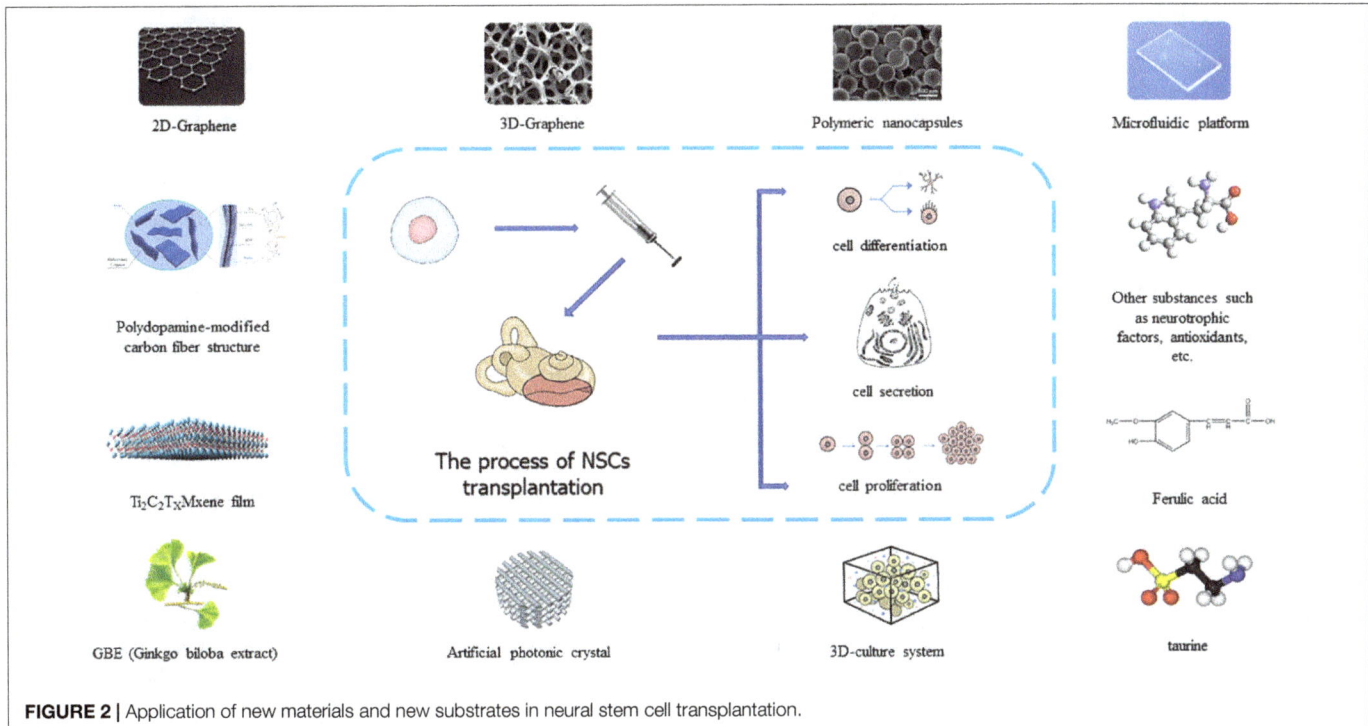

FIGURE 2 | Application of new materials and new substrates in neural stem cell transplantation.

stimulation (Yang et al., 2013; Ankam et al., 2015). Besides these new materials, anisotropic inverse opal is a material that regulates the behavior of neural stem cells by changing their surface morphology. Compared with isotropic inverse opal, special 3D (3-dimensional) porous structure of anisotropic inverse opal can make neural stem cell spheres have stronger proliferation ability, more orderly cell arrangement, better directional differentiation, and a significantly higher dendritic complexity index (DCI) (Xia et al., 2020). The use of a 3D culture system can simulate the inner ear microenvironment and promote the complete formation of stem cells into a functional structure of the inner ear (Chang et al., 2020). When neural stem cells are implanted in the inner ear to treat auditory diseases, different materials can be selected according to different treatment requirements (**Figure 2**). To date, extensive research has been carried out on the main processes of neural stem cell acquisition, implantation, and postoperative inner ear functional recovery. However, there are still unresolved problems related to tumorigenicity, targeted growth, and cell survival rate after implantation. Therefore, more precise and effective optimization of treatment methods is needed in the future.

CONCLUSION

At present, great progress has been made in the research on endogenous and exogenous neural stem cells in the treatment of auditory diseases. A large number of studies have covered the acquisition, induction, and implantation of neural stem cells, and the restoration of auditory function after implantation. Neural stem cells are implanted into the inner ear to replace and supplement hair cells or spiral ganglion cells, to promote the renewal and proliferation of residual cells and to restore or rebuild the neuron network, so as to achieve the recovery of auditory function (**Figure 1**). This is a valuable and promising treatment method for auditory diseases. However, there are still unknown factors in the inner ear implantation of neural stem cells, such as tumorigenicity and immune rejection. Moreover, functional recovery after implantation has not reached a satisfactory level for clinical application. In the future, research on inner ear stem cells will discover new materials and regulatory genes or proteins, which will promote the clinical application of neural stem cells.

AUTHOR CONTRIBUTIONS

ZH, YD, YM, and XX searched and read related literature, summarized the data in the field, and wrote the manuscript. ZH, RC, and XC guided the writing and review of the manuscript. All authors contributed to the article and approved the submitted version.

REFERENCES

Aburto, M. R., Magariños, M., Leon, Y., Varela-Nieto, I., and Sanchez-Calderon, H. (2012). AKT signaling mediates IGF-I survival actions on otic neural progenitors. *PLoS One* 7:e30790. doi: 10.1371/journal.pone.0030790

Akil, O., Seal, R. P., Burke, K., Wang, C., Alemi, A., During, M., et al. (2012). Restoration of hearing in the VGLUT3 knockout mouse using virally mediated gene therapy. *Neuron* 75, 283–293. doi: 10.1016/j.neuron.2012.05.019

Ankam, S., Lim, C. K., and Yim, E. K. (2015). Actomyosin contractility plays a role in MAP2 expression during nanotopography-directed neuronal differentiation of human embryonic stem cells. *Biomaterials* 47, 20–28. doi: 10.1016/j.biomaterials.2015.01.003

Bengoa-Vergniory, N., and Kypta, R. M. (2015). Canonical and noncanonical Wnt signaling in neural stem/progenitor cells. *Cell. Mol. Life Sci.* 72, 4157–4172. doi: 10.1007/s00018-015-2028-6

Bermingham, N. A., Hassan, B. A., Price, S. D., Vollrath, M. A., Ben-Arie, N., Eatock, R. A., et al. (1999). Math1: an essential gene for the generation of inner ear hair cells. *Science* 284, 1837–1841. doi: 10.1126/science.284.5421.1837

Beurg, M., Fettiplace, R., Nam, J. H., and Ricci, A. J. (2009). Localization of inner hair cell mechanotransducer channels using high-speed calcium imaging. *Nat. Neurosci.* 12, 553–558. doi: 10.1038/nn.2295

Bjorklund, A., and Parmar, M. (2020). Neuronal replacement as a tool for basal ganglia circuitry repair: 40 years in perspective. *Front. Cell. Neurosci.* 14:146. doi: 10.3389/fncel.2020.00146

Bodson, M., Breuskin, I., Lefebvre, P., and Malgrange, B. (2010). Hair cell progenitors: identification and regulatory genes. *Acta Otolaryngol.* 130, 312–317. doi: 10.1080/00016480903121057

Bogaerts, S., Douglas, S., Corlette, T., Pau, H., Saunders, D., McKay, S., et al. (2008). Microsurgical access for cell injection into the mammalian cochlea. *J. Neurosci. Methods* 168, 156–163. doi: 10.1016/j.jneumeth.2007.09.016

Brigande, J. V., and Heller, S. (2009). Quo vadis, hair cell regeneration? *Nat. Neurosci.* 12, 679–685. doi: 10.1038/nn.2311

Chai, R., Xia, A., Wang, T., Jan, T. A., Hayashi, T., Bermingham-McDonogh, O., et al. (2011). Dynamic expression of Lgr5, a Wnt target gene, in the developing and mature mouse cochlea. *J. Assoc. Res. Otolaryngol.* 12, 455–469. doi: 10.1007/s10162-011-0267-2

Chandrasekhar, S. S., Tsai Do, B. S., Schwartz, S. R., Bontempo, L. J., Faucett, E. A., Finestone, S. A., et al. (2019). Clinical practice guideline: sudden hearing loss (update). *Otolaryngol. Head Neck Surg.* 161 (1_suppl), S1–S45. doi: 10.1177/0194599819859885

Chang, H. T., Heuer, R. A., Oleksijew, A. M., Coots, K. S., Roque, C. B., Nella, K. T., et al. (2020). An engineered three-dimensional stem cell niche in the inner ear by applying a nanofibrillar cellulose hydrogel with a sustained-release neurotrophic factor delivery system. *Acta Biomater.* 108, 111–127. doi: 10.1016/j.actbio.2020.03.007

Chen, Y., Zhang, S., Chai, R., and Li, H. (2019). Hair cell regeneration. *Adv. Exp. Med. Biol.* 1130, 1–16. doi: 10.1007/978-981-13-6123-4_1

Chen, Z. B., Pu, M. M., Yao, J., Cao, X., and Cheng, L. (2018). [Screening of microRNAs targeting Notch signaling pathway implicated in inner ear development and the role of microRNA-384-5p]. *Zhonghua Er Bi Yan Hou Tou Jing Wai Ke Za Zhi* 53, 830–837. doi: 10.3760/cma.j.issn.1673-0860.2018.11.007

Choi, K. A., and Hong, S. (2017). Induced neural stem cells as a means of treatment in Huntington's disease. *Expert Opin. Biol. Ther.* 17, 1333–1343. doi: 10.1080/14712598.2017.1365133

Chonko, K. T., Jahan, I., Stone, J., Wright, M. C., Fujiyama, T., Hoshino, M., et al. (2013). Atoh1 directs hair cell differentiation and survival in the late embryonic mouse inner ear. *Dev. Biol.* 381, 401–410. doi: 10.1016/j.ydbio.2013.06.022

Clarke, D. L., Johansson, C. B., Wilbertz, J., Veress, B., Nilsson, E., Karlstrom, H., et al. (2000). Generalized potential of adult neural stem cells. *Science* 288, 1660–1663. doi: 10.1126/science.288.5471.1660

Cole, L. K., Le Roux, I., Nunes, F., Laufer, E., Lewis, J., and Wu, D. K. (2000). Sensory organ generation in the chicken inner ear: contributions of bone morphogenetic protein 4, serrate1, and lunatic fringe. *J. Comp. Neurol.* 424, 509–520. doi: 10.1002/1096-9861(20000828)424:3<509::aid-cne8>3.0.co;2-q

Corwin, J. T., and Cotanche, D. A. (1988). Regeneration of sensory hair cells after acoustic trauma. *Science* 240, 1772–1774. doi: 10.1126/science.3381100

Cox, B. C., Chai, R., Lenoir, A., Liu, Z., Zhang, L., Nguyen, D. H., et al. (2014). Spontaneous hair cell regeneration in the neonatal mouse cochlea in vivo. *Development* 141, 816–829. doi: 10.1242/dev.103036

Daudet, N., and Lewis, J. (2005). Two contrasting roles for Notch activity in chick inner ear development: specification of prosensory patches and lateral inhibition of hair-cell differentiation. *Development* 132, 541–551. doi: 10.1242/dev.01589

Ding, Y., Meng, W., Kong, W., He, Z., and Chai, R. (2020). The role of FoxG1 in the inner ear. *Front. Cell Dev. Biol.* 8:614954. doi: 10.3389/fcell.2020.614954

Dufner-Almeida, L. G., Cruz, D. B. D., Mingroni Netto, R. C., Batissoco, A. C., Oiticica, J., and Salazar-Silva, R. (2019). Stem-cell therapy for hearing loss: are we there yet? *Braz. J. Otorhinolaryngol.* 85, 520–529. doi: 10.1016/j.bjorl.2019.04.006

Gale, J. E., Marcotti, W., Kennedy, H. J., Kros, C. J., and Richardson, G. P. (2001). FM1-43 dye behaves as a permeant blocker of the hair-cell mechanotransducer channel. *J. Neurosci.* 21, 7013–7025.

Gao, L., Xu, W., Li, T., Chen, J., Shao, A., Yan, F., et al. (2018). Stem cell therapy: a promising therapeutic method for intracerebral hemorrhage. *Cell Transplant.* 27, 1809–1824. doi: 10.1177/0963689718773363

Géléoc, G. S., and Holt, J. R. (2014). Sound strategies for hearing restoration. *Science* 344:1241062. doi: 10.1126/science.1241062

Griesinger, C. B., Richards, C. D., and Ashmore, J. F. (2002). Fm1-43 reveals membrane recycling in adult inner hair cells of the mammalian cochlea. *J. Neurosci.* 22, 3939–3952.

Guo, R., Zhang, S., Xiao, M., Qian, F., He, Z., Li, D., et al. (2016). Accelerating bioelectric functional development of neural stem cells by graphene coupling: implications for neural interfacing with conductive materials. *Biomaterials* 106, 193–204. doi: 10.1016/j.biomaterials.2016.08.019

Han, F., Bi, J., Qiao, L., and Arancio, O. (2020). Stem cell therapy for Alzheimer's disease. *Adv. Exp. Med. Biol.* 1266, 39–55. doi: 10.1007/978-981-15-4370-8_4

Han, S., Sun, J., He, S., Tang, M., and Chai, R. (2019). The application of graphene-based biomaterials in biomedicine. *Am. J. Transl. Res.* 11, 3246–3260.

Han, Z., Wang, C. P., Cong, N., Gu, Y. Y., Ma, R., and Chi, F. L. (2017). Therapeutic value of nerve growth factor in promoting neural stem cell survival and differentiation and protecting against neuronal hearing loss. *Mol. Cell Biochem.* 428, 149–159. doi: 10.1007/s11010-016-2925-5

Hayashi, Y., Lin, H. T., Lee, C. C., and Tsai, K. J. (2020). Effects of neural stem cell transplantation in Alzheimer's disease models. *J. Biomed. Sci.* 27:29. doi: 10.1186/s12929-020-0622-x

Huang, L., and Zhang, L. (2019). Neural stem cell therapies and hypoxic-ischemic brain injury. *Prog. Neurobiol.* 173, 1–17. doi: 10.1016/j.pneurobio.2018.05.004

Iguchi, F., Nakagawa, T., Tateya, I., Kim, T. S., Endo, T., Taniguchi, Z., et al. (2003). Trophic support of mouse inner ear by neural stem cell transplantation. *Neuroreport* 14, 77–80. doi: 10.1097/00001756-200301200-00015

Izumikawa, M., Minoda, R., Kawamoto, K., Abrashkin, K. A., Swiderski, D. L., Dolan, D. F., et al. (2005). Auditory hair cell replacement and hearing improvement by Atoh1 gene therapy in deaf mammals. *Nat. Med.* 11, 271–276. doi: 10.1038/nm1193

Jeyakumar, A., Francis, D., and Doerr, T. (2006). Treatment of idiopathic sudden sensorineural hearing loss. *Acta Otolaryngol.* 126, 708–713. doi: 10.1080/00016480500504234

Jiang, D., Du, J., Zhang, X., Zhou, W., Zong, L., Dong, C., et al. (2016). miR-124 promotes the neuronal differentiation of mouse inner ear neural stem cells. *Int. J. Mol. Med.* 38, 1367–1376. doi: 10.3892/ijmm.2016.2751

Jiao, Q., Li, X., An, J., Zhang, Z., Chen, X., Tan, J., et al. (2017). Cell-cell connection enhances proliferation and neuronal differentiation of rat embryonic neural stem/progenitor cells. *Front. Cell. Neurosci.* 11:200. doi: 10.3389/fncel.2017.00200

Kanzaki, S. (2018). Gene delivery into the inner ear and its clinical implications for hearing and balance. *Molecules* 23:2507. doi: 10.3390/molecules23102507

Kanzaki, S., Toyoda, M., Umezawa, A., and Ogawa, K. (2020). Application of mesenchymal stem cell therapy and inner ear regeneration for hearing loss: a review. *Int. J. Mol. Sci.* 21:5764. doi: 10.3390/ijms21165764

Kiernan, A. E. (2013). Notch signaling during cell fate determination in the inner ear. *Semin. Cell Dev. Biol.* 24, 470–479. doi: 10.1016/j.semcdb.2013.04.002

Kiernan, A. E., Pelling, A. L., Leung, K. K., Tang, A. S., Bell, D. M., Tease, C., et al. (2005). Sox2 is required for sensory organ development in the mammalian inner ear. *Nature* 434, 1031–1035. doi: 10.1038/nature03487

Koehler, K. R., Mikosz, A. M., Molosh, A. I., Patel, D., and Hashino, E. (2013). Generation of inner ear sensory epithelia from pluripotent stem cells in 3D culture. *Nature* 500, 217–221. doi: 10.1038/nature12298

Lang, H. (2016). "Loss, degeneration, and preservation of the spiral ganglion neurons and their processes," in *The Primary Auditory Neurons of the Mammalian Cochlea. Springer Handbook of Auditory Research*, Vol. 52, eds A. Dabdoub, B. Fritzsch, A. Popper, and R. Fay (New York, NY: Springer), 229–262. doi: 10.1007/978-1-4939-3031-9_8

Lang, H., Schulte, B. A., Goddard, J. C., Hedrick, M., Schulte, J. B., Wei, L., et al. (2008). Transplantation of mouse embryonic stem cells into the cochlea of an auditory-neuropathy animal model: effects of timing after injury. *J. Assoc. Res. Otolaryngol.* 9, 225–240. doi: 10.1007/s10162-008-0119-x

Li, M., Guo, K., and Ikehara, S. (2014). Stem cell treatment for Alzheimer's disease. *Int. J. Mol. Sci.* 15, 19226–19238. doi: 10.3390/ijms151019226

Li, X., Aleardi, A., Wang, J., Zhou, Y., Andrade, R., and Hu, Z. (2016). Differentiation of spiral ganglion-derived neural stem cells into functional synaptogenetic neurons. *Stem Cells Dev.* 25, 803–813. doi: 10.1089/scd.2015.0345

Lindvall, O. (2015). Treatment of Parkinson's disease using cell transplantation. *Philos. Trans. R Soc. Lond. B Biol. Sci.* 370:20140370. doi: 10.1098/rstb.2014.0370

Liu, G., David, B. T., Trawczynski, M., and Fessler, R. G. (2020). Advances in pluripotent stem cells: history, mechanisms, technologies, and applications. *Stem Cell Rev. Rep.* 16, 3–32. doi: 10.1007/s12015-019-09935-x

Liu, Q., Chen, P., and Wang, J. (2014). Molecular mechanisms and potentials for differentiating inner ear stem cells into sensory hair cells. *Dev. Biol.* 390, 93–101. doi: 10.1016/j.ydbio.2014.03.010

Liu, R., Zhao, L., Cong, T., and Yang, S. (2016). Research and development of stem cell therapy for deafness. *Chin. J. Otol.* 14, 6–9.

Liu, Z., Owen, T., Fang, J., and Zuo, J. (2012). Overactivation of Notch1 signaling induces ectopic hair cells in the mouse inner ear in an age-dependent manner. *PLoS One* 7:e34123. doi: 10.1371/journal.pone.0034123

Marsh, S. E., and Blurton-Jones, M. (2017). Neural stem cell therapy for neurodegenerative disorders: the role of neurotrophic support. *Neurochem. Int.* 106, 94–100. doi: 10.1016/j.neuint.2017.02.006

Matsui, J. I., Parker, M. A., Ryals, B. M., and Cotanche, D. A. (2005). Regeneration and replacement in the vertebrate inner ear. *Drug Discov. Today* 10, 1307–1312. doi: 10.1016/S1359-6446(05)03577-4

Mellado Lagarde, M. M., Wan, G., Zhang, L., Gigliello, A. R., McInnis, J. J., Zhang, Y., et al. (2014). Spontaneous regeneration of cochlear supporting cells after neonatal ablation ensures hearing in the adult mouse. *Proc. Natl. Acad. Sci. U.S.A.* 111, 16919–16924. doi: 10.1073/pnas.1408064111

Menendez, L., Trecek, T., Gopalakrishnan, S., Tao, L., Markowitz, A. L., Yu, H. V., et al. (2020). Generation of inner ear hair cells by direct lineage conversion of primary somatic cells. *Elife* 9:e55249. doi: 10.7554/eLife.55249

Miska, J., and Lesniak, M. S. (2015). Neural stem cell carriers for the treatment of glioblastoma multiforme. *EBioMedicine* 2, 774–775. doi: 10.1016/j.ebiom.2015.08.022

Mizutari, K., Fujioka, M., Hosoya, M., Bramhall, N., Okano, H. J., Okano, H., et al. (2013). Notch inhibition induces cochlear hair cell regeneration and recovery of hearing after acoustic trauma. *Neuron* 77, 58–69. doi: 10.1016/j.neuron.2012.10.032

Morrison, A., Hodgetts, C., Gossler, A., Hrabé de Angelis, M., and Lewis, J. (1999). Expression of delta1 and serrate1 (Jagged1) in the mouse inner ear. *Mech. Dev.* 84, 169–172. doi: 10.1016/s0925-4773(99)00066-0

Moser, T., and Starr, A. (2016). Auditory neuropathy-neural and synaptic mechanisms. *Nat. Rev. Neurol.* 12, 135–149. doi: 10.1038/nrneurol.2016.10

Moser, T., Predoehl, F., and Starr, A. (2013). Review of hair cell synapse defects in sensorineural hearing impairment. *Otol. Neurotol.* 34, 995–1004. doi: 10.1097/MAO.0b013e3182814d4a

Muller, U., and Barr-Gillespie, P. G. (2015). New treatment options for hearing loss. *Nat. Rev. Drug Discov.* 14, 346–365. doi: 10.1038/nrd4533

Nacher-Soler, G., Garrido, J. M., and Rodriguez-Serrano, F. (2019). Hearing regeneration and regenerative medicine: present and future approaches. *Arch. Med. Sci.* 15, 957–967. doi: 10.5114/aoms.2019.86062

Nayagam, B. A., Muniak, M. A., and Ryugo, D. K. (2011). The spiral ganglion: connecting the peripheral and central auditory systems. *Hear. Res.* 278, 2–20. doi: 10.1016/j.heares.2011.04.003

Neves, J., Kamaid, A., Alsina, B., and Giraldez, F. (2007). Differential expression of Sox2 and Sox3 in neuronal and sensory progenitors of the developing inner ear of the chick. *J. Comp. Neurol.* 503, 487–500. doi: 10.1002/cne.21299

Ojha, S., Henderson, A., Bennett, W., and Clark, M. (2020). Sudden sensorineural hearing loss and bedside phone testing: a guide for primary care. *Br. J. Gen. Pract.* 70, 144–145. doi: 10.3399/bjgp20X708761

Oshima, K., Grimm, C. M., Corrales, C. E., Senn, P., Martinez Monedero, R., Geleoc, G. S., et al. (2007). Differential distribution of stem cells in the auditory and vestibular organs of the inner ear. *J. Assoc. Res. Otolaryngol.* 8, 18–31. doi: 10.1007/s10162-006-0058-3

Oshima, K., Senn, P., and Heller, S. (2009). Isolation of sphere-forming stem cells from the mouse inner ear. *Methods Mol. Biol.* 493, 141–162. doi: 10.1007/978-1-59745-523-7_9

Ottersen, O. P., Takumi, Y., Matsubara, A., Landsend, A. S., Laake, J. H., and Usami, S. (1998). Molecular organization of a type of peripheral glutamate synapse: the afferent synapses of hair cells in the inner ear. *Prog. Neurobiol.* 54, 127–148. doi: 10.1016/s0301-0082(97)00054-3

Ouyang, T., Meng, W., Li, M., Hong, T., and Zhang, N. (2020). Recent advances of the Hippo/YAP signaling pathway in brain development and glioma. *Cell. Mol. Neurobiol.* 40, 495–510. doi: 10.1007/s10571-019-00762-9

Perny, M., Ting, C. C., Kleinlogel, S., Senn, P., and Roccio, M. (2017). Generation of otic sensory neurons from mouse embryonic stem cells in 3D culture. *Front. Cell. Neurosci.* 11:409. doi: 10.3389/fncel.2017.00409

Prosser, H. M., Rzadzinska, A. K., Steel, K. P., and Bradley, A. (2008). Mosaic complementation demonstrates a regulatory role for myosin VIIa in actin dynamics of stereocilia. *Mol. Cell Biol.* 28, 1702–1712. doi: 10.1128/MCB.01282-07

Raft, S., Koundakjian, E. J., Quinones, H., Jayasena, C. S., Goodrich, L. V., Johnson, J. E., et al. (2007). Cross-regulation of Ngn1 and Math1 coordinates the production of neurons and sensory hair cells during inner ear development. *Development* 134, 4405–4415. doi: 10.1242/dev.009118

Roccio, M., and Edge, A. S. B. (2019). Inner ear organoids: new tools to understand neurosensory cell development, degeneration and regeneration. *Development* 146:dev177188. doi: 10.1242/dev.177188

Sage, C., Huang, M., Vollrath, M. A., Brown, M. C., Hinds, P. W., Corey, D. P., et al. (2006). Essential role of retinoblastoma protein in mammalian hair cell development and hearing. *Proc. Natl. Acad. Sci. U.S.A.* 103, 7345–7350. doi: 10.1073/pnas.0510631103

Schimmang, T. (2007). Expression and functions of FGF ligands during early otic development. *Int. J. Dev. Biol.* 51, 473–481. doi: 10.1387/ijdb.072334ts

Seyyedi, M., Viana, L. M., and Nadol, J. B. Jr. (2014). Within-subject comparison of word recognition and spiral ganglion cell count in bilateral cochlear implant recipients. *Otol. Neurotol.* 35, 1446–1450. doi: 10.1097/MAO.0000000000000443

Shi, F., and Edge, A. S. (2013). Prospects for replacement of auditory neurons by stem cells. *Hear. Res.* 297, 106–112. doi: 10.1016/j.heares.2013.01.017

Shin, S. R., Li, Y. C., Jang, H. L., Khoshakhlagh, P., Akbari, M., Nasajpour, A., et al. (2016). Graphene-based materials for tissue engineering. *Adv. Drug Deliv. Rev.* 105(Pt B), 255–274. doi: 10.1016/j.addr.2016.03.007

Stachler, R. J., Chandrasekhar, S. S., Archer, S. M., Rosenfeld, R. M., Schwartz, S. R., Barrs, D. M., et al. (2012). Clinical practice guideline: sudden hearing loss. *Otolaryngol. Head Neck Surg.* 146(3 Suppl.), S1–S35. doi: 10.1177/0194599812436449

Steel, K. P., and Kros, C. J. (2001). A genetic approach to understanding auditory function. *Nat. Genet.* 27, 143–149. doi: 10.1038/84758

Susanto, E., Marin Navarro, A., Zhou, L., Sundström, A., van Bree, N., Stantic, M., et al. (2020). Modeling SHH-driven medulloblastoma with patient iPS cell-derived neural stem cells. *Proc. Natl. Acad. Sci. U.S.A.* 117, 20127–20138. doi: 10.1073/pnas.1920521117

Trounson, A., and McDonald, C. (2015). Stem cell therapies in clinical trials: progress and challenges. *Cell Stem Cell* 17, 11–22. doi: 10.1016/j.stem.2015.06.007

Tucci, D. L., Farmer, J. C. Jr., Kitch, R. D., and Witsell, D. L. (2002). Treatment of sudden sensorineural hearing loss with systemic steroids and valacyclovir. *Otol. Neurotol.* 23, 301–308. doi: 10.1097/00129492-200205000-00012

Udovichenko, I. P., Gibbs, D., and Williams, D. S. (2002). Actin-based motor properties of native myosin VIIa. *J. Cell Sci.* 115(Pt 2), 445–450.

Vieira, M. S., Santos, A. K., Vasconcellos, R., Goulart, V. A. M., Parreira, R. C., Kihara, A. H., et al. (2018). Neural stem cell differentiation into mature neurons: mechanisms of regulation and biotechnological applications. *Biotechnol. Adv.* 36, 1946–1970. doi: 10.1016/j.biotechadv.2018.08.002

Wang, T., Chai, R., Kim, G. S., Pham, N., Jansson, L., Nguyen, D. H., et al. (2015). Lgr5+ cells regenerate hair cells via proliferation and direct transdifferentiation in damaged neonatal mouse utricle. *Nat. Commun.* 6:6613. doi: 10.1038/ncomms7613

Wang, Z., Jiang, H., Yan, Y., Wang, Y., Shen, Y., Li, W., et al. (2006). Characterization of proliferating cells from newborn mouse cochleae. *Neuroreport* 17, 767–771. doi: 10.1097/01.wnr.0000215781.22345.8b

Waqas, M., Gao, S., Us-Salam, I., Ali, M. K., Ma, Y., and Li, W. (2018). Inner ear hair cell protection in mammals against the noise-induced cochlear damage. *Neural Plast.* 2018:3170801. doi: 10.1155/2018/3170801

Waqas, M., Us-Salam, I., Bibi, Z., Wang, Y., Li, H., Zhu, Z., et al. (2020). Stem cell-based therapeutic approaches to restore sensorineural hearing loss in mammals. *Neural Plast.* 2020:8829660. doi: 10.1155/2020/8829660

Warchol, M. E. (2011). Sensory regeneration in the vertebrate inner ear: differences at the levels of cells and species. *Hear. Res.* 273, 72–79. doi: 10.1016/j.heares.2010.05.004

Weissman, J. L. (1996). Hearing loss. *Radiology* 199, 593–611. doi: 10.1148/radiology.199.3.8637972

White, P. M., Doetzlhofer, A., Lee, Y. S., Groves, A. K., and Segil, N. (2006). Mammalian cochlear supporting cells can divide and trans-differentiate into hair cells. *Nature* 441, 984–987. doi: 10.1038/nature04849

Wilson, B. S., Tucci, D. L., Merson, M. H., and O'Donoghue, G. M. (2017). Global hearing health care: new findings and perspectives. *Lancet* 390, 2503–2515. doi: 10.1016/S0140-6736(17)31073-5

Wu, X., Zou, S., Wu, F., He, Z., and Kong, W. (2020). Role of microRNA in inner ear stem cells and related research progress. *Am. J. Stem Cells* 9, 16–24.

Xia, L., Shang, Y., Chen, X., Li, H., Xu, X., Liu, W., et al. (2020). Oriented neural spheroid formation and differentiation of neural stem cells guided by anisotropic inverse opals. *Front. Bioeng. Biotechnol.* 8:848. doi: 10.3389/fbioe.2020.00848

Xia, M., Ma, J., Sun, S., Li, W., and Li, H. (2019). The biological strategies for hearing re-establishment based on the stem/progenitor cells. *Neurosci. Lett.* 711:134406. doi: 10.1016/j.neulet.2019.134406

Xiang, M., Gan, L., Li, D., Chen, Z. Y., Zhou, L., O'Malley, B. W. Jr., et al. (1997). Essential role of POU-domain factor Brn-3c in auditory and vestibular hair cell development. *Proc. Natl. Acad. Sci. U.S.A.* 94, 9445–9450. doi: 10.1073/pnas.94.17.9445

Xiao, J., Yang, R., Biswas, S., Zhu, Y., Qin, X., Zhang, M., et al. (2018). Neural stem cell-based regenerative approaches for the treatment of multiple sclerosis. *Mol. Neurobiol.* 55, 3152–3171. doi: 10.1007/s12035-017-0566-7

Xu, Y. P., Shan, X. D., Liu, Y. Y., Pu, Y., Wang, C. Y., Tao, Q. L., et al. (2016). Olfactory epithelium neural stem cell implantation restores noise-induced hearing loss in rats. *Neurosci. Lett.* 616, 19–25. doi: 10.1016/j.neulet.2016.01.016

Yang, K., Jung, K., Ko, E., Kim, J., Park, K. I., Kim, J., et al. (2013). Nanotopographical manipulation of focal adhesion formation for enhanced differentiation of human neural stem cells. *ACS Appl. Mater. Interfaces* 5, 10529–10540. doi: 10.1021/am402156f

Yang, Y., Zhang, Y., Chai, R., and Gu, Z. (2018). Designs of biomaterials and microenvironments for neuroengineering. *Neural Plast.* 2018:1021969. doi: 10.1155/2018/1021969

Yi, T. H., and Dong, M. M. (2010). Neural stem cells and inner ear hearing loss and restoration. *Zhongguo Zuzhi Gong. Yanjiu Linchuang Kangfu* 14, 5085–5089.

Zhai, S., Shi, L., Wang, B. E., Zheng, G., Song, W., Hu, Y., et al. (2005). Isolation and culture of hair cell progenitors from postnatal rat cochleae. *J. Neurobiol.* 65, 282–293. doi: 10.1002/neu.20190

Zhang, P. Z., He, Y., Jiang, X. W., Chen, F. Q., Chen, Y., Shi, L., et al. (2013). Stem cell transplantation via the cochlear lateral wall for replacement of degenerated spiral ganglion neurons. *Hear. Res.* 298, 1–9. doi: 10.1016/j.heares.2013.01.022

Zhang, S., Qiang, R., Dong, Y., Zhang, Y., Chen, Y., Zhou, H., et al. (2020a). Hair cell regeneration from inner ear progenitors in the mammalian cochlea. *Am. J. Stem Cells* 9, 25–35.

Zhang, S., Zhang, Y., Dong, Y., Guo, L., Zhang, Z., Shao, B., et al. (2020b). Knockdown of Foxg1 in supporting cells increases the trans-differentiation of supporting cells into hair cells in the neonatal mouse cochlea. *Cell. Mol. Life Sci.* 77, 1401–1419. doi: 10.1007/s00018-019-03291-2

Zhao, Y., Wang, Y., Wang, Z., Liu, H., Shen, Y., Li, W., et al. (2006). Sonic hedgehog promotes mouse inner ear progenitor cell proliferation and hair cell generation in vitro. *Neuroreport* 17, 121–124. doi: 10.1097/01.wnr.0000198439.44636.49

Zheng, L., Sekerková, G., Vranich, K., Tilney, L. G., Mugnaini, E., and Bartles, J. R. (2000). The deaf jerker mouse has a mutation in the gene encoding the espin actin-bundling proteins of hair cell stereocilia and lacks espins. *Cell* 102, 377–385. doi: 10.1016/s0092-8674(00)00042-8

Zhou, W., Du, J., Jiang, D., Wang, X., Chen, K., Tang, H., et al. (2018). microRNA183 is involved in the differentiation and regeneration of Notch signalingprohibited hair cells from mouse cochlea. *Mol. Med. Rep.* 18, 1253–1262. doi: 10.3892/mmr.2018.9127

Zhu, H., Chen, J., Guan, L., Xiong, S., and Jiang, H. (2018). The transplantation of induced pluripotent stem cells into the cochleae of mature mice. *Int. J. Clin. Exp. Pathol.* 11, 4423–4430.

Zhu, Q., and Lu, P. (2020). Stem cell transplantation for amyotrophic lateral sclerosis. *Adv. Exp. Med. Biol.* 1266, 71–97. doi: 10.1007/978-981-15-4370-8_6

Endolymphatic Hydrops is a Marker of Synaptopathy Following Traumatic Noise Exposure

Ido Badash[1], Patricia M. Quiñones[1], Kevin J. Oghalai[2], Juemei Wang[1], Christopher G. Lui[3], Frank Macias-Escriva[1], Brian E. Applegate[1,2] and John S. Oghalai[1,2]*

[1]Caruso Department of Otolaryngology-Head and Neck Surgery, Keck School of Medicine of the University of Southern California, Los Angeles, CA, United States, [2]Viterbi School of Engineering, University of Southern California, Los Angeles, CA, United States, [3]Department of Otolaryngology-Head and Neck Surgery, Northwestern University Feinberg School of Medicine, Chicago, IL, United States

*Correspondence:
John S. Oghalai
Oghalai@usc.edu

After acoustic trauma, there can be loss of synaptic connections between inner hair cells and auditory neurons in the cochlea, which may lead to hearing abnormalities including speech-in-noise difficulties, tinnitus, and hyperacusis. We have previously studied mice with blast-induced cochlear synaptopathy and found that they also developed a build-up of endolymph, termed endolymphatic hydrops. In this study, we used optical coherence tomography to measure endolymph volume in live CBA/CaJ mice exposed to various noise intensities. We quantified the number of synaptic ribbons and postsynaptic densities under the inner hair cells 1 week after noise exposure to determine if they correlated with acute changes in endolymph volume measured in the hours after the noise exposure. After 2 h of noise at an intensity of 95 dB SPL or below, both endolymph volume and synaptic counts remained normal. After exposure to 2 h of 100 dB SPL noise, mice developed endolymphatic hydrops and had reduced synaptic counts in the basal and middle regions of the cochlea. Furthermore, round-window application of hypertonic saline reduced the degree of endolymphatic hydrops that developed after 100 dB SPL noise exposure and partially prevented the reduction in synaptic counts in the cochlear base. Taken together, these results indicate that endolymphatic hydrops correlates with noise-induced cochlear synaptopathy, suggesting that these two pathologic findings have a common mechanistic basis.

Keywords: hidden hearing loss, acoustic trauma, ribbon synapse, cochlear synaptopathy, endolymphatic hydrops

INTRODUCTION

Acoustic trauma is the most common preventable cause of hearing loss, and it has been suggested that 12% or more of the world population is at risk for noise-induced loss of hearing (Alberti et al., 1979; Le et al., 2017). Research in mice, guinea pigs, and rhesus macaques has shown that even moderate noise exposure levels previously thought to cause only temporary threshold shifts can result in immediate and irreversible loss of the synaptic connections between inner hair cells (IHCs) and cochlear nerve fibers (Kujawa and Liberman, 2009; Jensen et al., 2015; Kujawa and Liberman, 2015; Liberman et al., 2015; Valero et al., 2017). As most of the nerve fibers affected by this change have high thresholds and low spontaneous rates of firing, the loss of ribbon synapses does not elevate behavioral auditory thresholds or auditory brainstem response (ABR) thresholds until it becomes extreme. This phenomenon has thus been called hidden hearing loss, since it would not be detected on traditional hearing tests (Liberman et al., 2016). While some studies suggest that cochlear synaptopathy is not common in humans (Prendergast et al., 2017; Guest et al., 2019a; Guest et al., 2019b), other studies argue that it contributes to a variety of hearing abnormalities including speech-in-noise difficulties, tinnitus and hyperacusis (Felder and Schrott-Fischer, 1995; Roberts et al., 2010; Hickox and Liberman, 2014; Viana et al., 2015; Liberman and Kujawa, 2017).

Noise-induced damage to auditory nerve dendrites is caused by excess release of glutamate, the neurotransmitter responsible for afferent signaling between hair cells and auditory neurons (Spoendlin, 1971; Robertson, 1983; Choi and Rothman, 1990; Pujol et al., 1993; Puel et al., 1998; Kim et al., 2019a). We have previously studied mice exposed to blast pressure waves and found widespread cochlear synaptopathy 1 week after the blast (Kim et al., 2018a). Using optical coherence tomography (OCT) to image the mouse cochlea non-invasively right after the blast, we also identified a build-up of fluid within the scala media, known as endolymphatic hydrops. Interestingly, treating the endolymphatic hydrops with hypertonic saline also reduced cochlear synaptopathy. Thus, although these data do not prove that endolymphatic hydrops causes cochlear synaptopathy, they suggest that they may be related.

Here, we sought to better assess this relationship by using a non-blast noise exposure protocol that permitted us to better titrate the level of the acoustic trauma. We examined the relationship between noise intensity, endolymph volume, and synapse loss, and found that endolymphatic hydrops correlates with the loss of IHC ribbons and postsynaptic densities (PSDs). Moreover, we showed that noise-induced endolymphatic hydrops and loss of cochlear synapses could be mitigated through the round window application of hypertonic saline, further suggesting that these two processes have a common mechanistic basis.

MATERIALS AND METHODS

Animals
All experiments were performed according to protocols approved by the Institutional Animal Care and Use Committee at the University of Southern California. We used a total of 59 CBA/CaJ mice that were 4- to 6-weeks old. Anesthesia consisted of a combination of ketamine (100 mg/kg) and xylazine (10 mg/kg).

Noise Exposure
Our noise exposure protocol has been previously published (Liu et al., 2011; Xia et al., 2013). Briefly, awake mice were placed inside a plastic cage with custom-built subdivisions made from chicken wire, such that each animal had its own area to freely move about. This allowed exposure of up to four mice simultaneously. The cage was fitted with a roof also made from chicken wire and placed inside a wooden box with speakers built into the lid. White noise that was bandpass filtered between 8 and 16 kHz was delivered to the mice for 2 h. The noise intensity was monitored using a ¼″ Brüel & Kjaer microphone and was consistent throughout the cage and over the course of the 2 h exposure within the range of ±2 decibel (dB) sound pressure level (SPL). Mice designated as controls were placed in the exact same experimental environment as the noise-exposed mice for 2 h but without noise delivered through the speakers.

In Vivo OCT Imaging
After noise or sham exposure, 21 of the 59 mice underwent cochlear imaging to measure endolymph volume, as previously described (Kim et al., 2018a). Anesthetized mice were positioned on a heating pad to maintain a core body temperature of 37°C, and additional doses of anesthesia were administered throughout the experiment to maintain sedation. The skull was exposed and glued to a head-holder with dental cement. A ventrolateral approach was used to surgically access the left middle ear bulla, which was opened carefully by microdissection to access the apical turn of the cochlea without disturbing the otic capsule. Our custom-built OCT system has been previously described (Dewey et al., 2019). Two-dimensional imaging of the cochlear duct was performed by repeatedly scanning the optical beam to collect cross-sectional images in the x and z dimensions. To quantify endolymph volume, we collected a volume stack of cross-sectional images of the cochlea, moving the y position in 2 µm steps over a 300-µm length of the basement membrane (150 cross-sections per mouse). The orientation of the mouse cochlea from our surgical approach and angle of the OCT scanning laser allowed us to image a limited portion of the apical turn centered at the 9 kHz location, which we know from previous studies in which we measured vibratory tuning curves at this cochlear position (Gao et al., 2014; Lee et al., 2015; Lee et al., 2016; Dewey et al., 2018; Dewey et al., 2019). We were able to collect images along an approximately 300-µm length of the cochlear duct at this location, and then used Imaris software (Bitplane, Concord, MA) to render 3D images from this volume stack. We removed 75-µm segments on both ends of the volume stack to select an identical 150-µm segment of the scala media from each sample, as we have previously reported (Kim et al., 2018a). The volume of this 150-µm long chamber was measured though a built-in feature within Imaris using a calculated voxel size based on the scanning parameters of the laser. A cochleogram showing the location of the 300-µm region where OCT was used to image the cochlea, and the 150-µm subsection of this region where endolymph volume of the scala media was measured, is included in **Supplementary Figure S1**.

Immunofluorescence and Cochlear Dissection
Thirty-eight of the 59 mice were assessed for cochlear synaptopathy. Following noise or sham exposure, these mice were returned to the animal facility for routine care. Our methods of immunofluorescence have been previously reported (Kim et al., 2018a). One week after noise or sham exposure, the mice were euthanized with isofluorane and both cochleae were extracted. We opened a fenestra in the apex and perfused 4% paraformaldehyde through the round window.

Following this, we immersed the cochlea in 4% paraformaldehyde solution at room temperature for 30 min. After washing with PBS, the cochlea was decalcified by immersing in a 0.5 M EDTA solution (pH 8) for 6 h at room temperature, and again washed in PBS.

The sensory epithelium was then dissected into apical, middle, and basal sections in a manner similar to the whole mount dissection technique reported by Montgomery and Cox (2016). The average lengths and variances of these segments were measured and converted into percentages of the total cochlear length. These percentages were correlated with their respective tonotopic frequencies based on the cochlear place-frequency maps described by Müller et al. (2005) and Viberg and Canlon (2004). The apical and middle segments each measured 1.9 ± 0.1 mm (mean ± standard error), and the basal segment measured 1.8 ± 0.05 mm. Approximately 10 ± 5% of the cochlea, corresponding to the hook region, was damaged due to limitations of the dissection and not included in our analysis. Assuming the CBA/CaJ cochlea ranges from 5 kHz at the apex to 80 kHz at the base (Viberg and Canlon, 2004; Müller et al., 2005), then the apical segment corresponds to the frequency range of $5 - 11.5 \pm 0.5$ kHz, the middle segment corresponds to the frequency range of $11.5 \pm 0.5 - 26 \pm 2$ kHz, and the base segment corresponds to the frequency range of $26 \pm 2 - 60 \pm 8$ kHz. The average tonotopic frequencies and percentages of total cochlear length from the base associated with the apical, middle and base segments are shown in the cochleogram in **Supplementary Figure S1**.

Dissected cochlear tissues were incubated in blocking solution (5% donkey serum, 0.1% Triton X-100, and 1.0% BSA in PBS) for 1 h at room temperature. Samples were incubated with primary antibodies diluted in the same blocking solution for 2 days at 4°C followed by a 2 h incubation at 37°C. The primary antibody solution contained mouse anti-CtBP2 IgG (1:200; 612044 (Lot: 8172904), BD Biosciences) and rabbit anti-Homer IgG (1:800; 160003 (Lot: 1–43), Synaptic Systems). After washing in PBST (0.1% Triton X-100 in PBS) the tissues were incubated with a secondary antibody solution diluted in 0.1% Triton X-100 and 0.1% BSA in PBS for 1 h at room temperature. The secondary antibodies were donkey anti-mouse IgG conjugated with Alexa Fluor 488 (1:500; A21202, Invitrogen) and donkey anti-rabbit IgG conjugated with Alexa Fluor 546 (1:500; A10040, Invitrogen). Alexa Fluor 647-conjugated phalloidin (1:200; A22287, Invitrogen) was added with the secondary antibody solution. After washing in PBS, the tissues were mounted on glass slides using Fluoromount-G with DAPI (00-4959-52, Invitrogen). Slides were kept overnight at 4°C before imaging with an upright confocal microscope (Zeiss LSM 800) using a 63X objective (1.4 N.A.) to generate z-stacks.

Identification and Co-Localization of synaptic Ribbons and Postsynaptic Densities

The number of IHCs, outer hair cells (OHCs), CtBP2-labeled synaptic ribbons, and Homer-labeled PSDs were counted using custom image processing software written in MATLAB (R2021a, The MathWorks Inc., Natick, MA). The number of IHCs and OHCs were counted manually by visual inspection of hair cell nuclei in each z-stack. Automated counts of ribbons and PSDs were then performed (**Supplementary Figure S2**). First, the background was developed by running the images through a 1.4 μm median filter to remove all objects at or below the size of ribbons and PSDs. The original images were passed through a 0.35 μ median filter to eliminate speckle noise, and the background was subtracted from these images to isolate the ribbon- and PSD-sized objects. Ribbons and PSDs were identified by picking only those objects that were more intense than a threshold level selected by eye. The program then grouped these objects by X, Y, and Z coordinates, with each group signifying a single ribbon or density. Structures which were shorter than 0.48 μm were deemed not tall enough to be ribbons or PSDs and were removed by the program. Co-localization of ribbons and PSDs was performed using the X, Y, and Z coordinates of these structures, such that nearby structures within 2 μm of each other were identified as a pair. Ribbons that were not paired with a corresponding PSD were determined to be orphan ribbons. All counts were verified and adjusted based on visual inspection by two blinded investigators acting independently. If there were any discrepancies between the final counts of the two independent reviewers, these were resolved by the senior author after independent, blinded review.

Application of Solutions to the Round Window Membrane

Of the 24 mice undergoing *in vivo* OCT imaging after noise or sham exposure, in 6 mice we surgically opened the middle ear bulla under anesthesia as described above and applied either hypertonic saline (6,000 mOsm/kg) or normotonic saline (307 mOsm/kg) to fill the bulla and cover the round window membrane. The solution was drawn up using a rolled Kimwipe and re-applied every 15 min in order to maintain the desired osmolality. The solution was also withdrawn and re-applied every time an image or volume stack was captured using OCT.

Thirteen of the 38 mice that were to be used for immunolabeling experiments were anesthetized immediately following noise or sham exposure and underwent round-window application of either hypertonic or normotonic saline. We pierced a small hole in the tympanic membrane under microscopic guidance and filled the middle ear space with the test solution through the perforation until fluid appeared in the ear canal. Only left ears were treated. Mice were maintained under anesthesia for 5.5 h from the time of intratympanic injection while lying with the left ear up to keep the test solution in contact with the round window membrane. Additional test solution was instilled into the ear every 15 min in order to maintain the desired osmolality.

Normotonic saline (307 mOsm/kg) was composed of 150 mM NaCl and 20 mM HEPES. Hypertonic saline (6,000 mOsm/kg) was composed of 2,990 mM NaCl and 20 mM HEPES. For both solutions, the pH was adjusted to 7.4 using a benchtop pH meter and either 1 M NaOH or 1 M HCl. The osmolality of normotonic saline was verified using a freezing pressure osmometer (3,320,

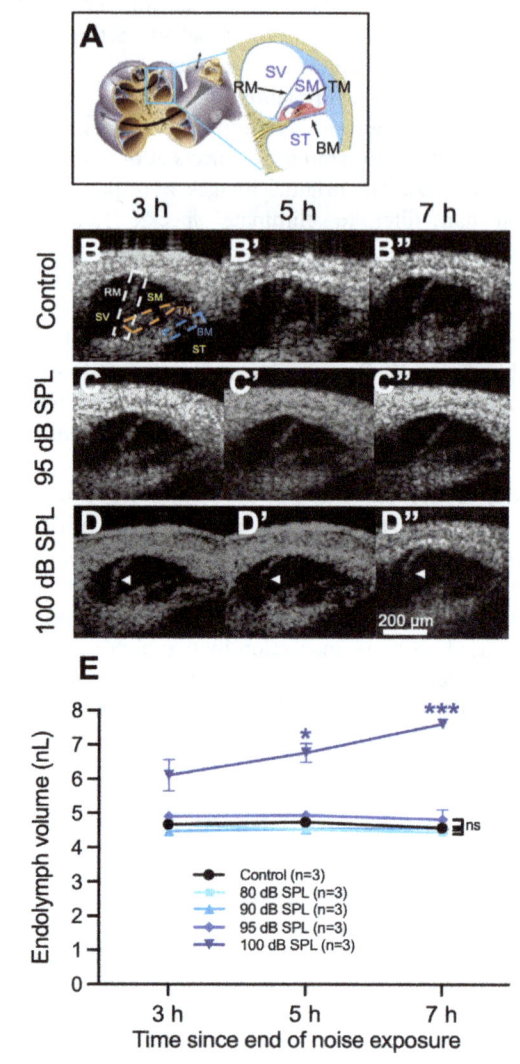

FIGURE 1 | Endolymphatic hydrops develops after 2 h of 100 decibel (dB) sound pressure level (SPL) noise exposure. **(A)** Diagram of the mouse cochlea indicating the location where optical coherence tomography (OCT) was performed within the apical turn. Locations of Reissner's membrane (RM), basilar membrane (BM), tectorial membrane (TM), scala vestibuli (SV), scala media (SM) and scala tympani (ST) are shown. **(B)** OCT images from a representative control mouse demonstrate normal endolymph volume and no change in the position of RM over time. Locations of the same structures from panel **(A)** are shown in the first panel. **(C)** OCT images from a mouse exposed to 95 dB SPL noise also demonstrate normal endolymph volume and no bulging of RM over time. **(D)** Endolymphatic hydrops is apparent at 3 h following 100 dB SPL noise exposure and progressively grows over the next 4 h. White arrow heads indicate the bowed position of RM. **(E)** Quantification of endolymph volume measured over time in mice exposed to 80, 90, 95, and 100 dB SPL as well as control mice that were not exposed to noise. Endolymph volume increased over time in mice exposed to 100 dB SPL and was significantly greater than control mice at 5 and 7 h following noise exposure. Endolymph volumes in mice exposed to lower noise intensity levels were not significantly different than in control mice. Endolymph volume represents the volume of the scala media over a segment of basement membrane that is 150 μm in length. Sample sizes are expressed in number of mice. Error bars indicate standard error. $*p < 0.05$, $***p < 0.001$.

Advanced Instruments). The osmolality of the hypertonic solution could only be predicted based on its constituents, as its osmolality exceeded the upper threshold of the osmometer (2000 mOsm/kg).

Statistical Analysis

Statistical analysis and data plotting was performed using GraphPad Prism (version 8.0.2, GraphPad Software Inc., La Jolla, CA). All data sets were tested for the presence of a normal distribution using the Shapiro-Wilk test for normality. Changes in endolymph volume across time between different noise intensities and treatment conditions were compared using repeated measures two-way ANOVA with the Geisser-Greenhouse correction and post-hoc Tukey multiple comparisons test. Ribbons, PSDs, and orphan ribbon counts in the base, middle and apex of the cochlea were compared between different noise intensities and treatment conditions using two-way ANOVA with post-hoc Tukey multiple comparisons test. Sum of squares calculations were performed as part of the two-way ANOVA to correct for imbalances caused by unequal sample sizes among groups (Landsheer and van den Wittenboer, 2015; Glantz et al., 2016; GraphPad Statistics Guide, 2021). All tests were two tailed, and a p value of <0.05 was considered statistically significant. In cases where the p values calculated from two-way ANOVA were statistically significant, only the p values for single-pair comparisons from the post-hoc Tukey multiple comparisons test are reported. All means are presented with standard errors and sample sizes. The results of all statistical tests performed in this study are provided in **Supplementary Tables S1–9**.

RESULTS

100 dB SPL 2-h Noise Exposure Produces Endolymphatic Hydrops

First, we titrated the level of acoustic trauma to determine the threshold for developing endolymphatic hydrops. We subjected cohorts of mice to 2 h of sham exposure (control, no noise) or noise exposure at an intensity of 80, 90, 95, or 100 dB SPL and serially imaged the apical turn of the cochlea *in vivo* using OCT. Reissner's membrane (RM), the basilar membrane (BM), and the tectorial membrane (TM) could all be resolved in the resulting cross-sectional image of the cochlea (**Figures 1A,B**). We anesthetized mice 2 h after the noise exposure was completed and used ~1 h to dissect and prepare the mouse. We then imaged the apical turn of the cochlea from 3–7 h after the noise exposure. Thus, the total anesthetic time was limited to 5 h.

In unexposed control mice and those exposed to noise intensity levels of 80, 90, or 95 dB SPL, there were no changes in the position of RM over time (**Figures 1B,C, Supplementary Movie S1**). In contrast, mice exposed to 100 dB SPL noise had progressive bulging of RM over time consistent with an increase in endolymph volume, termed endolymphatic hydrops (**Figure 1D, Supplementary Movie S2**).

We then quantified endolymph volume in these cohorts of mice (**Figure 1E**). Endolymph volume increased by 24.6 ± 7.8%

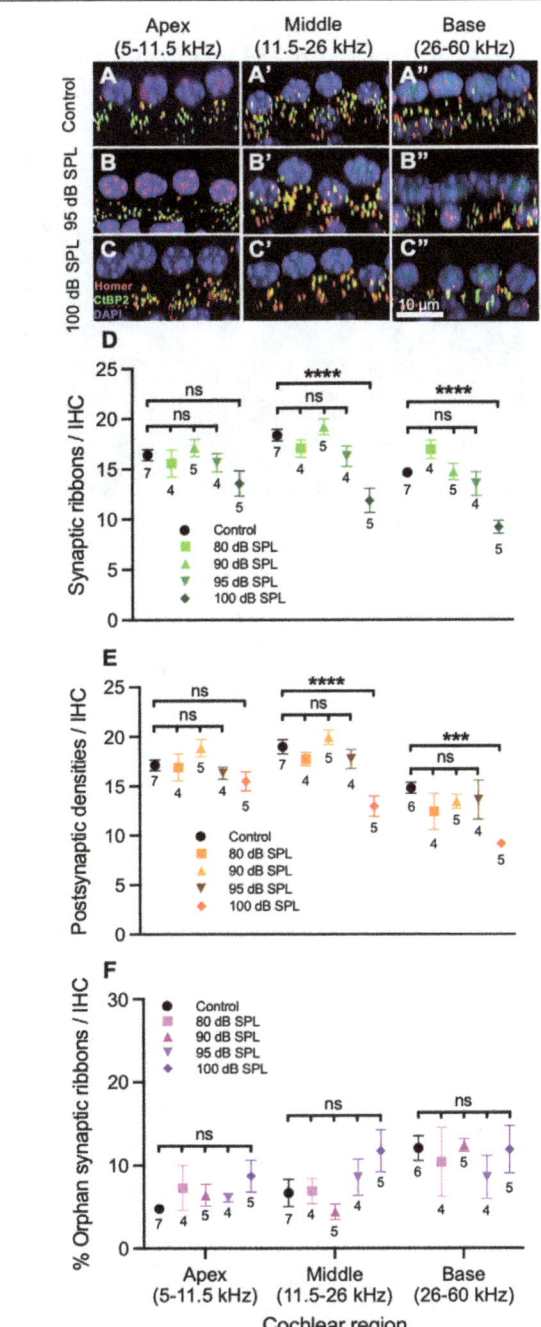

FIGURE 2 | Sound intensity affects degree of inner hair cell (IHC) synapse loss following 2 h noise exposure. **(A–C)** Representative sections from the organ of Corti of mice 7 days after noise or sham exposure (control) displaying 4 IHC nuclei and associated ribbons as well as postsynaptic densities (PSDs). Immunolabeling was performed to visualize IHC ribbons (CtBP2, green), PSDs (Homer, red) and nuclei (DAPI, blue). Control mice **(A)** had a similar number of ribbons and PSDs when compared to mice exposed to 95 decibel (dB) sound pressure level (SPL) **(B)**. **(C)** A reduction in the number of ribbons and PSDs can be seen in the middle and basal cochlear regions of mice exposed to 100 dB SPL. **(D)** Quantification of ribbons per IHC. Mice exposed to 100 dB SPL noise had reduced numbers of ribbons per IHC in the middle and base of the cochlea when compared with control, unexposed mice. There were no significant differences in ribbons per IHC
(Continued)

FIGURE 2 | between control mice and those exposed to 80, 90, or 95 dB SPL in any region of the cochlea. **(E)** Quantification of PSDs per IHC. Mice exposed to 100 dB SPL had reduced numbers of PSDs per IHC in the middle and base of the cochlea when compared with control, unexposed mice. There were no significant differences in PSDs per IHC between control mice and those exposed to 80, 90, or 95 dB SPL in any region of the cochlea. **(F)** Comparison of the percentage of orphan ribbons (without an associated PSD) per IHC between mice exposed to different noise intensities. There were no significant differences in the percentage of orphan ribbons per IHC between control mice and those exposed to 80, 90, 95 or 100 dB SPL in any region of the cochlea. Data points represent means and error bars indicate standard error. Sample sizes are displayed under each data point and expressed in number of mice. All ribbon, PSD, and percentage of orphan ribbon counts per IHC represent averages of both the right and left ears when available. ns = not significant, ***$p < 0.001$, ****$p < 0.0001$.

between 3 and 7 h after noise exposure in mice exposed to 100 dB SPL, while no such increase was observed in unexposed control mice or those exposed to 80, 90, or 95 dB SPL noise. Furthermore, endolymph volume was significantly greater in mice exposed to 100 dB SPL compared with unexposed control mice at 5 h (6.8 ± 0.3 nL, $n = 3$ vs. 4.7 ± 0.04 nL, $n = 3$, $p = 0.0496$) and 7 h (7.6 ± 0.1 nL, $n = 3$ vs. 4.6 ± 0.1 nL, $n = 3$, $p = 0.0006$) following noise exposure. By contrast, there were no significant differences in endolymph volume between control mice and those exposed to noise intensities lower than 100 dB SPL at any time point (**Supplementary Table S1**).

100 dB SPL 2-h Noise Exposure Induces Inner Hair Cell Cochlear Synaptopathy

To assess for cochlear synaptopathy, we counted the number of ribbons, PSDs, and percentage of orphan ribbons per IHC 7 days after noise exposure. This was done by immunolabeling for CtBP2, a marker for the presynaptic hair cell ribbon, Homer, a PSD scaffold protein, and DAPI, a counterstain for nuclear DNA (**Figure 2**). On gross visual inspection, control mice had a similar number of ribbons and PSDs per IHC when compared to mice exposed to 95 dB SPL throughout the cochlea (**Figures 2A,B**), while a reduction in the number of these structures was seen in the middle and basal turns of the cochlea in mice exposed to 100 dB SPL (**Figure 2C**).

Next, we quantified the synaptic ribbons, PSDs, and percentage of orphan ribbons per IHC (**Figures 2D–F**). In the middle of the cochlea, the number of ribbons and PSDs per IHC in mice exposed to 100 dB SPL noise were 11.9 ± 1.2, $n = 5$ and 12.9 ± 1.0, $n = 5$, respectively, compared with 18.4 ± 0.6 ribbons, $n = 7$ and 19.0 ± 0.7 PSDs, $n = 7$ in unexposed control mice ($p < 0.0001$ for both ribbons and PSDs per IHC). By contrast, there were no significant differences in the numbers of ribbons or PSDs per IHC between control mice and those exposed to lower noise intensity levels (**Supplementary Tables S2, 3**). In the base of the cochlea, there were also significant reductions in the number of ribbons (9.2 ± 0.7, $n = 5$) and PSDs (9.1 ± 0.1, $n = 5$) per IHC in mice exposed to 100 dB SPL compared with control mice (14.6 ± 0.5 ribbons, $n = 7$ and 14.8 ± 0.6 PSDs, $n = 6$; $p < 0.0001$ for ribbons and $p = 0.0002$ for PSDs per IHC). Ribbons and PSDs per IHC in the base of the cochlea did not differ significantly between

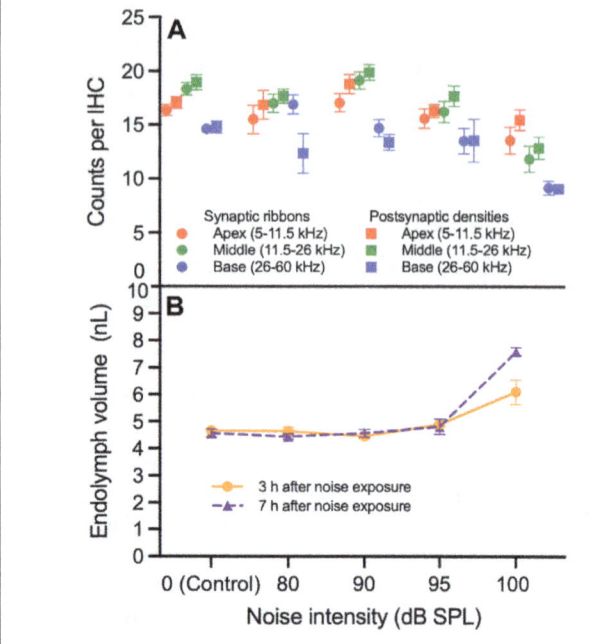

FIGURE 3 | Correlation between synapse loss and endolymphatic hydrops as a function of noise intensity. **(A)** The numbers of synaptic ribbons and postsynaptic densities (PSDs) per inner hair cell (IHC) in the apex, middle and base of the cochlea do not progressively decrease between 0 (control) and 95 decibel (dB) sound pressure level (SPL) noise exposure. Between 95 and 100 dB SPL noise exposure, ribbons and PSDs per IHC decrease in the middle and base of the cochlea more sharply than in the apex. **(B)** Endolymph volume is relatively stable between 0 and 95 dB SPL at 3 and 7 h after noise exposure. Between 95 and 100 dB SPL noise exposure, endolymph volume increases; this increase is sharpest 7 h after noise exposure. Data points represent means and error bars indicate standard error. All ribbon and PSD counts per IHC represent averages of both the right and left ears when available. Endolymph volume represents the volume of the scala media over a segment of basement membrane that is 150 μm in length.

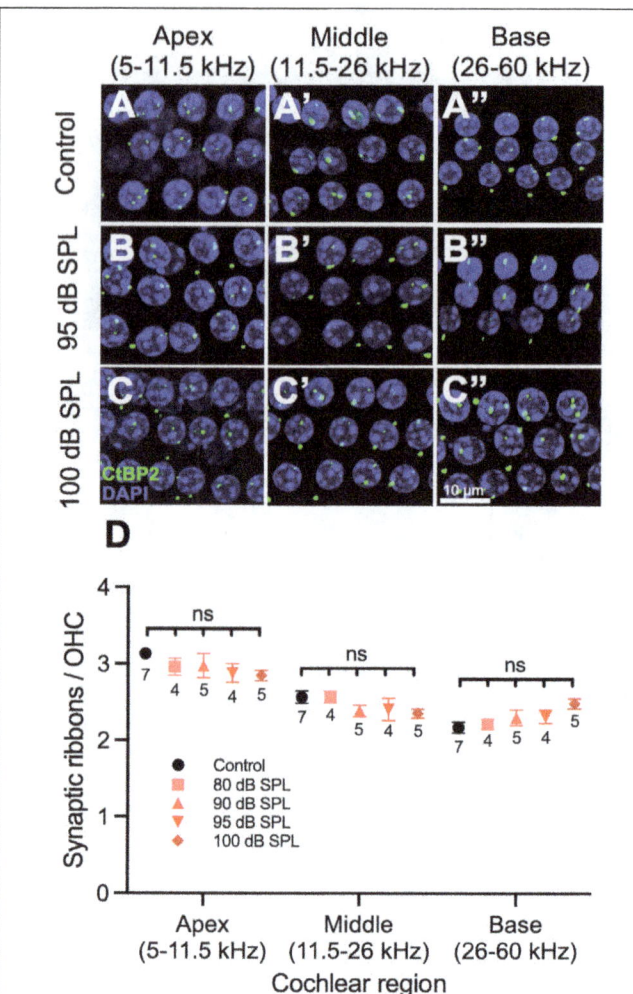

FIGURE 4 | 2 h noise exposure has no effect on outer hair cell (OHC) ribbons. **(A–C)** Representative sections from the organ of Corti of mice 7 days after noise or sham exposure (control) displaying 3 rows of 4 OHC nuclei and associated ribbons. Immunolabeling was performed to visualize OHC ribbons (CtBP2, green) as well as nuclei (DAPI, blue). Control mice **(A)**, mice exposed to 95 decibel (dB) sound pressure level SPL **(B)**, and mice exposed to 100 dB SPL **(C)** had similar numbers of ribbons per OHC. **(D)** Quantification of ribbons per OHC. There were no significant differences in the number of ribbons per OHC between mice exposed to 80, 90, 95, 100 dB SPL and control mice in any region of the cochlea. Data points represent means and error bars indicate standard error. Sample sizes are displayed under each data point and expressed in number of mice. All ribbon counts per OHC represent averages of both the right and left ears when available. ns = not significant.

control mice and those exposed to lower noise intensities. In the cochlear apex, there were no significant differences in ribbons or PSDs per IHC between mice exposed to any noise intensity level and controls. **Figure 3** displays the inverse relationship between endolymph volume and ribbon synapses in the middle and base of the cochlea as noise intensity increases. Of note, the percentage of orphan ribbons per IHC did not significantly differ between unexposed control mice and those exposed to any noise intensity level, including 100 dB SPL, in any region of the cochlea (**Supplementary Table S4**).

100 dB SPL Noise Exposure Does Not Cause Synaptopathy in Outer Hair Cells

We also counted synaptic ribbons in OHCs 7 days after noise exposure (**Figure 4**). There were no significant differences in ribbons per OHC between mice exposed to any noise intensity level and unexposed control mice in the apex, middle or base of the cochlea (**Supplementary Table S5**). PSDs were not assessed in OHC, since prior studies have shown that approximately half of Homer-immunolabeled PSDs in the OHC region are not associated with ribbons and would therefore not correlate with the presence of noise-induced synaptopathy (Martinez-Monedero et al., 2016).

Round Window Application of Hypertonic Saline Reduces Endolymphatic Hydrops

We have previously shown that round window application of a hypertonic solution reduces endolymph volume, whereas hypotonic solutions increase it (Kim et al., 2018a).

Control mice that were not exposed to noise demonstrated no bowing of RM over time (**Figure 5A**), whereas mice exposed to 100 dB SPL without round window solution application developed posttraumatic endolymphatic hydrops with outward bowing of RM (**Figure 5B**). Round window application of normotonic saline (307 mOsm/kg) had no impact on endolymphatic hydrops when compared with untreated mice (**Figure 5C**), while noise-exposed mice treated with hypertonic saline (6,000 mOsm/kg) showed a reduction of endolymphatic hydrops with decreased outward bowing of RM toward the scala vestibuli when compared with noise-exposed mice that were untreated or those treated with normotonic saline (**Figure 5D**).

Quantification of endolymph volume for each treatment condition was then performed (**Figure 5E**). Endolymph volume increased by 13.0 ± 4.4% between 3 and 7 h after noise exposure in mice treated with hypertonic saline after exposure to 100 dB SPL. Mice treated with hypertonic saline had significantly reduced endolymph volume 7 h after 100 dB SPL noise exposure (6.0 ± 0.1 nL, $n = 3$) when compared with untreated mice (7.6 ± 0.1 nL, $n = 3$, $p = 0.0047$), although no difference was observed at 3 and 5 h (**Supplementary Table S6**). The volume of endolymph in noise-exposed mice treated with hypertonic saline was still significantly elevated compared with unexposed control mice at the 5 h (5.6 ± 0.1 nL, $n = 3$ vs. 4.7 ± 0.04 nL, $n = 3$, $p = 0.01$) and 7 h (6.0 ± 0.1 nL, $n = 3$ vs. 4.6 ± 0.1 nL, $n = 3$, $p = 0.0057$) time points. Endolymph volume was not significantly different at any time point following 100 dB SPL noise exposure between untreated mice and those treated with normotonic saline.

Round Window Application of Hypertonic Saline in Noise-Exposed Ears Reduces Inner Hair Cell Synapse Loss in the Cochlear Base

Given that hypertonic saline ameliorates endolymphatic hydrops, we next sought to determine if it has any effect on noise-induced cochlear synaptopathy. We applied this solution to the left ears of mice through an intratympanic injection immediately following 100 dB SPL noise exposure. The untreated right ear served as one control, left ears treated with normotonic saline after noise exposure comprised another control group, and a final set of controls consisted of mice that were not exposed to noise. We counted the number of synaptic ribbons and PSDs per IHC 7 days after noise exposure as before. We did not count OHC ribbons or PSDs since we already showed that this noise exposure protocol did not alter the number of OHC synapses.

On visual inspection, it appeared that in the apical and middle regions of the cochlea there were no differences in the numbers of ribbons and PSDs per IHC between noise-exposed, untreated ears and those treated with normotonic or hypertonic saline (**Figures 6A–C**). More cochlear synapses per IHC were present in the cochlear base of noise-exposed ears treated with hypertonic saline compared with untreated ears and those treated with normotonic saline. The overall numbers of cochlear synapses were similar between noise-exposed and control ears in the apex but reduced in the middle and base of the cochlea in noise-exposed ears when compared with control ears.

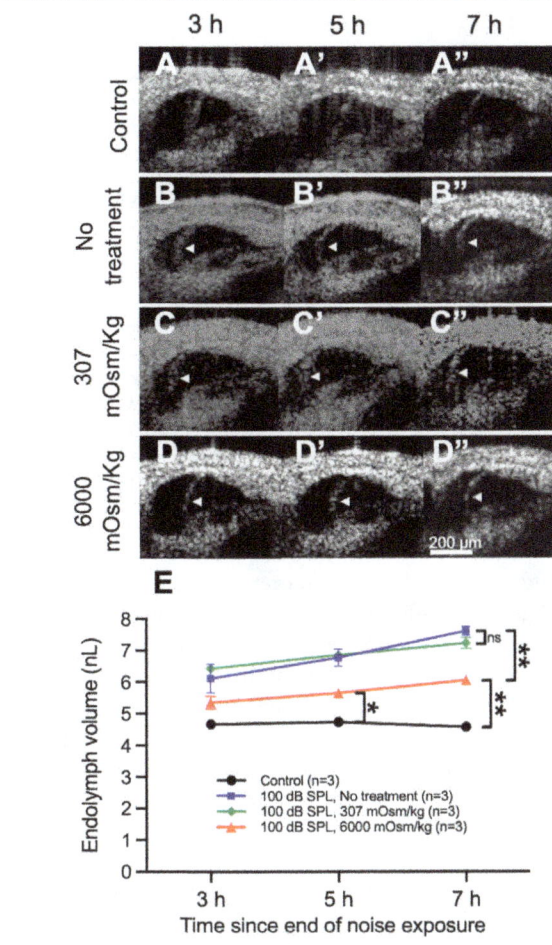

FIGURE 5 | Osmotic treatment partially reduces the degree of endolymphatic hydrops that develops after 2 h of 100 decibel (dB) sound pressure level (SPL) noise exposure. **(A)** Control mice that were not exposed to noise had no change in endolymph volume over time and demonstrated no bowing of Reissner's membrane (RM). **(B)** Noise-exposed mice without round window solution application (no treatment) developed posttraumatic endolymphatic hydrops with outward bowing of RM. White arrow heads indicate the bowed position of RM. **(C)** Round window application of normotonic saline (307 mOsm/kg) had no impact on endolymphatic hydrops. **(D)** Noise-exposed mice treated with hypertonic saline (6,000 mOsm/kg) showed a reduction of endolymphatic hydrops with decreased bowing of RM toward the scala vestibuli when compared with noise-exposed mice that were untreated or those treated with normotonic saline. **(E)** Quantification of endolymph volume over time in mice exposed to 100 dB SPL noise after undergoing round window application of hypertonic saline, normotonic saline, or no treatment, as well as unexposed control mice. Endolymph volume in noise-exposed mice treated with hypertonic saline was reduced compared with untreated mice and elevated compared with unexposed control mice at 7 h following the end of noise exposure. Endolymph volume in noise-exposed mice treated with normotonic saline was not significantly different than in noise-exposed untreated mice at any time point. Endolymph volume represents the volume of the scala media over a segment of basement membrane that is 150 μm in length. Sample sizes are expressed in number of mice. Error bars indicate standard error. ns = not significant, $*p < 0.05$, $**p < 0.01$.

Here, we tested whether the application of hypertonic saline reduces endolymph volume following 100 dB SPL 2-h noise exposure.

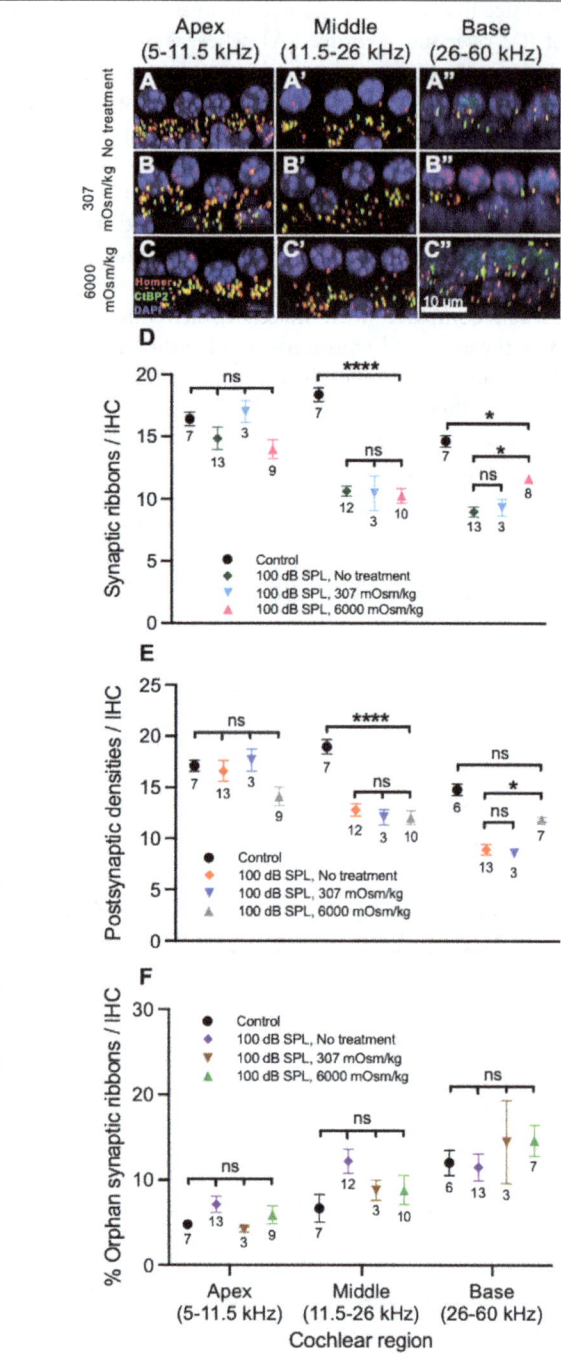

FIGURE 6 | Quantification of ribbons per IHC. Mouse ears treated with hypertonic saline had increased numbers of ribbons per IHC when compared with untreated ears in the base of the cochlea. There were no significant differences between untreated ears and those treated with hypertonic saline in the apex or middle of the cochlea. There were also no significant differences between untreated ears and those treated with normotonic saline in any region of the cochlea. **(E)** Quantification of PSDs per IHC. Mouse ears treated with hypertonic saline had increased numbers of PSDs per IHC when compared with untreated ears in the base of the cochlea. There were no significant differences between untreated ears and those treated with hypertonic saline in the apex or middle of the cochlea. There were also no significant differences between untreated ears and those treated with normotonic saline in any region of the cochlea. **(F)** Comparison of the percentage of orphan ribbons (without an associated PSD) per IHC between different treatment groups. There were no significant differences in the percentage of orphan ribbons per IHC between mice treated with hypertonic saline, normotonic saline, untreated mice and control, unexposed mice in any region of the cochlea. Data points represent means and error bars indicate standard error. Sample sizes are displayed under each data point and expressed in number of mice. ns = not significant, *$p < 0.05$, ****$p < 0.0001$.

FIGURE 6 | Osmotic treatment partially rescues synapse loss after 2 h of 100 decibel (dB) sound pressure level (SPL) noise exposure. **(A–C)** Representative sections from the organ of Corti of mice 7 days after 100 dB SPL noise exposure displaying 4 inner hair cell (IHC) nuclei and associated ribbons as well as postsynaptic densities (PSDs). Immunolabeling was performed to visualize IHC ribbons (CtBP2, green), PSDs (Homer, red) and nuclei (DAPI, blue). Right ears received no treatment **(A)**, while left ears received either normotonic saline (307 mOsm/kg) **(B)** or hypertonic saline (6,000 mOsm/kg) application to the middle ear after noise exposure **(C)**. More ribbons and PSDs per IHC are present in the cochlear base of ears treated with hypertonic saline (6,000 mOsm/kg) compared with ears treated with normotonic saline (307 mOsm/kg) and untreated ears (no treatment). **(D)**
(Continued)

Quantification of these structures was then performed as before (**Figures 6D–F**). Compared with control ears, there were significant reductions in the numbers of ribbons and PSDs per IHC in the middle of the cochlea among all groups exposed to 100 dB SPL noise (**Supplementary Tables S7, 8**). There were no significant differences in ribbons or PSDs per IHC in the middle of the cochlea when noise-exposed ears treated with hypertonic saline (10.3 ± 0.6 ribbons, $n = 10$ and 12.0 ± 0.7 PSDs, $n = 10$) were compared with untreated ears (10.6 ± 0.4 ribbons, $n = 12$ and 12.8 ± 0.6 PSDs, $n = 12$; $p = 0.9692$ for ribbons and $p = 0.8661$ for PSDs per IHC). There were also no significant differences in the numbers of ribbons and PSDs per IHC between untreated ears and those treated with normotonic saline (10.5 ± 1.4 ribbons, $n = 3$ and 12.1 ± 0.8 PSDs, $n = 3$; $p = 0.9991$ for ribbons and $p = 0.9594$ for PSDs per IHC) in the middle of the cochlea. In the base of the cochlea, there were significant reductions in the number of ribbons per IHC among all groups exposed to 100 dB SPL noise when compared with control ears. PSDs per IHC were only significantly reduced in untreated ears (8.9 ± 0.5, $n = 13$) and those treated with normotonic saline (8.5 ± 0.4, $n = 3$) when compared with controls (14.8 ± 0.6, $n = 6$; $p < 0.0001$ for comparison with untreated ears and $p = 0.001$ for comparison with ears treated with normotonic saline), while PSDs per IHC in ears treated with hypertonic saline after noise exposure (11.9 ± 0.2, $n = 7$) were not significantly different than controls ($p = 0.1001$). Most notably, noise-exposed ears treated with hypertonic saline had a significantly greater number of ribbons (11.6 ± 0.3, $n = 8$) and PSDs per IHC (11.9 ± 0.2, $n = 7$) in the base compared with untreated ears (9.0 ± 0.4 ribbons, $n = 13$ and 8.9 ± 0.5 PSDs, $n = 13$; $p = 0.0132$ for ribbons and $p = 0.0315$ for PSDs per IHC). Compared with controls, ears which were treated with hypertonic saline after exposure to 100 dB SPL nose had a 20.5 ± 3.5% reduction in ribbons and 19.8 ± 3.9% reduction in PSDs per IHC in the base of the cochlea. By comparison, ears that did not undergo treatment after 100 dB SPL noise exposure had a 38.7 ± 4.4% reduction in ribbons and 39.8 ± 5.8% reduction in PSDs per IHC compared with controls. There were no significant differences in the numbers of ribbons and PSDs between ears treated with normotonic saline and untreated ears in the base of the cochlea. In the apex, ribbon and PSD per IHC counts did not significantly differ between control ears and those exposed to 100 dB SPL, including untreated ears and those treated with hypertonic or normotonic saline. Additionally, the percentage of orphan ribbons per IHC did not significantly differ between any of the experimental groups in the apex, middle or base of the cochlea (**Supplementary Table S9**).

DISCUSSION

Endolymphatic Hydrops and Inner Hair Cell Synaptopathy Occur at Similar Noise Intensity Thresholds

Herein, we demonstrate that a threshold level of traumatic noise exposure exists. Above this threshold, both endolymphatic hydrops and cochlear synaptopathy develop. Below this threshold, neither develops. This finding suggests that endolymphatic hydrops and cochlear synaptopathy may derive through a common mechanism. Furthermore, it argues that endolymphatic hydrops may develop via an "all-or-none" mechanism following prolonged noise exposure. One potential mechanism is that a large amount of noise-induced stereociliary damage may be necessary before the ability of stereociliary mechanoelectrical transduction (MET) channels to uptake potassium becomes less than the secretion of potassium into the endolymph by the stria vascularis (Wangemann, 2002; Zdebik et al., 2009; Salt and Plontke, 2010). Once this point is reached, potassium buildup occurs, leading to osmotic influx of water into the endolymph and the development of endolymphatic hydrops (Kim et al., 2018a).

In support of this mechanism, we have previously shown that Tecta$^{C1509G/C1509G}$ mutant mice, in which the tectorial membrane is elevated off the cochlear epithelium, have increased endolymph volume compared with CBA/CaJ mice and do not develop excess endolymphatic hydrops in response to blast exposure (Xia et al., 2010; Kim et al., 2018a). We postulated that this is because the lack of static displacement of OHC stereociliary bundles by the tectorial membrane reduces potassium uptake through MET channels, increasing endolymph volume in these mice. After blast exposure, the tectorial membrane does not shear OHC stereocilia because it is detached from the organ of Corti, so endolymph volume does not increase further. It is possible that similar findings would also be observed in TMC1 mutant mice, or any other mouse mutant that has impaired MET channel currents (Kawashima et al., 2011; Fettiplace, 2016; Beurg et al., 2019).

Using our noise exposure protocol, we found that the threshold for the formation of endolymphatic hydrops, between 95–100 dB SPL, mirrors the threshold for noise-induced cochlear synaptopathy in CBA/CaJ mice. The sharp demarcation between synaptopathic and non-synaptopathic noise intensities is supported by a study from Jensen et al. (2015), which showed that 6-week old mice exposed to 2 h of 94 dB SPL noise developed a temporary threshold shift (TTS) without a corresponding loss of IHC ribbons, while those exposed to 97 dB SPL developed TTS and synaptopathy throughout the basal half of the cochlea. Hickox and Liberman (2014) similarly found that in 16–18 week old CBA/CaJ mice, a 100 dB SPL noise exposure reliably produced cochlear synaptopathy, whereas a 94 dB SPL stimulus did not, despite the fact that both produced a TTS of 40 dB SPL. While the reason for the sharp cutoff between synaptopathic and non-synaptopathic noise intensities is still unknown, our results argue that the development of endolymphatic hydrops plays a role, since both endolymphatic hydrops and cochlear synaptopathy have similar thresholds. Importantly, while our results demonstrate that endolymphatic hydrops is associated with cochlear synaptopathy following noise exposure, no conclusion about a causative relationship between endolymphatic hydrops and loss of synapses can be made based on the experiments performed in this study. Still, these results indicate that endolymphatic hydrops may be used as a surrogate marker for the loss of IHC ribbon synapses following prolonged noise exposure just as it does after blast trauma (Kim et al., 2018a).

Endolymphatic Hydrops is not Correlated with Changes in the Number of Inner Hair Cell Orphan Ribbons or Outer Hair Cell Ribbons

Of note, we found no change in the percentage of IHC orphan ribbons 1 week after traumatic noise exposure. This finding is consistent with the results of prior studies, which have shown that while the number of orphans may increase and remain increased in number for at least 24 hours after noise trauma, most IHC ribbons are once again paired with postsynaptic elements by 1 week post-exposure in both CBA/CaJ (Liberman et al., 2015; Suzuki et al., 2016) and C57BL/6J mice (Kim et al., 2019a). The number of orphan ribbons in our study was larger than has been reported in prior studies on noise-exposed CBA/CaJ mice, which is likely due to the less robust labelling of Homer when compared with CtBP2 in our experiments (Liberman et al., 2015; Suzuki et al., 2016). Our results also indicated that there was no significant change in the number of ribbons per OHC 1 week after noise exposure, a finding supported by similar results observed by Zhao et al. (2021). Although we did not investigate the localization of ribbons relative to the nucleus of OHCs, a recent study noted an increase in ribbons at the OHC synaptic pole after traumatic noise exposure, despite finding no change in the total number of ribbons per OHC after noise (Wood et al., 2021). Thus, while our previous work showed that blast exposure results in the loss of OHC ribbons, it appears that cochlear trauma from noise exposure of approximately 100 dB SPL is not sufficient to cause a reduction in OHC ribbon numbers (Kim et al., 2018a; Wood et al., 2021; Zhao et al., 2021).

Round Window Application of Hypertonic Saline Decreases Endolymphatic Hydrops and Partially Prevents the Loss of Inner Hair Cell Synapses After Traumatic Noise Exposure

Round window application of hypertonic saline decreased the degree of endolymphatic hydrops that developed following prolonged noise exposure when compared with untreated mice. The mechanism behind this effect is based on the principle of osmotic stabilization, which we have previously shown to be effective in reducing endolymphatic hydrops following blast exposure (Kim et al., 2018a). The hypertonic saline creates an osmotic gradient across the round window membrane, which drives water efflux from the perilymph. This efflux then creates a second osmotic gradient between perilymph and endolymph across RM, leading to water efflux from the scala media and a reduction in endolymph volume (Goycoolea, 2001; Duan and Zhi-qiang, 2009; Kim et al., 2018a). Importantly, endolymphatic hydrops still developed following round window application of hypertonic saline in our study, but to a lesser degree than in untreated mice. This may be because the rate of efflux driven by hypertonic saline and resorption of potassium by the damaged apical transduction channels is not sufficient to completely overcome the secretion of potassium by the stria vascularis and corresponding influx of water into the endolymph.

Nonetheless, we found that hypertonic saline treatment was able to partially rescue the loss of ribbons and PSDs in the base of the cochlea. This further supports the notion that endolymphatic hydrops may be a reliable surrogate marker for noise-induced synaptopathy since a reduction in endolymphatic hydrops was associated with a corresponding increase in cochlear synapses. The reason that hypertonic saline rescued synaptic loss in the base of the cochlea may be either through the reduction of endolymphatic hydrops, reduction of auditory dendrite terminal bouton swelling, or both. If endolymphatic hydrops contributes to synaptopathy by overstimulating IHCs and leading to glutamate excitotoxicity, then reducing the severity of endolymphatic hydrops would reduce the loss of ribbons (Kim et al., 2018a). Alternatively, the hypertonic solution may reduce postsynaptic terminal bouton swelling independent of its effect on endolymphatic hydrops. Glutamate excitotoxicity results in swelling of auditory nerve postsynaptic boutons by activating ligand-gated ion channels, causing a toxic entry of ions and water into the terminal bouton (Mayer and Westbrook, 1987; Choi and Rothman, 1990; Pujol and Puel, 1999; Kim et al., 2019a; Hu et al., 2020). Morphological studies have demonstrated that swelling, disorganization and damage of type I postsynaptic nerve terminals in the region of their synaptic contact with IHCs follows noise exposure, and this likely precedes synaptic breakdown and a corresponding loss of ribbons within IHCs (Spoendlin, 1971; Robertson, 1983; Puel et al., 1998). Therefore, the osmotic gradient established between postsynaptic boutons and the surrounding perilymph through round window application of hypertonic saline may be capable of reducing the toxic swelling of synaptic boutons following glutamate excitotoxicity, thus preventing destruction of the synapse and protecting IHC ribbons (Kim et al., 2018a). Therefore, endolymphatic hydrops and synaptopathy may occur by separate mechanisms, yet both appear to be activated at similar sound intensity thresholds between 95 and 100 dB SPL and affected by changes in perilymph osmolarity.

In the absence of noise exposure, the correlation between endolymphatic hydrops and synaptopathy is less clear. While we have previously shown that lowering perilymph osmolarity through round-window application of hypotonic saline causes the development of endolymphatic hydrops and a loss of synapses throughout the cochlea of CBA/CaJ mice (Kim et al., 2018a), Valenzuela et al. found that endolymphatic sac ablation in guinea pigs, which has been shown to cause histologically measurable endolymphatic hydrops by 30 postoperative days (Lee et al., 2020), did not result in a corresponding loss of cochlear synapses (Valenzuela et al., 2020). Unlike our prior study (Kim et al., 2018a), Valenzuela et al. did not visualize endolymphatic hydrops directly in live animals. Nonetheless, the lack of a clear relationship between endolymphatic hydrops and cochlear synaptopathy in the absence of noise exposure suggests that endolymphatic hydrops may only be a reliable surrogate marker for cochlear synaptopathy after noise trauma, although further research on this topic is needed.

In the Cochlear Apex, Endolymphatic Hydrops and Inner Hair Cell Synaptopathy did not Correlate

Differences in IHC sensitivity to acoustic trauma or scala media distensibility throughout the cochlea may explain the discrepancy between the location of endolymphatic hydrops and the pattern of noise-induced cochlear synaptopathy identified in our study. Based on the orientation of the mouse cochlea and the angle of the OCT scanning laser, only the apical turn of the cochlea could be imaged, corresponding to the 9 kHz location on the cochlear tonotopic map. While endolymphatic hydrops was observed in the apex of the cochlea in response to 100 dB SPL noise exposure, loss of IHC synapses occurred throughout the middle and base of the cochlea and spared the apical region. This pattern of noise-induced synapse loss is well established and may be due to the increased sensitivity of IHCs in the basal half of the cochlea to acoustic trauma, possibly due to decreased levels of glutathione and increased susceptibility to reactive oxygen species (Sha et al., 2001; Hickox and Liberman, 2014; Liberman et al., 2015; Kim et al., 2019a). Alternatively, the discrepancy between the locations of endolymphatic hydrops and synaptopathy may be due to differences in the distensibility of the scala media between the apex, middle and base of the cochlea. The cochlear apex is the most distensible segment of the cochlea, partially driven by the reduced stiffness and widening of the basilar membrane in this segment (Kimura and Schuknecht, 1965; Lichtenhan et al., 2017). The greater distensibility of the apical sensory structures may make them less susceptible to pressure build-up from increased endolymph volume, thus protecting IHC synapses in this location from overstimulation, glutamate excitotoxicity and synaptopathy.

Applications to Acoustic Trauma in Humans

That endolymphatic hydrops is a marker of synaptopathy following traumatic noise exposure could lead to potential novel techniques for detecting noise-induced cochlear synaptopathy in humans. In animals, cochlear synaptopathy can be diagnosed via the suprathreshold amplitude of wave 1 of the ABR (Bramhall et al., 2018). In humans, however, intersubject variability in ABR amplitude due to small signal-to-noise ratios and variability in head size, tissue conductivity, and electrode resistance limit the diagnostic utility of this technique (Nikiforidis et al., 1993; Liberman et al., 2016). The ratio of summating potential to action potential and the middle ear reflex have recently been suggested to be more reliable metrics for cochlear synaptopathy than ABR amplitudes in humans (Liberman et al., 2016; Wojtczak et al., 2017; Valero et al., 2018). Here, we showed that noise exposures with intensities sufficient to produce cochlear synaptopathy also result in endolymphatic hydrops which can be detected using OCT. Although the use of OCT for cochlear imaging is currently not performed in humans, an OCT device that images the cochlea through the ear canal may allow translation of this technology to humans (Monroy et al., 2017; Kim et al., 2018b; Kim et al., 2019b; Burwood et al., 2019; Lui et al., 2021).

A second application of our results is that hypertonic saline may be used to partially rescue IHC ribbon loss in the base of the cochlea following traumatic noise exposure. Intratympanic injections are relatively simple procedures that can be performed in the office, and round window delivery of medications is routinely performed for other otologic conditions, including the use of intratympanic steroids for sudden sensorineural hearing loss (Patel et al., 2019). While other treatment modalities have been suggested for the treatment of cochlear synaptopathy following acoustic trauma, including intratympanic application of neutrophin 3 for regeneration of cochlear synapses and inhibition of AMP-activated protein kinase, a mediator of cochlear synaptopathy, using siRNA-silencing techniques and administration of competitive inhibitors, these therapies are likely to require substantial time and research to prove their efficacy (Hill et al., 2016; Suzuki et al., 2016; Hu et al., 2020). An advantage of hypertonic saline is that it is commonly used in the nasal passageways to treat sinus disease. The middle ear, being an extension of the sinuses, is likely to be considered a safe space to apply hypertonic saline. Our results suggest that osmotic treatment could be investigated as a therapy for acute noise exposure, such as after being exposed to a gunshot, firecracker, or airbag deployment. It is important to note, however, that the absence of auditory metrics in our study should limit its interpretations to only the assessment of physical damage to the cochlea.

ETHICS STATEMENT

The animal study was reviewed and approved by the Institutional Animal Care and Use Committee at the University of Southern California.

AUTHOR CONTRIBUTIONS

IB: Conducted experiments, analyzed data, created figures and videos, wrote manuscript; PQ: Designed study, conducted experiments, analyzed data, edited figures, videos and manuscript; KO: Designed software, analyzed data, created figures, wrote manuscript; JW: Established materials and methods, conducted experiments, edited figures, videos and manuscript; CL: Conducted experiments, analyzed data, edited figures, videos and manuscript; FM-E: Designed software, established materials and methods, edited figures, videos and manuscript; BA: Designed study, designed software, established materials and methods, edited figures, videos and manuscript; JO: Designed study, designed software, established materials and methods, analyzed data, edited figures, videos, and manuscript. All authors have read and contributed to the article and approved the final submitted manuscript.

ACKNOWLEDGMENTS

We would like to thank Thomas Maierhofer for his assistance with the statistical analyses performed in this study.

SUPPLEMENTARY MATERIAL

Supplementary Movie S1 | Time-lapse series of optical coherence tomography cross-sectional images demonstrating no change in the position of Reissner's membrane over time following exposure to 95 decibel sound pressure level noise. Time since the end of noise exposure is displayed in the bottom right corner.

Supplementary Movie S2 | Time-lapse series of optical coherence tomography cross-sectional images demonstrating progressive bowing of Reissner's membrane over time (endolymphatic hydrops) following exposure to 100 decibel sound pressure level noise. Time since the end of noise exposure is displayed in the bottom right corner.

Supplementary Figure S1 | Cochleogram showing the average frequency ranges and percentages of total cochlear length from the base associated with the apical, middle and base segments, as well as the location where optical coherence tomography (OCT) was performed. Red dots indicate 10% intervals along the length of the cochlea, with 0% corresponding to the basal-most cochlear location. The base segment corresponds to the frequency range of 60 ± 8 – 26 ± 2 kHz (10.0% to 39.0% of total cochlear length), the middle segment corresponds to the frequency range of 26 ± 2 – 11.5 ± 0.5 kHz (39.0% to 69.3% of total cochlear length), and the apical segment corresponds to the frequency range of 11.5 ± 0.5 – 5 kHz (69.3% to 100.0% of total cochlear length). The hook region, corresponding to the frequency range of 80 – 60 ± 8 kHz (0.0 to 10.0% of total cochlear length), was not analyzed as it is easily injured during dissection. The 300-μm region where OCT was performed to image the cochlea, centered around the 9 kHz location, is marked (75.7%-80.3% of total cochlear length). Also shown is the 150-μm subsection of this region where endolymph volume of the scala media was measured.

Supplementary Figure S2 | Automatic method for detecting, mapping, and counting ribbons and postsynaptic densities (PSDs). **(A)** Image of inner hair cells (IHCs) with CtBP2-labeled ribbons shown in green and Homer-labeled PSDs in red. Magnified image of a co-localized ribbon and PSD is shown in the bottom left corner. **(B)** From the CtBP2-labeled image, a 2D median filter of ±1.4 μm removes most of the smaller features of the image and just leaves the background. **(C)** A median filter of ±0.35 μm is used to smooth out the original data and reduce speckle noise. **(D)** Structures the size of ribbons are isolated by subtracting **(B)** from **(C)**. **(F)** Ribbons are identified by selecting only those structures with an intensity above a set threshold and with a height in the z-direction >0.48 μm (ribbons marked by blue circles). This same process is repeated for the Homer-labeled image to count PSDs.

REFERENCES

Alberti, P. W., Symons, F., and Hyde, M. L. (1979). Occupational Hearing LossThe Significance of Asymmetrical Hearing Thresholds. *Acta Oto-Laryngologica.* 87, 255–263. doi:10.3109/00016487909126417

Beurg, M., Barlow, A., Furness, D. N., and Fettiplace, R. (2019). A Tmc1 Mutation Reduces Calcium Permeability and Expression of Mechanoelectrical Transduction Channels in Cochlear Hair Cells. *Proc. Natl. Acad. Sci. USA* 116, 20743–20749. doi:10.1073/pnas.1908058116

Bramhall, N. F., Konrad-Martin, D., and McMillan, G. P. (2018). Tinnitus and Auditory Perception After a History of Noise Exposure: Relationship to Auditory Brainstem Response Measures. *Ear Hear* 39, 881e894.

Burwood, G. W. S., Fridberger, A., Wang, R. K., and Nuttall, A. L. (2019). Revealing the Morphology and Function of the Cochlea and Middle Ear with Optical Coherence Tomography. *Quant. Imaging Med. Surg.* 9, 858–881. doi:10.21037/qims.2019.05.10

Choi, D. W., and Rothman, S. M. (1990). The Role of Glutamate Neurotoxicity in Hypoxic-Ischemic Neuronal Death. *Annu. Rev. Neurosci.* 13, 171–182. doi:10.1146/annurev.ne.13.030190.001131

Dewey, J. B., Applegate, B. E., and Oghalai, J. S. (2019). Amplification and Suppression of Traveling Waves along the Mouse Organ of Corti: Evidence for Spatial Variation in the Longitudinal Coupling of Outer Hair Cell-Generated Forces. *J. Neurosci.* 39, 1805–1816. doi:10.1523/JNEUROSCI.2608-18.2019

Dewey, J. B., Xia, A., Müller, U., Belyantseva, I. A., Applegate, B. E., and Oghalai, J. S. (2018). Mammalian Auditory Hair Cell Bundle Stiffness Affects Frequency Tuning by Increasing Coupling along the Length of the Cochlea. *Cel Rep.* 23, 2915–2927. doi:10.1016/j.celrep.2018.05.024

Duan, M.-l., and Zhi-qiang, C. (2009). Permeability of Round Window Membrane and its Role for Drug Delivery: Our Own Findings and Literature Review. *J. Otology* 4, 34–43. doi:10.1016/S1672-2930(09)50006-2

Felder, E., and Schrott-Fischer, A. (1995). Quantitative Evaluation of Myelinated Nerve Fibres and Hair Cells in Cochleae of Humans with Age-Related High-Tone Hearing Loss. *Hearing Res.* 91, 19–32. doi:10.1016/0378-5955(95)00158-1

Fettiplace, R. (2016). Is TMC1 the Hair Cell Mechanotransducer Channel?. *Biophysical J.* 111, 3–9. doi:10.1016/j.bpj.2016.05.032

Gao, S. S., Wang, R., Raphael, P. D., Moayedi, Y., Groves, A. K., Zuo, J., et al. (2014). Vibration of the Organ of Corti within the Cochlear apex in Mice. *J. Neurophysiol.* 112, 1192–1204. doi:10.1152/jn.00306.2014

Glantz, S. A., Slinker, B. K., and Neilands, T. B. (2016). *Primer of Applied Regression and Analysis of Variance.* Third Edition. New York: McGraw-Hill Education.

Goycoolea, M. V. (2001). Clinical Aspects of Round Window Membrane Permeability under Normal and Pathological Conditions. *Acta Oto-Laryngologica* 121, 437–447. doi:10.1080/000164801300366552

GraphPad Statistics Guide (2021). How Prism Computes Two-Way ANOVA. Available at: https://www.graphpad.com/guides/prism/latest/statistics/how_prism_computes_two-way_anova.htm (Accessed October 1, 2021).

Guest, H., Munro, K. J., and Plack, C. J. (2019a). Acoustic Middle-Ear-Muscle-Reflex Thresholds in Humans with Normal Audiograms: No Relations to Tinnitus, Speech Perception in Noise, or Noise Exposure. *Neuroscience* 407, 75–82. doi:10.1016/j.neuroscience.2018.12.019

Guest, H., Munro, K. J., Prendergast, G., and Plack, C. J. (2019b). Reliability and Interrelations of Seven Proxy Measures of Cochlear Synaptopathy. *Hearing Res.* 375, 34–43. doi:10.1016/j.heares.2019.01.018

Hickox, A. E., and Liberman, M. C. (2014). Is Noise-Induced Cochlear Neuropathy Key to the Generation of Hyperacusis or Tinnitus?. *J. Neurophysiol.* 111, 552–564. doi:10.1152/jn.00184.2013

Hill, K., Yuan, H., Wang, X., and Sha, S.-H. (2016). Noise-Induced Loss of Hair Cells and Cochlear Synaptopathy Are Mediated by the Activation of AMPK. *J. Neurosci.* 36, 7497–7510. doi:10.1523/JNEUROSCI.0782-16.2016

Hu, N., Rutherford, M. A., and Green, S. H. (2020). Protection of Cochlear Synapses from Noise-Induced Excitotoxic Trauma by Blockade of Ca^{2+}-Permeable AMPA Receptors. *Proc. Natl. Acad. Sci. USA* 117, 3828–3838. doi:10.1073/pnas.1914247117

Jensen, J. B., Lysaght, A. C., Liberman, M. C., Qvortrup, K., and Stankovic, K. M. (2015). Immediate and Delayed Cochlear Neuropathy after Noise Exposure in Pubescent Mice. *PLoS One* 10, e0125160. doi:10.1371/journal.pone.0125160

Kawashima, Y., Géléoc, G. S. G., Kurima, K., Labay, V., Lelli, A., Asai, Y., et al. (2011). Mechanotransduction in Mouse Inner Ear Hair Cells Requires Transmembrane Channel-like Genes. *J. Clin. Invest.* 121, 4796–4809. doi:10.1172/JCI60405

Kim, J., Xia, A., Grillet, N., Applegate, B. E., and Oghalai, J. S. (2018a). Osmotic Stabilization Prevents Cochlear Synaptopathy after Blast Trauma. *Proc. Natl. Acad. Sci. USA* 115, E4853–E4860. doi:10.1073/pnas.1720121115

Kim, K. X., Payne, S., Yang-Hood, A., Li, S.-Z., Davis, B., Carlquist, J., et al. (2019a). Vesicular Glutamatergic Transmission in Noise-Induced Loss and Repair of Cochlear Ribbon Synapses. *J. Neurosci.* 39, 4434–4447. doi:10.1523/jneurosci.2228-18.2019

Kim, W., Kim, S., Huang, S., Oghalai, J. S., and Applegate, B. E. (2019b). Picometer Scale Vibrometry in the Human Middle Ear Using a Surgical Microscope Based Optical Coherence Tomography and Vibrometry System. *Biomed. Opt. Express* 10, 4395–4410. doi:10.1364/BOE.10.004395

Kim, W., Kim, S., Oghalai, J. S., and Applegate, B. E. (2018b). Endoscopic Optical Coherence Tomography Enables Morphological and Subnanometer Vibratory Imaging of the Porcine Cochlea through the Round Window. *Opt. Lett.* 43, 1966–1969. doi:10.1364/OL.43.001966

Kimura, R. S., and Schuknecht, H. F. (1965). Membranous Hydrops in the Inner Ear of the guinea Pig after Obliteration of the Endolymphatic Sac. *Orl* 27, 343–354. doi:10.1159/000274693

Kujawa, S. G., and Liberman, M. C. (2009). Adding Insult to Injury: Cochlear Nerve Degeneration after "Temporary" Noise-Induced Hearing Loss. *J. Neurosci.* 29, 14077–14085. doi:10.1523/jneurosci.2845-09.2009

Kujawa, S. G., and Liberman, M. C. (2015). Synaptopathy in the Noise-Exposed and Aging Cochlea: Primary Neural Degeneration in Acquired Sensorineural Hearing Loss. *Hearing Res.* 330, 191–199. doi:10.1016/j.heares.2015.02.009

Landsheer, J. A., and van den Wittenboer, G. (2015). Unbalanced 2 X 2 Factorial Designs and the Interaction Effect: A Troublesome Combination. *PLoS One* 10, e0121412. doi:10.1371/journal.pone.0121412

Le, T. N., Straatman, L. V., Lea, J., and Westerberg, B. (2017). Current Insights in Noise-Induced Hearing Loss: A Literature Review of the Underlying Mechanism, Pathophysiology, Asymmetry, and Management Options. *J. Otolaryngol. - Head Neck Surg.* 46, 41. doi:10.1186/s40463-017-0219-x

Lee, C., Valenzuela, C. V., Goodman, S. S., Kallogjeri, D., Buchman, C. A., and Lichtenhan, J. T. (2020). Early Detection of Endolymphatic Hydrops Using the Auditory Nerve Overlapped Waveform (ANOW). *Neuroscience* 425, 251–266. doi:10.1016/j.neuroscience.2019.11.004

Lee, H. Y., Raphael, P. D., Park, J., Ellerbee, A. K., Applegate, B. E., and Oghalai, J. S. (2015). Noninvasive In Vivo Imaging Reveals Differences between Tectorial Membrane and Basilar Membrane Traveling Waves in the Mouse Cochlea. *Proc. Natl. Acad. Sci. USA* 112 (10), 3128–3133. doi:10.1073/pnas.1500038112

Lee, H. Y., Raphael, P. D., Xia, A., Kim, J., Grillet, N., Applegate, B. E., et al. (2016). Two-Dimensional Cochlear Micromechanics Measured In Vivo Demonstrate Radial Tuning within the Mouse Organ of Corti. *J. Neurosci.* 36, 8160–8173. doi:10.1523/jneurosci.1157-16.2016

Liberman, L. D., Liberman, M. C., and Liberman, M. C. (2015). Dynamics of Cochlear Synaptopathy after Acoustic Overexposure. *Jaro* 16, 205–219. doi:10.1007/s10162-015-0510-3

Liberman, M. C., Epstein, M. J., Cleveland, S. S., Wang, H., and Maison, S. F. (2016). Toward a Differential Diagnosis of Hidden Hearing Loss in Humans. *PLoS One* 11, e0162726. doi:10.1371/journal.pone.0162726

Liberman, M. C., and Kujawa, S. G. (2017). Cochlear Synaptopathy in Acquired Sensorineural Hearing Loss: Manifestations and Mechanisms. *Hearing Res.* 349, 138–147. doi:10.1016/j.heares.2017.01.003

Lichtenhan, J. T., Lee, C., Dubaybo, F., Wenrich, K. A., and Wilson, U. S. (2017). The Auditory Nerve Overlapped Waveform (ANOW) Detects Small Endolymphatic Manipulations that May Go Undetected by Conventional Measurements. *Front. Neurosci.* 11, 405. doi:10.3389/fnins.2017.00405

Liu, C. C., Gao, S. S., Yuan, T., Steele, C., Puria, S., and Oghalai, J. S. (2011). Biophysical Mechanisms Underlying Outer Hair Cell Loss Associated with a Shortened Tectorial Membrane. *Jaro* 12, 577–594. doi:10.1007/s10162-011-0269-0

Lui, C. G., Kim, W., Dewey, J. B., Macías-Escrivá, F. D., Ratnayake, K., Oghalai, J. S., et al. (2021). *In Vivo* functional Imaging of the Human Middle Ear with a Hand-Held Optical Coherence Tomography Device. *Biomed. Opt. Express* 12, 5196–5213. doi:10.1364/boe.430935

Martinez-Monedero, R., Liu, C., Weisz, C., Vyas, P., Fuchs, P. A., and Glowatzki, E. (2016). GluA2-Containing AMPA Receptors Distinguish Ribbon-Associated from Ribbonless Afferent Contacts on Rat Cochlear Hair Cells. *eNeuro* 3, ENEURO.0078-16.2016. doi:10.1523/ENEURO.0078-16.2016

Mayer, M. L., and Westbrook, G. L. (1987). Cellular Mechanisms Underlying Excitotoxicity. *Trends Neurosciences* 10, 59–61. doi:10.1016/0166-2236(87)90023-3

Monroy, G. L., Won, J., Spillman, D. R., Dsouza, R., and Boppart, S. A. (2017). Clinical Translation of Handheld Optical Coherence Tomography: Practical Considerations and Recent Advancements. *J. Biomed. Opt.* 22, 1–30. doi:10.1117/1.JBO.22.12.121715

Montgomery, S. C., and Cox, B. C. (2016). Whole Mount Dissection and Immunofluorescence of the Adult Mouse Cochlea. *JoVE* 107, 53561. doi:10.3791/53561

Müller, M., Hünerbein, K. v., Hoidis, S., and Smolders, J. W. T. (2005). A Physiological Place-Frequency Map of the Cochlea in the CBA/J Mouse. *Hearing Res.* 202, 63–73. doi:10.1016/j.heares.2004.08.011

Nikiforidis, G. C., Koutsojannis, C. M., Varakis, J. N., and Goumas, P. D. (1993). Reduced Variance in the Latency and Amplitude of the Fifth Wave of Auditory Brain Stem Response after Normalization for Head Size. *Ear and Hearing* 14, 423–428. doi:10.1097/00003446-199312000-00008

Patel, J., Szczupak, M., Rajguru, S., Balaban, C., and Hoffer, M. E. (2019). Inner Ear Therapeutics: An Overview of Middle Ear Delivery. *Front. Cel. Neurosci.* 13, 261. doi:10.3389/fncel.2019.00261

Prendergast, G., Millman, R. E., Guest, H., Munro, K. J., Kluk, K., Dewey, R. S., et al. (2017). Effects of Noise Exposure on Young Adults with Normal Audiograms II: Behavioral Measures. *Hearing Res.* 356, 74–86. doi:10.1016/j.heares.2017.10.007

Puel, J.-L., Ruel, J., d'Aldin, C. G., and Pujol, R. (1998). Excitotoxicity and Repair of Cochlear Synapses after Noise-Trauma Induced Hearing Loss. *Neuroreport* 9, 2109–2114. doi:10.1097/00001756-199806220-00037

Pujol, R., Puel, J.-L., D'aldin, C. G., and Eybalin, M. (1993). Pathophysiology of the Glutamatergic Synapses in the Cochlea. *Acta Oto-Laryngologica* 113, 330–334. doi:10.3109/00016489309135819

Pujol, R., and Puel, J.-L. (1999). Excitotoxicity, Synaptic Repair, and Functional Recovery in the Mammalian Cochlea: A Review of Recent Findings. *Ann. N. Y Acad. Sci.* 884, 249–254. doi:10.1111/j.1749-6632.1999.tb08646.x

Roberts, L. E., Eggermont, J. J., Caspary, D. M., Shore, S. E., Melcher, J. R., and Kaltenbach, J. A. (2010). Ringing Ears: The Neuroscience of Tinnitus. *J. Neurosci.* 30, 14972–14979. doi:10.1523/JNEUROSCI.4028-10.2010

Robertson, D. (1983). Functional Significance of Dendritic Swelling after Loud Sounds in the Guinea Pig Cochlea. *Hearing Res.* 9, 263–278. doi:10.1016/0378-5955(83)90031-x

Salt, A. N., and Plontke, S. K. (2010). Endolymphatic Hydrops: Pathophysiology and Experimental Models. *Otolaryngologic Clin. North America* 43, 971–983. doi:10.1016/j.otc.2010.05.007

Sha, S.-H., Taylor, R., Forge, A., and Schacht, J. (2001). Differential Vulnerability of Basal and Apical Hair Cells Is Based on Intrinsic Susceptibility to Free Radicals. *Hearing Res.* 155, 1–8. doi:10.1016/s0378-5955(01)00224-6

Spoendlin, H. (1971). Primary Structural Changes in the Organ of Corti after Acoustic Overstimulation. *Acta Oto-Laryngologica* 71, 166–176. doi:10.3109/00016487109125346

Suzuki, J., Corfas, G., and Liberman, M. C. (2016). Round-Window Delivery of Neurotrophin 3 Regenerates Cochlear Synapses after Acoustic Overexposure. *Sci. Rep.* 6, 24907. doi:10.1038/srep24907

Valenzuela, C. V., Lee, C., Mispagel, A., Bhattacharyya, A., Lefler, S. M., Payne, S., et al. (2020). Is Cochlear Synapse Loss an Origin of Low-Frequency Hearing Loss Associated with Endolymphatic Hydrops?. *Hearing Res.* 398, 108099. doi:10.1016/j.heares.2020.108099

Valero, M. D., Burton, J. A., Hauser, S. N., Hackett, T. A., Ramachandran, R., and Liberman, M. C. (2017). Noise-induced Cochlear Synaptopathy in Rhesus Monkeys (*Macaca mulatta*). *Hearing Res.* 353, 213–223. doi:10.1016/j.heares.2017.07.003

Valero, M. D., Hancock, K. E., Maison, S. F., and Liberman, M. C. (2018). Effects of Cochlear Synaptopathy on Middle-Ear Muscle Reflexes in Unanesthetized Mice. *Hearing Res.* 363, 109–118. doi:10.1016/j.heares.2018.03.012

Viana, L. M., O'Malley, J. T., Burgess, B. J., Jones, D. D., Oliveira, C. A. C. P., Santos, F., et al. (2015). Cochlear Neuropathy in Human Presbycusis: Confocal Analysis of Hidden Hearing Loss in post-mortem Tissue. *Hearing Res.* 327, 78–88. doi:10.1016/j.heares.2015.04.014

Viberg, A., and Canlon, B. (2004). The Guide to Plotting a Cochleogram. *Hearing Res.* 197, 1–10. doi:10.1016/j.heares.2004.04.016

Wangemann, P. (2002). K+ Cycling and the Endocochlear Potential. *Hearing Res.* 165, 1–9. doi:10.1016/s0378-5955(02)00279-4

Wojtczak, M., Beim, J. A., and Oxenham, A. J. (2017). Weak Middle-Ear-Muscle Reflex in Humans with Noise-Induced Tinnitus and Normal Hearing May Reflect Cochlear Synaptopathy. *eNeuro* 4, ENEURO.0363-17.2017. doi:10.1523/ENEURO.0363-17.2017

Wood, M. B., Nowak, N., Mull, K., Goldring, A., Lehar, M., and Fuchs, P. A. (2021). Acoustic Trauma Increases Ribbon Number and Size in Outer Hair Cells of the Mouse Cochlea. *Jaro* 22, 19–31. doi:10.1007/s10162-020-00777-w

Xia, A., Gao, S. S., Yuan, T., Osborn, A., Bress, A., Pfister, M., et al. (2010). Deficient Forward Transduction and Enhanced Reverse Transduction in the Alpha Tectorin C1509G Human Hearing Loss Mutation. *Dis. Model. Mech.* 3, 209–223. doi:10.1242/dmm.004135

Xia, A., Song, Y., Wang, R., Gao, S. S., Clifton, W., Raphael, P., et al. (2013). Prestin Regulation and Function in Residual Outer Hair Cells after Noise-Induced Hearing Loss. *PLoS One* 8, e82602. doi:10.1371/journal.pone.0082602

Zdebik, A. A., Wangemann, P., and Jentsch, T. J. (2009). Potassium Ion Movement in the Inner Ear: Insights from Genetic Disease and Mouse Models. *Physiology* 24, 307–316. doi:10.1152/physiol.00018.2009

Zhao, H.-B., Zhu, Y., and Liu, L.-M. (2021). Excess Extracellular K+ Causes Inner Hair Cell Ribbon Synapse Degeneration. *Commun. Biol.* 4, 24. doi:10.1038/s42003-020-01532-w

Treatment With Calcineurin Inhibitor FK506 Attenuates Noise-Induced Hearing Loss

Zu-Hong He[†], Song Pan[†], Hong-Wei Zheng[†], Qiao-Jun Fang, Kayla Hill and Su-Hua Sha*

Department of Pathology and Laboratory Medicine, Medical University of South Carolina, Charleston, SC, United States

*Correspondence:
Su-Hua Sha
shasu@musc.edu

[†]These authors have contributed equally to this work

Attenuation of noise-induced hair cell loss and noise-induced hearing loss (NIHL) by treatment with FK506 (tacrolimus), a calcineurin (CaN/PP2B) inhibitor used clinically as an immunosuppressant, has been previously reported, but the downstream mechanisms of FK506-attenuated NIHL remain unknown. Here we showed that CaN immunolabeling in outer hair cells (OHCs) and nuclear factor of activated T-cells isoform c4 (NFATc4/NFAT3) in OHC nuclei are significantly increased after moderate noise exposure in adult CBA/J mice. Consequently, treatment with FK506 significantly reduces moderate-noise-induced loss of OHCs and NIHL. Furthermore, induction of reactive oxygen species (ROS) by moderate noise was significantly diminished by treatment with FK506. In agreement with our previous finding that autophagy marker microtubule-associated protein light chain 3B (LC3B) does not change in OHCs under conditions of moderate-noise-induced permanent threshold shifts, treatment with FK506 increases LC3B immunolabeling in OHCs after exposure to moderate noise. Additionally, prevention of NIHL by treatment with FK506 was partially abolished by pretreatment with LC3B small interfering RNA. Taken together, these results indicate that attenuation of moderate-noise-induced OHC loss and hearing loss by FK506 treatment occurs not only *via* inhibition of CaN activity but also through inhibition of ROS and activation of autophagy.

Keywords: noise-induced hearing loss, calcineurin inhibitor, nuclear factor of activated T-cells isoform c4, reactive oxygen species, autophagy

INTRODUCTION

Noise-induced hearing loss (NIHL) acquired from military duty, industrial occupations, and recreation and leisure activities is the most common occupational disease in the US and probably worldwide (Neitzel and Fligor, 2019; Themann and Masterson, 2019). Loss of sensory hair cells in the cochlea, with outer hair cells (OHCs) being more vulnerable than inner hair cells (IHCs), has been well documented in humans and various animal models as a cause of permanent threshold shifts (PTS or permanent hearing loss) (Sha and Schacht, 2017; Wang and Puel, 2018). Although the molecular events occurring after noise exposure are highly complex, the notion of overload of calcium in the endolymph and hair cells, accumulation of reactive oxygen species (ROS), and increased cytokines contributing to the pathogenesis of noise-induced loss of sensory hair cells is well accepted (Ikeda and Morizono, 1988; Fridberger et al., 1998; Ohlemiller et al., 1999; Yamashita et al., 2004; Fujioka et al., 2006; Chen et al., 2012; Hill et al., 2016; Dhukhwa et al., 2019; Fettiplace and Nam, 2019).

Calcineurin (CaN/PP2B) belongs to the protein phosphatase 2B family of Ca^{2+}/calmodulin-dependent protein phosphatases and is activated by binding between Ca^{2+} and calmodulin (Hashimoto et al., 1990; Morioka et al., 1999). The activation of CaN may contribute to hair cell death as treatment with CaN inhibitor FK506 (tacrolimus) attenuates noise and aminoglycoside-induced hair cell loss and hearing loss (Minami et al., 2004; Uemaetomari et al., 2005; Bas et al., 2012), but the underlying mechanisms are not fully understood. FK506 forms a complex with binding protein FKBP12 (FK506-binding protein), which binds to a common composite surface made up of residues from the catalytic subunit of CaN (Ke and Huai, 2003) and, in turn, inhibits CaN activity. Nuclear factor of activated T-cells (NFAT), a downstream target of CaN, is an attractive candidate as the executor of CaN's detrimental effects. Five NFAT family members, NFAT1 (NFATp or NFATc2), NFAT2 (NFATc1), NFAT3 (NFATc4), NFAT4 (NFATc3 or NFATx), and NFAT5, have been identified (Rao et al., 1997; Crabtree and Olson, 2002). Following increases in intracellular Ca^{2+}, NFATs are dephosphorylated by CaN and subsequently form a complex with CaN that is translocated from the cytoplasm to the nucleus (Shibasaki et al., 1996). Several *in-vivo* experiments show that the use of constitutively active CaN leads to the translocation of NFAT3 into the nuclei in the brain following ischemia (Shioda et al., 2006, 2007), in Alzheimer's disease (Abdul et al., 2009), and in neuronal apoptosis (Shioda et al., 2007). Therefore, NFAT3 can be used as a marker of CaN activity.

Recently, a report showed that *Nfatc3* (*NFAT3*) deficiency in mice attenuates ototoxicity by suppressing TNF-mediated hair cell apoptosis (Zhang et al., 2019). In fact, overproduction of both ROS and cytokines has been well documented in noise trauma with loss of OHCs (Yamane et al., 1995; Shi et al., 2003; Yamashita et al., 2005; Fujioka et al., 2006; Le Prell et al., 2007; Dhukhwa et al., 2019; Fetoni et al., 2019; Frye et al., 2019). It is speculated that ROS and inflammation have a complex interplay (Fetoni et al., 2019). Additionally, autophagy dysfunction has been suggested to induce several pathological states, like cancer, inflammation, neurodegenerative diseases, and metabolic disorders (Levine and Kroemer, 2008; Arroyo et al., 2013; Ryter et al., 2014). In the inner ear, the lower levels of oxidative stress induced by temporary threshold shift (TTS) noise exposure or lower doses of aminoglycoside treatment inhibit apoptosis and promote hair cell survival *via* autophagy (Yuan et al., 2015; He et al., 2017). On the other hand, excessive activation of autophagy may induce cell death (Kroemer and Levine, 2008; Bandyopadhyay et al., 2014; Wu et al., 2020b).

Interestingly, FK506 also activates the autophagy system by binding to the V-ATPase catalytic subunit A in neuronal cells (Kim et al., 2017; Wang et al., 2017). Autophagy, as a major cellular self-protection mechanism, plays a role in adapting cells and organs to changing micro-environments by eliminating intracellular components and potentially harmful molecules and organelles. Therefore, we speculate that treatment with FK506 not only inhibits CaN but also inhibits ROS and activates autophagy for prevention of NIHL.

In this study, we investigated the attenuation of noise-induced OHC loss and hearing loss by FK506 *via* inhibition of CaN activity and ROS accumulation and the promotion of autophagy using immunohistochemistry and small interfering RNA silencing (siRNA) techniques in adult CBA/J mice. In agreement with previous results (Minami et al., 2004; Uemaetomari et al., 2005; Bas et al., 2012), our data support the notion that treatment with FK506 prevents NIHL.

MATERIALS AND METHODS
Animals
Male CBA/J mice at 10 weeks of age were purchased from The Jackson Laboratory. All mice had free access to water and a regular mouse diet (irradiated lab diet #5V75) and were kept at $22 \pm 1°C$ under a standard 12:12-h light–dark cycle to acclimate for at least 1 week before conducting baseline auditory brainstem response (ABR) measurements. CBA/J mice at the age of 12 weeks were exposed to noise. The mice were euthanized 2 weeks after auditory functional measurement for hair cell morphological analysis or 1–3 h after noise exposure for immunolabeling of protein expression in OHCs. All mice were specific pathogen-free and housed in the animal facility with controlled noise levels [below 60 dB sound pressure level (SPL)] in the Children's Research Institute at the Medical University of South Carolina. All research protocols were approved by the Institutional Animal Care and Use Committee at MUSC (protocol # IACUC-2019-00752). Animal care was under the supervision of the Division of Laboratory Animal Resources at MUSC. A randomized two- to three-animal block allocation was employed to assign animals to different experimental groups with three to four repetitions for each experiment. No animals were excluded or died during the experiments.

Noise Exposure
Unrestrained male CBA/J male mice at the age of 12 weeks (one mouse per stainless steel wire cage, $\sim 9\ cm^3$) were exposed to broadband noise (BBN) with a frequency spectrum of 2–20 kHz at 101–103 dB SPL for 2 h to induce permanent threshold shifts (PTS) at 16 and 32 kHz with loss of OHCs by 14 days after the noise exposure, referred to as our moderate-PTS-noise conditions. The mice were exposed to BBN at 106–108 dB SPL for 2 h to induce severe permanent threshold shifts (sPTS) at 8, 16, and 32 kHz with loss of sensory hair cells including both OHCs and IHCs by 14 days after the noise exposure, referred to as our sPTS-noise conditions. Noise exposures were conducted in the morning (between 9 and 11 a.m.) to avoid confounding influences of circadian rhythm on hearing function.

Abbreviations: ABR, auditory brainstem response; CaN/PP2B, calcineurin; DMSO, dimethyl sulfoxide; FK506, tacrolimus; FKBP12, FK506-binding protein; GFP, green fluorescent protein; IHC, inner hair cell; IP, intraperitoneal; LC3B, microtubule-associated protein light chain 3B; LC3-GFP mice, green fluorescent protein (GFP)-LC3 transgenic mice; NFATc4/NFAT3, nuclear factor of activated T-cells isoform c4; NIHL, noise-induced hearing loss; OHCs, outer hair cells; PBS, phosphate-buffered saline; PBS-T, PBS with 0.1% Tween 20; PTS, permanent threshold shifts; sPTS, severe permanent threshold shifts; SDS-PAGE, sodium dodecyl sulfate polyacrylamide gel electrophoresis; siControl, scrambled small interfering RNA; siLC3B, LC3B small interfering RNA; SPL, sound pressure level; TDT, Tucker-Davis Technologies; TTS, temporary threshold shifts.

The sound exposure chamber was fitted with a loudspeaker (model 2450H + 2385A; JBL) driven by a power amplifier (model XLS 202D; Crown Audio) fed from a CD player (model CD-200; Tascam TEAC American). Audio CD sound files were created and equalized with audio editing software (Audition 3; Adobe Systems, Inc.). The background sound intensity of the environment surrounding the cages was 65 dB as measured with a sound level meter (model 1200; Quest Technologies). Noise sound pressure level calibration was performed immediately before each exposure session. The sound levels were calibrated with a Bruel and Kjaer condenser microphone, allowing precise calibration and monitoring of the sound exposure. The noise level varied by a maximum of 1–2 dB across the measured sites within the exposure chamber. The sound levels for noise exposure were measured with a sound level meter at multiple locations within the sound chamber to ensure uniformity of the sound field and measured before and after exposure to ensure stability. Control mice were kept in silence (without use of the loudspeaker) within the same chamber for 2 h.

Drug Administration *via* Intra-Peritoneal Route

FK506 (tacrolimus, #F4679) was purchased from Sigma-Aldrich, dissolved in dimethyl sulfoxide (DMSO) as a stock solution (20 mg/ml), and stored at −20°C. The stock solution was diluted with 0.9% saline solution immediately before injections. Initially, we tested two doses of FK506 (3 and 5 mg/kg) for prevention of NIHL based on prior literature (Uemaetomari et al., 2005). Since 5 mg/kg of FK506 attenuated NIHL, we used 5 mg/kg for the rest of the experiments. For immunohistochemistry, each animal received a total of three intraperitoneal (IP) injections of FK506 at a dose of 5 mg/kg per injection. The vehicle control mice received the same volume of DMSO (0.1%) in saline. Three IP injections were administered 24 h before, 1 h before, and immediately after the noise exposure. The mice used for the experiments to observe the effects of treatment on ABR thresholds received two additional IP injections on the day following the noise exposure (a.m. and p.m.).

Auditory Brainstem Response Measurements

ABRs were measured before and 2 weeks after the noise exposure. The mice were anesthetized with an IP injection of a mixture of ketamine (100 mg/kg) and xylazine (10 mg/kg). After anesthesia, the mice were placed in a sound-isolated and electrically shielded booth (Acoustic Systems). Body temperature was monitored and maintained near 37°C with a heating pad. Acoustic stimuli were delivered monaurally to a Beyer earphone attached to a customized plastic speculum inserted into the ear canal. Subdermal electrodes were inserted at the vertex of the skull (active), mastoid region under the left ear, and mastoid region under the right ear (ground). ABRs were measured at 8, 16, and 32 kHz. Tucker-Davis Technologies (TDT) System III hardware and SigGen/Biosig software were used to present the stimuli (15-ms-duration tone bursts with 1-ms rise–fall time) and record the response. Up to 1,024 responses were averaged for each stimulus level. ABR wave II was used to determine the ABR thresholds for each frequency. Thresholds were determined for each frequency by reducing the intensity in 10-dB increments and then in 5-dB steps near the threshold until no organized responses were detected. Thresholds were estimated between the lowest stimulus level where a response was observed and the highest level without response. All ABR measurements were conducted by the same experimenter. The ABR values were assigned by an expert who was blinded to the treatment conditions.

Intra-Tympanic Delivery of LC3B siRNA *in vivo*

LC3B siRNA (siLC3B, Thermofisher, 4390771) or scrambled siRNA (siControl, Thermofisher, 4390844) was delivered locally *via* intra-tympanic application as previously described (Chen et al., 2013; Oishi et al., 2013). Briefly, after anesthesia, a retroauricular incision (left ear) was made to approach the temporal bone. The otic bulla was identified ventral to the facial nerve, and a shallow hole was made in the thin part of the otic bulla with a 30-G needle and enlarged with a dental drill to a diameter of 2 mm in order to visualize the round window. A customized sterile micro-medical tube was inserted into the hole just above the round window niche (RWN) to slowly deliver 10 µl (0.6 µg) of pre-designed siLC3B or siControl to completely fill the mouse RWN. After the siRNA was delivered, the hole was covered with the surrounding muscle. Finally, the skin incision was closed with tissue adhesive. The animal was allowed to rest in surgical position for an additional 30–60 min before waking from anesthesia. About 72 h after siRNA delivery, the animals were exposed to noise for 2 h. Based on our previous experiments, local intra-tympanic delivery of siRNA results in a temporary elevation of thresholds that completely recovers to baseline after 48 h (Oishi et al., 2013; Zheng et al., 2014; Yuan et al., 2015). Therefore, noise exposure was performed near 72 h after siRNA delivery.

Immunocytochemistry for Cochlear Surface Preparations

We have followed a procedure as previously described in detail (Fang et al., 2019). Briefly, the temporal bones were removed and perfused locally with a solution of 4% paraformaldehyde in phosphate-buffered saline (PBS), pH 7.4, and kept in this fixative overnight at 4°C. Between each step, the cochlear samples were washed at least three times with PBS for 5–10 min each wash. After decalcification with 4% sodium ethylenediaminetetraacetic acid solution (adjusted with HCl to pH 7.4) for 3 days at 4°C, the cochleae were micro-dissected into three turns (apex, middle, and base) and adhered to 10-mm round coverslips (Microscopy Products for Science and Industry, #260367) with Cell-Tak (BD Biosciences, #354240). The specimens were first permeabilized in 2% Triton X-100 solution and then blocked with 10% normal goat serum for 30 min each step at room temperature, followed by incubation with primary antibodies: monoclonal mouse anti-calcineurin (BD Biosciences #610260), monoclonal rabbit anti-NFAT3 at 1:50 (Sigma-Aldrich #SAB4501982), rabbit polyclonal anti-4 hydroxynonenal (4-HNE) at 1:100 (Abcam, #46545), and rabbit anti-LC3B at 1:200 (Cell Signaling Technology, #2775) at 4°C for 48 h. The specimens were then incubated with the Alexa-Fluor-488-conjugated or Alexa-Fluor-594-conjugated secondary antibody at a concentration of 1:200 at 4°C overnight and followed by incubation with propidium iodide (PI) or phalloidin for 1 h at room temperature in darkness. Control incubations were routinely processed without primary antibody treatments.

Surface preparations for counting of hair cells were incubated with Myosin-VIIa (Proteus Biosciences, #25-6790, 1:200) at 4°C overnight and then incubated overnight at 4°C with secondary antibody (biotinylated goat anti-rabbit) at a 1:100 dilution. The specimens were then incubated in ABC solution (Vector Laboratories, PK-4001) overnight followed by incubation in 3,3′-diaminobenzidine (DAB) for 3 h as necessary for sufficient staining intensity. Finally, the specimens were washed to stop the DAB reaction.

After at least three final washes with PBS, all immunolabeling samples (already on round coverslips) were mounted by adding 8 μl mounting agent (Fluoro-gel with Tris buffer, Electron Microscopy Sciences, #17985-10), sandwiched with another round coverslip, and placed on a microscope slide. Finally, the edges were sealed with nail polish. The immunolabeled images were taken with a ×63-magnification lens under identical Z-stack conditions using Zeiss LSM 880.

Semi-quantification of the Immunolabeling Signals From Outer Hair Cells or Outer Hair Cell Nuclei of Surface Preparations

Immunohistochemistry is well-accepted as a semi-quantitative methodology when used with careful consideration of the utility and semi-quantitative nature of these assays (Taylor and Levenson, 2006; Walker, 2006). Immunolabeling for CaN, NFAT3, 4-HNE, and LC3B was semi-quantified from original confocal images with eight-bit grayscale values, each taken with a ×63-magnification lens under identical conditions and equal parameter settings for laser gains and photomultiplier tube gains within linear ranges of the fluorescence using Image J software (National Institutes of Health, Bethesda, MD). The cochleae from the different groups were fixed and immunolabeled simultaneously with identical solutions and processed in parallel. All surface preparations were counterstained with phalloidin (green) or propidium iodide (red) to identify the comparable parts of the OHC or OHC nuclei in confocal images. The regions of interest of individual OHCs or OHC nuclei were outlined with the circle tool based on phalloidin or PI staining. The immunolabeling in grayscale in OHCs was measured in the upper basal region of surface preparations (corresponding to sensitivity to 22–32 kHz) in 0.12-mm segments, each containing about 60 OHCs. The intensity of the background was subtracted, and the average grayscale intensity per cell was then calculated. For each repetition, the relative grayscale value was determined by normalizing the ratio to control. Since there were no significant changes in all assessed immunolabeling in the apex and middle regions of cochlear OHC or OHC nuclei when assessed 1–3 h after the completion of the noise exposure, we performed only semi-quantification of the immunolabeling signals from OHC or OHC nuclei in the basal turn (corresponding to sensitivity to 22–32 kHz). This procedure provided semi-quantitative measurements that are not confounded by protein expression in other cell types of the cochlea.

Hair Cell Counts

Images from the apex through the base of the Myosin-VIIa-labeled and DAB-stained surface preparations were captured using a ×20 lens on a Zeiss microscope. The lengths of the cochlear epithelia were measured and recorded in millimeters. Mapping of frequencies as a function of distance along the entire length of the cochlear spiral was calculated with the equation [d (%) = 156.5 − 82.5 × log (f)] from Müller's paper (Muller et al., 2005). The results are in agreement with the literature (Viberg and Canlon, 2004). OHCs were counted from the apex to the base along the entire length of the mouse cochlear epithelium. The percentage of hair cell loss in each 0.5-mm length of epithelium was plotted as a function of the cochlear length as a cytocochleogram (Zheng et al., 2014).

Cell Culture, LC3B Silencing, and Protein Extraction

HEI-OC1, an inner ear cell line, was kindly provided by Dr. Federico Kalinec at UCLA Health. HEI-OC1 cells were seeded in six-well dishes to about 2×10^5 cells/well and cultivated in Dulbecco's modified Eagle's medium (DMEM, Invitrogen, #11965-084) containing 4.5 g/l glucose and 10% fetal bovine serum (FBS) (Fisher Scientific, #16000044) in a humidified incubator (33°C, 10% CO_2, 95% humidity). For LC3B siRNA transfection into cells, the same LC3B siRNA (Thermofisher, 4390771) or scrambled siRNA Control (Thermofisher, 4390844) was used as in *in vivo* experiments. Lipofectamine™ RNAIMAX Reagent (Invitrogen, 13778075) was used for the transfection. The cells were seeded in six-well dishes and cultivated in DMEM containing FBS until reaching 70% confluence; the medium was then replaced with serum-free DMEM before transfection. The cells were transfected with siLC3B or siControl according to the manufacturer's instructions. The transfections lasted for 6 h, and the medium was replaced with fresh DMEM containing FBS and cultured for another 42 h. The cells were digested with 0.25% trypsin. The collected cells were transferred to a 15-ml conical tube (Corning, #430052) and centrifuged at $500 \times g$ for 5 min, the medium was decanted, and the cells were washed with 1 ml of PBS (Invitrogen, #20012). After removing the PBS, total protein was extracted using RIPA buffer (Sigma-Aldrich, #R0278) contained phosphatase inhibitor (Sigma-Aldrich, #04906845001) following the provided instructions. Finally, total protein was stored at −80°C after quantification. In this study, the HEI-OC1 cells used were between 10 and 20 culture passages.

Western Blot Analysis

Protein samples (30 μg) were separated by sodium dodecyl sulfate–polyacrylamide gel electrophoresis. After electrophoresis, the proteins were transferred onto a nitrocellulose membrane (Pierce) and blocked with 5% solution of nonfat dry milk in PBS−0.1% Tween 20 (PBS-T). The membranes were incubated with monoclonal rabbit anti-LC3B (Cell Signaling Technology,

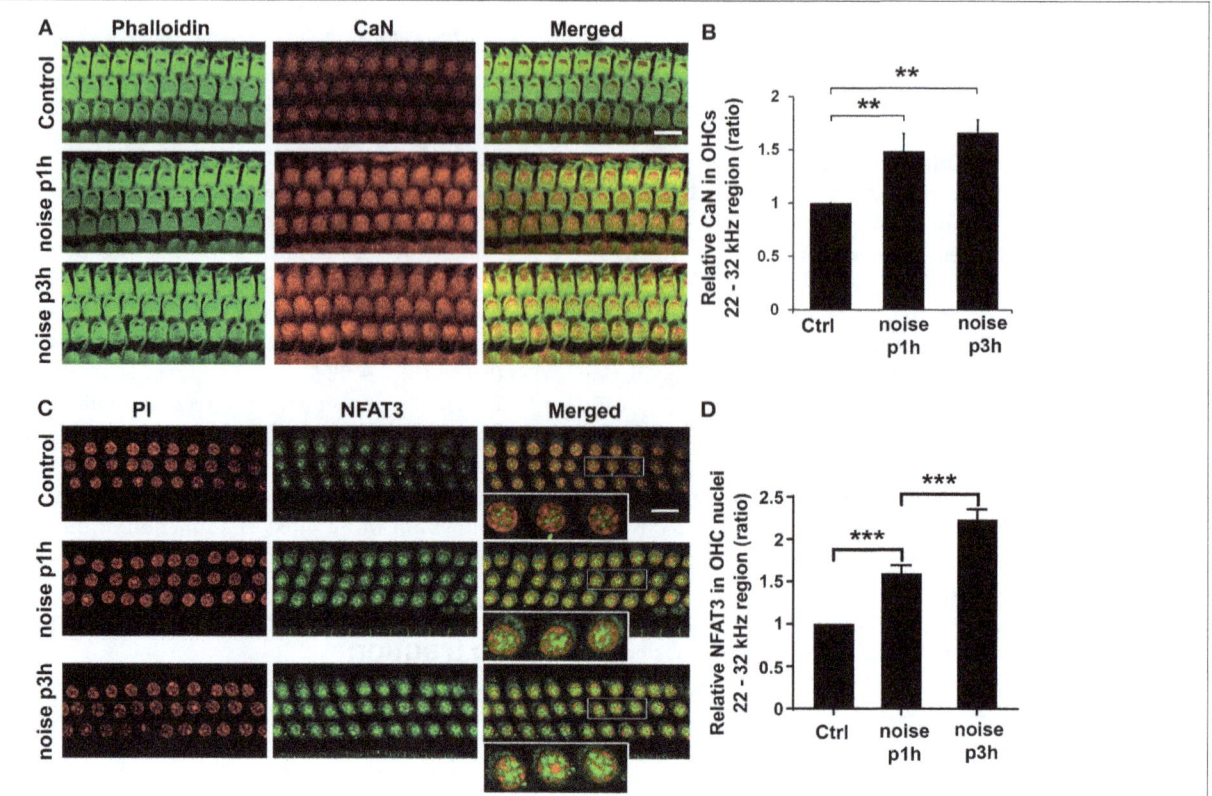

FIGURE 1 | Noise exposure increases CaN in outer hair cells (OHCs) and NFAT3 in OHC nuclei. **(A)** Surface preparations of the cochlear epithelium show that immunolabeling for CaN (red) in OHCs was stronger in noise-exposed mice examined 1 and 3 h after the completion of exposure compared to control mice without exposure. Green, phalloidin-labeled sensory hair cells. Images were taken from the basal turn corresponding to sensitivity to 22–32 kHz, and each figure is representative of five individual mice for each condition. Scale bar = 10 μm. **(B)** Quantification of relative CaN immunolabeling intensity in grayscale in OHCs normalized to control mice confirms significant increases. Data are presented as means ± SD; $n = 5$ for each condition with one ear analyzed per mouse; $^{**}p < 0.01$. **(C)** Surface preparations show that NFAT3 immunolabeling was stronger in OHC nuclei 1 h after, followed by an even greater increase 3 h after exposure. For better visualization, three OHC nuclei were enlarged of the merged panels. This figure is representative of one ear per mouse in five individual mice in each group. Scale bar = 10 μm. **(D)** Quantification of NFAT3 immunolabeling intensity in grayscale in OHC nuclei confirms a significant increase 1 h after and a further increase 3 h after exposure. Data are presented as means ± SD; $n = 5$ for each condition, $^{***}p < 0.001$.

#3868, 1:200) at 4°C overnight and then washed three times (10 min each) with PBS-T buffer. The membranes were then incubated with the appropriate secondary antibody at a concentration of 1:2,500 for 1 h at room temperature. Following extensive washing of the membrane, the immunoblot bands were visualized by SuperSignal West Dura Extended Duration Substrate or Pierce® ECL Western Blotting Substrate (Thermo Scientific). The membranes were then stripped and relabeled for GAPDH (Cell Signaling Tech., #5174, 1:3,000) as a sample loading control.

Western blot bands were scanned by the LI-COR Odyssey Fc imaging system and analyzed using Image J software. First, the background staining density for each band was subtracted from the band density. Next, the probing protein/GAPDH ratio was calculated from the band densities run on the same gel to normalize for differences in protein loading. Finally, the difference in the ratio of the control and experimental bands was tested for statistical significance.

Statistical Analyses

Data were analyzed using SYSTAT 8.0 and GraphPad 5.0 software for Windows. Biological sample sizes were determined based on the variability of measurements and the magnitude of the differences between groups as well as experience from our previous studies, with stringent assessments of difference. Data of OHC loss along the length of the cochlear spiral were analyzed with one-way repeated-measures analysis of variance (ANOVA) with *post hoc* tests using SYSTAT 8.0. The rest of the analyses were done using GraphPad 5.0. Differences with multiple comparisons were evaluated by one-way ANOVA with multiple comparisons. Differences for single-pair comparisons were analyzed using two-tailed unpaired Student's *t*-tests. Data for relative ratios of single-pair comparisons were analyzed with one-sample *t*-tests. A *p*-value <0.05 was considered statistically significant. Data are presented as means ± SD or SEM based on the sample size and variability within groups. Sample sizes are indicated for each figure.

TABLE 1 | *Post-hoc* analysis of outer hair cell loss (**Figure 2E**).

Groups	Distance from apex (mm)	p-value	Symbol
100 dB + DMSO vs. 100 dB + FK506	3.5	$p = 0.369$	ns
	4	$p = 0.034$	*
	4.5	$p = 0.000$	***
	5	$p = 0.000$	***

$* < 0.05, *** < 0.001$.

without exposure (**Figure 1A**). A semi-quantitative analysis of CaN immunolabeling intensity converted to grayscale in OHCs showed a statistically significant increase, with a ratio of control to 1 and 3 h post-exposure of 1:1.48 ($t_4 = 6.6388, p = 0.0027$) and 1:1.60, respectively ($t_4 = 12.8305, p = 0.0002$, **Figure 1B**). Although the immunolabeling for CaN remained stably elevated 3 h after exposure, there was no difference between 1 and 3 h post-exposure. Immunolabeling for NFAT3 in OHC nuclei appeared stronger and more punctate 1 and 3 h after exposure (**Figure 1C**). Semi-quantification of immunolabeling for NFAT3 (converted to grayscale) in OHC nuclei increased when examined 1 h after ($t_3 = 6.3, p = 0.0078$) and continued to increase 3 h after ($t_6 = 4.1, p = 0.0065$) the exposure (**Figure 1D**). These results support the notion that NFAT3 acts as an indicator of CaN activity.

Treatment With FK506 Attenuates Noise-Induced Hearing Loss and Outer Hair Cell Loss

Based on prior literature (Uemaetomari et al., 2005), we tested two doses (3 and 5 mg/kg) of FK506 against NIHL in our preliminary studies, and both doses of FK506 attenuated PTS. Since the 5-mg/kg dose offered stronger reduction of NIHL, we used 5 mg/kg for all the FK506 experiments. Auditory thresholds of four groups (DMSO alone, FK506 alone, DMSO + noise, and FK506 + noise) at 8, 16, and 32 kHz were measured 5 days before (baseline) and 2 weeks after moderate-PTS-noise exposure, with significant differences at 16 [$F_{(3, 34)} = 162.4, p < 0.0001$] and 32 kHz [$F_{(3, 34)} = 149, p < 0.0001$], but not at 8 kHz [$F_{(3, 37)} = 1, p = 0.38$], as analyzed by one-way ANOVA. Noise exposure significantly increased the auditory threshold shifts at 16 ($p < 0.0001$) and 32 kHz ($p < 0.0001$) compared to control mice without exposure (**Figure 2A**). Treatment with FK506 significantly attenuated noise-induced PTS at both 16 ($p < 0.0001$) and 32 kHz ($p < 0.0001$) (**Figure 2A**). Additionally, DMSO alone as the vehicle did not attenuate moderate-PTS-noise-induced auditory threshold shifts. The auditory thresholds of mice treated with FK506 alone did not differ from those of control mice treated with the vehicle control (DMSO) alone.

To confirm the protective effect of FK506 against moderate-noise-induced hearing loss, we counted the number of OHCs on surface preparations labeled with Myosin-VIIa and stained with DAB. Noise-induced OHC loss was significantly attenuated

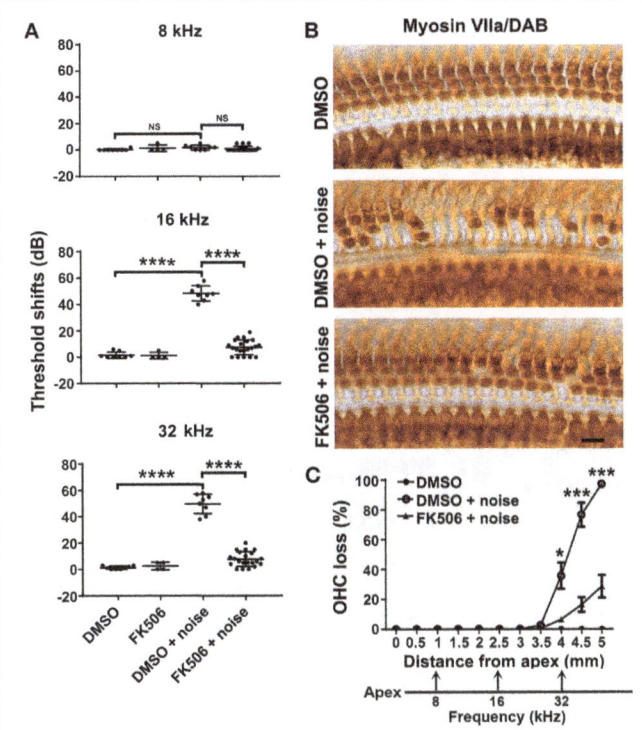

FIGURE 2 | Treatment with FK506 prevents noise-induced outer hair cell (OHC) loss and hearing loss. **(A)** Treatment with FK506 significantly attenuates noise-induced auditory threshold shifts at 16 and 32 kHz measured 14 days after exposure. FK506 alone and vehicle control (dimethyl sulfoxide, DMSO) alone do not alter auditory threshold shifts. Data are presented as individual points measured in the left ears with means ± SD for each group; ****$p < 0.0001$; ns, not significant. **(B)** Representative images show Myosin-VIIa-labeled and 3,3′-diaminobenzidine-stained surface preparations from three groups: DMSO without noise, DMSO + noise, and FK506 + noise. Images were taken from the basal turn around 4.5 mm from the apex. Scale bar = 10 µm. **(C)** The percentage of cochlear OHC loss assessed 14 days after noise exposure, with OHC loss beginning around 3.5 mm from the apex and increasing until reaching 100% OHC loss in the basal region (5 mm from the apex). Treatment with FK506 significantly reduced noise-induced OHC loss. DMSO alone without noise exposure had no effect on hair cell loss. The distances along the cochlear spiral correlating with the frequencies 8, 16, and 32 kHz are indicated. Data are presented as means ± SEM for the left ears; DMSO only: $n = 6$, DMSO + noise: $n = 9$, FK506 + noise: $n = 6$; *$p < 0.05$, ***$p < 0.0001$.

RESULTS

Noise Increases Immunolabeling for CaN in Outer Hair Cells and NFAT3 in Outer Hair Cell Nuclei

To determine whether CaN and NFAT3 are linked to noise-induced outer hair cell death, we first assessed the expression of CaN and NFAT3 in sensory hair cells in response to PTS noise because NFAT, a downstream target of CaN, is an attractive candidate for the pathogenesis of the underlying detrimental effects of CaN (Shioda et al., 2006, 2007). Immunolabeling for CaN (red) on surface preparations increased in OHCs 1 and 3 h after noise exposure compared to control mice

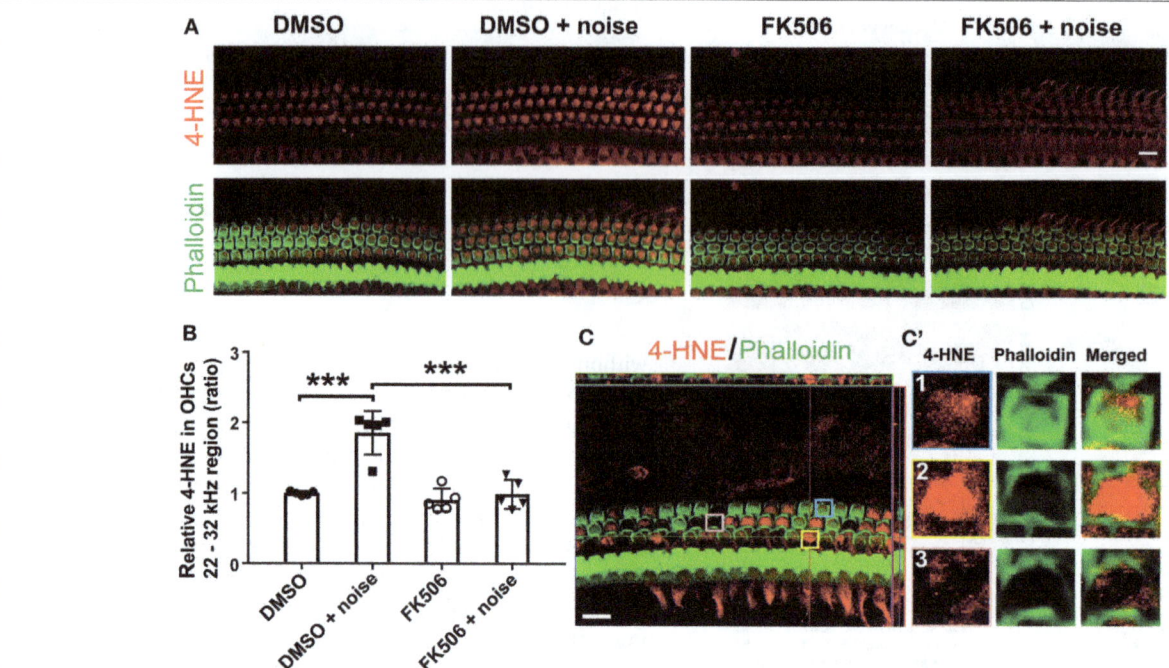

FIGURE 3 | Treatment with FK506 blocks the induction of lipid peroxidation product 4-HNE by noise. **(A)** Surface preparations show immunolabeling for 4-HNE (red) in outer hair cells (OHCs) assessed 3 h after the completion of exposure. Noise-increased 4-HNE is inhibited by treatment with FK506. Green, phalloidin labeling of sensory hair cells. Images were taken from the basal turn corresponding to sensitivity to 22–32 kHz, and each figure is representative of five individual mice for each condition. Scale bar = 10 μm. **(B)** Quantification of relative 4-HNE immunolabeling intensity in grayscale in OHCs normalized to dimethyl sulfoxide control mice confirms inhibition by treatment with FK506. Data are presented as individual points with means ± SD; each condition was examined in one ear per mouse; ***$p < 0.001$. **(C)** This representative image shows very strong 4-HNE immunolabeling in structurally damaged OHCs assessed 3 h after exposure. The image was taken from the lower basal turn corresponding to sensitivity to 45 kHz. **(C′)** For better visualization, three OHCs were enlarged and presented in the right panels with intact OHCs (1), structurally damaged OHCs (2), and scars of lost OHCs (3). This figure is representative of five individual animals per group. Scale bar = 10 μm.

by treatment with FK506 (**Figure 2B**). Counts of the total number of missing OHCs along the entire length of the cochlear spiral showed that the loss of OHCs followed a base-to-apex gradient, with OHC loss beginning 3.5 mm from the apex and increasing to complete OHC loss in the base of the cochlear epithelium. Treatment with FK506 significantly reduced the noise-induced OHC loss as analyzed by repeated-measures ANOVA followed by *post-hoc* tests [$F_{(1,12)} = 35.207$, $p = 0.000$; for detailed *post-hoc* values, see **Table 1** for **Figure 2C**]. In the basal portion 5 mm from the apex, OHC loss was reduced from 100 to about 20% (**Figure 2C**).

Furthermore, to test if treatment with FK506 can attenuate hearing loss from even stronger noise insults, we evaluated FK506 against sPTS-noise conditions. In agreement with our previous data, sPTS-noise exposure induced auditory threshold shifts at all three tested frequencies (8, 16, and 32 kHz), with loss of both OHCs and IHCs 14 days after exposure. Treatment with FK506 significantly attenuated sPTS at only 8 kHz ($t_{12} = 2.865$, $p = 0.0142$), but not at 16 and 32 kHz (data not shown). These results suggest that treatment with FK506 can significantly attenuate noise-induced hearing loss in a noise-intensity-dependent manner. The potency of preventive effects was reduced with increasing noise-exposure intensity.

Treatment With FK506 Diminishes Noise-Induced Accumulation of ROS

Accumulation of ROS in noise-induced OHC death is well documented in the literature, including in publications from our lab and others, through evaluation of markers of lipid peroxidation and protein nitration with 4-HNE and 3-NT, respectively (Yamashita et al., 2004; Fetoni et al., 2015; Wu et al., 2020a). To test whether treatment with FK506 prevents NIHL *via* inhibition of noise-induced accumulation of ROS, we assessed immunolabeling for 4-HNE, a lipid peroxidation product and a consequence of ROS formation acting as a surrogate marker for ROS, in OHCs 3 h after moderate-PTS-noise exposure. In agreement with previous reports, noise exposure increased immunolabeling for 4-HNE in basal turn OHCs, and this increase was significantly inhibited by treatment with FK506 (**Figure 3A**). Semi-quantitative analysis of immunolabeling for 4-HNE in grayscale in OHCs in the basal turn corresponding to sensitivity to 22–32 kHz confirmed a significant increase after exposure ($t_8 = 6.233$, $p = 0.0003$), whereas treatment with FK506 significantly inhibited noise-increased 4-HNE ($t_8 = 5.243$, $p = 0.0008$, **Figure 3B**). Treatment with FK506 alone showed similar levels as those of DMSO alone. Additionally, noise exposure did not increase immunolabeling for 4-HNE in OHCs in the apical and middle turns. It is worth mentioning that we

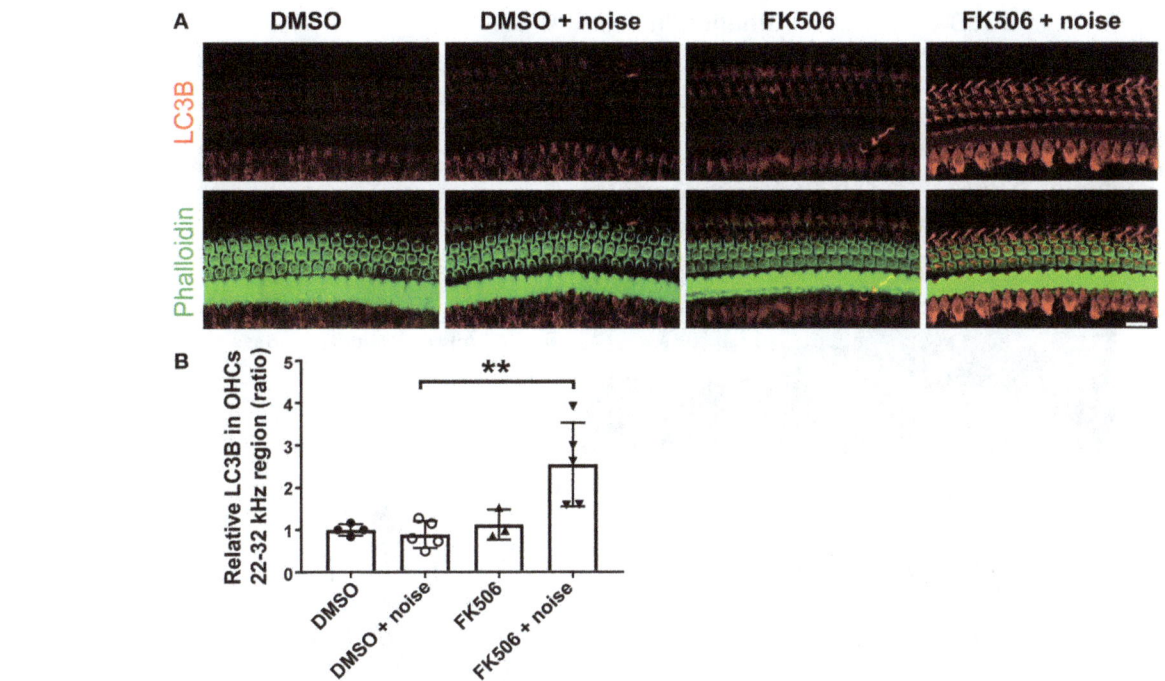

FIGURE 4 | Treatment with FK506 increases LC3B in outer hair cells (OHCs). **(A)** Surface preparations show that immunolabeling for LC3B (red) in OHCs was increased after treatment with FK506 when assessed 3 h after the completion of noise exposure. Green, phalloidin labeling of sensory hair cells. Images were taken from the basal turn corresponding to sensitivity to 22–32 kHz, and each figure is representative of three to five individual mice for each condition. Scale bar = 10 μm. **(B)** Quantification of relative LC3B immunolabeling intensity in grayscale in OHCs normalized to dimethyl sulfoxide control mice confirms enhancement by treatment with FK506. Data are presented as individual points with means ± SD; each condition was examined in one ear per mouse; **$p < 0.01$.

did observe OHC loss 3 h after the PTS-noise exposure in the lower basal turn (about 4.5–5 mm from the apex). In this region, immunolabeling for 4-HNE was extremely strong in structurally damaged OHCs, but not in scars of lost OHCs (**Figures 3C,C′**, enlarged OHCs in the right panel).

Treatment With FK506 Activates Autophagy in Cochlear Outer Hair Cells

Based on the literature, FK506 activates the autophagy system (Kim et al., 2017; Wang et al., 2017). To determine if autophagy plays a role in the prevention of noise-induced hearing loss by treatment with FK506, we assessed immunolabeling for LC3B in OHCs 3 h after moderate-PTS-noise exposure. In agreement with our previous publication (Yuan et al., 2015), noise exposure (DMSO + noise) did not change the levels of LC3B in OHCs compared to DMSO control mice without exposure when assessed 3 h after exposure, whereas treatment with FK506 increased immunolabeling for LC3B in OHCs in the basal turn compared to noise exposure alone (FK506 + moderate PTS noise vs. DMSO + moderate PTS noise; **Figure 4A**). Semi-quantitative analysis confirmed significant changes in the basal turn corresponding to sensitivity to 22–32 kHz ($t_8 = 3.570$, $p = 0.0073$, **Figure 4B**). There were no differences in LC3B expression in OHCs between the three groups (DMSO alone, FK506 alone, and DMSO + moderate PTS noise). These data indicate that treatment with FK506 induces autophagy after noise exposure.

Inhibition of Autophagy by Silencing LC3B Reduces the Protective Effect of FK506 Against Noise-Induced Hearing Loss and Outer Hair Cell Loss

To confirm if autophagy is involved in the protective effects of FK506, we took advantage of LC3B siRNA techniques to reduce the expression of LC3B in OHCs and then evaluated the protective effect of FK506 against PTS-noise-induced auditory threshold shifts and hair cell loss. Based on our previous results, we selected the 0.6-μg dose of siLC3B or siControl delivered onto the RWN of the left ear of each mouse via intra-tympanic application (Oishi et al., 2013; Yuan et al., 2015). Immunolabeling for LC3B in OHCs on surface preparations was assessed nearly 72 h after siLC3B delivery (**Figure 5A**). Semi-quantification of the relative immunolabeling for LC3B converted to grayscale in OHCs of the apical, middle, and basal turns showed around 50% reduction compared to that of the siControls (apex: $t_6 = 10.13$, $p < 0.0001$; middle: $t_6 = 10.66$, $p < 0.0001$; base: $t_6 = 6.228$, $p = 0.0008$, **Figure 5B**). Additionally, we transfected siLC3B to HEI-OC1 cells and analyzed silencing efficiency by Western blot (**Figure 5C**). Densitometry analysis of both LC3B-I and LC3B-II bands together showed about 50% reduction after silencing with siLC3B ($p = 0.0095$, **Figure 5D**). In agreement with our previous

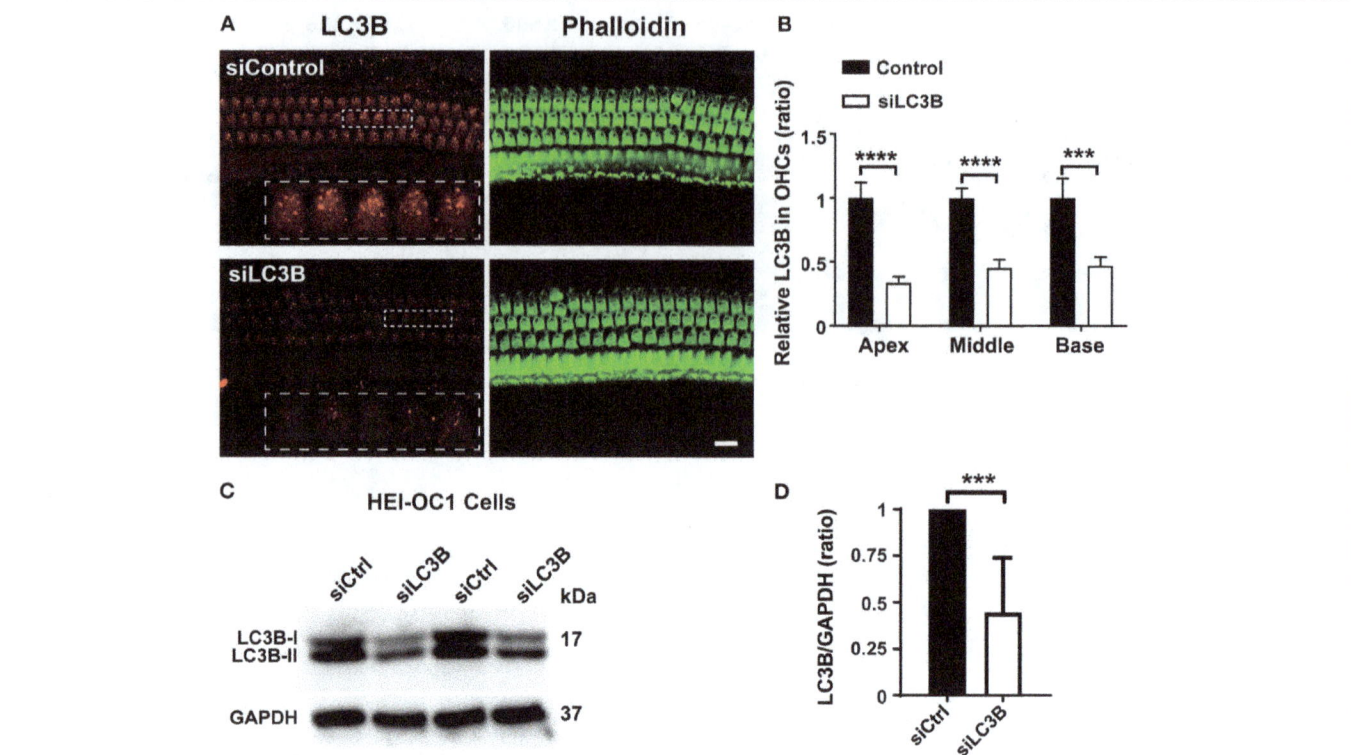

FIGURE 5 | Downregulation of LC3B by LC3B-siRNA both *in vivo* and *in vitro*. (A) Surface preparations immunolabeled with LC3B reveal decreased immunolabeling for LC3B (red) in outer hair cells (OHCs) assessed 72 h after the intra-tympanic delivery of LC3B-siRNA. The representative images were taken from the basal turn corresponding to sensitivity to 22–32 kHz. The apical and middle turns showed a similar attenuation of LC3B. Green, phalloidin staining for sensory hair cells. Scale bar = 10 μm. (B) Quantification of LC3B immunolabeling intensity in grayscale in OHCs in the apical (corresponding to sensitivity to 8 kHz), middle (corresponding to sensitivity to 16 kHz), and basal turns (corresponding to 22–32 kHz) confirms a significant decrease. Data are presented as means ± SD, $n = 4$; ***$p < 0.001$, ****$p < 0.0001$. (C) Representative blots show that the protein levels of LC3B decreased after 48 h of transfection with the LC3B-siRNA in cells compared to the control group transfected with scrambled siRNA (siCtrl). GAPDH serves as a sample loading control. (D) Semi-quantification of the band density (both LC3B I and II) confirms a significant decrease. Data are presented as means ± SD; $n = 4$, ***$p < 0.001$.

results (Yuan et al., 2015), pretreatment with siLC3B only mildly increased moderate-PTS-noise-induced auditory threshold shifts at 16 kHz by less than 10 dB measured 14 days after exposure, with no effect seen at 32 kHz compared to mice treated with siControl. There was no exacerbation of loss of OHCs with pretreatment of siLC3B after moderate PTS-noise exposure. Additionally, there were no differences in auditory threshold shifts between these three groups (moderate PTS noise, surgery + moderate PTS noise, and siControl + moderate PTS noise) when application of surgery or administration of siControl was performed 72 h before exposure to noise. Finally, after 72 h of siRNA pretreatment (left ears), both siControl and siLC3B mice received identical FK506 (5 mg/kg) treatment and noise exposure as described in **Figure 2**. The auditory threshold shifts (left ears) of mice pretreated with siLC3B were 10 dB greater at 16 ($t_8 = 3.004$, $p = 0.017$) and 32 kHz ($t_8 = 2.362$, $p = 0.046$) than those of the siControl mice (**Figures 6A–C**). To confirm that treatment with FK506 prevented NIHL in these mice, we assessed right-ear auditory threshold shifts in both groups. In agreement with our results described in **Figure 2**, the right-ear auditory threshold shifts of both groups were similar to the previous treatment with FK506 and significantly attenuated NIHL at both 16 ($p < 0.0001$) and 32 kHz ($p < 0.0001$).

Furthermore, counting OHCs along the entire cochlear spiral showed that pretreatment with siLC3B significantly decreased the protective effects of FK506 against OHC loss. In the siLC3B group, noise-induced OHC loss increased in the basal portions between 3.5 and 5 mm from the apex by repeated-measures ANOVA [$F_{(1, 11)} = 45.040$, $p = 0.000$; for detailed *post-hoc* values, see **Table 2** for **Figure 6D**]. At 5 mm from the apex, the siLC3B group showed around 80% OHC loss compared to 30% loss with the siControl mice (**Figure 6D**). These results indicate that, when autophagy was inhibited by pretreatment with siLC3B, the protective effect of FK506 was partially blocked, indicating that the activation of autophagy is involved in the mechanism of FK506 protection.

DISCUSSION

Consistent with and building upon previous reports (Minami et al., 2004; Uemaetomari et al., 2005), our results show that

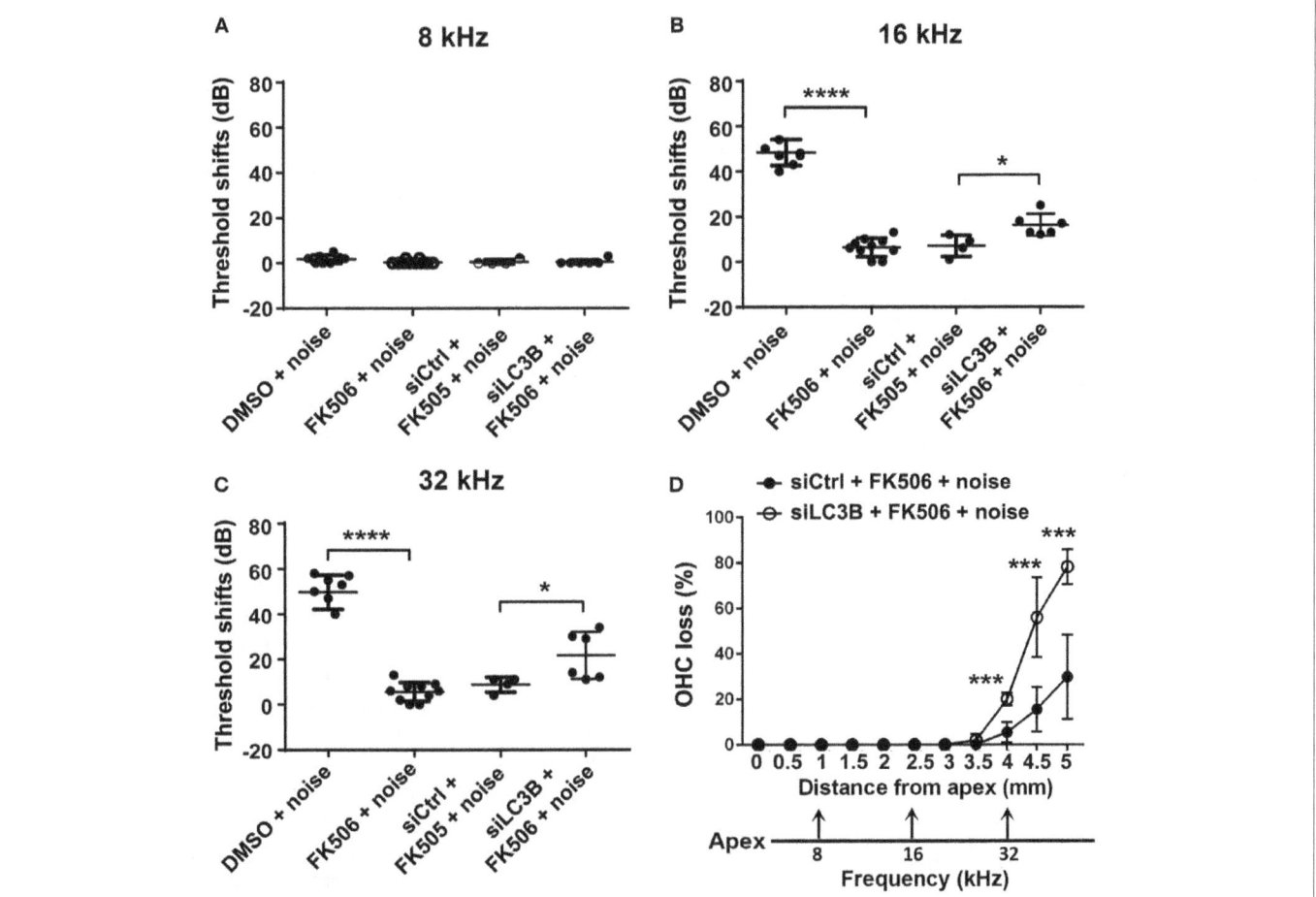

FIGURE 6 | Inhibition of autophagy reduces the protective effects of FK506 against noise-induced hearing loss and auditory outer hair cell (OHC) loss. **(A–C)** Pretreatment with siLC3B reduces the protective effect of FK506 at 16 and 32 kHz when assessed 14 days after exposure. Noise does not induce auditory threshold shifts at 8 kHz. Data are presented as individual points for each mouse and means ± SD for each group; $*p < 0.05$, $****p < 0.0001$. **(D)** Quantitative analysis of loss of OHCs along the entire cochlear spiral shows that the reduction of OHC loss by treatment with FK506 was partially diminished by pretreatment with siLC3B assessed 14 days after exposure. The distances along the cochlear spiral correlating with the frequencies 8, 16, and 32 kHz are indicated. Data are presented as means ± SD. siControl + FK506 + noise, $n = 4$; siLC3B + FK506 + noise, $n = 6$; $**p < 0.01$, $****p < 0.0001$.

treatment with the CaN antagonist FK506 attenuates noise-induced loss of OHCs and, consequently, NIHL in adult CBA/J mice. Additionally, attenuation of moderate-PTS-noise-induced hair cell loss and hearing loss by FK506 is significantly stronger than treatment with autophagy agonist rapamycin or antioxidant N-acetylcysteine (NAC) as evaluated in our previous report (Yuan et al., 2015). CaN is activated by a sustained elevation in intracellular calcium levels, which has been shown to be a consequence of traumatic noise exposure (Fridberger et al., 1998; Oliver et al., 2001). In our study, the expression of NFAT3 in OHC nuclei is significantly increased in a time-dependent fashion after exposure to moderate PTS noise, in agreement with the notion that the NFAT transcription factor family can be activated by CaN. OHC death, as a consequence of increased nuclear NFAT3, is compatible with an earlier report that application of an NFAT inhibitor on explants attenuates gentamicin-induced hair cell death (Bodmer et al., 2016) and is in line with the recent report showing that *Nfatc3* (*NFAT3*)

deficiency in mice attenuates ototoxicity by suppressing TNF-mediated hair cell apoptosis (Zhang et al., 2019). NFAT forms a cooperative complex with AP-1 or other bZIP proteins through its binding site (Macián et al., 2001). The cooperation of NFAT with AP-1 is required for the transcription of several different genes, including IL-3, IFN-γ, and FasL, and plays an important role in immune responses and determining cell fate (Rao et al., 1997; Macián et al., 2001).

In fact, ROS and inflammation may interplay (Fetoni et al., 2019), as accumulation of both ROS and cytokines has been well documented in noise-induced OHC death (Yamane et al., 1995; Shi et al., 2003; Yamashita et al., 2005; Fujioka et al., 2006; Le Prell et al., 2007; Dhukhwa et al., 2019; Fetoni et al., 2019; Frye et al., 2019). Our results support this notion as we show that the lipid peroxidation product 4-HNE, acting as a surrogate marker for ROS, is highly expressed in damaged OHCs in the basal turn after noise exposure that induces high-frequency hearing loss, while treatment with FK506 inhibits noise-induced accumulation of 4-HNE. Additionally, our previous publication demonstrated that the levels of autophagy in OHCs increase after TTS-noise exposure where no OHC loss occurred, while the levels of autophagy marker LC3B remain close to that of the unexposed control mice after moderate-PTS-noise and even after sPTS-noise exposure (Yuan et al., 2015). Consistent with those findings, our current results show no changes in LC3B in OHCs after moderate-PTS-noise exposure. However, treatment with FK506 activates autophagy as indicated by an increased expression of LC3B in OHCs in the basal turn concurrent with attenuation of NIHL. Indeed lower levels of ROS have the ability to induce cellular defense pathways such as autophagy as seen in brain injury and cortical neuron apoptosis and optic nerve degeneration (Rodriguez-Muela et al., 2012; Wang et al., 2012). The current results support our previous conclusion that low levels of oxidative stress caused by exposure to TTS-noise activate autophagy, which inhibits cell apoptosis and prevents hair cell loss by inhibiting the accumulation of ROS. On the other hand, moderate PTS noise and sPTS noise induce excessive oxidative stress, which may trigger cell death pathways, leading to sensory hair cell death (He et al., 2017; Wu et al., 2020b). Furthermore, this notion is supported by the fact that inhibition of autophagy by siLC3B pre-treatment reduces the protective effect of FK506 against noise-induced loss of OHCs and hearing function. FK506 has previously been reported to be an activator of autophagy. FK506 can activate the translocation of TFEB from the cytoplasm into the nucleus by binding to ATP6V1A and then induce autophagy (Kim et al., 2017). Such a mechanism of FK506 action is in line with studies showing that treatment with FK506 increases the survival rate of myocardial cells *via* activation of the autophagy pathway (Wang et al., 2017) and is consistent with the general notion that activation of autophagy plays an important role in cellular survival, particularly in stress conditions such as starvation and oxidative stress (Mizushima et al., 2008; Esclatine et al., 2009; Rabinowitz and White, 2010). Our current results delineate that pretreatment with siLC3B mildly reduces the protective effects of FK506 against noise-induced OHC loss and hearing loss. This result is consistent with our previous data showing that pretreatment with siLC3B increased moderate-PTS-noise-induced auditory threshold shifts only minimally, by about 10 dB, compared with mice treated with siControl (Yuan et al., 2015), i.e., autophagy promotes sensory hair cell survival only slightly under certain conditions. This conclusion is supported by the fact that pharmacological activation of autophagy alone is insufficient to counteract ROS generation after moderate-PTS-noise exposure (Yuan et al., 2015). Nevertheless, autophagy may play dual roles in both cell survival early after insults and cell death at later stages (Baehrecke, 2005), although we never observe activation of autophagy in sensory hair cells after moderate-PTS-noise or sPTS-noise exposure.

We should emphasize that attenuation of moderate-PTS-noise-induced hearing loss and hair cell loss by FK506 is significantly stronger than treatment with autophagy agonist rapamycin or antioxidant NAC (Yuan et al., 2015). Attenuation of moderate-PTS-noise-induced auditory threshold shifts at 16 and 32 kHz was on average 40 dB after treatment with FK506 compared to 10–15 dB with rapamycin or NAC treatment. Additionally, reduction of moderate-PTS-noise-induced loss of OHCs was roughly 50% higher with treatment with FK506 than treatment with rapamycin or NAC (Yuan et al., 2015). It is worth noting that exposure of 12-week-old CBA/J mice to moderate PTS noise induces permanent hearing loss with loss of OHCs; the damage is less severe than that from sPTS-noise conditions, which result in loss of both OHCs and IHCs. Treatment with FK506 prevents the majority of damage induced by exposure to moderate PTS noise but only mildly attenuates sPTS-noise-induced damage. This result agrees with the general concept that the more severe the damage, the harder it is to achieve physiologically meaningful protection. This fact could be related to the activation of multiple cell death pathways after exposure to higher-intensity sPTS noise, including the possibility that inhibition of apoptotic OHC death promotes necrotic-like cell death (Zheng et al., 2014). A more effective protection would require further understanding of noise-induced hearing loss pathways and focus on potentially synergistic protective effects. We are aware that moderate-PTS-noise-induced auditory threshold shifts may be influenced by numerous confounding factors, for instance, surgical opening of the middle ear that could activate protective (e.g., heat shock proteins) or damaging (e.g., cochlear inflammation) mechanisms. Appropriate controls are essential before drawing conclusions. In our experiments, noise exposure was performed 72 h after surgery on the left ears. Our results showed there were no differences in auditory thresholds between moderate PTS noise exposure and surgery plus moderate PTS noise exposure. In summary, our results are in agreement with the notion that the noise-induced increase in nuclear NFAT3 in OHCs is a downstream consequence of CaN activation and a target of FK506. Treatment with FK506 inhibits noise-accumulated ROS and promotes autophagy, suggesting that FK506 attenuates noise-induced trauma that occurs not only *via* inhibition of CaN activity but also through inhibition of ROS and activation of autophagy.

TABLE 2 | *Post-hoc* analysis of outer hair cell loss (**Figure 6D**).

Groups	Distance from apex (mm)	p-value	Symbol
siControl + 101 dB + FK506 vs. siLC3B + 101 dB + FK506	3.5	$p = 0.078$	ns
	4	$p = 0.000$	***
	4.5	$p = 0.000$	***
	5	$p = 0.0001$	***

*** < 0.001.

ETHICS STATEMENT

The animal study was reviewed and approved by the Institutional Animal Care and Use Committee at the Medical University of South Carolina.

AUTHOR CONTRIBUTIONS

S-HS designed research. Z-HH, SP, H-WZ, and Q-JF performed research. Z-HH, KH, and S-HS analyzed data and wrote the paper. All authors contributed to the article and approved the submitted version.

ACKNOWLEDGMENTS

We thank Dr. Jochen Schacht for his valuable comments on the manuscript. We also thank Andra Talaska for proofreading of the manuscript. All research protocols were approved by the Institutional Animal Care and Use Committee at the Medical University of South Carolina. Animal care was under the supervision of the Division of Laboratory Animal Resources at MUSC.

REFERENCES

Abdul, H. M., Sama, M. A., Furman, J. L., Mathis, D. M., Beckett, T. L., Weidner, A. M., et al. (2009). Cognitive decline in Alzheimer's disease is associated with selective changes in calcineurin/NFAT signaling. *J. Neurosci.* 29, 12957–12969. doi: 10.1523/JNEUROSCI.1064-09.2009

Arroyo, D. S., Soria, J. A., Gaviglio, E. A., Garciakeller, C., Cancela, L. M., Rodriguezgalan, M. C., et al. (2013). Toll-like receptor 2 ligands promote microglial cell death by inducing autophagy. *FASEB J.* 27, 299–312. doi: 10.1096/fj.12-214312

Baehrecke, E. H. (2005). Autophagy: dual roles in life and death? *Nat. Rev. Mol. Cell Biol.* 6, 505–510. doi: 10.1038/nrm1666

Bandyopadhyay, U., Nagy, M., Fenton, W. A., and Horwich, A. L. (2014). Absence of lipofuscin in motor neurons of SOD1-linked ALS mice. *Proc. Natl. Acad. Sci. U.S.A* 111, 11055–11060. doi: 10.1073/pnas.1409314111

Bas, E., Van De Water, T. R., Gupta, C., Dinh, J., Vu, L., Martinez-Soriano, F., et al. (2012). Efficacy of three drugs for protecting against gentamicin-induced hair cell and hearing losses. *Br. J. Pharmacol.* 166, 1888–1904. doi: 10.1111/j.1476-5381.2012.01890.x

Bodmer, D., Perkovic, A., Sekulic-Jablanovic, M., Wright, M. B., and Petkovic, V. (2016). Pasireotide prevents nuclear factor of activated T cells nuclear translocation and acts as a protective agent in aminoglycoside-induced auditory hair cell loss. *J. Neurochem.* 139, 1113–1123. doi: 10.1111/jnc.13880

Chen, F. Q., Zheng, H. W., Hill, K., and Sha, S. H. (2012). Traumatic noise activates rho-family GTPases through transient cellular energy depletion. *J. Neurosci.* 32, 12421–12430. doi: 10.1523/JNEUROSCI.6381-11.2012

Chen, F. Q., Zheng, H. W., Schacht, J., and Sha, S. H. (2013). Mitochondrial peroxiredoxin 3 regulates sensory cell survival in the cochlea. *PLoS ONE* 8:e61999. doi: 10.1371/journal.pone.0061999

Crabtree, G. R., and Olson, E. N. (2002). NFAT signaling: choreographing the social lives of cells. *Cell* 109(Suppl.), S67–S79. doi: 10.1016/S0092-8674(02)00699-2

Dhukhwa, A., Bhatta, P., Sheth, S., Korrapati, K., Tieu, C., Mamillapalli, C., et al. (2019). Targeting inflammatory processes mediated by TRPVI and TNF-alpha for treating noise-induced hearing loss. *Front. Cell. Neurosci.* 13:444. doi: 10.3389/fncel.2019.00444

Esclatine, A., Chaumorcel, M., and Codogno, P. (2009). Macroautophagy signaling and regulation. *Curr. Top. Microbiol. Immunol.* 335, 33–470. doi: 10.1007/978-3-642-00302-8_2

Fang, Q. J., Wu, F., Chai, R., and Sha, S. H. (2019). Cochlear surface preparation in the adult mouse. *J. Vis. Exp.* doi: 10.3791/60299

Fetoni, A. R., Paciello, F., Rolesi, R., Eramo, S. L., Mancuso, C., Troiani, D., et al. (2015). Rosmarinic acid up-regulates the noise-activated Nrf2/HO-1 pathway and protects against noise-induced injury in rat cochlea. *Free Radic. Biol. Med.* 85, 269–281. doi: 10.1016/j.freeradbiomed.2015.04.021

Fetoni, A. R., Paciello, F., Rolesi, R., Paludetti, G., and Troiani, D. (2019). Targeting dysregulation of redox homeostasis in noise-induced hearing loss: oxidative stress and ROS signaling. *Free Radic. Biol. Med.* 135, 46–59. doi: 10.1016/j.freeradbiomed.2019.02.022

Fettiplace, R., and Nam, J. H. (2019). Tonotopy in calcium homeostasis and vulnerability of cochlear hair cells. *Hear. Res.* 376, 11–21. doi: 10.1016/j.heares.2018.11.002

Fridberger, A., Flock, A., Ulfendahl, M., and Flock, B. (1998). Acoustic overstimulation increases outer hair cell Ca2+ concentrations and causes dynamic contractions of the hearing organ. *Proc. Natl. Acad. Sci. U.S.A.* 95, 7127–7132. doi: 10.1073/pnas.95.12.7127

Frye, M. D., Ryan, A. F., and Kurabi, A. (2019). Inflammation associated with noise-induced hearing loss. *J. Acoust. Soc. Am.* 146:4020. doi: 10.1121/1.5132545

Fujioka, M., Kanzaki, S., Okano, H. J., Masuda, M., Ogawa, K., and Okano, H. (2006). Proinflammatory cytokines expression in noise-induced damaged cochlea. *J. Neurosci. Res.* 83, 575–4583. doi: 10.1002/jnr.20764

Hashimoto, Y., Perrino, B. A., and Soderling, T. R. (1990). Identification of an autoinhibitory domain in calcineurin. *J. Biol. Chem.* 265, 1924–1927. doi: 10.1016/S0021-9258(19)39919-3

He, Z., Guo, L., Shu, Y., Fang, Q., Zhou, H., Liu, Y., et al. (2017). Autophagy protects auditory hair cells against neomycin-induced damage. *Autophagy* 13, 1884–1904. doi: 10.1080/15548627.2017.1359449

Hill, K., Yuan, H., Wang, X., and Sha, S. H. (2016). Noise-induced loss of hair cells and cochlear synaptopathy are mediated by the activation of AMPK. *J. Neurosci.* 36, 7497–7510. doi: 10.1523/JNEUROSCI.0782-16.2016

Ikeda, K., and Morizono, T. (1988). Calcium transport mechanism in the endolymph of the chinchilla. *Hear. Res.* 34, 307–311. doi: 10.1016/0378-5955(88)90010-X

Ke, H., and Huai, Q. (2003). Structures of calcineurin and its complexes with immunophilins-immunosuppressants. *Biochem. Biophys. Res. Commun.* 311, 1095–1102. doi: 10.1016/S0006-291X(03)01537-7

Kim, D., Hwang, H. Y., Kim, J. Y., Lee, J. Y., Yoo, J. S., Marko-Varga, G., et al. (2017). FK506, an Immunosuppressive drug, induces autophagy by binding to the V-ATPase catalytic subunit A in neuronal cells. *J. Proteome Res.* 16, 55–64. doi: 10.1021/acs.jproteome.6b00638

Kroemer, G., and Levine, B. (2008). Autophagic cell death: the story of a misnomer. *Nat. Rev. Mol. Cell. Biol.* 9, 1004–1010. doi: 10.1038/nrm2529

Le Prell, C. G., Yamashita, D., Minami, S. B., Yamasoba, T., and Miller, J. M. (2007). Mechanisms of noise-induced hearing loss indicate multiple methods of prevention. *Hear. Res.* 226, 22–43. doi: 10.1016/j.heares.2006.10.006

Levine, B., and Kroemer, G. (2008). Autophagy in the pathogenesis of disease. *Cell* 132:27. doi: 10.1016/j.cell.2007.12.018

Macián, F., López-Rodríguez, C., and Rao, A. (2001). Partners in transcription: NFAT and AP-1. *Oncogene* 20, 2476–2489. doi: 10.1038/sj.onc.1204386

Minami, S. B., Yamashita, D., Schacht, J., and Miller, J. M. (2004). Calcineurin activation contributes to noise-induced hearing loss. *J. Neurosci. Res.* 78, 383–392. doi: 10.1002/jnr.20267

Mizushima, N., Levine, B., Cuervo, A. M., and Klionsky, D. J. (2008). Autophagy fights disease through cellular self-digestion. *Nature* 451, 1069–1075. doi: 10.1038/nature06639

Morioka, M., Hamada, J., Ushio, Y., and Miyamoto, E. (1999). Potential role of calcineurin for brain ischemia and traumatic injury. *Prog. Neurobiol.* 58, 1–30. doi: 10.1016/S0301-0082(98)00073-2

Muller, M., von Hunerbein, K., Hoidis, S., and Smolders, J. W. (2005). A physiological place-frequency map of the cochlea in the CBA/J mouse. *Hear. Res.* 202, 63–73. doi: 10.1016/j.heares.2004.08.011

Neitzel, R. L., and Fligor, B. J. (2019). Risk of noise-induced hearing loss due to recreational sound: Review and recommendations. *J. Acoust. Soc. Am.* 146:3911. doi: 10.1121/1.5132287

Ohlemiller, K. K., Wright, J. S., and Dugan, L. L. (1999). Early elevation of cochlear reactive oxygen species following noise exposure. *Audiol. Neurootol.* 4, 229–3236. doi: 10.1159/000013846

Oishi, N., Chen, F. Q., Zheng, H. W., and Sha, S. H. (2013). Intra-tympanic delivery of short interfering RNA into the adult mouse cochlea. *Hear. Res.* 296, 36–41. doi: 10.1016/j.heares.2012.10.011

Oliver, D., Ludwig, J., Reisinger, E., Zoellner, W., Ruppersberg, J. P., and Fakler, B. (2001). Memantine inhibits efferent cholinergic transmission in the cochlea by blocking nicotinic acetylcholine receptors of outer hair cells. *Mol. Pharmacol.* 60, 183–189. doi: 10.1124/mol.60.1.183

Rabinowitz, J. D., and White, E. (2010). Autophagy and metabolism. *Science* 330, 1344–1348. doi: 10.1126/science.1193497

Rao, A., Luo, C., and Hogan, P. G. (1997). Transcription factors of the NFAT family: regulation and function. *Annu. Rev. Immunol.* 15, 707–747. doi: 10.1146/annurev.immunol.15.1.707

Rodriguez-Muela, N., Germain, F., Marino, G., Fitze, P. S., and Boya, P. (2012). Autophagy promotes survival of retinal ganglion cells after optic nerve axotomy in mice. *Cell Death Differ.* 19, 162–169. doi: 10.1038/cdd.2011.88

Ryter, S. W., Mizumura, K., and Choi, A. M. (2014). The impact of autophagy on cell death modalities. *Int. J. Cell Biol.* 2014:502676. doi: 10.1155/2014/502676

Sha, S. H., and Schacht, J. (2017). Emerging therapeutic interventions against noise-induced hearing loss. *Expert Opin. Invest. Drugs* 26, 85–96. doi: 10.1080/13543784.2017.1269171

Shi, X., Dai, C., and Nuttall, A. L. (2003). Altered expression of inducible nitric oxide synthase (iNOS) in the cochlea. *Hear. Res.* 177, 43–52. doi: 10.1016/S0378-5955(02)00796-7

Shibasaki, F., Price, E. R., Milan, D., and McKeon, F. (1996). Role of kinases and the phosphatase calcineurin in the nuclear shuttling of transcription factor NF-AT4. *Nature* 382, 370–373. doi: 10.1038/382370a0

Shioda, N., Han, F., Moriguchi, S., and Fukunaga, K. (2007). Constitutively active calcineurin mediates delayed neuronal death through Fas-ligand expression via activation of NFAT and FKHR transcriptional activities in mouse brain ischemia. *J. Neurochem.* 102, 1506–1517. doi: 10.1111/j.1471-4159.2007.04600.x

Shioda, N., Moriguchi, S., Shirasaki, Y., and Fukunaga, K. (2006). Generation of constitutively active calcineurin by calpain contributes to delayed neuronal death following mouse brain ischemia. *J. Neurochem.* 98, 310–320. doi: 10.1111/j.1471-4159.2006.03874.x

Taylor, C. R., and Levenson, R. M. (2006). Quantification of immunohistochemistry–issues concerning methods, utility and semiquantitative assessment II. *Histopathology* 49, 411–424. doi: 10.1111/j.1365-2559.2006.02513.x

Themann, C. L., and Masterson, E. A. (2019). Occupational noise exposure: a review of its effects, epidemiology, and impact with recommendations for reducing its burden. *J. Acoust. Soc. Am.* 146:3879. doi: 10.1121/1.5134465

Uemaetomari, I., Tabuchi, K., Hoshino, T., and Hara, A. (2005). Protective effect of calcineurin inhibitors on acoustic injury of the cochlea. *Hear. Res.* 209, 86–90. doi: 10.1016/j.heares.2005.06.010

Viberg, A., and Canlon, B. (2004). The guide to plotting a cochleogram. *Hear. Res.* 197, 1–10. doi: 10.1016/j.heares.2004.04.016

Walker, R. A. (2006). Quantification of immunohistochemistry–issues concerning methods, utility and semiquantitative assessment I. *Histopathology* 49, 406–410. doi: 10.1111/j.1365-2559.2006.02514.x

Wang, J., and Puel, J. L. (2018). Toward cochlear therapies. *Physiol. Rev.* 98, 2477–2522. doi: 10.1152/physrev.00053.2017

Wang, Y., Lu, J., Cheng, W., Gao, R., Yang, L., and Yang, Z. (2017). FK506 protects heart function via increasing autophagy after myocardial infarction in mice. *Biochem. Biophys. Res. Commun.* 493:S0006291X17319368. doi: 10.1016/j.bbrc.2017.09.155

Wang, Z., Shi, X. Y., Yin, J., Zuo, G., Zhang, J., and Chen, G. (2012). Role of autophagy in early brain injury after experimental subarachnoid hemorrhage. *J. Mol. Neurosci.* 46, 192–202. doi: 10.1007/s12031-011-9575-6

Wu, F., Xiong, H., and Sha, S. (2020a). Noise-induced loss of sensory hair cells is mediated by ROS/AMPKalpha pathway. *Redox Biol.* 29:101406. doi: 10.1016/j.redox.2019.101406

Wu, J., Ye, J., Kong, W., Zhang, S., and Zheng, Y. (2020b). Programmed cell death pathways in hearing loss: a review of apoptosis, autophagy and programmed necrosis. *Cell Prolif.* 53:e12915. doi: 10.1111/cpr.12915

Yamane, H., Nakai, Y., Takayama, M., Iguchi, H., Nakagawa, T., and Kojima, A. (1995). Appearance of free radicals in the guinea pig inner ear after noise-induced acoustic trauma. *Eur. Arch. Otorhinolaryngol.* 252, 504–508. doi: 10.1007/BF02114761

Yamashita, D., Jiang, H. Y., Le Prell, C. G., Schacht, J., and Miller, J. M. (2005). Post-exposure treatment attenuates noise-induced hearing loss. *Neuroscience* 134, 633–642. doi: 10.1016/j.neuroscience.2005.04.015

Yamashita, D., Jiang, H. Y., Schacht, J., and Miller, J. M. (2004). Delayed production of free radicals following noise exposure. *Brain Res.* 1019, 201–209. doi: 10.1016/j.brainres.2004.05.104

Yuan, H., Wang, X., Hill, K., Chen, J., Lemasters, J., Yang, S. M., et al. (2015). Autophagy attenuates noise-induced hearing loss by reducing oxidative stress. *Antioxid. Redox Signal.* 22:1308. doi: 10.1089/ars.2014.6004

Zhang, Y., Chen, D., Zhao, L., Li, W., Ni, Y., Chen, Y., et al. (2019). Nfatc4 deficiency attenuates ototoxicity by suppressing Tnf-mediated hair cell apoptosis in the mouse cochlea. *Front. Immunol.* 10:1660. doi: 10.3389/fimmu.2019.01660

Zheng, H. W., Chen, J., and Sha, S. H. (2014). Receptor-interacting protein kinases modulate noise-induced sensory hair cell death. *Cell Death Dis.* 5:e1262. doi: 10.1038/cddis.2014.177

Syndromic Deafness Gene *ATP6V1B2* Controls Degeneration of Spiral Ganglion Neurons Through Modulating Proton Flux

Shiwei Qiu[1,2†], Weihao Zhao[1,3†], Xue Gao[4†], Dapeng Li[5], Weiqian Wang[1], Bo Gao[1], Weiju Han[1], Shiming Yang[1*], Pu Dai[1*], Peng Cao[6*] and Yongyi Yuan[1*]

[1] Department of Otolaryngology, Head and Neck Surgery, Institute of Otolaryngology, Genetic Testing Center for Deafness, Chinese PLA General Hospital; National Clinical Research Center for Otolaryngologic Diseases; Key Lab of Hearing Impairment Science of Ministry of Education; Key Lab of Hearing Impairment Prevention and Treatment of Beijing, Beijing, China, [2] The Institute of Audiology and Balance Science, Artificial Auditory Laboratory of Jiangsu Province, Xuzhou Medical University, Xuzhou, China, [3] Department of Otolaryngology General Hospital of Tibet Military Region, Lhasa, China, [4] Department of Otolaryngology, PLA Rocket Force Characteristic Medical Center, Beijing, China, [5] Department of Neurobiology, School of Basic Medical Sciences, Beijing Key Laboratory of Neural Regeneration and Repair, Advanced Innovation Center for Human Brain Protection, Capital Medical University, Beijing, China, [6] National Institute of Biological Sciences, Beijing, China

*Correspondence:
Shiming Yang
yangsm301@263.net
Pu Dai
daipu301@vip.sina.com
Peng Cao
caopeng@nibs.ac.cn
Yongyi Yuan
yyymzh@163.com

[†] These authors have contributed equally to this work

ATP6V1B2 encodes the V1B2 subunit in V-ATPase, a proton pump responsible for the acidification of lysosomes. Mutations in this gene cause DDOD syndrome, DOORS syndrome, and Zimmermann–Laband syndrome, which share overlapping feature of congenital sensorineural deafness, onychodystrophy, and different extents of intellectual disability without or with epilepsy. However, the underlying mechanisms remain unclear. To investigate the pathological role of mutant *ATP6V1B2* in the auditory system, we evaluated auditory brainstem response, distortion product otoacoustic emissions, in a transgenic line of mice carrying c.1516 C > T (p.Arg506*) in *Atp6v1b2*, *Atp6v1b2*$^{Arg506*/Arg506*}$. To explore the pathogenic mechanism of neurodegeneration in the auditory pathway, immunostaining, western blotting, and RNAscope analyses were performed in *Atp6v1b2*$^{Arg506*/Arg506*}$ mice. The *Atp6v1b2*$^{Arg506*/Arg506*}$ mice showed hidden hearing loss (HHL) at early stages and developed late-onset hearing loss. We observed increased transcription of *Atp6v1b1* in hair cells of *Atp6v1b2*$^{Arg506*/Arg506*}$ mice and inferred that *Atp6v1b1* compensated for the *Atp6v1b2* dysfunction by increasing its own transcription level. Genetic compensation in hair cells explains the milder hearing impairment in *Atp6v1b2*$^{Arg506*/Arg506*}$ mice. Apoptosis activated by lysosomal dysfunction and the subsequent blockade of autophagic flux induced the degeneration of spiral ganglion neurons and further impaired the hearing. Intraperitoneal administration of the apoptosis inhibitor, BIP-V5, improved both phenotypical and pathological outcomes in two live mutant mice. Based on the pathogenesis underlying hearing loss in *Atp6v1b2*-related syndromes, systemic drug administration to inhibit apoptosis might be an option for restoring the function of spiral ganglion neurons and promoting hearing, which provides a direction for future treatment.

Keywords: syndromic hearing loss, *Atp6v1b2*, lysosome, apoptosis, function compensation

INTRODUCTION

V-ATPase is a multi-subunit enzyme complex also known as the vacuolar H^+-ATPase. This proton pump is mainly responsible for the acidification of lysosomes and other membrane-bound compartments (Beyenbach and Wieczorek, 2006). V-ATPase comprises a peripheral V1 domain catalyzing ATP hydrolysis and a membrane integral V0 domain involved in proton translocation (Beyenbach and Wieczorek, 2006; Mindell, 2012). The V1 domain includes at least eight different subunits (A-H), while the V0 domain includes six different subunits (a, d, e, c, c′, and c″). The loss of any subunit will disrupt the assembly of V-ATPase and affect lysosome acidification, which could lead to various disorders (Ma et al., 2011).

ATP6V1B2, which encodes the V1B2 subunit in V-ATPase, is the causative gene for dominant deafness-onychodystrophy syndrome (DDOD syndrome, MIM: 124480) (Yuan et al., 2014); deafness, onychodystrophy, osteodystrophy, intellectual disability, and seizures syndrome (DOORS syndrome, MIM: 220500) (Beauregard-Lacroix et al., 2020); and Zimmermann-Laband syndrome (ZLS, MIM: 135500) (Kortüm et al., 2015). These syndromes share the symptoms of congenital sensorineural deafness, onychodystrophy, and different extents of intellectual disability without or with epilepsy. *ATP6V1B2* c.1516 C > T, p.Arg506*, was identified in all families with DDOD syndrome (Yuan et al., 2014; Menendez et al., 2017). To investigate the pathological role of mutant *ATP6V1B2* in the neurosensory system, we generated a transgenic line of mice carrying c.1516 C > T (p.Arg506*) in *Atp6v1b2*, $Atp6v1b2^{Arg506*/Arg506*}$ (homozygous mutant), and identified that the mutant mice displayed obvious cognitive defects for which impairment in the hippocampal CA1 region might be the pathological basis (Zhao et al., 2019). The interaction between the V1B2 and V1E subunits was found to be weaker in $Atp6v1b2^{Arg506*/Arg506*}$ mice than in wild-type (WT) mice, indicating that the assembly of V-ATPase was affected by the mutation (Zhao et al., 2019). In another prior study, when pIRES2-EGFP-*ATP6V1B2* WT and pIRES2-EGFP-*ATP6V1B2* c.1516 C > T mutant plasmids were transfected into HEK293 cells, the lysosomal pH was increased, revealing the reduced acidification in the lysosome caused by the c.1516 C > T mutation (Yuan et al., 2014). Lysosomes, as scavengers of living cells, play a critical role in cellular metabolism. An abnormal lysosomal pH will cause dysfunctional macromolecule degradation and lead to lysosomal storage diseases. Loss of the V-ATPase subunits in the *Drosophila* fat body cells resulted in an abnormal pH in the lysosomal lumen, causing an accumulation of non-functional lysosomes and leading to a blockade of autophagic flux (Mauvezin et al., 2015). Additionally, abnormalities in autophagy caused by V-ATPase defects are associated with neurodegenerative diseases (Peric and Annaert, 2015; Cerri and Blandini, 2019).

Whether the *Atp6v1b2* c.1516 C > T mutation results in autophagic dysfunction and leads to abnormal auditory function remains unanswered. However, the $Atp6v1b2^{Arg506*/Arg506*}$ mice displayed normal auditory brainstem response (ABR) thresholds before 24 weeks of age (Zhao et al., 2019), while in the patients with *ATP6V1B2*-related syndromes, the hearing loss is congenital and severe. Genetic compensation can be induced by non-sense mutations that could occur between homologous genes (Ma et al., 2019). Two highly homologous genes encode V1B subunits: *ATP6V1B1* and *ATP6V1B2*. The B2 subunit of V-ATPase was shown to functionally substitute for the B1 subunit (Paunescu et al., 2007). Therefore, we speculate that genetic compensation might be responsible for the phenotype of $Atp6v1b2^{Arg506*/Arg506*}$ mice.

Herein, we performed long-term studies on hearing in $Atp6v1b2^{Arg506*/Arg506*}$ mice, investigated the pathogenic mechanism of neurodegeneration in the auditory pathway, and confirmed the genetic compensation in $Atp6v1b2^{Arg506*/Arg506*}$ mice to explain the difference between hearing impairments observed in patients and those produced in this mouse model.

MATERIALS AND METHODS

Animals

$Atp6v1b2^{Arg506*/Arg506*}$ mice were generated in the C57BL/6 strain background by Shanghai Model Organisms Center, Inc., (Shanghai, China), as described in detail previously (Zhao et al., 2019). Heterozygous (HE) mutant mice were crossed to generate homozygous $Atp6v1b2^{Arg506*/Arg506*}$ (HO) mutant mice, and WT littermates were used as controls. Male WT and $Atp6v1b2^{Arg506*/Arg506*}$ (HO) mutant mice were tested.

Bax Inhibitor Peptide V5 Treatment

The concentration of Bax inhibitor peptide V5 (BIP-V5) was adjusted to 100 µmol/L with saline. Starting from 4 weeks after birth, mice ($n = 8$) were injected intraperitoneally at a dose of 10 µL/g body weight once weekly until 40 weeks after birth. In addition, WT ($n = 8$) and $Atp6v1b2^{Arg506*/Arg506*}$ ($n = 8$) control mice were injected intraperitoneally with saline alone.

ABR Analysis

Hearing was evaluated in WT and $Atp6v1b2^{Arg506*/Arg506*}$ mice at the age of 4, 12, 20, 28, 36, and 40 weeks ($n = 6$ per genotype and age group). In brief, the stimuli of ABR included click and tone-burst (1, 2, 4, 8, 16, 24, and 32 kHz) and were presented from 90 to 10 dB SPL. Amplitude and latency of ABR wave I were analyzed for 90 dB SPL click stimuli.

Immunostaining

Inner ear tissues were dissected and fixed in 4% paraformaldehyde for 1–2 h at room temperature or for 12 h at 4°C, followed by decalcification in 10% EDTA (pH = 7.2) at 4°C for 5 days. For cryosections, the calcium-depleted cochlea tissues were placed into a 30% sucrose solution for dehydration. Serial sections were cut at 10 µm thickness. For basilar membrane with organ of Corti, cochlea ducts were dissected.

The primary antibodies used were as follows: rabbit anti-Myo7a (Proteus Biosciences, Ramona, CA, United States, 1:300), mouse anti-Ctbp2 (BD Biosciences, San Jose, CA, United States, 1:200), chicken anti-NFH (AB5539, EMD Millipore, Billerica, MA, United States, 1:500), rabbit anti-beta III tubulin (ab230847, Abcam, United Kingdom, 1:500), rabbit anti-cleaved caspase-3

(9661, Cell Signaling Technology, Boston, MA, United States, 1:500), rat anti-MBP (MAB386, EMD Millipore, Billerica, MA, United States, 1:500), rabbit anti-caspase-3 (ab4051, Abcam, United Kingdom, 1:500), rat anti-LAMP1 (ab25245, Abcam, United Kingdom, 1:500), rabbit anti-Bax (ab199677, Abcam, United Kingdom, 1:500), rabbit anti-BCL2 (12789-1-AP, Proteintech, Chicago, IL, United States, 1:500), rabbit anti-LC3B (ab48394, Abcam, United Kingdom, 1:500), rabbit anti-TOM20 (SC-11415, CiteAB, Santa Cruz, CA, United States, 1:500), and mouse anti-cytochrome C (556432, BD Pharmingen, United States, 1:500). The secondary antibodies used were as follows: goat anti-rabbit IgG (A-11008, Thermo Fisher Scientific, Waltham, MA, United States, 1:500), goat anti-mouse IgG (A-10684, Thermo Fisher Scientific, Waltham, MA, United States, 1:500), goat anti-rat IgG (A-11077, Thermo Fisher Scientific, Waltham, MA, United States, 1:500), and goat anti-chicken IgY (A-21449, Thermo Fisher Scientific, Waltham, MA, United States, 1:500). Nuclei were labeled with DAPI.

Confocal Laser Scanning Microscopy

Confocal z-stacks (0.3 μm step size) of cochlea tissues were taken using either a Zeiss LSM800 or a Leica SP8 microscope. ImageJ software (version 1.46, NIH, MD, United States) was used for image processing of z-stacks. All immunofluorescence images shown in this study are representative of at least three individual mice in each group.

Western Blotting

The cochlea tissues were quickly removed from mice and cryo-milled in RIPA lysis buffer and centrifuged. The supernatants were collected, and the protein concentration was detected using the BCA protein assay kit (PI23227, Thermo Fisher Scientific, Waltham, MA, United States). Then equal amounts of protein sample were separated by 12% Tris/Glycine SDS-PAGE and transferred to a polyvinylidene difluoride membrane. The primary antibodies used were the same as those used for immunostaining analysis. The experiments were independently repeated three times.

Transmission Electron Microscopy

Mice were perfused intracardially with 4% paraformaldehyde (in 0.1 M phosphate buffer). Cochleae were then isolated and postfixed with 1.5% paraformaldehyde and 2.5% glutaraldehyde, followed by decalcification in 10% EDTA at 4°C for 5 days and osmification in 1% osmium tetroxide. Then the samples were dehydrated in ethanol and embedded in araldite resin. After resin solidification, semi-thin sections were made stained for localization. Then ultra-thin sections, uranium dioxide acetate saturated and lead citrate were stained respectively. Transmission electron microscopy (TEM) was performed using a Jeol 1400-plus electron microscope (JEM-1400, JEDL, Tokyo). Multiple non-overlapping regions of the ANF cross-sections were imaged at ×3,400 magnification. All images of semi-thin sections and electron microscopy sections shown are representative of at least three individual mice in each group.

RNAscope

Cochleae of 4-week-old mice were perfused and decalcified. After freezing the tissues in OCT compound with dry ice or liquid nitrogen, they were stored in an airtight container at −80°C. Before tissue sectioning, the tissue blocks were placed at −20°C for at least 1 h in a cryostat. The blocks were then sectioned to 7 μm. After air drying the slides for 20 min at −20°C, the RNAscope experiment was performed as previously described (Shrestha et al., 2018; Sun et al., 2018). The following probes for RNA binding were used: Mm-Atp6v1b1 (#804281, Advanced Cell Diagnostics, United States) and Mm-Atp6v1b1-C2 (#804291-C2, Advanced Cell Diagnostics). The sections were imaged using a confocal microscope.

Statistical Analysis

Statistical analyses were performed using Microsoft Excel and SPSS (18.0). Statistical differences were analyzed using t-test. The data are represented as the mean ± SEM. Densitometric analysis in the western blotting experiment was performed using the ImageJ software. P values less than 0.05 were considered to indicate statistical significance.

RESULTS

$Atp6v1b2^{Arg506*/Arg506*}$ Mice Begin to Develop Hidden Hearing Loss at 12 Weeks and Develop Hearing Loss at 28 Weeks After Birth

Mice were phenotyped using ABR at 4–40 weeks of age. The ABR waveform in mice is composed of five peaks, corresponding to electrical signals generated by different components of the peripheral and central auditory pathway (**Figure 1A**). The ABR at 4, 20, and 40 weeks, which represent the early, middle, and aged stages of $Atp6v1b2^{Arg506*/Arg506*}$ mice, are shown in **Figures 1B–D**. The ABR of the mice at other ages are shown in **Supplementary Figures 1A–C**. The thresholds for $Atp6v1b2^{Arg506*/Arg506*}$ mice did not differ significantly from those of WT mice at 4, 12, and 20 weeks. $Atp6v1b2^{Arg506*/Arg506*}$ mice presented hidden hearing loss (HHL) at 12 and 20 weeks with lower P1 amplitudes and a longer latency than WT mice (**Figures 1C,D** and **Supplementary Figures 1B,C**). From 28 weeks, $Atp6v1b2^{Arg506*/Arg506*}$ mice showed progressive HL and increased ABR thresholds compared with WT mice (70 dB SPL average, **Supplementary Figure 1A**). However, DPOAE threshold of 4–32 kHz showed no significant difference between $Atp6v1b2^{Arg506*/Arg506*}$ (4 kHz: 41.67 ± 3.33, 8 kHz: 38.33 ± 1.67, 16 kHz: 43.33 ± 3.33, 32 kHz: 65 ± 5.77, $n = 3$) and WT mice (4 kHz: 40 ± 2.89, 8 kHz: 38.33 ± 4.41, 16 kHz: 45 ± 5.77, 32 kHz: 68.33 ± 3.33, $n = 3$) (T-test, $P > 0.05$, **Supplementary Figure 1D**) at 6 months, which indicated the normal function of outer hair cells (OHCs).

No morphological changes of the organ of Corti between WT and $Atp6v1b2^{Arg506*/Arg506*}$ mice were observed (**Figure 2B**), also indicating that hearing loss in $Atp6v1b2^{Arg506*/Arg506*}$ mice was not related to hair cell loss. The synaptic density

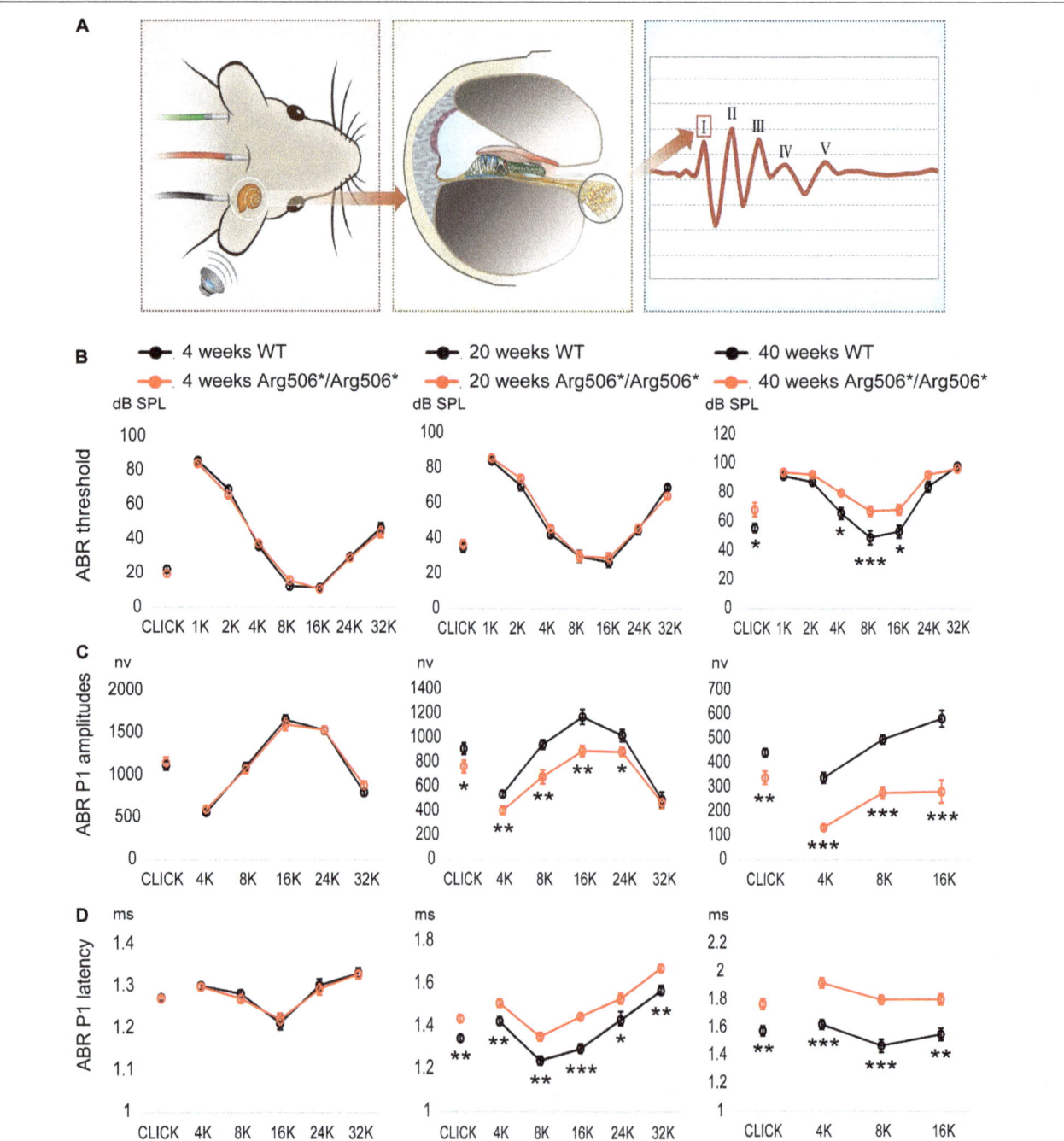

FIGURE 1 | Progressive hearing impairment with increasing age in $Atp6v1b2^{Arg506*/Arg506*}$ mice. **(A)** Auditory brainstem responses (ABR) were recorded to evaluate the hearing in mice. After acoustic stimulation, the recording electrode recorded five waveforms, of which peak I (P1) was derived from spiral ganglion neurons in the mouse cochlea. The hearing thresholds were defined as the lowest sound intensity that elicited identifiable waves. **(B)** ABR thresholds (shown in ordinate) to click and to 1, 2, 4, 8, 16, 24, and 32 kHz (shown in abscissa) tone-burst stimuli were compared between WT and $Atp6v1b2^{Arg506*/Arg506*}$ mice. At 4 weeks and 20 weeks, ABR thresholds showed no significant difference between WT and $Atp6v1b2^{Arg506*/Arg506*}$ mice. At 40 weeks, ABR thresholds to click and to 4, 8, and 16 kHz stimuli were significantly higher in $Atp6v1b2^{Arg506*/Arg506*}$ than in WT mice. **(C)** ABR P1 amplitudes (shown in ordinate) were compared between WT and $Atp6v1b2^{Arg506*/Arg506*}$ mice. There was no significant difference at 4 weeks. At 20 weeks, $Atp6v1b2^{Arg506*/Arg506*}$ mice had significantly lower peaks to click and to 4, 8, 16, and 24 kHz tone-burst stimuli than WT mice. At 40 weeks, $Atp6v1b2^{Arg506*/Arg506*}$ mice had significantly lower peaks to click and to 4, 8, and 16 kHz tone-burst stimuli than WT mice. **(D)** ABR P1 latencies (shown in ordinate) stimulated by different sound types (shown in abscissa) with the same sound intensity (90 dB SPL) were compared between WT and $Atp6v1b2^{Arg506*/Arg506*}$ mice. There was no significant difference at 4 weeks. At 20 weeks, $Atp6v1b2^{Arg506*/Arg506*}$ mice showed significantly longer latencies to click and to 4, 8, 16, 24 and 32 kHz tone-burst stimuli than WT mice. At 40 weeks, $Atp6v1b2^{Arg506*/Arg506*}$ mice showed significantly longer latencies to click and to 4, 8, and 16 kHz tone-burst stimuli than WT mice. The t-test was performed to evaluate statistical significance; n represents the number of test ears, n = 6 for each group; * denotes $P < 0.05$, ** denotes $P < 0.01$, *** denotes $P < 0.001$. Data are described as mean ± SEM (standard error of mean).

in $Atp6v1b2^{Arg506*/Arg506*}$ mice did not differ significantly from that in WT mice at different ages (**Supplementary Figure 2**). Interestingly, although the auditory nerve fibers of $Atp6v1b2^{Arg506*/Arg506*}$ mice did not change significantly at 4 weeks, the myelin sheath covering the auditory nerve fibers decreased at 20 weeks (**Figures 2C,D**). We labeled the unmyelinated nerve fibers in the osseous spiral lamina (OSL) of mouse cochlea with the NFH antibody (**Supplementary Figures 3A–F**). In the cochlea of $Atp6v1b2^{Arg506*/Arg506*}$ mice at 20 weeks, parts of auditory nerve fibers in the OSL stained positive for NFH, indicating the presence of auditory nerve fiber demyelination (**Supplementary Figures 3C,F**), which was consistent with myelin stain results (**Figures 2C,D**). To further clarify the changes in myelination of the nerve fibers, we performed TEM to observe the morphology of the myelin sheath in mice at 4, 12, and 20 weeks of age (**Supplementary Figures 3G–L**). $Atp6v1b2^{Arg506*/Arg506*}$ mice showed vacuolar-like changes in the myelin sheath of auditory nerve fibers in the OSL at 4 weeks, but the myelin sheath was still wrapped around the nerve fibers (**Supplementary Figure 3J**). Demyelination was observed in the auditory nerve fibers of $Atp6v1b2^{Arg506*/Arg506*}$ mice at 12 and 20 weeks (**Supplementary Figures 3K,L**). These changes did not appear in WT mice (**Supplementary Figures 3G–I**). The above results indicate that demyelination of cochlear auditory nerve fibers was the pathological basis for HHL in $Atp6v1b2^{Arg506*/Arg506*}$ mice.

In addition, the number of SGNs decreased significantly in $Atp6v1b2^{Arg506*/Arg506*}$ mice compared to that in WT mice at 40 weeks (**Figures 2E,F**). The excitation of type I SGNs is caused by the action potential of IHCs and is further transmitted to the neuronal body, type II SGNs connect the OHCs and are mainly responsible for receiving signals from the OHCs (**Figure 2A**). Another special feature of type II SGNs is that the cell bodies and the nerve fibers that connect the OHCs are unmyelinated. By labeling type II nerve fibers with NFH antibody, we found that the number of type II nerve fibers connecting the OHCs was reduced in $Atp6v1b2^{Arg506*/Arg506*}$ mice at 28 weeks (**Supplementary Figures 1E,F**). In summary, the decrease in SGNs was the cause of hearing loss in the aged $Atp6v1b2^{Arg506*/Arg506*}$ mice.

Atp6v1b2 c.1516C > T Causes Abnormal Autophagy, Which Leads to Apoptosis of the SGNs in $Atp6v1b2^{Arg506*/Arg506*}$ Mice

Western blotting results revealed increased LC3-II in the cochlea of $Atp6v1b2^{Arg506*/Arg506*}$ mice (**Figure 3B**), indicating that autophagosomes accumulated in the cytoplasm. In $Atp6v1b2^{Arg506*/Arg506*}$ mice, autophagosomes increased in the SGNs (**Figure 3A**). However, in the organ of Corti, there was no significant difference between WT and $Atp6v1b2^{Arg506*/Arg506*}$ mice (**Supplementary Figure 4A**). To evaluate if this increase in autophagosomes in the SGNs could be explained by a fusion barrier between autophagosomes and lysosomes or the abnormal degradation of the lysosome, we performed TEM analysis. The results showed high levels of substrates in the autophagic lysosomes of the SGNs in $Atp6v1b2^{Arg506*/Arg506*}$ mice (**Figure 4A**), indicating that autophagosomes could fuse with the lysosomes. However, the proportion of autolysosomes increased in the SGNs of $Atp6v1b2^{Arg506*/Arg506*}$ mice (**Figure 4B**), suggesting that the substrates in the lysosomal cavity could not be effectively degraded, which further made it difficult for autophagosomes to enter lysosomes. Thus, we speculated that abnormal lysosomal degradation was the cause of the autophagosome accumulation in the cytoplasm of the SGNs.

Immunofluorescence analysis revealed that cytochrome C was released from the mitochondria to the cytosol of the SGNs of $Atp6v1b2^{Arg506*/Arg506*}$ mice (**Figure 3C**). Western blotting results showed that in the cochlea of $Atp6v1b2^{Arg506*/Arg506*}$ mice, the ratio of Bcl-2 to Bax was reduced significantly compared with that in WT mice (**Figure 3D**). Results showed that cleaved caspase-3 in the inner ear of $Atp6v1b2^{Arg506*/Arg506*}$ mice increased significantly (**Figure 3F**). To further verify the exact area of apoptosis, immunofluorescence staining was performed. The results showed that in the cochlea of $Atp6v1b2^{Arg506*/Arg506*}$ mice, apoptosis was mostly observed in the spiral ganglia (**Figure 3E**), and no excessive apoptosis was identified in the organ of Corti (**Supplementary Figure 4C**).

These data suggested that in the inner ear of $Atp6v1b2^{Arg506*/Arg506*}$ mice, disequilibrium of the acidic environment in the lysosomes and autophagosome accumulation in the cytoplasm led to a decrease in the ratio of Bcl-2 to Bax, which further increased the outer membrane permeability of the mitochondria and induced the release of cytochrome C and activation of caspase-3.

BIP-V5 Improves Phenotypical and Pathological Outcomes in $Atp6v1b2^{Arg506*/Arg506*}$ Mice

During the process of BIP-V5 administration, four mice in the $Atp6v1b2^{Arg506*/Arg506*}$-BIP-V5 group died, thus affecting the statistics of the experimental data. We observed that the hearing threshold was restored in two out of four $Atp6v1b2^{Arg506*/Arg506*}$ mice treated with BIP-V5, and they had better ABR waveforms (**Supplementary Figure 5**), suggesting a potential role of BIP-V5 in improving the hearing of mutant mice. After BIP-V5 intervention, the expression of Bax (**Supplementary Figure 6**) and the release of cytochrome C (**Supplementary Figure 7C**) in the mitochondria of the cochlea were significantly reduced. In addition, immunostaining and western blotting results showed that active caspase-3 (**Supplementary Figures 6,7D**) in the cochlea of $Atp6v1b2^{Arg506*/Arg506*}$ mice was reduced and the number of SGNs (**Supplementary Figure 7A**) increased significantly with BIP-V5 intervention, but lysosomal function evaluated by autophagosomes was not significantly changed (**Supplementary Figures 6,7B**).

Genetic Compensation Exists in the Hair Cells of $Atp6v1b2^{Arg506*/Arg506*}$ Mice

Clinically, patients diagnosed with *ATP6V1B2*-related syndromes have congenital severe to profound sensorineural hearing loss (Yuan et al., 2014; Menendez et al., 2017; Beauregard-Lacroix et al., 2020); however, the hearing of $Atp6v1b2^{Arg506*/Arg506*}$ mice

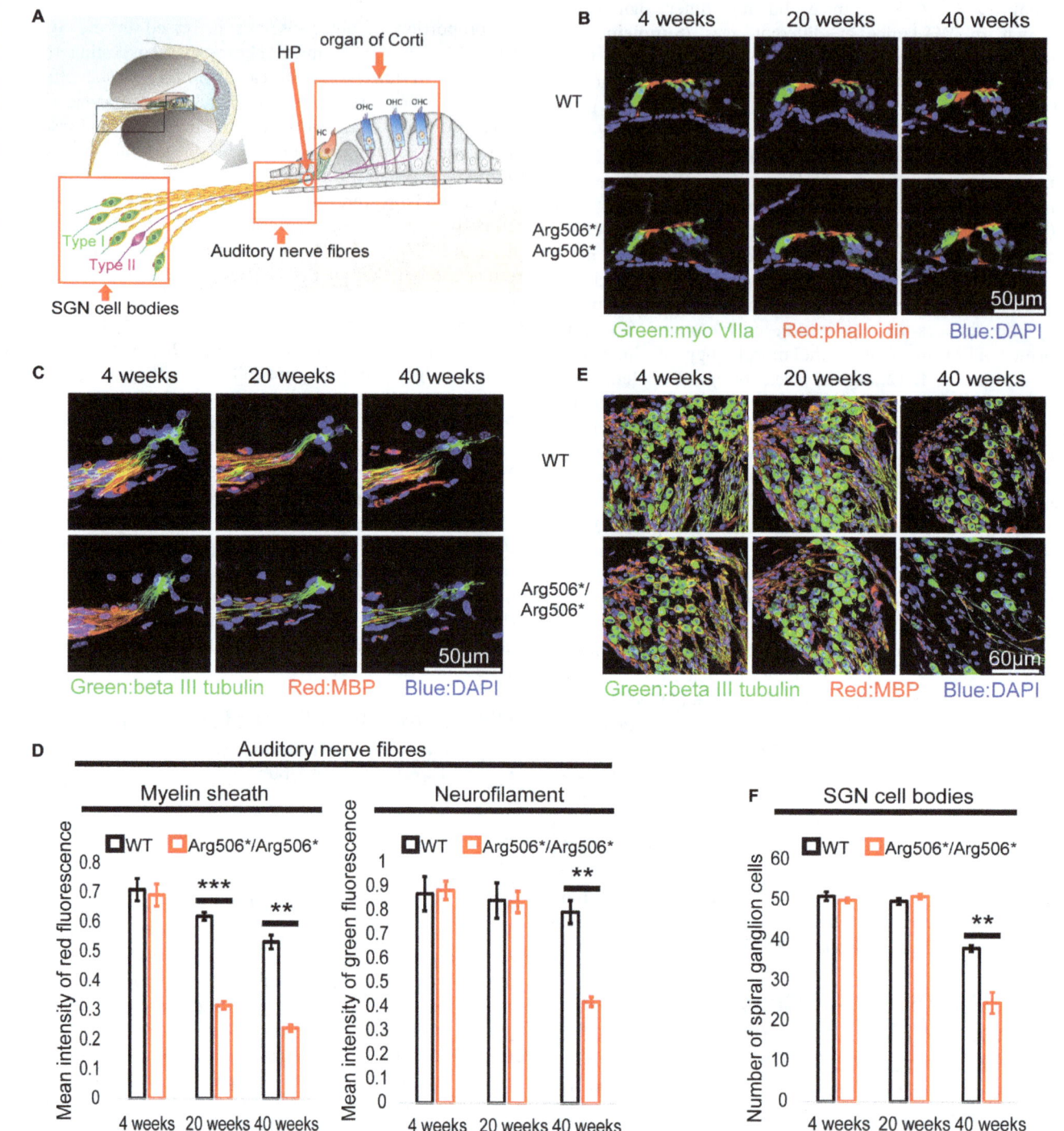

FIGURE 2 | Abnormal morphology in the cochlea of $Atp6v1b2^{Arg506*/Arg506*}$ mice at different postnatal ages of 4, 20, and 40 weeks. **(A)** Illustration of the cochlear architecture. The three areas within the red frame (from left to right): spiral ganglion neuron (SGN) cell bodies, auditory nerve fibers, and organ of Corti. **(B)** There is no obvious difference in the morphology of organ of Corti between WT and $Atp6v1b2^{Arg506*/Arg506*}$ mice. Phalloidin, MyoVIIa, and DAPI are markers of hair cell cilia, inner/outer hair cells, and nuclei, respectively. The experiments were repeated three times. **(C)** Representative images of auditory nerve fibers for WT and $Atp6v1b2^{Arg506*/Arg506*}$ mice. **(D)** Statistical results of the red and green fluorescence intensities for panel **(C)**. The intensity of red fluorescence (myelin) decreased significantly at 20 and 40 weeks in $Atp6v1b2^{Arg506*/Arg506*}$ mice. The intensity of green fluorescence (nerve fibers) decreased significantly at 40 weeks in $Atp6v1b2^{Arg506*/Arg506*}$ mice. **(E)** Representative images of SGN cell bodies of WT and $Atp6v1b2^{Arg506*/Arg506*}$ mice. **(F)** Statistical results of the number of SGN cell bodies for panel **(E)**. The number of SGN cell bodies decreased significantly in $Atp6v1b2^{Arg506*/Arg506*}$ mice compared to that in WT mice at 40 weeks. The myelin sheath, nerve fibers, and nuclei are labeled with red (MBP), green (beta III tubulin), and blue (DAPI) fluorescence, respectively. The t-test was performed to evaluate the statistical significance. Each group included three mice, and one slice for each mouse was processed. ** denotes $P < 0.01$, *** denotes $P < 0.001$. Data are described as mean ± SEM (standard error of mean). HP, habenula perforate.

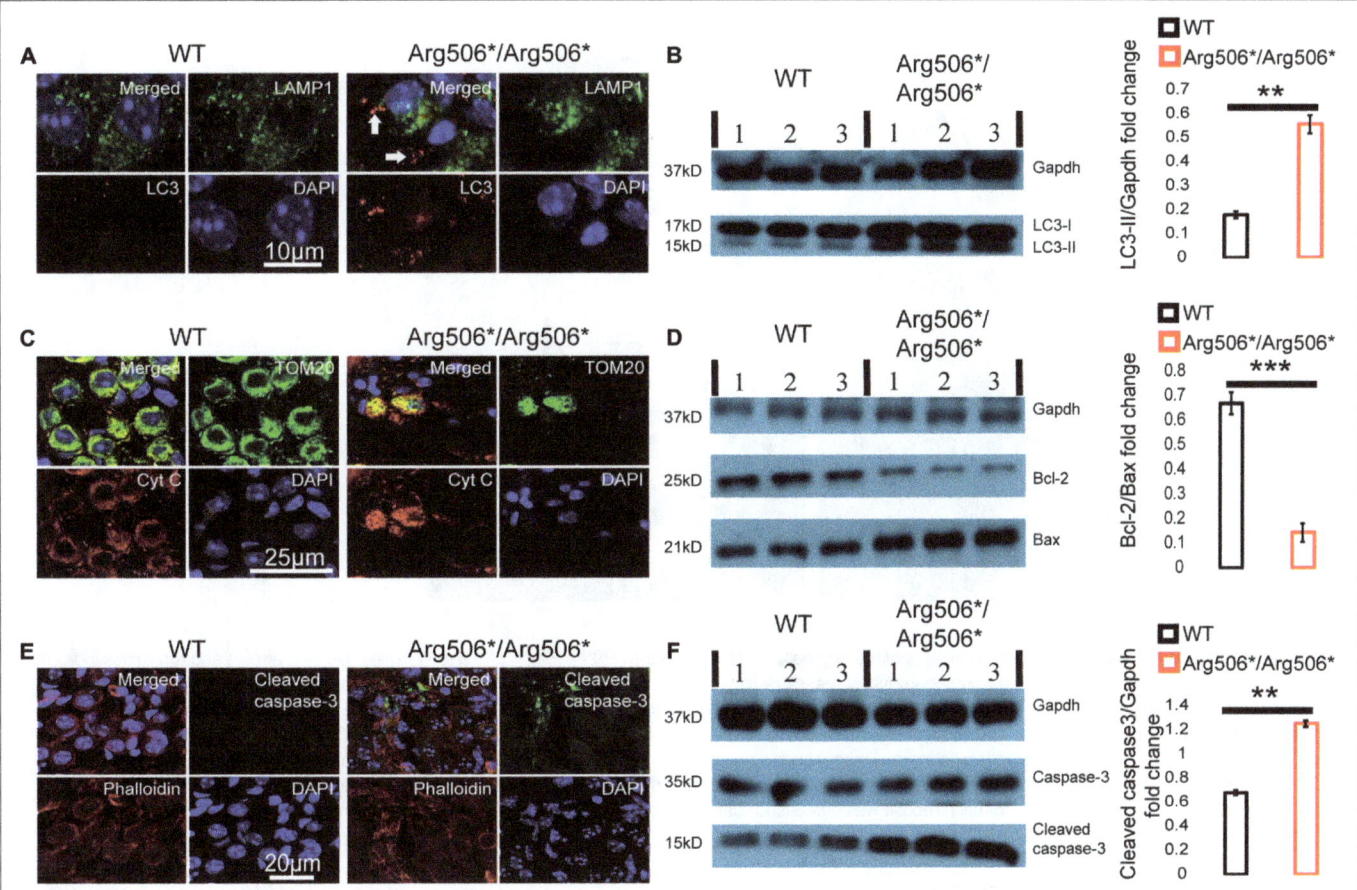

FIGURE 3 | Abnormal autophagy and apoptosis activated by cytochrome C in the spiral ganglion neurons (SGNs) of $Atp6v1b2^{Arg506*/Arg506*}$ mice. **(A)** Representative images of immunostaining showed that autophagosomes labeled with LC3 (white arrows) were present in large numbers as dots in the SGNs of $Atp6v1b2^{Arg506*/Arg506*}$ mice. **(B)** Left: Western blotting results showed that LC3-II increased in the cochlea of $Atp6v1b2^{Arg506*/Arg506*}$ mice compared with that in the cochlea of WT mice. LC3-II can be used to estimate the extent of autophagy. Right: Statistical results of gray value for western blotting. The ratio of LC3-II/Gapdh in the cochlea of $Atp6v1b2^{Arg506*/Arg506*}$ mice was significantly higher than that in the cochlea of WT mice (** denotes $P < 0.01$ by t-test; $n = 3$ for each group). **(C)** The release of cytochrome C from the mitochondria into the cytosol of the SGNs in $Atp6v1b2^{Arg506*/Arg506*}$ mice is shown. Mitochondria are labeled with TOM20 (green). Cytochrome C is labeled as red. In WT mice, cytochrome C remains in the mitochondria and no red signal was observed in the cytosol of the SGNs. In $Atp6v1b2^{Arg506*/Arg506*}$ mice, cytochrome C was observed both in the mitochondria and the cytosol of the SGNs, indicating its release from mitochondria. **(D)** Left: Western blotting results showed that in the cochlea of $Atp6v1b2^{Arg506*/Arg506*}$ mice, Bcl-2 decreased significantly compared with that in the cochlea of WT mice. Right: Statistical results of gray value for western blotting (*** denotes $P < 0.001$ by t-test; $n = 3$ for each group). **(E)** More pronounced positive signal for cleaved caspase-3 in the region of SGNs of $Atp6v1b2^{Arg506*/Arg506*}$ mice was identified. Phalloidin is a high-affinity filamentous actin (F-actin) marker, which is used to mark the cytoskeleton. **(F)** Left: Western blotting results showed that cleaved caspase-3 increased in the cochlea of $Atp6v1b2^{Arg506*/Arg506*}$ mice compared with that in the cochlea of WT mice. Right: Statistical results of gray value for western blotting. The ratio of cleaved caspase-3/Gapdh in the cochlea of $Atp6v1b2^{Arg506*/Arg506*}$ mice was significantly higher than that in the cochlea of WT mice. ** denotes $P < 0.01$. $n = 3$ for each group. Data are described as mean ± SEM (standard error of mean). Cyt C, cytochrome C.

was quite different. To verify whether functional compensation occurs in the cochlea of $Atp6v1b2^{Arg506*/Arg506*}$ mice, we determined the $Atp6v1b2$ and $Atp6v1b1$ transcription levels and localization in the cochlea of mice at 4 weeks by RNAscope and found that the RNA level of $Atp6v1b2$ was down-regulated in both the SGNs and hair cells in $Atp6v1b2^{Arg506*/Arg506*}$ mice compared with that in WT mice, indicating that the transcription level of $Atp6v1b2$ decreased or that the RNA was excessively degraded. In $Atp6v1b2^{Arg506*/Arg506*}$ mice, the transcription level of $Atp6v1b1$ significantly increased in the hair cells but not in the SGNs. These results suggested that $Atp6v1b1$ may compensate for the loss of $Atp6v1b2$ function in the hair cells (**Figures 5A,B**).

DISCUSSION

The manifestation of normal auditory thresholds but reduced suprathreshold amplitude of the sound-evoked compound action potential of SGNs, shown as peak I of the ABR waveform, is defined as HHL (Kujawa and Liberman, 2009; Bharadwaj et al., 2014; Mehraei et al., 2016). The pathological mechanisms of HHL are complicated and are not yet fully understood. The electrophysiological results showed that $Atp6v1b2^{Arg506*/Arg506*}$ mice younger than 20 weeks did not have an elevated ABR threshold but had lower P1 amplitudes and longer P1 latencies than WT mice, similar to patients with HHL

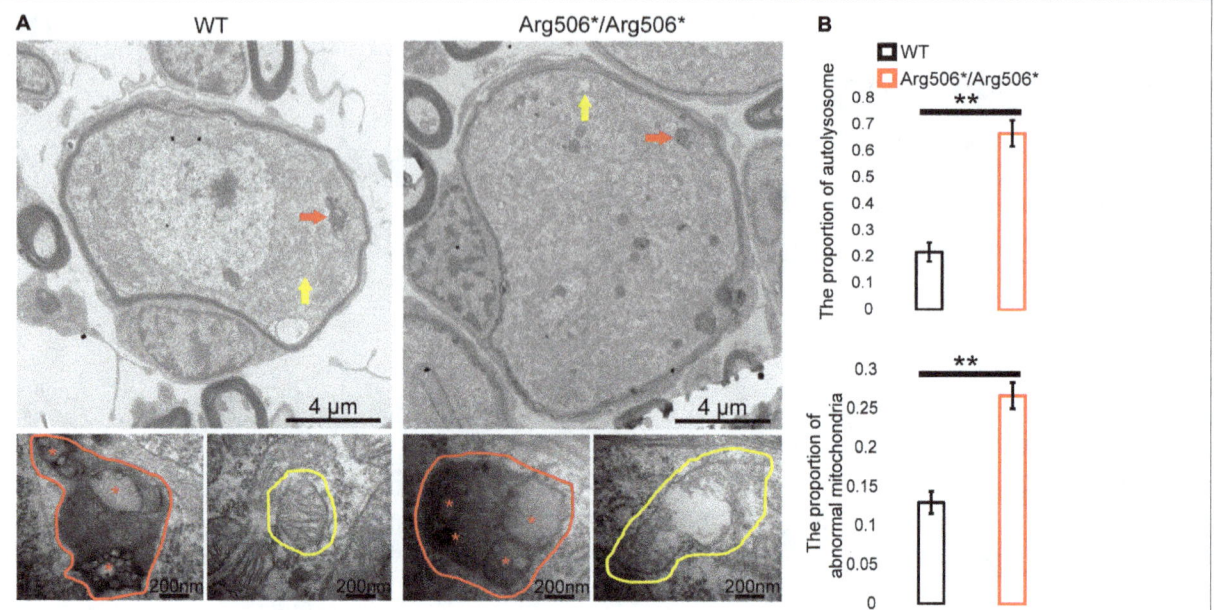

FIGURE 4 | Transmission electron microscopy images of the organelles of SGNs in $Atp6v1b2^{Arg506*/Arg506*}$ and WT mice. **(A)** Red arrows and red circles indicate the locations and enlarged views of a typical autophagy lysosome, respectively. Yellow arrows and yellow circles indicate the locations and enlarged views of mitochondria, respectively. In $Atp6v1b2^{Arg506*/Arg506*}$ mice, increased degraded substrates indicated by red asterisks in the autophagy lysosomes of the spiral ganglion neurons (SGNs) were observed, and some of the mitochondria appeared swollen. Most of the mitochondria in the SGNs showed normal morphology in WT mice. **(B)** The percentage of autolysosomes and abnormal mitochondria significantly increased in $Atp6v1b2^{Arg506*/Arg506*}$ mice. The t-test was performed to evaluate statistical significance. The percentage of autolysosomes in lysosomes and the percentage of abnormal mitochondria were manually determined. Each group included three mice, and one slice for each mouse was processed. Data are described as mean ± SEM (standard error of mean). ** denotes $P < 0.01$.

(Mehraei et al., 2016). Current studies suggest that risk factors associated with HHL include a noisy environment (Liu H. et al., 2019), aging (Fischer et al., 2019), and ototoxic drugs (Liu et al., 2015). LOHL (late-onset hearing loss) is defined as hearing loss that is not present at birth but is identified at a later period. Both environmental and hereditary factors influence the development of LOHL. Clinically, there is no early diagnostic indicator for LOHL until hearing loss is detected. HHL and LOHL are regarded as two diseases with different pathogeneses (Song et al., 2020). We proposed that (1) the $Atp6v1b2^{Arg506*/Arg506*}$ mouse model could be used as a natural model for HHL and LOHL; (2) patients with LOHL may have HHL early in life, and it is important for those who have been diagnosed with HHL to be cautious of risk factors such as noise, ototoxic drugs, etc. to avoid further hearing impairment.

Abnormalities in ribbon synaptic density and demyelination of the auditory nerve fibers have been identified as causes of HHL (Liberman and Kujawa, 2017; Wan and Corfas, 2017). In our study, we identified that HHL in $Atp6v1b2^{Arg506*/Arg506*}$ mice was caused by demyelination of nerve fibers but not the ribbon synaptic density. Schwann cells are essential for the formation of nodes of Ranvier, which is a special structure along the myelinated fibers where voltage-gated sodium channels and potassium channels accumulate for regeneration of action potentials and fast synchronous transmission of electrical signals. This phenomenon explains why nerve fibers with myelin sheaths can conduct action potentials more quickly and efficiently than nerve fibers without myelin sheaths (Rasband and Peles, 2015).

Damage or loss of cells from the auditory pathway in the cochlea, such as IHCs and/or OHCs, supporting cells and SGNs, is a pathological feature of LOHL (Vreugde et al., 2002; Liu et al., 2016; Cheng et al., 2019; Gao et al., 2019; Han et al., 2020; Zhang S. et al., 2020; Zhang Y. et al., 2020; Chen et al., 2021). HCs are highly specialized cells attached to the basement membrane in the organ of Corti in the cochlea, and mainly function in transduce the sound mechanical vibration into the electrical signal (He et al., 2017, 2020, 2021; Tan et al., 2019; Jiang et al., 2020; Zhong et al., 2020; Zhou et al., 2020). These cells have hair-like protrusions (stereocilia) embedded in the tectorial membrane (Wang et al., 2017; Liu Y. et al., 2019; Qi et al., 2019, 2020; Cheng et al., 2021; Fu et al., 2021; Zhang et al., 2021). Incoming soundwaves distort the basement membrane, and the resulting mechanical distortion of the stereocilia is transduced into neural signals that are conveyed through the SGNs to the auditory regions of the brain (Ding et al., 2020; Guo et al., 2020; Jiang et al., 2020; Qian et al., 2020; Liu et al., 2021; Lv et al., 2021; Yuan et al., 2021). Improved culture system of SGNs facilitates the study of physiology and pathophysiology, and promotes identification of potential therapeutic targets for SGNs protection and regeneration (Guo et al., 2016, 2019, 2020; Waqas et al., 2017; Yan et al., 2018; Liu W. et al., 2019; Liu et al., 2021). In this study, $Atp6v1b2^{Arg506*/Arg506*}$ mice developed demyelination of nerve fibers, followed by loss of nerve fibers and SGN cell bodies. This process appears to be neurodegenerative. However, the cochlear hair cells of $Atp6v1b2^{Arg506*/Arg506*}$ mice were morphologically normal.

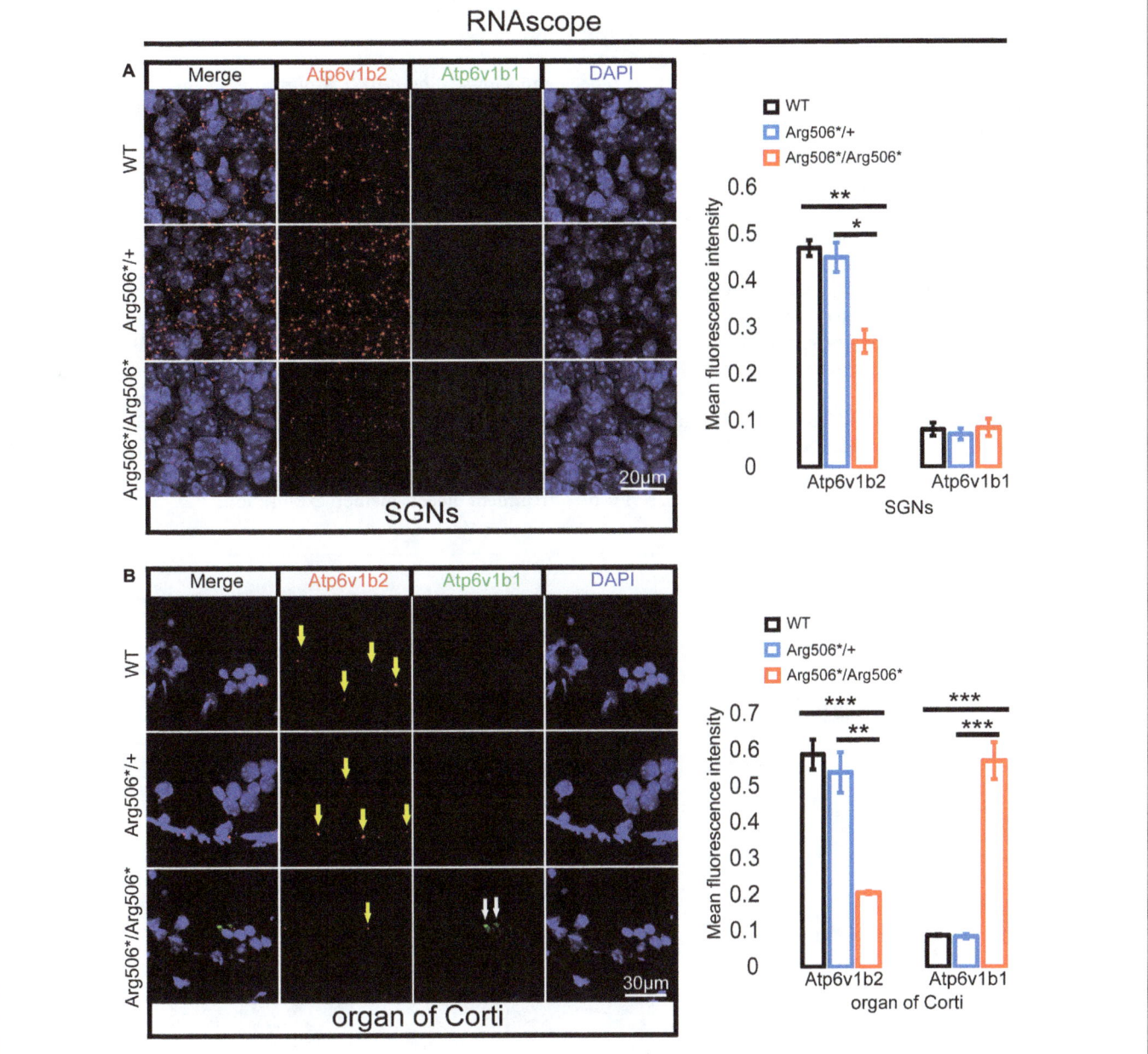

FIGURE 5 | Increased transcription of *Atp6v1b1* occurs in the hair cells of *Atp6v1b2*$^{Arg506*/Arg506*}$ mice. **(A)** Representative images and quantification of RNAscope results in the spiral ganglion neurons (SGNs). The mean fluorescence intensity of *Atp6v1b2* RNA in *Atp6v1b2*$^{Arg506*/Arg506*}$ mice was significantly lower than that in WT and *Atp6v1b2*$^{Arg506*/+}$ mice. No *Atp6v1b1* RNA was found in the SGNs. **(B)** Representative images and quantification of RNAscope results in the organ of Corti. *Atp6v1b2* RNA decreased in *Atp6v1b2*$^{Arg506*/Arg506*}$ mice compared with that in WT and *Atp6v1b2*$^{Arg506*/+}$ mice (yellow arrow). There was no significant difference in the mean fluorescence intensity of *Atp6v1b2* RNA between WT and *Atp6v1b2*$^{Arg506*/+}$ mice. *Atp6v1b1* RNA was found in the hair cells of *Atp6v1b2*$^{Arg506*/Arg506*}$ mice (white arrow) but not in the hair cells of WT and *Atp6v1b2*$^{Arg506*/+}$ mice. $n = 3$ for each group. * denotes $P < 0.05$, ** denotes $P < 0.01$ and *** denotes $P < 0.001$. Data are described as mean ± SEM (standard error of mean).

Hearing loss in patients with DDOD syndrome is primarily treated by cochlear implantation. However, although the implanted cochlea worked well, clinical follow-up of DDOD syndrome patients with cochlear implantation revealed that their language rehabilitation was unsatisfactory. Our findings regarding the pathological changes in SGNs and mild learning and memory problems in DDOD syndrome patients (Zhao et al., 2019) could explain this clinical puzzle.

V-ATPase has two main effects on the organelle: maintaining the acidic environment of the organelles and participating in and regulating the fusion between vesicle-type organelles, such as the fusion between lysosomes and autophagosomes (Colacurcio and Nixon, 2016). We have demonstrated that abnormalities in the assembly of the subunits of V-ATPase occurred in *Atp6v1b2*$^{Arg506*/Arg506*}$ mice, which affects the transfer of hydrogen ions into the lysosome (Yuan et al., 2014;

Zhao et al., 2019). In this study, we observed the presence of metabolic substrates inside lysosomes, which indicated there might be no fusion barrier between lysosomes and autophagosomes in $Atp6v1b2^{Arg506*/Arg506*}$ mice. The degradation of lysosomes depends on the presence of multiple hydrolases, and the activity of these hydrolases requires an acidic environment (De Duve, 1957; Saftig and Haas, 2016). We found abnormal degradation of metabolic substrates in lysosomes of the SGNs in $Atp6v1b2^{Arg506*/Arg506*}$ mice as a result of the abnormal acidic environment and the affected activity of the hydrolases in the lysosomes. In addition, redundant autophagosomes were observed outside the lysosomes in the SGNs of $Atp6v1b2^{Arg50*/Arg506*}$ mice, indicating that high levels of undegraded substrates in the lysosomes affected the normal process of autophagic flow (Colacurcio and Nixon, 2016).

We observed an increase in caspase-3, the ultimate initiator of apoptosis, in the SGNs and Schwann cells of $Atp6v1b2^{Arg506*/Arg506*}$ mice, which suggested that lysosomal dysfunction induced apoptosis. Mitochondrial dysfunction and premature termination of cell cycle occur when a series of lysosomal functional abnormalities present, such as increased intraluminal pH value, abnormal degradation, and excessive accumulation of exogenous substrate for lysosomes (Hughes and Gottschling, 2012; Molin and Demir, 2014; Ruckenstuhl et al., 2014). Cell damage triggers degradation of the Bcl-2 family of proteins, which in turn activates Bax. Activated Bax/Bak complexes bind to and reduce the permeability of the mitochondrial membrane, resulting in cytochrome C release to the cytosol. Cytochrome C induces apoptosome formation, which can directly activate caspase-3 (Kroemer et al., 2007; Galluzzi et al., 2012; Ilmarinen et al., 2014).

Next, we evaluated whether treatment with the Bax inhibitor BIP-V5 could ameliorate the hearing loss in the mutant mice. After 36-week systemic administration of BIP-V5, auditory function and pathological changes improved in two out of four $Atp6v1b2^{Arg506*/Arg506*}$-BIP-V5 mice, which further verifies that apoptosis induces the degeneration of SGNs and further impaired the hearing. As the reason for mortality was unknown in 50% (four out of eight) of the treated mice, the safety of BIP-V5 treatment needs further exploration. Bax plays an important

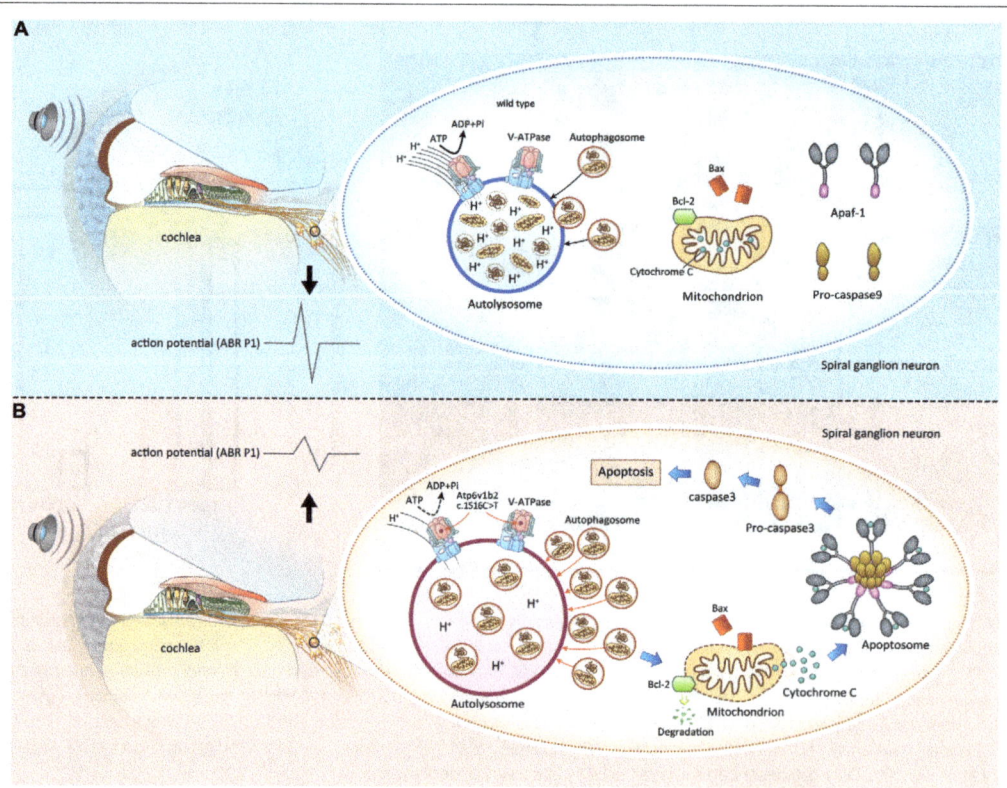

FIGURE 6 | Apoptosis induced by lysosome dysfunction and autophagic flux block in spiral ganglion neurons (SGNs) causes hearing impairment in $Atp6v1b2^{Arg506*/Arg506*}$ mice. **(A)** In WT mice, V-ATPases in the SGNs maintain the acidic environment by pumping protons into the lumen of lysosomes. It is a process that requires ATP hydrolysis. When autophagosomes enter the lysosomes, the intracellular components carried by autophagosomes are degraded. The magnitude of peak I (P1) amplitudes of ABR correlates with the number and synchronous firing rate of the SGN fibers. **(B)** $Atp6v1b2$ c.1516 C > T affects the assembly of V-ATPases and their role in pumping protons into the lumen of lysosomes. Thus, the pH in the lysosomes increases, and the activity of acid hydrolases decreases. Under this circumstance, the autophagosomes are not effectively degraded and they accumulate in the lysosomes, which further affects the entrance of other autophagosomes. When the anti-apoptotic member of Bcl-2 family, Bcl-2, detects the acid environment disequilibrium in the lysosomes and autophagosome accumulation within the cytoplasm, it itself degrades, which in turn activates Bax/Bak complexes. Bax binds to and decreases the permeability of the mitochondrial membrane, leading to cytochrome C release. Cytochrome C binds to its partner Apaf-1 to induce the formation of a caspase-9-activating protein complex known as an apoptosome, which directly activates caspase-3, the ultimate initiator of the apoptosis process. Once apoptosis occurs in the SGNs, the hearing is impaired.

role in programmed cell death or apoptosis and contributes to maintenance of normal psychological functions of various organs. *Atp6v1b2* gene is highly expressed in the inner ear and central nervous system of mice (Yue et al., 2014), and we presented the Arg506* mutation might induce Bax-mediated apoptosis. Therefore, administration of BIP-V5 to inhibit Bax is a reasonable way to maintain normal apoptosis in the inner ear and central nervous system. However, *Atp6v1b2* gene is rarely expressed in some organs such as the adrenal gland, intestine, stomach, liver, etc. and the mutation has minimal effect on Bax. In this case, intervention of Bax is likely to disrupt the normal physiological functions of these organs and lead to abnormalities (Kanauchi et al., 2002; Anagnostopoulos et al., 2005; Zhou et al., 2017; Al Humayed et al., 2020). Therefore, although intraperitoneal administration can control the apoptosis of spiral ganglion cells to a certain extent, it also has serious side effects on other important organs, and even leads to death. Topical administration of the inner ear might avoid the high mortality caused by intraperitoneal administration in mice, but this also brings an additional problem: the mice require long-term drug intervention, and routine operation of multiple cochlear administrations in mice can damage the structure of the inner ear, thus affecting hearing. Therefore, in order to achieve the purpose of hearing recovery by targeted drug intervention in the inner ear of mice, it is crucial to explore a new surgical method in the future.

Patients with *ATP6V1B2*-related syndromes showed severe congenital sensorineural hearing loss, which was not consistent with the milder hearing phenotype of $Atp6v1b2^{Arg506*/Arg506*}$ mice despite the presence of the same type of mutation (Menendez et al., 2017). Based on the finding that hair cells were not affected in $Atp6v1b2^{Arg506*/Arg506*}$ mice, we hypothesized the presence of genetic compensation. Genetic compensation was already shown between isoforms of V-ATPases. For example, compensation exists between *Atp6v1g1* and *Atp6v1g2*, both of which encode the V1G subunit. The V1G subunit plays an important role in the nervous system. Defects in the V1G subunit can lead to cognitive disorders. However, $Atp6v1g2^{-/-}$ mice did not show any developmental defects or obvious behavioral abnormalities until adulthood, which is considered to be associated with the upregulation of *Atp6v1g1* in the mouse brain (Kawamura et al., 2015).

The V1B subunits of the V-ATPase are encoded by *Atp6v1b2* and *Atp6v1b1*. *Atp6v1b2* mRNA is ubiquitously expressed in mouse tissues, including the inner ears. *Atp6v1b1* is mainly expressed in the kidney, epididymis, eyes, and inner ears (Tian et al., 2017). The B2 subunit of V-ATPase was shown to compensate for the function of the B1 subunit of V-ATPase in the renal medullary intercalated cells of B1-deficient mice (Paunescu et al., 2007). In this study, we observed increased transcription of *Atp6v1b1* in hair cells of $Atp6v1b2^{Arg506*/Arg506*}$ mice and inferred that *Atp6v1b1* compensated for the *Atp6v1b2* dysfunction by increasing its own transcription level. Genetic compensation in hair cells explains the milder hearing impairment in $Atp6v1b2^{Arg506*/Arg506*}$ mice. The mechanism of elevated transcription may be due to an enhancement in the promoter region of the gene by trimethylation (El-Brolosy et al., 2019; Ma et al., 2019). However, if a mutation occurs only at the transcriptome level and not at the DNA level, this compensatory mechanism will not be activated (Rossi et al., 2015; Ma et al., 2019). This finding was verified by our previous work: when we injected morpholinos designed to knock down *Atp6v1b2* mRNA in the cochlea of mice, the hair cells were damaged, and the mice showed severe hearing loss (Yuan et al., 2014). In addition, the cognitive and memory impairment in $Atp6v1b2^{Arg506*/Arg506*}$ mice was verified to be caused by apoptosis in the hippocampus (**Supplementary Figure 8**). We speculated that the function of *Atp6v1b2* gene is more important or more specific both in the SGNs and the central nervous system than in the hair cells, and thus it might not be fully compensated by other genes, or that defect of *Atp6v1b2* does not induce functional compensation in the regions of SGNs and hippocampus.

CONCLUSION

Based on the findings of this study and our previous studies, we elucidated the pathogenesis of *Atp6v1b2* defects as follows: (1) the mutation causes dysfunctional assembly between V-ATPase V1 subunits, and H^+ transfer to lysosomes is decreased, which leads to an increased pH value; (2) disequilibrium in the acidic environment of the lysosome further affects the function of acid-dependent hydrolytic enzymes, resulting in the accumulation of degradation substrates; (3) the Bcl-2 family detects abnormal lysosome autophagy and then induces the release of cytochrome C from the mitochondria; and (4) apoptosis occurs in SGNs, affecting hearing function (**Figure 6**).

ETHICS STATEMENT

The animal study was reviewed and approved by the institutional animal care and use committee of the Chinese PLA General Hospital.

AUTHOR CONTRIBUTIONS

SQ, WZ, and YY drafted the manuscript. SQ and WZ participated in the construction and analysis of *Atp6v1b2* c.1516C > T knockin mice and performed western blotting, electron microscopy, RNAscope, and BIP-V5 treatment. DL and BG carried out the experiments of immunohistochemistry. XG and WW performed the auditory evaluation and statistical analysis. YY and PD conceived the study. PC, SY, and WH participated in its design and coordination. All authors read and approved the final manuscript.

SUPPLEMENTARY MATERIAL

Supplementary Figure 1 | $Atp6v1b2^{Arg506*/Arg506*}$ mice show HHL at 12 weeks and LOHL at 28 weeks. **(A)** ABR thresholds in mice aged 12 and 28 weeks. At 12 weeks, ABR thresholds showed no significant difference between WT and

$Atp6v1b2^{Arg506*/Arg506*}$ mice. At 28 weeks, ABR thresholds of 4 and 8 kHz stimulations were significantly lower in WT than in $Atp6v1b2^{Arg506*/Arg506*}$ mice. **(B)** ABR P1 amplitudes in mice aged 12 and 28 weeks. $Atp6v1b2^{Arg506*/Arg506*}$ mice at 12 and 28 weeks had lower peaks to click as well as 4, 8, and 16 kHz stimulations than WT mice. **(C)** ABR P1 latencies in mice aged 12 and 28 weeks. At 12 weeks, $Atp6v1b2^{Arg506*/Arg506*}$ mice showed longer latencies to 16 and 24 kHz stimulations than WT mice. At 28 weeks, $Atp6v1b2^{Arg506*/Arg506*}$ mice showed significantly longer latencies to click as well as 4, 8, and 16 kHz stimulations than WT mice. The t-test was used to evaluate statistical significance; n represents the number of test ears, $n = 6$ for each group; * denotes $P < 0.05$, ** denotes $P < 0.01$, *** denotes $P < 0.001$. Data were described as mean ± SEM (standard error of mean). **(D)** DPOAE thresholds of $Atp6v1b2^{Arg506*/Arg506*}$ and WT mice at 6 months after birth. The acoustic frequency was set to 4~32kHz, and the acoustic intensity was set to gradually decrease from 80 dB SPL until reliable DPOAE signal could not be extracted. The lowest intensity of extracted DPOAE signal was taken as the threshold value of DPOAE at this frequency. The t-test was used to evaluate statistical significance; n represents the number of test ears, $n = 3$ for each group; $P > 0.05$. Data were described as mean ± SEM (standard error of mean). **(E)** Representative images of type II auditory nerve fibers in WT and $Atp6v1b2^{Arg506*/Arg506*}$ mice at high magnification. Green fluorescence represents type II auditory nerve fibers labeled by NFH (neurofilament heavy polypeptide) antibody; these nerve fibers are connected to outer hair cells. The experiments were repeated three times. **(F)** Statistical results of type II auditory nerve fibers in panel **(E)**. The t-test was used to evaluate statistical significance; $n = 3$ for each group. * denotes $P < 0.05$. Data are described as mean ± SEM (standard error of mean).

Supplementary Figure 2 | Ribbon synapse density is not affected in the cochlea of $Atp6v1b2^{Arg506*/Arg506*}$ mice. **(A–C)** Representative images of ribbon synapses immunostained with Ctbp2 (green) and DAPI (blue) in WT and $Atp6v1b2^{Arg506*/Arg506*}$ mice aged 4 **(A)**, 12 **(B)**, and 20 **(C)** weeks. The IHC nuclei were also labeled due to the nuclear expression of Ctbp2. The labeled dots represent ribbon synapses between IHCs and auditory nerve fibers. **(D–F)** Quantitative analysis of ribbon synapses per IHC field in the cochlea regions of 8, 16, and 32 kHz; $n = 5$ for each group. Data are described as mean ± SEM (standard error of mean). IHC: inner hair cell.

Supplementary Figure 3 | $Atp6v1b2^{Arg506*/Arg506*}$ mice show demyelination in the osseous spiral lamina. **(A–F)** Basilar membrane of the cochlea immunostained for NFH (neurofilament heavy polypeptide, green), which preferentially stains unmyelinated axons. In the cochlea of $Atp6v1b2^{Arg506*/Arg506*}$ mice, ANFs (auditory nerve fibers) in the OSL (osseous spiral lamina) were labeled with NFH [**(F)**, red arrows] at 20 weeks, indicating the presence of ANF demyelination. This staining was absent in WT mice **(C)**. **(G–L)** Transmission electron microscopy of mouse cochlea. Representative images showed a few vacuoles in the myelin of $Atp6v1b2^{Arg506*/Arg506*}$ mice at 4 weeks [**(J)**, white arrows]. Demyelination occurred occasionally in ANFs of $Atp6v1b2^{Arg506*/Arg506*}$ mice at 12 weeks [**(K)**, yellow arrow]. Demyelinated ANFs were more common in $Atp6v1b2^{Arg506*/Arg506*}$ mice at 20 weeks [**(L)**, blue arrows]. These features were not observed in WT mice **(G–I)**. The experiments were repeated three times.

Supplementary Figure 4 | No autophagy and apoptosis in the organ of Corti activated by cytochrome C were observed in $Atp6v1b2^{Arg506*/Arg506*}$ mice. **(A)** Representative images of immunostaining showed no increase in the number of autophagosomes labeled with LC3 in the organ of Corti of $Atp6v1b2^{Arg506*/Arg506*}$ mice compared with that of WT mice. **(B)** Compared with WT mice, no cytochrome C was released from the mitochondria into the cytosol in the organ of Corti of $Atp6v1b2^{Arg506*/Arg506*}$ mice. **(C)** No obvious cleaved caspase-3 in the organ of Corti of $Atp6v1b2^{Arg506*/Arg506*}$ mice was identified compared with that of WT mice.

Supplementary Figure 5 | BIP-V5 was effective in improving the auditory function of $Atp6v1b2^{Arg506*/Arg506*}$ mice. ABR waveforms of click, 4, 8, and 16 kHz in one $Atp6v1b2^{Arg506*/Arg506*}$ mouse are shown. The sound intensity (dB SPL), which was used to stimulate the mice, successively decreased from high to low. The minimum sound intensity that can stimulate the mice to produce ABR waveforms was considered the hearing threshold of the mice.

Supplementary Figure 6 | Western blotting analysis of the proteins of the cytochrome C-caspase-3 apoptosis pathway in the cochlea of $Atp6v1b2^{Arg506*/Arg506*}$ mice after BIP-V5 administration. Western blotting showed that after BIP-V5 administration, Bax was effectively inhibited and Bcl-2 level was increased, which could have prevented the permeabilization of the mitochondrial membrane and the release of cytochrome C. As a result, cleaved caspase-3 levels reduced.

Supplementary Figure 7 | BIP-V5 administration increased the number of SGNs in the cochlea of $Atp6v1b2^{Arg506*/Arg506*}$ mice. **(A)** The number of SGNs in the cochlea of $Atp6v1b2^{Arg506*/Arg506*}$ mice increased after BIP-V5 administration. **(B)** The number of LC3-labeled autophagosomes in the SGNs of $Atp6v1b2^{Arg506*/Arg506*}$ mice was significantly increased (white arrow) compared with that of WT mice, and no obvious decrease was observed after BIP-V5 administration. **(C)** BIP-V5 reduced the release of cytochrome C from the mitochondria of SGNs in the cochlea of $Atp6v1b2^{Arg506*/Arg506*}$ mice. **(D)** BIP-V5 reduced the activation of caspase-3 in SGNs of $Atp6v1b2^{Arg506*/Arg506*}$ mice.

Supplementary Figure 8 | More pronounced positive signal for cleaved caspase-3 in the region of hippocampus of $Atp6v1b2^{Arg506*/Arg506*}$ mice was identified.

REFERENCES

Al Humayed, S., Al-Hashem, F., Haidara, M. A., El Karib, A. O., Kamar, S. S., Amin, S. N., et al. (2020). Resveratrol pretreatment ameliorates p53-bax axis and augments the survival biomarker B-cell lymphoma 2 modulated by paracetamol overdose in a rat model of acute liver injury. *Pharmacology* 105, 39–46. doi: 10.1159/000502632

Anagnostopoulos, G. K., Stefanou, D., Arkoumani, E., Sakorafas, G., Pavlakis, G., Arvanitidis, D., et al. (2005). Bax and Bcl-2 protein expression in gastric precancerous lesions: immunohistochemical study. *J. Gastroenterol. Hepatol.* 20, 1674–1678. doi: 10.1111/j.1440-1746.2005.04057.x

Beauregard-Lacroix, E., Pacheco-Cuellar, G., Ajeawung, N. F., Tardif, J., Dieterich, K., Dabir, T., et al. (2020). DOORS syndrome and a recurrent truncating ATP6V1B2 variant. *Genet. Med.* 23, 149–154. doi: 10.1038/s41436-020-00950-9

Beyenbach, K. W., and Wieczorek, H. (2006). The V-type H+ ATPase: molecular structure and function, physiological roles and regulation. *J. Exp. Biol.* 209, 577–589.

Bharadwaj, H. M., Verhulst, S., Shaheen, L., Liberman, M. C., and Shinn-Cunningham, B. G. (2014). Cochlear neuropathy and the coding of supra-threshold sound. *Front. Syst. Neurosci.* 8:26. doi: 10.3389/fnsys.2014.00026

Cerri, S., and Blandini, F. (2019). Role of autophagy in Parkinson's disease. *Curr. Med. Chem.* 26, 3702–3718.

Chen, Y., Gu, Y., Li, Y., Li, G. L., Chai, R., Li, W., et al. (2021). Generation of mature and functional hair cells by co-expression of Gfi1, Pou4f3, and Atoh1 in the postnatal mouse cochlea. *Cell Rep.* 35:109016. doi: 10.1016/j.celrep.2021.109016

Cheng, C., Hou, Y., Zhang, Z., Wang, Y., Lu, L., Zhang, L., et al. (2021). Disruption of the autism-related gene Pak1 causes stereocilia disorganization, hair cell loss, and deafness in mice. *J. Genet. Genomics* 48, 324–332. doi: 10.1016/j.jgg.2021.03.010

Cheng, C., Wang, Y., Guo, L., Lu, X., Zhu, W., Muhammad, W., et al. (2019). Age-related transcriptome changes in Sox2+ supporting cells in the mouse cochlea. *Stem Cell Res. Ther.* 10:365.

Colacurcio, D. J., and Nixon, R. A. (2016). Disorders of lysosomal acidification–the emerging role of v-ATPase in aging and neurodegenerative disease. *Ageing Res. Rev.* 32, 75–88. doi: 10.1016/j.arr.2016.05.004

De Duve, C. (1957). [The lysosomes: a novel group of cytoplasmic granules]. *J. Physiol. (Paris)* 49, 113–115.

Ding, Y., Meng, W., Kong, W., He, Z., and Chai, R. (2020). The role of FoxG1 in the inner ear. *Front. Cell Dev. Biol* 8:614954. doi: 10.3389/fcell.2020.614954

El-Brolosy, M. A., Kontarakis, Z., Rossi, A., Kuenne, C., Gunther, S., Fukuda, N., et al. (2019). Genetic compensation triggered by mutant mRNA degradation. *Nature* 568, 193–197. doi: 10.1038/s41586-019-1064-z

Fischer, N., Johnson Chacko, L., Glueckert, R., and Schrott-Fischer, A. (2019). Age-dependent changes in the Cochlea. *Gerontology* 66, 33–39.

Fu, X., An, Y., Wang, H., Li, P., Lin, J., Yuan, J., et al. (2021). Deficiency of Klc2 induces low-frequency sensorineural hearing loss in C57BL/6 J mice and human. *Mol. Neurobiol.* 58, 4376–4391.

Galluzzi, L., Vitale, I., Abrams, J. M., Alnemri, E. S., Baehrecke, E. H., Blagosklonny, M. V., et al. (2012). Molecular definitions of cell death subroutines: recommendations of the nomenclature committee on cell death 2012. *Cell Death Differ.* 19, 107–120.

Gao, S., Cheng, C., Wang, M., Jiang, P., Zhang, L., Wang, Y., et al. (2019). Blebbistatin inhibits neomycin-induced apoptosis in hair cell-like HEI-OC-1 cells and in cochlear hair cells. *Front. Cell. Neurosci.* 13:590. doi: 10.3389/fncel.2019.00590

Guo, R., Ma, X., Liao, M., Liu, Y., Hu, Y., Qian, X., et al. (2019). Development and application of cochlear implant-based electric-acoustic stimulation of spiral ganglion neurons. *ACS Biomater. Sci. Eng.* 5, 6735–6741.

Guo, R., Xiao, M., Zhao, W., Zhou, S., Hu, Y., Liao, M., et al. (2020). 2D Ti3C2TxMXene couples electrical stimulation to promote proliferation and neural differentiation of neural stem cells. *Acta Biomater.* S1742-7061(20)30749-2.

Guo, R., Zhang, S., Xiao, M., Qian, F., He, Z., Li, D., et al. (2016). Accelerating bioelectric functional development of neural stem cells by graphene coupling: implications for neural interfacing with conductive materials. *Biomaterials* 106, 193–204. doi: 10.1016/j.biomaterials.2016.08.019

Han, S., Xu, Y., Sun, J., Liu, Y., Zhao, Y., Tao, M., et al. (2020). Isolation and analysis of extracellular vesicles in a Morpho butterfly wing-integrated microvortex biochip. *Biosens. Bioelectron.* 154:112073. doi: 10.1016/j.bios.2020.112073

He, Z., Guo, L., Shu, Y., Fang, Q., Zhou, H., Liu, Y., et al. (2017). Autophagy protects auditory hair cells against neomycin-induced damage. *Autophagy* 13, 1884–1904. doi: 10.1080/15548627.2017.1359449

He, Z. H., Li, M., Fang, Q. J., Liao, F. L., Zou, S. Y., Wu, X., et al. (2021). FOXG1 promotes aging inner ear hair cell survival through activation of the autophagy pathway. *Autophagy* 19, 1–22.

He, Z. H., Zou, S. Y., Li, M., Liao, F. L., Wu, X., Sun, H. Y., et al. (2020). The nuclear transcription factor FoxG1 affects the sensitivity of mimetic aging hair cells to inflammation by regulating autophagy pathways. *Redox Biol.* 28:101364. doi: 10.1016/j.redox.2019.101364

Hughes, A. L., and Gottschling, D. E. (2012). An early age increase in vacuolar pH limits mitochondrial function and lifespan in yeast. *Nature* 492, 261–265. doi: 10.1038/nature11654

Ilmarinen, P., Moilanen, E., and Kankaanranta, H. (2014). Mitochondria in the center of human eosinophil apoptosis and survival. *Int. J. Mol. Sci.* 15, 3952–3969. doi: 10.3390/ijms15033952

Jiang, P., Zhang, S., Cheng, C., Gao, S., Tang, M., Lu, L., et al. (2020). The roles of exosomes in visual and auditory systems. *Front. Bioeng. Biotechnol.* 8:525. doi: 10.3389/fbioe.2020.00525

Kanauchi, H., Wada, N., Clark, O. H., and Duh, Q. Y. (2002). Apoptosis regulating genes, bcl-2 and bax, and human telomerase reverse transcriptase messenger RNA expression in adrenal tumors: possible diagnostic and prognostic importance. *Surgery* 132, 1021–1026. discussion 1026-1027. doi: 10.1067/msy.2002.128616

Kawamura, N., Sun-Wada, G. H., and Wada, Y. (2015). Loss of G2 subunit of vacuolar-type proton transporting ATPase leads to G1 subunit upregulation in the brain. *Sci. Rep.* 5:14027.

Kortum, F., Caputo, V., Bauer, C. K., Stella, L., Ciolfi, A., Alawi, M., et al. (2015). Mutations in KCNH1 and ATP6V1B2 cause zimmermann-laband syndrome. *Nat. Genet.* 47, 661–667. doi: 10.1038/ng.3282

Kroemer, G., Galluzzi, L., and Brenner, C. (2007). Mitochondrial membrane permeabilization in cell death. *Physiol. Rev.* 87, 99–163. doi: 10.1152/physrev.00013.2006

Kujawa, S. G., and Liberman, M. C. (2009). Adding insult to injury: cochlear nerve degeneration after "temporary" noise-induced hearing loss. *J. Neurosci.* 29, 14077–14085. doi: 10.1523/jneurosci.2845-09.2009

Liberman, M. C., and Kujawa, S. G. (2017). Cochlear synaptopathy in acquired sensorineural hearing loss: manifestations and mechanisms. *Hear. Res.* 349, 138–147. doi: 10.1016/j.heares.2017.01.003

Liu, H., Lu, J., Wang, Z., Song, L., Wang, X., Li, G. L., et al. (2019). Functional alteration of ribbon synapses in inner hair cells by noise exposure causing hidden hearing loss. *Neurosci. Lett.* 707:134268. doi: 10.1016/j.neulet.2019.05.022

Liu, K., Chen, D., Guo, W., Yu, N., Wang, X., Ji, F., et al. (2015). Spontaneous and partial repair of ribbon synapse in cochlear inner hair cells after ototoxic withdrawal. *Mol. Neurobiol.* 52, 1680–1689. doi: 10.1007/s12035-014-8951-y

Liu, L., Chen, Y., Qi, J., Zhang, Y., He, Y., Ni, W., et al. (2016). Wnt activation protects against neomycin-induced hair cell damage in the mouse cochlea. *Cell Death Dis.* 7:e2136. doi: 10.1038/cddis.2016.35

Liu, W., Xu, L., Wang, X., Zhang, D., Sun, G., Wang, M., et al. (2021). PRDX1 activates autophagy via the PTEN-AKT signaling pathway to protect against cisplatin-induced spiral ganglion neuron damage. *Autophagy* 12, 1–23. doi: 10.1080/15548627.2021.1905466

Liu, W., Xu, X., Fan, Z., Sun, G., Han, Y., Zhang, D., et al. (2019). Wnt signaling activates TP53-induced glycolysis and apoptosis regulator and protects against cisplatin-induced spiral ganglion neuron damage in the mouse cochlea. *Antioxid. Redox Signal.* 30, 1389–1410. doi: 10.1089/ars.2017.7288

Liu, Y., Qi, J., Chen, X., Tang, M., Chu, C., Zhu, W., et al. (2019). Critical role of spectrin in hearing development and deafness. *Sci. Adv.* 5:eaav7803. doi: 10.1126/sciadv.aav7803

Lv, J., Fu, X., Li, Y., Hong, G., Li, P., Lin, J., et al. (2021). Deletion of Kcnj16 in mice does not alter auditory function. *Front. Cell Dev. Biol.* 9:630361. doi: 10.3389/fcell.2021.630361

Ma, B., Xiang, Y., and An, L. (2011). Structural bases of physiological functions and roles of the vacuolar H(+)-ATPase. *Cell. Signal.* 23, 1244–1256. doi: 10.1016/j.cellsig.2011.04.003

Ma, Z., Zhu, P., Shi, H., Guo, L., Zhang, Q., Chen, Y., et al. (2019). PTC-bearing mRNA elicits a genetic compensation response via Upf3a and COMPASS components. *Nature* 568, 259–263. doi: 10.1038/s41586-019-1057-y

Mauvezin, C., Nagy, P., Juhasz, G., and Neufeld, T. P. (2015). Autophagosome-lysosome fusion is independent of V-ATPase-mediated acidification. *Nat. Commun.* 6:7007.

Mehraei, G., Hickox, A. E., Bharadwaj, H. M., Goldberg, H., Verhulst, S., Liberman, M. C., et al. (2016). Auditory brainstem response latency in noise as a marker of cochlear synaptopathy. *J. Neurosci.* 36, 3755–3764. doi: 10.1523/jneurosci.4460-15.2016

Menendez, I., Carranza, C., Herrera, M., Marroquin, N., Foster, J. II, Cengiz, F. B., et al. (2017). Dominant deafness-onychodystrophy syndrome caused by an ATP6V1B2 mutation. *Clin. Case Rep.* 5, 376–379. doi: 10.1002/ccr3.761

Mindell, J. A. (2012). Lysosomal acidification mechanisms. *Annu. Rev. Physiol.* 74, 69–86. doi: 10.1146/annurev-physiol-012110-142317

Molin, M., and Demir, A. B. (2014). Linking peroxiredoxin and vacuolar-ATPase functions in calorie restriction-mediated life span extension. *Int. J. Cell Biol.* 2014:913071.

Paunescu, T. G., Russo, L. M., Da Silva, N., Kovacikova, J., Mohebbi, N., Van Hoek, A. N., et al. (2007). Compensatory membrane expression of the V-ATPase B2 subunit isoform in renal medullary intercalated cells of B1-deficient mice. *Am. J. Physiol. Renal Physiol.* 293, F1915–F1926.

Peric, A., and Annaert, W. (2015). Early etiology of Alzheimer's disease: tipping the balance toward autophagy or endosomal dysfunction? *Acta Neuropathol.* 129, 363–381. doi: 10.1007/s00401-014-1379-7

Qi, J., Liu, Y., Chu, C., Chen, X., Zhu, W., Shu, Y., et al. (2019). A cytoskeleton structure revealed by super-resolution fluorescence imaging in inner ear hair cells. *Cell Discov.* 5:12.

Qi, J., Zhang, L., Tan, F., Liu, Y., Chu, C., Zhu, W., et al. (2020). Espin distribution as revealed by super-resolution microscopy of stereocilia. *Am. J. Transl. Res.* 12, 130–141.

Qian, F., Wang, X., Yin, Z., Xie, G., Yuan, H., Liu, D., et al. (2020). The slc4a2b gene is required for hair cell development in zebrafish. *Aging (Albany NY)* 12, 18804–18821. doi: 10.18632/aging.103840

Rasband, M. N., and Peles, E. (2015). The nodes of ranvier: molecular assembly and maintenance. *Cold Spring Harb. Perspect. Biol.* 8:a020495. doi: 10.1101/cshperspect.a020495

Rossi, A., Kontarakis, Z., Gerri, C., Nolte, H., Holper, S., Kruger, M., et al. (2015). Genetic compensation induced by deleterious mutations but not gene knockdowns. *Nature* 524, 230–233. doi: 10.1038/nature14580

Ruckenstuhl, C., Netzberger, C., Entfellner, I., Carmona-Gutierrez, D., Kickenweiz, T., Stekovic, S., et al. (2014). Lifespan extension by methionine restriction requires autophagy-dependent vacuolar acidification. *PLoS Genet.* 10:e1004347.

Saftig, P., and Haas, A. (2016). Turn up the lysosome. *Nat. Cell Biol.* 18, 1025–1027. doi: 10.1371/journal.pgen.1004347

Shrestha, B. R., Chia, C., Wu, L., Kujawa, S. G., Liberman, M. C., and Goodrich, L. V. (2018). Sensory Neuron diversity in the inner ear is shaped by activity. *Cell* 174, 1229–1246.e17.

Song, M. H., Jung, J., Rim, J. H., Choi, H. J., Lee, H. J., Noh, B., et al. (2020). Genetic inheritance of late-onset, down-sloping hearing loss and its implications for auditory rehabilitation. *Ear Hear.* 41, 114–124. doi: 10.1097/aud.0000000000000734

Sun, S., Babola, T., Pregernig, G., So, K. S., Nguyen, M., Su, S. M., et al. (2018). Hair cell mechanotransduction regulates spontaneous activity and spiral ganglion subtype specification in the auditory system. *Cell* 174, 1247–1263.e15.

Tan, F., Chu, C., Qi, J., Li, W., You, D., Li, K., et al. (2019). AAV-ie enables safe and efficient gene transfer to inner ear cells. *Nat. Commun.* 10:3733.

Tian, C., Gagnon, L. H., Longo-Guess, C., Korstanje, R., Sheehan, S. M., Ohlemiller, K. K., et al. (2017). Hearing loss without overt metabolic acidosis in ATP6V1B1 deficient MRL mice, a new genetic model for non-syndromic deafness with enlarged vestibular aqueducts. *Hum. Mol. Genet.* 26, 3722–3735. doi: 10.1093/hmg/ddx257

Vreugde, S., Erven, A., Kros, C. J., Marcotti, W., Fuchs, H., Kurima, K., et al. (2002). Beethoven, a mouse model for dominant, progressive hearing loss DFNA36. *Nat. Genet.* 30, 257–258. doi: 10.1038/ng848

Wan, G., and Corfas, G. (2017). Transient auditory nerve demyelination as a new mechanism for hidden hearing loss. *Nat. Commun.* 8:14487.

Wang, Y., Li, J., Yao, X., Li, W., Du, H., Tang, M., et al. (2017). Loss of CIB2 causes profound hearing loss and abolishes mechanoelectrical transduction in mice. *Front. Mol. Neurosci.* 10:401. doi: 10.3389/fnmol.2017.00401

Waqas, M., Sun, S., Xuan, C., Fang, Q., Zhang, X., Islam, I. U., et al. (2017). Bone morphogenetic protein 4 promotes the survival and preserves the structure of flow-sorted Bhlhb5+ cochlear spiral ganglion neurons in vitro. *Sci. Rep.* 7:3506.

Yan, W., Liu, W., Qi, J., Fang, Q., Fan, Z., Sun, G., et al. (2018). A three-dimensional culture system with matrigel promotes purified spiral ganglion neuron survival and function in vitro. *Mol. Neurobiol.* 55, 2070–2084. doi: 10.1007/s12035-017-0471-0

Yuan, T. F., Dong, Y., Zhang, L., Qi, J., Yao, C., Wang, Y., et al. (2021). Neuromodulation-based stem cell therapy in brain repair: recent advances and future perspectives. *Neurosci. Bull.* 37, 735–745. doi: 10.1007/s12264-021-00667-y

Yuan, Y., Zhang, J., Chang, Q., Zeng, J., Xin, F., Wang, J., et al. (2014). De novo mutation in ATP6V1B2 impairs lysosome acidification and causes dominant deafness-onychodystrophy syndrome. *Cell Res.* 24, 1370–1373. doi: 10.1038/cr.2014.77

Yue, F., Cheng, Y., Breschi, A., Vierstra, J., Wu, W., Ryba, T., et al. (2014). A comparative encyclopedia of DNA elements in the mouse genome. *Nature* 515, 355–364.

Zhang, S., Dong, Y., Qiang, R., Zhang, Y., Zhang, X., Chen, Y., et al. (2021). Characterization of strip1 expression in mouse cochlear hair cells. *Front. Genet.* 12:625867. doi: 10.3389/fgene.2021.625867

Zhang, S., Zhang, Y., Dong, Y., Guo, L., Zhang, Z., Shao, B., et al. (2020). Knockdown of Foxg1 in supporting cells increases the trans-differentiation of supporting cells into hair cells in the neonatal mouse cochlea. *Cell Mol. Life Sci.* 77, 1401–1419. doi: 10.1007/s00018-019-03291-2

Zhang, Y., Zhang, S., Zhang, Z., Dong, Y., Ma, X., Qiang, R., et al. (2020). Knockdown of Foxg1 in Sox9+ supporting cells increases the trans-differentiation of supporting cells into hair cells in the neonatal mouse utricle. *Aging (Albany NY)* 12, 19834–19851. doi: 10.18632/aging.104009

Zhao, W., Gao, X., Qiu, S., Gao, B., Gao, S., Zhang, X., et al. (2019). A subunit of V-ATPases, ATP6V1B2, underlies the pathology of intellectual disability. *EBioMedicine* 45, 408–421. doi: 10.1016/j.ebiom.2019.06.035

Zhong, Z., Fu, X., Li, H., Chen, J., Wang, M., Gao, S., et al. (2020). Citicoline protects auditory hair cells against neomycin-induced damage. *Front. Cell Dev. Biol.* 8:712. doi: 10.3389/fcell.2020.00712

Zhou, H., Qian, X., Xu, N., Zhang, S., Zhu, G., Zhang, Y., et al. (2020). Disruption of Atg7-dependent autophagy causes electromotility disturbances, outer hair cell loss, and deafness in mice. *Cell Death Dis.* 11:913.

Zhou, X., Li, Y., Li, Z., Cao, Y., Wang, F., and Li, C. (2017). Effect of dietary zinc on morphological characteristics and apoptosis related gene expression in the small intestine of Bama miniature pigs. *Acta Histochem.* 119, 235–243. doi: 10.1016/j.acthis.2017.01.006

N-Acetylcysteine Combined with Dexamethasone Treatment Improves Sudden Sensorineural Hearing Loss and Attenuates Hair Cell Death Caused by ROS Stress

Xue Bai[†], Sen Chen[†], Kai Xu[†], Yuan Jin, Xun Niu, Le Xie, Yue Qiu, Xiao-Zhou Liu and Yu Sun*

Department of Otorhinolaryngology, Union Hospital, Tongji Medical College, Huazhong University of Science and Technology, Wuhan, China

*Correspondence:
Yu Sun
sunyu@hust.edu.cn

[†]*These authors have contributed equally to this work*

Sudden sensorineural hearing loss (SSNHL) is a common emergency in the world. Increasing evidence of imbalance of oxidant–antioxidant were found in SSNHL patients. Steroids combined with antioxidants may be a potential strategy for the treatment of SSNHL. In cochlear explant experiment, we found that N-acetylcysteine (NAC) combined with dexamethasone can effectively protect hair cells from oxidative stress when they were both at ineffective concentrations alone. A clinic trial was designed to explore whether oral NAC combined with intratympanic dexamethasone (ITD) as a salvage treatment has a better therapeutic effect. 41 patients with SSNHL were randomized to two groups. 23 patients in control group received ITD therapy alone, while 18 patient s in NAC group were treated with oral NAC and ITD. The patients were followed-up on day 1st (initiation of treatment) and day 14th. Overall, there was no statistical difference in final pure-tone threshold average (PTA) improvement between those two groups. However, a significant hearing gain at 8,000 Hz was observed in NAC group. Moreover, the hearing recovery rates of NAC group is much higher than that in control group. These results demonstrated that oral NAC in combination with ITD therapy is a more effective therapy for SSNHL than ITD alone.

Keywords: sudden sensorineural hearing loss, hair cell, ROS, N-acetylcysteine, steroid

INTRODUCTION

Sudden sensorineural hearing loss (SSNHL) is considered one of the most common emergencies in clinical practice. In the United States, SSNHL is thought to affect between 5–27 in 100,000 individuals, with about 66,000 new cases per year (Alexander and Harris, 2013; Chandrasekhar et al., 2019). In Japan, there are 60.9 cases per 100,000 population diagnosed with SSNHL annually (Nakashima et al., 2014). Further epidemiological investigations have shown that the incidence of SSNHL is increasing globally (Michel, 2011; Kitoh et al., 2020). Currently, high-dose systemic steroid treatment is used as the first-line treatment of SSNHL (Chandrasekhar et al., 2019;

Kitoh et al., 2020). However, approximately 50% of patients experience no or limited hearing improvement after systemic steroid treatment (Hunchaisri et al., 2010; Tong et al., 2020). Therefore, those patients with limited hearing improvement (less than 10–20 dB) are considered to have refractory sudden hearing loss (RSHL) (Hunchaisri et al., 2010; Ferri et al., 2012). Although intratympanic dexamethasone (ITD) therapy has been recommended as a salvage treatment for RSHL or after failure of systemic steroid treatment (Moon et al., 2011; Berjis et al., 2016; Sun et al., 2018), its efficacy remains unsatisfactory (Li et al., 2015). It is therefore necessary to devise new strategies for SSNHL.

Steroids combined with another therapy is a common strategy for the treatment of SSNHL. In the United States, hyperbaric oxygen therapy (HBOT) combined with ITD is one option for salvage therapy (Chandrasekhar et al., 2019). Meanwhile, prostaglandin E1 combined with steroids has been recommended by Japanese clinicians for severe to profound SSNHL (Kitoh et al., 2020). Pharmacologically, combination therapy has unique advantages, with potential synergistic effects to achieve better therapeutic outcomes. Recently, antioxidants have been removed from the list of interventions that the American Clinical Practice Guidelines for SSNHL (published in 2019) recommend against using (Chandrasekhar et al., 2019). Although no explanation is given for this change, it indicates that antioxidants may have potential value in the treatment of SSNHL.

To date, a wide variety of antioxidants have been used in the treatment of SSNHL, but their effects remain controversial. Previous studies showed that different combinations or single vitamins (used as antioxidants, vitamin A, C, or E) combined with a steroid were more beneficial for patients with SSNHL (Joachims et al., 2003; Hatano et al., 2008; Kang et al., 2013; Kaya et al., 2015). Similarly, a clinical trial showed that a zinc supplement may enhance the hearing recovery of SSNHL patients by reducing oxidative stress of the cochlea (Yang et al., 2011). However, another study did not find any convincing benefits of a zinc supplement (Niran et al., 2015). Although evidence of an oxidant–antioxidant imbalance was found in SSNHL patients, the therapeutic targets of antioxidants and the mechanism of their interaction with steroids are still difficult to fully elucidate (Jarosław et al., 2019; Ozdamar et al., 2019). Therefore, how to select the effective antioxidant for SSNHL has become a puzzled problem to be solved.

N-acetylcysteine (NAC), as a precursor of glutathione (GSH) and a limiting factor in the process of GSH synthesis, is one of the antioxidants commonly used in the inner ear (Duan et al., 2004; Pathak et al., 2015; Tillinger et al., 2018). It has been clinically proven to be effective as a single therapy in the treatment of SSNHL or cisplatin-induced hearing loss (Riga et al., 2013; Chen and Young, 2016). For initial treatment, combination therapy with corticosteroids plus L-NAC is associated with improved hearing compared to corticosteroids alone (Angeli et al., 2012). Moreover, addition of NAC has been shown to increase glucocorticoid sensitivity in a mouse model of steroid-resistant asthma (Eftekhari et al., 2013). These studies indicate that NAC and steroids may enhance treatment efficacy through synergistic action. Combining a steroid with NAC may be a potential alternative to salvage therapy of SSNHL or RSHL. To prove our hypothesis, *in vitro* experiments were performed to verify whether NAC and steroid have a synergistic effect on oxidative stress injury. In addition, a clinical trial was designed to compare the therapeutic efficacy of ITD with that of ITD combined with NAC in the salvage therapy of SSNHL.

MATERIALS AND METHODS

Culture of Cochlear Explants and Drug Treatments

C57BL/6 mice at P3 were decapitated after anesthesia, then the cochlear basilar membrane was carefully isolated from the cochlea in transparent Hank's balanced salt solution (PB180321, ProCell, Wuhan, China). The cochlear basilar membrane containing the organ of Corti was transferred onto a collagen gel matrix. A 15 µL droplet of a 9:1:1 rat tail collagen (Type 1-4236, BD Biosciences, Franklin Lakes, NJ, United States), 10 × Basal Medium Eagle (BME; B9638, Sigma-Aldrich, St. Louis, MO, United States), 2% sodium carbonate (P1110, Solarbio, Beijing, China) mixture was placed on the surface of a 35-mm culture dish and allowed to gel for approximately 30 min at 37°C. Afterward, 1.3 mL medium consisting of 1 × BME (41010109, Gibco, Carlsbad, CA, United States) containing 1% bovine serum albumin (A8020, Solarbio), 10% glutamine (G7513, Sigma-Aldrich), 5 mg/mL glucose and 10,000 U/mL penicillin G (P3414, Sigma-Aldrich) were added to the culture dish. The cochlear explants were placed as a flat preparation on the surface of the collagen gel, and the surface of the basilar membrane was exactly even with the culture medium. All explants were incubated overnight at 37°C in an atmosphere of 5% CO_2. On the following day, the culture medium was removed, the explants of the cochlea for primary culture were treated with fresh medium containing drugs for 24 h *in vitro*, then subjected to immunofluorescent staining. The cochlear explants were divided into four groups and were exposed to 160 U/L glucose oxidase (GO; G3660, Sigma-Aldrich; GO group), 160 U/L GO together with 50 µg/mL dexamethasone (GO + Dex group), 160 U/L GO with 5 mM NAC (A7250, Sigma-Aldrich; GO + NAC group), or 160 U/L GO together with 5 mM NAC and 50 µg/mL dexamethasone (GO + Dex + NAC group). The cochlear explants (n = 3–5 in each group) were incubated at 37°C in 5% CO_2 for 24 h and then harvested for further experiments.

Cochlear Tissue Preparation and Fluorescent Labeling

The cochlear explants were fixed in 4% paraformaldehyde in 0.01 M PBS for 1 h at room temperature. After washing three times in 0.01 M PBS, explants were stained with DAPI (C1005, Beyotime Institute of Biotechnology, Jiangsu, China) and phalloidin (0.05 mg/mL, P5282, Sigma-Aldrich) for 10 min each. Images were captured with a laser scanning confocal microscope (Nikon, Tokyo, Japan). Three regions from the apical, middle, and basal turns of the stretched cochlear explants were scanned using a ×60 magnification lens.

Clinical Study Design and Patients

This clinical trial was carried out between March 2017 and March 2019 at the Department of Otorhinolaryngology of Wuhan Union hospital. Eligible subjects were patients with at least 30 dB hearing loss in three contiguous frequencies that had occurred over a course of 3 days, with available previous audiometry data. All patients had a normal otoscopic exam and tympanograms and had not responded to initial treatment. The hearing thresholds of patients were measured at 250–8,000 Hz. Exclusion criteria for the study were: Subjects older than 60 years old (to rule out potential presbycusis); patients with completely hearing loss at 4,000 and 8,000 Hz; patients with Meniere's disease or other recognized pathologies of SSHL, such as genetic causes, acoustic trauma, previous otologic surgery and so on; any contraindication for the use of NAC and steroids, such as pregnancy or hypertension; MRI scan finding acoustic neuroma or other retrocochlear lesions; disease onset time of more than 14 days; incomplete medical records or inadequate follow-up. All individuals underwent medical history, physical examinations, and laboratory tests, as well as audiologic evaluations that included tympanometry and pure tone audiometry before diagnosis and therapy. All individuals were informed about the procedure and the possible risks. They all agreed to participate in this research and signed an informed consent form. This study was approved by the institutional review board of Wuhan Union hospital.

Therapy Protocol

After screening for eligibility, all subjects were randomly divided into two groups. Randomization was carried out by generating sequential random numbers using computer-based software. Every recruited individual received sequential random numbers placed in closed envelopes. All doctors and patients were aware of the allocation. The physicians that performed the pure tone audiometry and data analysis were kept blinded to the allocation.

All of the eligible subjects had received ITD injections and basic treatment for SSNHL, which included nourishing nerves and improving vascular microcirculation. All patients underwent hearing tests before treatment and 2 weeks later after treatment. The patients were treated by the senior physicians and received ITD administration alone in the control group. In the experimental groups (NAC groups), all patients routinely received combination therapy with ITD plus oral NAC. NAC (Conbe Biopharmaceutical Company, China) was given orally in the form of effervescent tablets at a dose of 600 mg two times daily for 2 weeks, starting with the with the first IT Dex therapy.

Measurement of Auditory Function

The audiometric data of all evaluable patients were analyzed. The pure-tone hearing thresholds were measured at 250, 500, 1,000, 2,000, 4,000, and 8,000 Hz. The pure-tone threshold average (PTA) was calculated by measuring the six-frequency average of the threshold value at 500, 1,000, 2,000, and 4,000 Hz. Thresholds that were not measurable because of the limit of the audiometric equipment were coded with the maximum level of the audiometer that was set at 120 dB (HL). Pure tone audiometry was performed before initiation of treatment and 2 weeks after initiation of treatment. The main end-point of this research was the final mean hearing improvement, which was regarded as the difference between initial and final PTA. PTA values were compared to assess the hearing recovery before and after treatment. According to the criteria in the guidelines for the diagnosis and treatment of sudden deafness of the Chinese society of otorhinolaryngology, "hearing improvement" was defined as more than 15 dB hearing gain, and "no improvement" as less than 15 dB hearing gain.

Cell Culture and Treatment

BxPC3 cells were cultured in high-glucose DMEM (11995500, Gibco) mixed with 5% volume of fetal bovine serum (11054001, Gibco) with antibiotics and incubated in 5% CO_2 at 37°C. The levels of ROS in cells were detected by staining with dichlorodihydrofluorescein diacetate (DCFH-DA; D6883, Sigma-Aldrich). The cells were exposed to 80 U/L glucose oxidase (GO, GO group) for 4 h. Cells after treatment were washed in pre-warmed PBS and stained with 10 μM DCFH-DA in serum-free DMEM for 30 min. The cell fluorescence intensity was measured by fluorescence microscopy.

Statistical Analysis

Efficacy was analyzed in all eligible patients. Descriptive statistics were used for the feature description. Paired samples t tests were used to compare the means of quantitative variables in the same group at different points in time. Independent samples t tests were used to compare the means of metric variables between two groups. Categorial variables were compared using Fisher's exact test or Chi-square test. A difference was considered to be statistically significant when the P value was less than 0.05. All statistical analyses were performed using the SPSS statistical software package (version 22.0; IBM SPSS Statistics for Windows, Armonk, NY, United States). The graphs were created using GraphPad Prism (version 8.2.1).

RESULTS

A Cochlear Explant Model of Oxidative Stress Injury Was Established to Verify the Oto-Protective Synergistic Effect of Dexamethasone Combined With NAC

In patients with SSNHL, some indirect evidence of oxidative stress injury has been found successively (Becatti et al., 2017; Jarosław et al., 2019). Therefore, a cochlear explant model of oxidative stress injury was adopted to explore the effects of combined therapy. In the BxPC3 cell line, 4 h of GO treatment significantly increased the intracellular ROS level. The green fluorescent signal in the GO group detected by DCFH-DA, a probe of reactive oxygen species, was much stronger than that of the control group (**Figures 1A–D**). Therefore, GO was used to increase the ROS level in cochlear explants. Compared to the control group (**Figures 1E–G**, $n = 3$), a

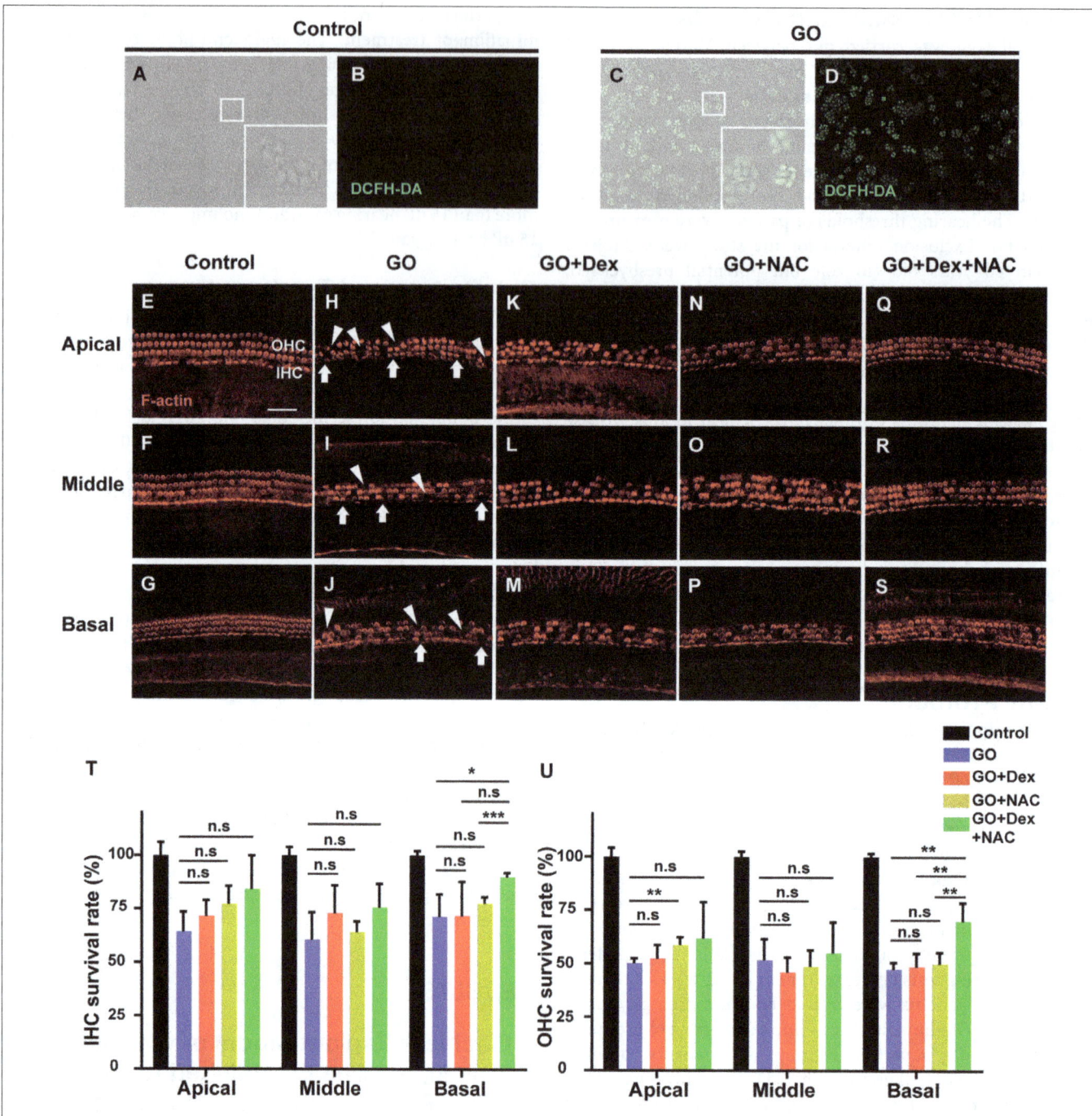

FIGURE 1 | The changes in the number of hair cells after drug treatment for 24 h in ROS models *in vitro* were measured by fluorescence. (A–D) The intracellular ROS level in BxPC3 cells was measured in control group and GO group, using a peroxide-sensitive fluorescent probe, DCFH-DA. White boxes in the lower left corner are magnified images. (E–S) Representative confocal images showing hair cells from the three turns of the cochlea labeled with F-actin (red) after culturing for 24 h. Images from the control group and the groups treated with GO, GO + Dex, GO + NAC, and GO + NAC + Dex are shown. White arrowheads indicate the missing of hair cells in three turns. (T) Comparison of the survival rate of inner hair cells in control, GO, GO + Dex, GO + NAC, and GO + NAC + Dex groups. (U) Comparison of the survival rate of outer hair cells in control, GO, GO + Dex, GO + NAC, and GO + NAC + Dex groups. GO, Glucose oxidase; IHCs, inner hair cells, OHCs, outer hair cells; Dex, dexamethasone; NAC, N-acetylcysteine. $*P < 0.05$, $**P < 0.01$, $***P < 0.001$, and n.s, no significant difference. Scale in panel E represents for 40 μm.

moderate degeneration of hair cells was observed in different turns of the GO group ($n = 4$). After 24 h of GO incubation, half of the outer hair cells (OHCs) had died, while 60.51–71.34% of inner hair cells (IHCs) survived (hair cell loss, white arrows and arrowheads, **Figures 1H–J**). A low concentration of dexamethasone (50 μg/mL) was added to GO-treated explants (GO + Dex group), and the results revealed that dexamethasone had no protective effect on hair cells at this concentration. The rates of OHC survival were 52.25 ± 6.46, 46.09 ± 6.97, and 48.64 ± 6.32% in the apical, middle and basal turns, respectively (GO + Dex group, $n = 5$). Meanwhile, approximately 70% of IHC survived in the GO + Dex group (**Figures 1K–M**). Similarly, a non-therapeutic concentration of NAC (5 mM) was also added to the GO-treated explant (GO + NAC group). In this group, the average OHC survival rates were 48.87–58.80% in different turns, while IHC survival rates fluctuated between 64.09 and 77.56% (**Figures 1N–P**). However, there was a statistically-significant difference in the OHC survival rate of the apical turn between the GO and GO + NAC groups (GO: 50.16 ± 2.36% vs. GO + NAC: 58.50 ± 3.54%, $P = 0.0042$). This improvement of OHC survival was fairly limited (less than 9%). Except for the above improvement, there was no statistically-significant difference in hair cell survival rates between the GO + NAC group and the GO group (**Figures 1T,U**). When Dex and NAC were both added to GO-treated cochlear explants ($n = 5$), the number of surviving IHCs or OHCs in the basal turn was significantly increased (**Figures 1Q–S**). Compared with the GO group, the survival rates of OHC and IHC in the basal turn of the GO + Dex + NAC group were significantly increased (OHC, 47.41 ± 3.20 vs. 69.85 ± 8.65%, $P = 0.0018$; IHC, 71.34 ± 10.56 vs. 90.00 ± 2.00%, $P = 0.0057$, **Figures 1T,U**).

Clinical Trial to Observe the Effectiveness of NAC Combined With Dexamethasone Therapy

There was a total of 64 patients who agreed to take part in this study. Of those, 14 were excluded for not conforming to eligibility criteria, consisting of three patients who had experienced symptoms for more than 14 days, one who had uncontrolled diabetes mellitus, one patient with a history of Meniere's disease, two patients who had not undergone any initial treatment at other hospitals, four patients who did not have hearing loss in five frequencies, and three participants who declined to take part. The remaining 50 patients who agreed to participate were randomized into two groups for further treatment and analysis. Of the 50 participants included, five were later excluded because of loss of contact from this clinical trial, and four patients were excluded owing to withdrawal of consent. Finally, overall 41 patients were included in our analysis. There were 23 patients in the control group, while 18 patients were analyzed in the NAC group (**Figure 2**).

All 41 patients were recruited at the Department of Otorhinolaryngology of Wuhan Union hospital. Sixteen of the patients were male (39.0%) and 25 were female (61.0%) with an average age of 38.5 ± 14.4 years (range: 14–60). Twenty-three (56.1%) participants were randomized to the control group, and 18 (43.9%) to the NAC group. The initial PTA of all patients was 64.1 ± 21.5 dB HL (66.25 ± 20.17 dB in the control group, 61.3 ± 22.8 dB in the NAC group). The post-treatment PTA of the control group was 54.7 ± 25.4 dB HL, while it was 42.2 ± 26.3 dB HL in the NAC group. For all patients, the mean duration of hospital treatment was 11.8 ± 4.7 days (11.8 ± 4.9 days in the control group; 12 ± 4.5 days in the NAC group). The mean PTA gain of all patients was 14.9 ± 15.5 dB (11.6 ± 17.8 dB in the control group; 19.0 ± 11.1 dB in the NAC group). No statistically-significant differences were found between the control and NAC groups concerning age, sex, days in hospital, initial PTA, final PTA, or mean PTA gain ($P > 0.05$, **Table 1**).

Figure 3 indicates the audiologic outcomes at different frequencies for all patients in the control and NAC groups. The hearing gains of the control group were 17.2 ± 18.5, 17.2 ± 20.7, 12.8 ± 16.1, 8.9 ± 17.6, 7.4 ± 24.1, and 6.1 ± 22.1 dB at 250, 500, 1,000, 2,000 4,000, and 8,000 Hz, respectively. These gains in the NAC group were 15.6 ± 18.5, 18.3 ± 13.7, 20.3 ± 10.8, 17.2 ± 12.6, 20.3 ± 16.6, and 20.8 ± 14.8 dB, respectively, at the corresponding frequencies. Compared with the control group, the mean gain of the NAC group was significantly different at 8,000 Hz ($P = 0.019$, Power = 0.854, **Figure 3G**). No statistically-significant differences were detected at any of the other frequencies ($P > 0.05$, **Figures 3A–F**).

In terms of hearing recovery (**Table 2**), any PTA gain (500–4,000 Hz) greater than 15 dB is considered effective. The percentage of patients who experienced effective recovery in the control group vs. the NAC group was 39.1% (9 of 23) vs. 72.2% (13 of 18). Thus there was a significant difference in the effective rate between control and NAC groups ($P = 0.035$, Pearson's chi-squared test).

DISCUSSION

Hair cells mainly function in transducing sound waves into the electric signals (Wang Y. et al., 2017; Liu Y. et al., 2019; Qi et al., 2019). Hearing loss could be caused by genetic factors,

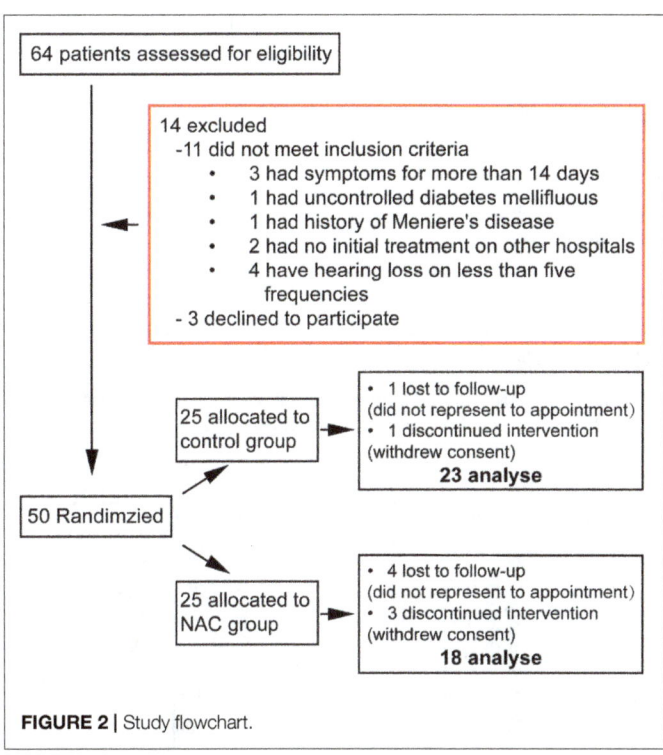

FIGURE 2 | Study flowchart.

TABLE 1 | Demographic and audiological features of patients in control group and NAC group.

	All (n = 41)	Control(n = 23)	NAC(n = 18)	P value
Age (years) (mean ± SD)	38.54 ± 14.35	41.96 ± 12.50	34.17 ± 15.69	0.08
Gender (male/female)	16: 25	8: 15	8: 10	0.54
Time in hospital (days) (mean ± SD)	11.88 ± 4.66	11.78 ± 4.88	12.00 ± 4.50	0.88
Initial PTA (dB) (mean ± SD)	64.05 ± 21.52	66.25 ± 20.72	61.25 ± 22.78	0.46
Final PTA (dB) (mean ± SD)	49.21 ± 26.20	54.67 ± 25.37	42.22 ± 26.26	0.24
Mean PTA gain (Db) (mean ± SD)	14.85 ± 15.54	11.57 ± 17.84	19.03 ± 11.09	0.17
ALT (U/T) (mean ± SD)	23.63 ± 16.08	23.52 ± 14.41	23.78 ± 18.43	0.96
Blood fat (Dyslipidemia/Ortholiposis)	19: 22	10: 13	9: 9	0.65
NLR (mean ± SD)	2.22 ± 1.16	2.12 ± 0.74	2.34 ± 1.57	0.57

PTA, pure tone audiometry; ALT, alanine transaminase; NLR, neutrophil-to-lymphocyte ratio; SD, standard deviation; NAC, N-acetylcysteine. PTA pure tone average at 500, 1,000, 2,000, and 4,000 Hz hearing thresholds.

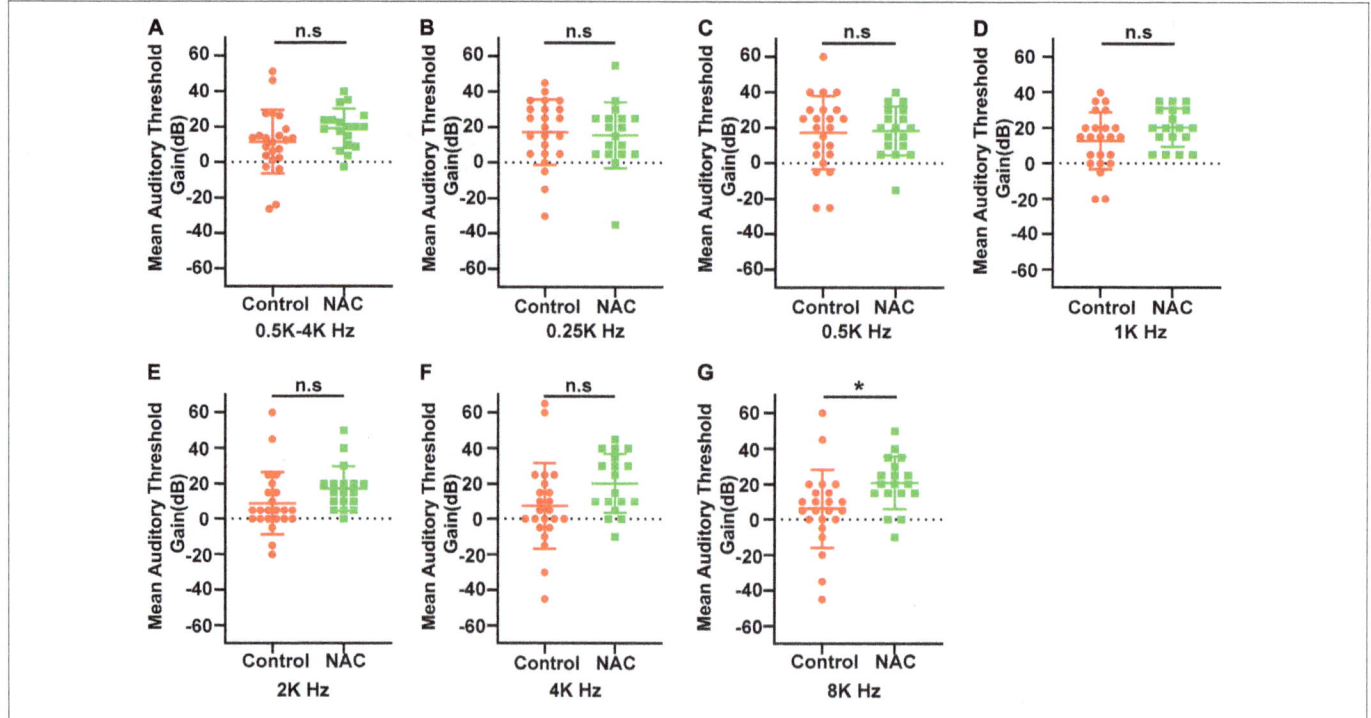

FIGURE 3 | (A) The mean hearing gain at 0.5–4k Hz in control and NAC groups. (B–G) The hearing gain at 0.25k (B), 0.5k (C), 1k (D), 2k (E), 4k (F), and 8k (G) Hz in two groups. *$P < 0.05$ and n.s, no significant difference.

aging, chronic cochlear infections, ototoxic drugs, and noise exposure (Zhu et al., 2018; Zhang Y. et al., 2019; Zhou et al., 2020). The reported mechanisms of hair cell damage mainly include mechanical shearing forces and oxidative damage to HCs (Liu et al., 2016; He et al., 2017; Li et al., 2018; Zhong et al., 2020), eventually induce apoptotic cell death in HCs, especially the outer HCs of the basal turn. The loss of sensory hair cells is irreversible in adult mammals. Although the neonatal cochlea has very limited hair cell regeneration ability, this regeneration ability is rapidly reduced with age (Wang et al., 2015; Zhang S. et al., 2019, 2020; Zhang Y. et al., 2020). It is still a controversy that the mechanism of SSNHL in the cochlea, Capaccio et al. (2012) had done a research indicating that the patients in SSNHL group had higher serum levels of ROS than in control group, therefore, researcher speculated that hearing loss in SSNHL may be due to antioxidant system failing to handle a sudden rise in ROS. There were studies indicating that excessive ROS, which was produced by noxious stimulation (such as noise, drug) in the cochlea, can destroy hair cell components by oxidizing molecules, such as DNA, proteins (Fechter, 2005; Li and Steyger, 2009). And the unbalance of antioxidant system can activate the programmed cell death pathway in cochlea, causing sensorineural hearing loss (Liu et al., 1998). Therefore, the GO model, a classical oxidative stress model, was used to set up a cochlear explant model of oxidative stress injury for studying SSNHL *in vitro* in our study. Our data show that NAC and dexamethasone have an obvious synergistic effect in the treatment of hair cell damage

TABLE 2 | Hearing improvements, respectively, in control and NAC group.

	Control group (n = 23)	NAC group (n = 18)
Hearing improvement (%)	9 (39%)	13 (72%)
No improvement (%)	14 (61%)	5 (28%)

$P = 0.035$.

induced by oxidative stress *in vitro*. There is plenty of evidence to suggest that NAC used as an antioxidant can attenuate hair cell degeneration or deafness *in vitro* or in different animal models of deafness (Kopke et al., 2000; Ohinata et al., 2003; Duan et al., 2004; Wang W. et al., 2017; Liu W. et al., 2019). Moreover, glucocorticoids have strong anti-inflammatory, antitoxic immunoregulatory effects. Some studies have reported that glucocorticoids can protect hair cells from a variety of adverse factors, such as noise and inflammation (Hirose et al., 2007; Haake et al., 2015; Müller et al., 2017). Evidence from animal and *in vitro* experiments suggests that hair cell protection may be one of the common therapeutic effects of NAC and glucocorticoid. In our *in vitro* experiments, the combination of NAC and glucocorticoids was effective in protecting hair cells, although they were administered at concentrations which were ineffective when used alone. Previous research suggests that NAC may be a steroid sensitizer which can help to treat steroid-resistant asthma in mice (Eftekhari et al., 2013). At present, we do not know whether the protection of hair cells is caused by NAC increasing the therapeutic effect of dexamethasone. However, this interesting finding has potential value for clinical application. It may help us overcome steroid-resistant SSNHL or achieve better results with smaller doses of drugs.

N-acetylcysteine combined with ITD therapy can significantly improve hearing loss at high frequency in SSHNL patients. A study by Machado et al. showed that ITD combined with oral prednisone and NAC can improve hearing loss at 4,000 Hz as initial therapy. However, it was not until 6 months later that there was a statistically-significant difference between the steroid alone group and the steroids + NAC group (Angeli et al., 2012). In our study, the onset of hearing loss of all patients was at more than 2 weeks. Therefore, a salvage therapy of ITD was adopted without oral steroids. Considering the safety of the drug, the oral dose of NAC was 600 mg two times daily in our design, which was half of the dose used in the study by Machado et al. Since we observed the protection of hair cells in the high frequency region *in vitro*, all the patients chosen in this study suffered hearing loss in the high frequency region (4,000 or 8,000 Hz). Our data showed that ITD combined with NAC as a salvage approach was found to significantly improve high-frequency hearing loss in patients with SSHNL.

The protective effect at high frequency may be caused by increasing the sensitivity of the inner ear to dexamethasone through oral NAC. When ITD is used in clinical practice, both injection dose and interval may affect the efficacy (Liebau et al., 2016). Recent studies found that the therapeutic effect of steroids on SSNHL can be significantly improved through use of a microcatheter with an electronic pump, near-continual transtympanic steroid perfusion or ITD administration using saturated Gelfoam (Chou et al., 2013; Li et al., 2013; Lundy et al., 2018). The above evidence suggested that increasing the amount and the effective time of steroids in the inner ear can significantly improve the therapeutic effect on SSNHL. However, the above method requires a complicated operation and corresponding equipment, making it difficult to popularize at present. Our finding, from another perspective, can achieve similar goals. We speculate that oral NAC may increase the effectiveness of steroids by reducing the minimum effective concentration or extending the effective duration. However, NAC may also help the hearing recovery of SSNHL patients through direct antioxidant effects.

Although there were some interesting findings, our study does have some limitations. Firstly, significant hearing improvement occurred only at high frequency. We and Machado et al. failed to observe any effect of this combination therapy on hearing improvement at low frequencies. Different doses of NAC and different methods of administration may need to be tried in the future. Secondly, the specific therapeutic mechanism of this combined therapy remains unknown. Although one study suggested that NAC alone can improve SSNHL, our *in vitro* experiment indicated that the synergistic effect of NAC and steroids may play a key role in protecting hair cells from oxidative stress. More evidence is needed to determine whether antioxidant therapy alone is effective against SSHNL. Finally, in our clinical trial, it was difficult to perform subgroup analysis of the different deafness types due to the limited numbers of patients. More extensive studies related to the associations between NAC and subtypes of SSNHL will be conducted with larger numbers of patients in future.

CONCLUSION

In this study, we found that NAC combined with dexamethasone may protect against hearing damage by protecting hair cells. The results of our clinical study suggest that the use of NAC in combination with ITD is beneficial in the 8,000 Hz frequency. Combined therapy of NAC and ITD can improve the hearing recovery rate of patients with SSNHL.

ETHICS STATEMENT

The studies involving human participants were reviewed and approved by the institutional review board of Wuhan Union hospital. Written informed consent to participate in this study was provided by the participants' legal guardian/next of kin. The animal study was reviewed and approved by the institutional review board of Wuhan Union hospital. Written informed consent was obtained from the owners for the participation of their animals in this study.

AUTHOR CONTRIBUTIONS

YS and SC conceived and designed the experiments. XB and KX performed the experiments *in vitro*. XB and XN collect the clinic data. YJ, LX, and YQ analyzed the data. XB, SC, and YS wrote the manuscript. All authors contributed to the article and approved the submitted version.

REFERENCES

Alexander, T. H., and Harris, J. P. (2013). Incidence of sudden sensorineural hearing loss. *Otol. Neurotol.* 34:1586. doi: 10.1097/MAO.0000000000000222

Angeli, S. I., Abi-Hachem, R. N., Vivero, R. J., Telischi, F. T., and Machado, J. J. L.-N. (2012). Acetylcysteine treatment is associated with improved hearing outcome in sudden idiopathic sensorineural hearing loss. *Acta Otolaryngol.* 132, 369–376. doi: 10.3109/00016489.2011.647359

Becatti, M., Marcucci, R., Mannucci, A., Gori, A. M., Giusti, B., Sofi, F., et al. (2017). Erythrocyte membrane fluidity alterations in sudden sensorineural hearing loss patients: the role of oxidative stress. *Thromb. Haemost.* 117, 2334–2345. doi: 10.1160/TH17-05-0356

Berjis, N., Soheilipour, S., Musavi, A., and Hashemi, S. M. (2016). Intratympanic dexamethasone injection vs methylprednisolone for the treatment of refractory sudden sensorineural hearing loss. *Adv. Biomed. Res.* 5:111. doi: 10.4103/2277-9175.184277

Capaccio, P., Pignataro, L., Gaini, L. M., Sigismund, P. E., Novembrino, C., De Giuseppe, R., et al. (2012). Unbalanced oxidative status in idiopathic sudden sensorineural hearing loss. *Eur. Arch. Otorhinolaryngol.* 269, 449–453. doi: 10.1007/s00405-011-1671-2

Chandrasekhar, S. S., Tsai Do, B. S., Schwartz, S. R., Bontempo, L. J., Faucett, E. A., Finestone, S. A., et al. (2019). Clinical practice guideline: sudden hearing loss (Update) executive summary. *Otolaryngol. Head Neck Surg.* 161, 195–210. doi: 10.1177/0194599819859883

Chen, C. H., and Young, Y. H. (2016). N-acetylcysteine as a single therapy for sudden deafness. *Acta Otolaryngol.* 137, 58–62. doi: 10.1080/00016489.2016.1214981

Chou, Y. F., Chen, P. R., Kuo, I. J., Yu, S. H., Wen, Y. H., and Wu, H. P. (2013). Comparison of intermittent intratympanic steroid injection and near-continual transtympanic steroid perfusion as salvage treatments for sudden sensorineural hearing loss. *Laryngoscope* 123, 2264–2269. doi: 10.1002/lary.23909

Duan, M., Qiu, J., Laurell, G. R., Olofsson, k, Counter, S. A., and Borg, E. (2004). Dose and time-dependent protection of the antioxidant N-L-acetylcysteine against impulse noise trauma. *Hear. Res.* 192, 1–9. doi: 10.1016/j.heares.2004.02.005

Eftekhari, P., Hajizadeh, S., Raoufy, M. R., Masjedi, M. R., and Foster, P. S. (2013). Preventive effect of N-acetylcysteine in a mouse model of steroid resistant acute exacerbation of asthma. *EXCLI J.* 12, 184–192.

Fechter, L. D. (2005). Oxidative stress: a potential basis for potentiation of noise-induced hearing loss. *Environ. Toxicol. Pharmacol.* 19, 543–546. doi: 10.1016/j.etap.2004.12.017

Ferri, E., Frisina, A., Fasson, A. C., Armato, E., Spinato, G., and Amadori, M. (2012). Intratympanic steroid treatment for idiopathic sudden sensorineural hearing loss after failure of intravenous therapy. *ISRN Otolaryngol.* 2012:647271. doi: 10.5402/2012/647271

Haake, S. M., Dinh, C. T., Chen, S., Eshraghi, A. A., and Water, T. R. V. D. (2015). Dexamethasone protects auditory hair cells against TNFalpha-initiated apoptosis via activation of PI3K/Akt and NFkappaB signaling. *Hear. Res.* 255, 22–32. doi: 10.1016/j.heares.2009.05.003

Hatano, M., Uramoto, N., Okabe, Y., Furukawa, M., and Makoto, I. (2008). Vitamin E and vitamin C in the treatment of idiopathic sudden sensorineural hearing loss. *Acta Otolaryngol.* 128, 116–121. doi: 10.1080/00016480701387132

He, Z., Guo, L., Shu, Y., Fang, Q., Zhou, H., Liu, Y., et al. (2017). Autophagy protects auditory hair cells against neomycin-induced damage. *Autophagy* 13, 1884–1904. doi: 10.1080/15548627.2017.1359449

Hirose, Y., Tabuchi, K., Oikawa, K., Murashita, H., and Hara, A. (2007). The effects of the glucocorticoid receptor antagonist RU486 and phospholipase A2 inhibitor quinacrine on acoustic injury of the mouse cochlea. *Neurosci. Lett.* 413, 63–67. doi: 10.1016/j.neulet.2006.11.029

Hunchaisri, N., Chantapant, S., and Srinangyam, N. (2010). Intratympanic dexamethasone for refractory sudden sensorineural hearing loss. *Chotmaihet Thangphaet* 93, 1406–1414.

Jarosław, P., Sutkowy, P., Piechocki, J., and Woźniak, A. (2019). Markers of oxidant-antioxidant equilibrium in patients with sudden sensorineural hearing loss treated with hyperbaric oxygen therapy. *Oxid. Med. Cell. Longev.* 2019:8472346. doi: 10.1155/2019/8472346

Joachims, H. Z., Segal, J., Golz, A., Netzer, A., and Goldenberg, D. (2003). Antioxidants in treatment of idiopathic sudden hearing loss. *Otol. Neurotol.* 24, 572–575. doi: 10.1097/00129492-200307000-00007

Kang, H. S., Park, J. J., Ahn, S. K., Hur, D. G., and Kim, H. Y. (2013). Effect of high dose intravenous vitamin C on idiopathic sudden sensorineural hearing loss: a prospective single-blind randomized controlled trial. *Eur. Arch. Oto Rhino Laryngol.* 270, 2631–2636. doi: 10.1007/s00405-012-2294-y

Kaya, H., Koç, A. K., Sayın, Ý, Güneş, S., Altıntaş, A., Yeğin, Y., et al. (2015). Vitamins A, C, and E and selenium in the treatment of idiopathic sudden sensorineural hearing loss. *Eur. Arch. Otorhinolaryngol.* 272, 1119–1125. doi: 10.1007/s00405-014-2922-9

Kitoh, R., Nishio, S. Y., and Usami, S. I. (2020). Treatment algorithm for idiopathic sudden sensorineural hearing loss based on epidemiologic surveys of a large Japanese cohort. *Acta Otolaryngol.* 140, 32–39. doi: 10.1080/00016489.2019.1687936

Kopke, R. D., Weisskopf, P. A., Boone, J. L., Jackson, R. L., Wester, D. C., Hoffer, M. E., et al. (2000). Reduction of noise-induced hearing loss using L-NAC and salicylate in the chinchilla. *Hear. Res.* 149, 138–146. doi: 10.1016/S0378-5955(00)00176-3

Li, H., Feng, G., Wang, H., and Feng, Y. (2015). Intratympanic steroid therapy as a salvage treatment for sudden sensorineural hearing loss after failure of conventional therapy: a meta-analysis of randomized. controlled trials. *Clin. Ther.* 37, 178–187. doi: 10.1016/j.clinthera.2014.11.009

Li, H., Song, Y., He, Z., Chen, X., Wu, X., Li, X., et al. (2018). Meclofenamic acid reduces reactive oxygen species accumulation and apoptosis, inhibits excessive autophagy, and protects hair cell-like HEI-OC1 cells from cisplatin-induced damage. *Front. Cell. Neurosci.* 12:139. doi: 10.3389/fncel.2018.00139

Li, H., and Steyger, P. S. (2009). Synergistic ototoxicity due to noise exposure and aminoglycoside antibiotics. *Noise Health* 11, 26–32. doi: 10.4103/1463-1741.45310

Li, L., Ren, J., Yin, T., and Liu, W. (2013). Intratympanic dexamethasone perfusion versus injection for treatment of refractory sudden sensorineural hearing loss. *Eur. Arch. Oto Rhino Laryngol.* 270, 861–867. doi: 10.1007/s00405-012-2061-0

Liebau, A., Pogorzelski, O., Salt, A. N., and Plontke, S. K. (2016). Hearing changes after intratympanically applied steroids for primary therapy of sudden hearing loss: a meta-analysis using mathematical simulations of drug delivery protocols. *Otol. Neurotol.* 38, 19–30. doi: 10.1097/MAO.0000000000001254

Liu, L., Chen, Y., Qi, J., Zhang, Y., He, Y., Ni, W., et al. (2016). Wnt activation protects against neomycin-induced hair cell damage in the mouse cochlea. *Cell Death Dis.* 7:e2136. doi: 10.1038/cddis.2016.35

Liu, W., Staecker, H., Stupak, H., Malgrange, B., Lefebvre, P., and Van De Water, T. R. (1998). Caspase inhibitors prevent cisplatin-induced apoptosis of auditory sensory cells. . *NeuroReport* 9, 2609–2614. doi: 10.1097/00001756-199808030-00034

Liu, W., Xu, X., Fan, Z., Sun, G., Han, Y., Zhang, D., et al. (2019). Wnt signaling activates TP53-Induced glycolysis and apoptosis regulator and protects against cisplatin-induced spiral ganglion neuron damage in the mouse cochlea. *Antioxid. Redox Signal.* 30, 1389–1410. doi: 10.1089/ars.2017.7288

Liu, Y., Qi, J., Chen, X., Tang, M., Chu, C., Zhu, W., et al. (2019). Critical role of spectrin in hearing development and deafness. *Sci. Adv.* 5:eaav7803. doi: 10.1126/sciadv.aav7803

Lundy, L., Karatayli Ozgursoy, S., and Kleindienst, S. (2018). Intratympanic dexamethasone via saturated gelfoam for idiopathic sudden sensorineural hearing loss. *Otolaryngol. Head Neck Surg.* 160, 361–363. doi: 10.1177/0194599818816306

Michel, O. (2011). The revised version of the german guidelines "sudden idiopathic sensorineural hearing loss". *Laryngo Rhino Otologie* 90, 290–293. doi: 10.1055/s-0031-1273721

Moon, I. S., Lee, J. D., Kim, J., Hong, S., and Lee, W. (2011). Intratympanic dexamethasone is an effective method as a salvage treatment in refractory sudden hearing loss. *Otol. Neurotol.* 32, 1432–1436. doi: 10.1097/MAO.0b013e318238fc43

Müller, M., Tisch, M., Maier, H., and Lwenheim, H. (2017). Reduction of permanent hearingloss by local glucocorticoid application : guinea pigs with acute acoustic trauma. *HNO* 65, 1–10. doi: 10.1007/s00106-016-0266-z

Nakashima, T., Sato, H., Gyo, K., Hato, N., Yoshida, T., Shimono, M., et al. (2014). Idiopathic sudden sensorineural hearing loss in Japan. *Acta Otolaryngol.* 134, 1158–1163. doi: 10.3109/00016489.2014.919406

Niran, H., Chantapant, S., and Sirirattanapan, J. (2015). Effectiveness of oral zinc supplementation in the treatment of idiopathic sudden sensorineural hearing loss (ISSNHL). *J. Med. Assoc. Thai.* 98, 400–407.

Ohinata, Y., Miller, J. M., and Schacht, J. (2003). Protection from noise-induced lipid peroxidation and hair cell loss in the cochlea. *Brain Res.* 966, 265–273. doi: 10.1016/S0006-8993(02)04205-1

Ozdamar, K., Sen, A., and Gonel, A. (2019). Assessment of oxidative stress in patients with sudden hearing loss: a non-randomized prospective clinical study. *Indian J. Otolaryngol. Head Neck Surg.* 71(Suppl 2), 1543–1548. doi: 10.1007/s12070-019-01623-z

Pathak, S., Stern, C., and Vambutas, A. N. - (2015). Acetylcysteine attenuates tumor necrosis factor alpha levels in autoimmune inner ear disease patients. *Immunol. Res.* 63, 236–245. doi: 10.1007/s12026-015-8696-3

Qi, J., Liu, Y., Chu, C., Chen, X., Zhu, W., Shu, Y., et al. (2019). A cytoskeleton structure revealed by super-resolution fluorescence imaging in inner ear hair cells. *Cell Discov.* 5:12. doi: 10.1038/s41421-018-0076-4

Riga, M. G., Chelis, L., Kakolyris, S., Papadopoulos, S., and Danielides, V. (2013). Transtympanic injections of N-acetylcysteine for the prevention of cisplatin-induced ototoxicity: a feasible method with promising efficacy. *Am. J. Clin. Oncol.* 36, 1–6. doi: 10.1097/COC.0b013e31822e006d

Sun, H., Qiu, X., Hu, J., and Ma, Z. (2018). Comparison of intratympanic dexamethasone therapy and hyperbaric oxygen therapy for the salvage treatment of refractory high-frequency sudden sensorineural hearing loss. *Am. J. Otolaryngol.* 39, 531–535. doi: 10.1016/j.amjoto.2018.06.004

Tillinger, J. A., Gupta, C., Ila, K., Ahmed, J., Mittal, J., Van De Water, T. R., et al. (2018). l-N-acetylcysteine protects outer hair cells against TNFalpha initiated ototoxicity in vitro. *Acta Otolaryngol.* 138, 676–684. doi: 10.1080/00016489.2018.1440086

Tong, B., Wang, Q., Dai, Q., Hellstrom, S., and Duan, M. (2020). Efficacy of various corticosteroid treatment modalities for the initial treatment of idiopathic sudden hearing loss: a prospective randomized controlled trial. *Audiol. Neurootol.* 26, 45–52. doi: 10.1159/000508124

Wang, T., Chai, R., Kim, G. S., Pham, N., Jansson, L., Nguyen, D. H., et al. (2015). Lgr5+ cells regenerate hair cells via proliferation and direct transdifferentiation in damaged neonatal mouse utricle. *Nat. Commun.* 6:6613. doi: 10.1038/ncomms7613

Wang, W., Li, D., Ding, X., Zhao, Q., Chen, J., Tian, K., et al. (2017). N-Acetylcysteine protects inner ear hair cells and spiral ganglion neurons from manganese exposure by regulating ROS levels. *Toxicol. Lett.* 279, 77–86. . . doi: 10.1016/j.toxlet.2017.07.903

Wang, Y., Li, J., Yao, X., Li, W., Du, H., Tang, M., et al. (2017). Loss of CIB2 causes profound hearing loss and abolishes mechanoelectrical transduction in mice. *Front. Mol. Neurosci.* 10:401. doi: 10.3389/fnmol.2017.00401

Yang, C. H., Ko, M. T., Peng, J. P., and Hwang, C. F. (2011). Zinc in the treatment of idiopathic sudden sensorineural hearing loss. *Laryngoscope* 121, 617–621. doi: 10.1002/lary.21291

Zhang, S., Liu, D., Dong, Y., Zhang, Z., Zhang, Y., Zhou, H., et al. (2019). Frizzled-9+ supporting cells are progenitors for the generation of hair cells in the postnatal mouse cochlea. *Front. Mol. Neurosci.* 12:184. doi: 10.3389/fnmol.2019.00184

Zhang, S., Qiang, R., Dong, Y., Zhang, Y., Chen, Y., Zhou, H., et al. (2020). Hair cell regeneration from inner ear progenitors in the mammalian cochlea. *Am. J. Stem Cells* 9, 25–35.

Zhang, Y., Li, W., He, Z., Wang, Y., Shao, B., Cheng, C., et al. (2019). Pre-treatment with fasudil prevents neomycin-induced hair cell damage by reducing the accumulation of reactive oxygen species. *Front. Mol. Neurosci.* 12:264. doi: 10.3389/fnmol.2019.00264

Zhang, Y., Zhang, S., Zhang, Z., Dong, Y., Ma, X., Qiang, R., et al. (2020). Knockdown of Foxg1 in Sox9+ supporting cells increases the transdifferentiation of supporting cells into hair cells in the neonatal mouse utricle. *Aging* 12, 19834–19851. doi: 10.18632/aging.104009

Zhong, Z., Fu, X., Li, H., Chen, J., Wang, M., Gao, S., et al. (2020). Citicoline protects auditory hair cells against neomycin-induced damage. *Front. Cell Dev. Biol.* 8:712. doi: 10.3389/fcell.2020.00712

Zhou, H., Qian, X., Xu, N., Zhang, S., Zhu, G., Zhang, Y., et al. (2020). Disruption of Atg7-dependent autophagy causes electromotility disturbances, outer hair cell loss, and deafness in mice. *Cell Death Dis.* 11:913. doi: 10.1038/s41419-020-03110-8

Zhu, C., Cheng, C., Wang, Y., Muhammad, W., Liu, S., Zhu, W., et al. (2018). Loss of ARHGEF6 causes hair cell stereocilia deficits and hearing loss in mice. *Front. Mol. Neurosci.* 11:362. doi: 10.3389/fnmol.2018.00362

CCDC154 Mutant Caused Abnormal Remodeling of the Otic Capsule and Hearing Loss in Mice

Kai Xu[1†], Xue Bai[1†], Sen Chen[1†], Le Xie[1], Yue Qiu[1], He Li[2]* and Yu Sun[1]*

[1] Department of Otorhinolaryngology, Union Hospital, Tongji Medical College, Huazhong University of Science and Technology, Wuhan, China,
[2] Department of Otolaryngology, The First Affiliated Hospital of Wenzhou Medical University, Wenzhou, China

*Correspondence:
He Li
lihewuyao@163.com
Yu Sun
sunyu@hust.edu.cn
†These authors have contributed equally to this work

Osteopetrosis is a rare inherited bone disease characterized by dysfunction of osteoclasts, causing impaired bone resorption and remodeling, which ultimately leads to increased bone mass and density. Hearing loss is one of the most common complications of osteopetrosis. However, the etiology and pathogenesis of auditory damage still need to be explored. In this study, we found that a spontaneous mutation of coiled-coil domain-containing 154 (CCDC154) gene, a new osteopetrosis-related gene, induced congenital deafness in mice. Homozygous mutant mice showed moderate to severe hearing loss, while heterozygous or wild-type (WT) littermates displayed normal hearing. Pathological observation showed that abnormal bony remodeling of the otic capsule, characterized by increased vascularization and multiple cavitary lesions, was found in homozygous mutant mice. Normal structure of the organ of Corti and no substantial hair cell or spiral ganglion neuron loss was observed in homozygous mutant mice. Our results indicate that mutation of the osteopetrosis-related gene CCDC154 can induce syndromic hereditary deafness in mice. Bony remodeling disorders of the auditory ossicles and otic capsule are involved in the hearing loss caused by CDCC154 mutation.

Keywords: CCDC154, otosclerosis, hearing loss, auditory ossicles, otic capsule

INTRODUCTION

Osteopetrosis is a rare bone disorder caused by the absence or dysfunction of osteoclasts. This leads to a marked increase in bone density due to defective bone resorption (Del Fattore et al., 2008). Osteoclast-mediated bone resorption plays a vital role in bone homeostasis, and perturbation of this process can lead to profound alterations in bone mass that have clinical relevance. In addition to skeletal lesions, patients with osteopetrosis are often also affected by neurological complications, notably hearing loss or visual impairment. Approximately 80% of patients with osteosclerosis develop hearing loss in childhood. Most deaf patients present with conductive deafness due to abnormalities of the auditory ossicles or temporal bone, while some present with sensorineural or mixed hearing loss (Stocks et al., 1998; Dozier et al., 2005). Most cases of osteosclerosis are caused by genetic mutations, but a few cases still lack an accurate molecular diagnosis (Sobacchi et al., 2013). These findings suggest that osteosclerosis-related genes are also involved in the formation and maintenance of normal hearing.

There are many animal models of osteosclerosis with hearing-related symptoms. The osteopetrotic mutation toothless (tl) rat exhibits auditory ossicle abnormalities and hearing loss due to the truncated *Csf1* gene (encoding colony-stimulating facter-1, CSF-1) and non-functional protein (Aharinejad et al., 1999; Van Wesenbeeck et al., 2002). Auditory brainstem and visual evoked potentials are both abnormal in CSF-1-deficient mice (Michaelson et al., 1996). Osteoprotegerin (OPG) is a key regulator of bone homeostasis. Mice lacking OPG show abnormal remodeling of the otic capsule and auditory ossicles induced by osteoclast hyperactivity (Zehnder et al., 2005; Kanzaki et al., 2006). Moreover, the absence of OPG in the inner ear causes demyelination of the cochlear nerve and sensorineural hearing loss (Kao et al., 2013).

The mammalian middle ear contains the most delicate bone structure, called the ossicular chain, which consists of the malleus, incus, and stapes. These ossicles transmit vibrations from the tympanic membrane through the oval window to the inner ear, where the vibrations are converted into electrical signals in the otic capsule of the temporal bone and transduced to the brain *via* auditory nerves (Frolenkov et al., 2004). Osteoclasts are essential for development of the bone structures of the middle ear (Mallo, 2001), and the absence of osteoclastic resorption perturbs the process of bone resorption in the auditory ossicles or the otic capsule, thus significantly affecting their morphology and function (Kanzaki et al., 2011). Therefore, abnormal osteoclasts may cause deafness by affecting the bone structure development of the middle and inner ears. A new spontaneous autosomal recessive osteopetrosis mouse strain was reported by Lu et al. (2009). A CCDC15 mutant was identified in this strain and the osteoclasts were deficient in bone resorption. These mice displayed an osteopetrotic phenotype, including lack of tooth roots, relatively pyknotic and much thinner cortical bone. However, whether the mutant mice had auditory system complications had not been explored. In this study, we evaluated hearing function in this mouse line. Furthermore, the pathology of the auditory ossicles and the inner ear was investigated. Abnormal bony remodeling due to disordered osteoclastic bone resorption was observed in the otic capsule of homozygous mutant mice which displayed congenital deafness with abnormal bony remodeling in the otic capsule and auditory ossicles. However, the morphology of the organ of Corti (OC) showed normal organization and there was no cell loss in the auditory sensory epithelium or the spiral ganglion neurons (SGNs). Our findings provide further support for a critical role of osteoclasts in the development of auditory ossicles and the otic capsule. Abnormal bony remodeling of the auditory ossicles and otic capsule due to deficient osteoclasts might be the potential cause of hearing loss in CCDC154 mutant mice.

MATERIALS AND METHODS

Mouse Model

Osteopetrosis mutant (ntl) mice were provided by Prof. Xin-Cheng Lu at Wenzhou Medical College. Homozygous mutant mice were generated by crossbreeding the heterozygous mutant mice. As reported previously (Lu et al., 2009; Liao et al., 2012), mouse genotyping was performed by PCR amplification of tail genomic DNA, using the following genotyping primers:

CCDC154-mutant: (F) -5′CAGTCATGGCAATGACAAACA-3′
CCDC154-mutant: (R) -5′CAGGAAGGACCTAGCAAGATA-3′
CCDC154-wild-type: (F)-5′TGGGGTGGGAGACTGGTTATGTGT-3′
CCDC154-wild-type: (R)-5′GTGGGGCCGCAGTTGTCAGAAG-3′.

All mice were raised in the specific-pathogen-free Experimental Animal Center of Huazhong University of Science and Technology. All experimental procedures were conducted in accordance with the policies of the Committee on Animal Research of Tongji Medical College, Huazhong University of Science and Technology.

Auditory Brainstem Response

Auditory brainstem response (ABR) was examined at P20. As we previously reported (Chen et al., 2018), mice ($n = 5$ in each group) were anesthetized by intraperitoneal injection with a mixture of ketamine (120 mg/kg) and chlorpromazine (20 mg/kg). Body temperature was maintained by placing the mice on an electric blanket. The recording electrode was placed at the vertex of the skull, and the reference electrode was placed at the tested ear, with an earth electrode placed at the contralateral ear. Tone bursts of 8, 16, 24, 32, and 40 kHz were generated and responses were recorded using a Tucker-Davis Technologies system (RZ6, Tucker-Davis Tech., Alachua, FL, United States). The responses were recorded as the average response to 1,024 stimuli and were recorded in decreasing 10 dB steps, which narrowed to 5 dB steps near the threshold. The lowest sound level that could be recognized was considered to be the auditory threshold.

Preparation and Morphological Examination of Auditory Ossicles

Mice were deeply anesthetized and then culled by cervical dislocation. The middle ear was exposed by dissection of the bulla, and then the malleus, incus, and stapes were carefully separated from the middle ear. The collected tissues were fixed in 4% paraformaldehyde at room temperature for 2 h. For frozen sections, after decalcification with disodium EDTA for 48 h, the auditory ossicles were dehydrated with sucrose and embedded in OCT overnight at 4°C. Sections with a thickness of 10 μm were cut for morphological examination. Hematoxylin-eosin (HE) staining was performed following standard protocols.

Cochlear Tissue Preparation and Immunofluorescent Labeling

Mice were deeply anesthetized and sacrificed at P20. The cochleae were carefully dissected from the temporal bones and fixed in 4% paraformaldehyde at room temperature for

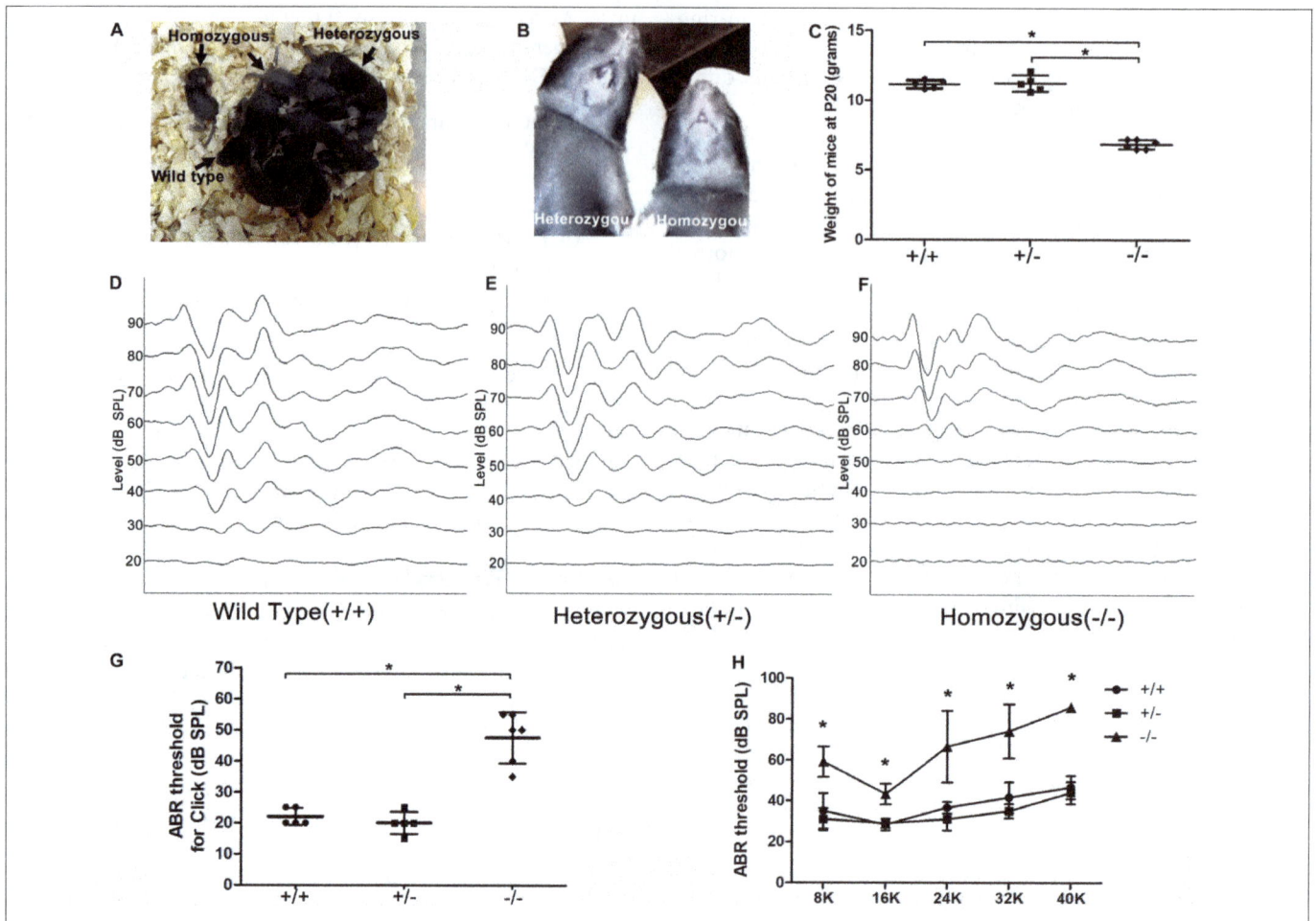

FIGURE 1 | Significant hearing loss was observed in the homozygous mutant mice. (A) A litter of CDCC mutant mice, homozygous mutant mice showed smaller body size compared to wild-type or heterozygous littermates. (B) Homozygous mutant mice displayed no tooth. (C) Comparison of the weight at P20 between the three groups (D–F) ABR-click waveforms in wild type (D), heterozygous (E), and homozygous mice (F), respectively. (G) Comparison of the ABR-click thresholds between the three groups. (H) Comparison of tone-burst thresholds in the three groups. *Significantly different from the control group ($P < 0.05$). All ABR tests were performed at P20.

1 h. For frozen sections, after decalcification with disodium EDTA for 48 h, the cochleae were dehydrated in 20 and 30% sucrose for 1.5 h each and then embedded in OCT overnight at 4°C. Modiolar sections with a thickness of 10 μm were cut for subsequent procedures as described previously (Zhou et al., 2016). For flattened cochlear preparations, each stretched cochlear preparation was carefully dissected from decalcifying cochleae in PBS. The sections or flattened cochlear preparations were incubated in a blocking solution of 10% donkey serum with 0.1% Triton X-100 for 1 h at room temperature, and then incubated with polyclonal rabbit anti-myosin 7a antibodies (1:500 dilution, 25–6,790, Proteus Biosciences, Ramona, CA, United States), or polyclonal goat anti-sox2 antibodies (1:200 dilution, AF2018, R&D systems, Minneapolis, MN, United States) diluted in PBS with 0.3% Triton X-100 overnight at 4°C. Samples were washed three times in PBS with 0.1% Tween-20 and then stained with Alexa Fluor 647 donkey anti-goat IgG or Alexa Fluor 488 donkey anti-rabbit IgG (1:200 dilution; ANT032 and ANT031, Antgene Biotechnology Company Ltd., Wuhan, China) for 2 h at room temperature. DAPI (C1005; Beyotime Biotechnology) and phalloidin (0.05 mg/mL; P5282; Sigma-Aldrich, St. Louis, MO, United States) were used for nuclear and F-actin staining. Images of each cochlea turn were obtained with a laser scanning confocal 408 microscope (Nikon, Tokyo, Japan).

Nissl Staining Analysis

Animals were deeply anesthetized and heart perfusion was performed with 4% paraformaldehyde in PBS. The brains were carefully removed and fixed in 4% paraformaldehyde overnight at room temperature, and then dehydrated sequentially through graded alcohol, and embedded in paraffin following a conventional protocol. Sections with a thickness of 5 μm were cut for Nissl staining. Transverse sections were deparaffinized with xylene, followed by rehydration in graded alcohol and immersion in 0.3% toluidine blue for 40 min at 60°C as described previously (Chen et al., 2015). The number of neurons in the V layer of the auditory cortex was counted.

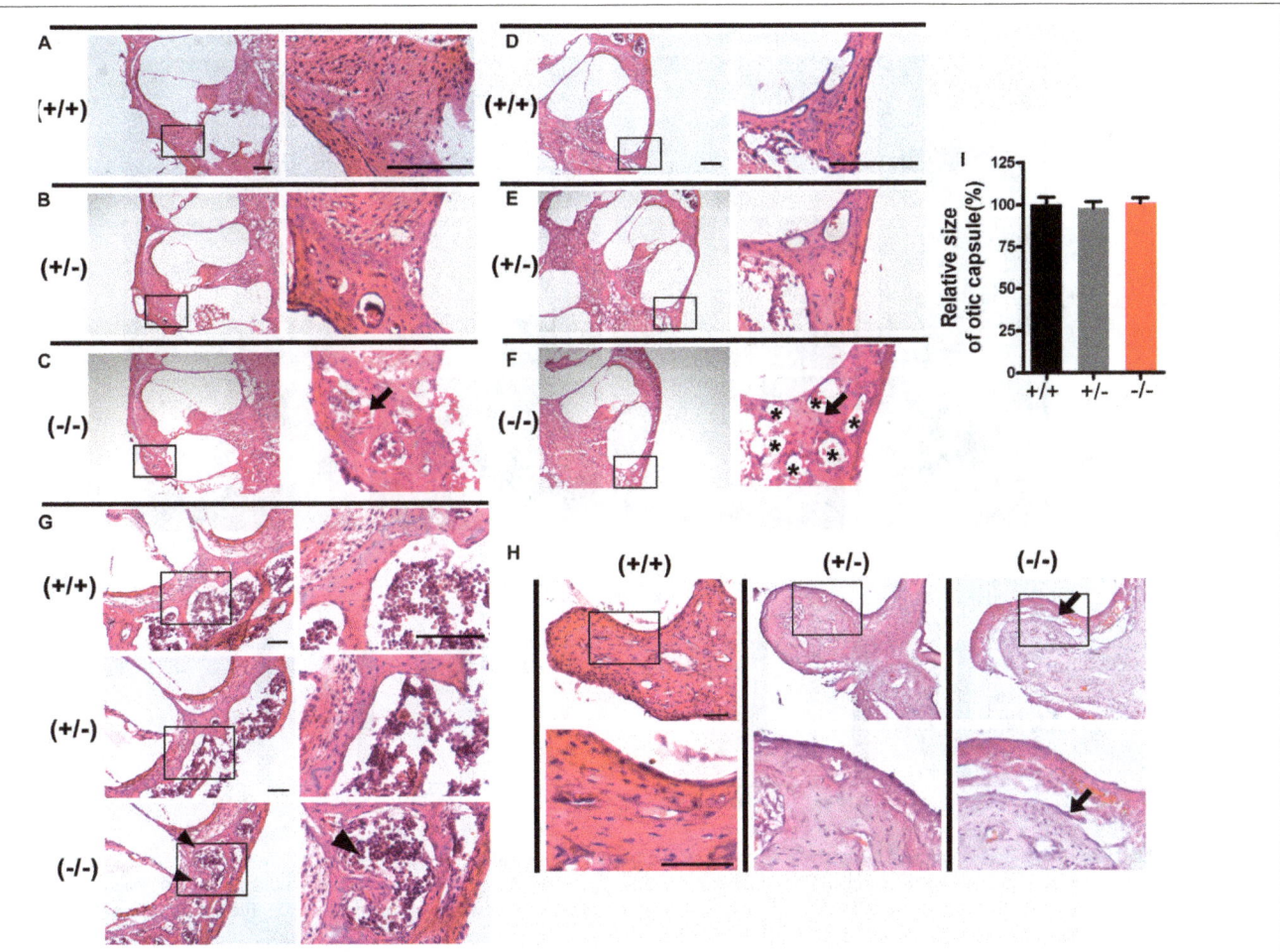

FIGURE 2 | Histological examination of the otic capsule and auditory ossicles in the mutant mice. **(A–C)** The basal turn of modiolar sections stained with hematoxylin-eosin (HE) in wild type **(A)**, heterozygous **(B)**, and homozygous **(C)** mutant mice, respectively. **(D–F)** The middle turn of otic capsule in wild type **(D)**, heterozygous **(E)**, and homozygous **(F)** mutant mice, respectively. Black arrows indicate the regions of abnormal bone remodeling in otic capsule from homozygous mutant mice **(C,F)**, Asterisks indicate the numerous large vascular channels **(F)**. **(G)** The apical turn of otic capsule in the three groups. Black arrowheads indicate the regions of abnormal bone remodeling and erodes the cartilage of otic capsule. **(H)** Representative images of malleus stained with hematoxylin-eosin (HE) from three groups. Black arrows indicate abnormal bone resorption and the bony cortex of the malleus was thickened in homozygous mutant mice. **(I)** Relative heights of the organ of Corti in the wild type and mutant mice. The scales in panels **(A,D,G,H)** represent 100 μm.

Data Analyses

All data are presented as means ± S.D. and were plotted by GraphPad Prism (Version 8.0, GraphPad Software Inc., La Jolla, CA, United States). The t-tests were performed using SPSS software (version 19, IBM SPSS Statistics, Armonk, NY, United States), and $P < 0.05$ was considered to be statistically significant.

RESULTS

Edentulism and Significant Hearing Loss Was Observed in the Homozygous Mutant Mice

The homozygous mutant mice had a smaller body size compared to wild-type (WT) or heterozygous littermates (**Figure 1A**) and no tooth eruption (**Figure 1B**). The homozygous mutant mice weighed only approximately half as much as the WT or heterozygous mutant mice at P20 (**Figure 1C**). ABR was tested at P18–20. The homozygous mutant mice showed hearing loss at all frequencies, while heterozygous or WT littermates displayed normal hearing ($n = 5$ mice in each group). The different ABR-click waveforms in the three groups are shown (**Figures 1D–F**). The minimum sound intensity to evoke a response (threshold) was $50.0 ± 5.5$ dB sound pressure level (SPL) in the homozygous mutant mice and $22.5 ± 2.5$ or $20.0 ± 3.2$ in the heterozygous or WT mice, respectively (**Figure 1G**, $P < 0.05$). ABR-click waveforms showed that there was obvious wave I–III at 70–90 dB SPL in homozygous mutant mice (**Figure 1F**). The thresholds of homozygous mutant mice at 8, 16, 24, 32, and 40 kHz were $62.0 ± 2.4$, $44.0 ± 14.9$, $72.0 ± 11.7$, $79.0 ± 5.8$, and $86.0 ± 2$ dB SPL, respectively. In comparison, the hearing thresholds of WT mice were $33.8 ± 6.5$, $27.5 ± 2.5$, $35.0 ± 3.5$, $41.3 ± 5.4$, and

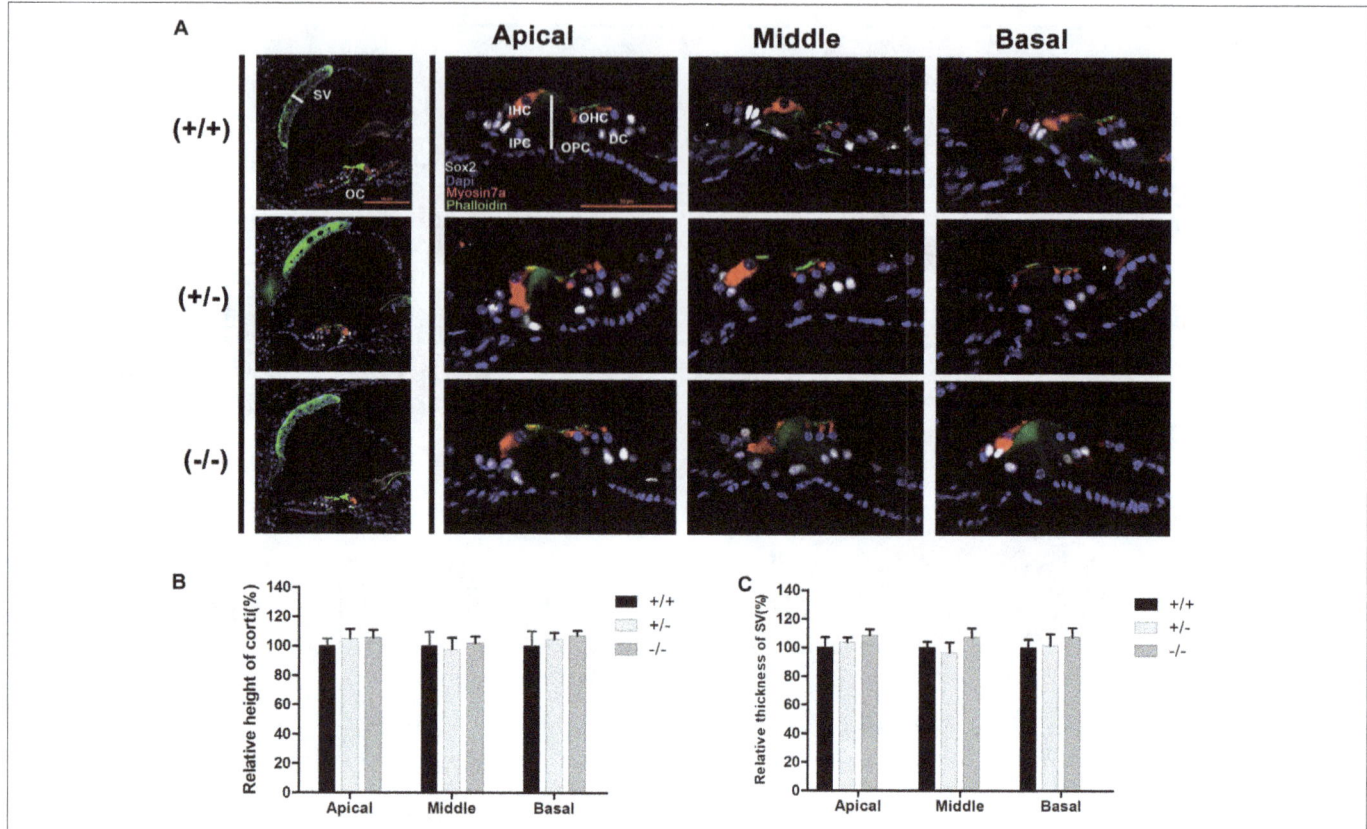

FIGURE 3 | There was no significant change in the cochlear morphology of the mutant mice. (A) Myosin7a (red) and Sox2 (white) immunolabeling showing the morphology of the organ of Corti and spiral ligament in different turns from the wild type, heterozygous and homozygous mutant mice. (B) Relative heights of the organ of Corti in the wild type and mutant mice. (C) Relative thickness of the organ of Corti in the wild type and mutant mice. The scales in panel (A) represent 50 μm.

47.5 ± 4.3 dB SPL respectively, at corresponding frequencies. Differences between the homozygous and WT animals were significant at all frequencies (**Figure 1H**, $P < 0.05$, one-way ANOVA).

Abnormal Structure of the Auditory Ossicles and Otic Capsule in the Mutant Mice

Disruption of transmission in the middle ear can also be associated with elevated ABR thresholds. The tympanic membrane and middle ear of mice were observed under an optical microscope after posterior auricular incision. The tympanic membrane and bulla were normal, there was no effusion in the tympanum and no evidence of infection was seen in mutant mice. To examine the morphology of the auditory ossicles, we isolated the malleus, incus, and stapes from the middle ear cavities. There were no significant structural differences of the malleus, incus or stapes in homozygous mutant mice compared with heterozygous or WT littermates. To further analyze the histological characteristics of the auditory ossicles and otic capsule in mutant mice, sections of auditory ossicles stained with HE showed increased active bone remodeling of the otic capsule in homozygous mutant mice compared with heterozygous or WT littermates. Notable features of the active bone remodeling included formation of well-defined hypercellular areas, abundant angiogenesis and cavitary lesions in the otic capsule showing bone resorption and deposition (**Figures 2C,F**), compared to the same area in the heterozygous or wild type (**Figures 2A,B,D,E**). Abnormal bone resorption and hypercellular erosion of the cartilage of the otic capsule in the apical turn were observed in homozygous mutant mice, while the cartilage in heterozygous or WT mice displayed intact boundaries (**Figure 2G**). However, the size of ear cartilage capsule of homozygous mutant mice was not significantly different, compared to heterozygous and WT mice (**Figure 2I**). Furthermore, the auditory ossicles also showed remodeling, as evidenced by abnormal bone resorption, and the bony cortex of the malleus was thickened in homozygous mutant mice (**Figure 2H**).

Normal Structure of the Organ of Corti and no Hair Cell Loss Were Observed in the Mutant Mice

Normal formation of the OC is essential for hearing development, and the tunnel of Corti usually opens completely in all

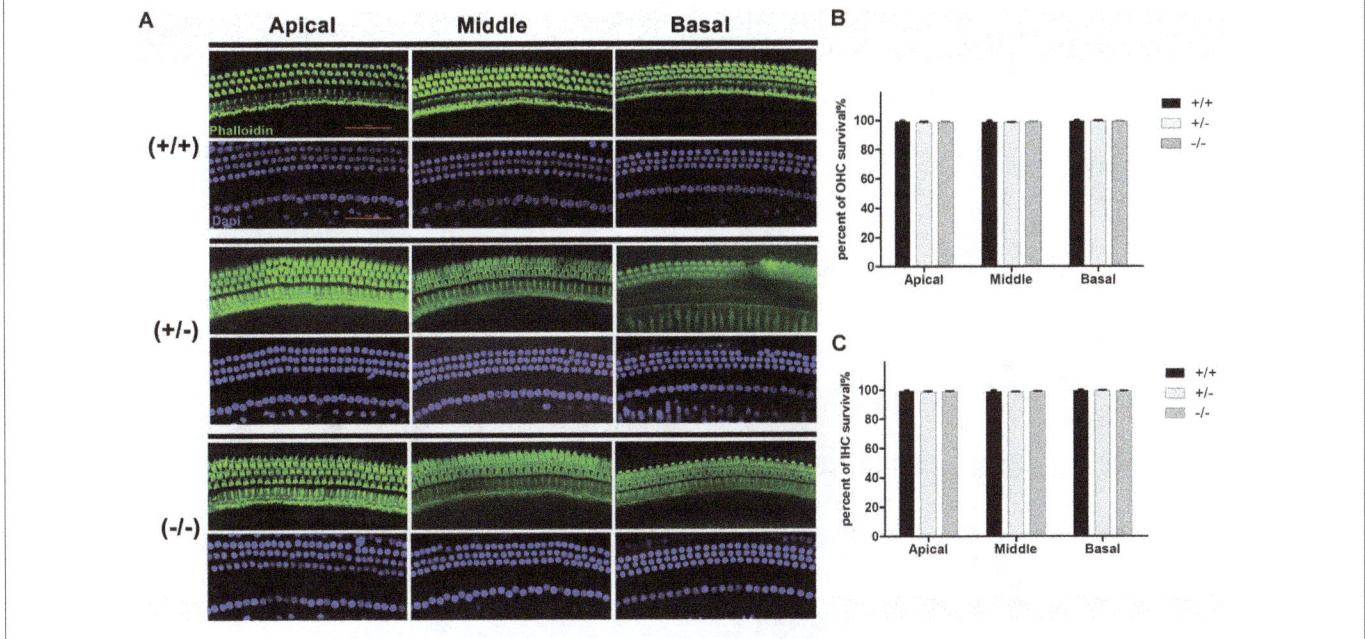

FIGURE 4 | There was no significant degeneration of hair cell in the mutant mice at P20. (A) Representative images of HCs (Phalloidin, green) in the apical, middle, and basal turn of basilar membrane from the wild type, heterozygous and homozygous mutant mice. (B) Quantifications of OHCs survival at specific cochlear locations in the different groups at P20. (C) Quantifications of IHCs survival at specific cochlear locations in the different groups at P20. The scales in panel (A) represent 50 μm.

turns at P8–P9 (Roth and Bruns, 1992a,b). Immunostaining of radial sections showed that the tunnel of Corti and the spiral ligament were well formed at P20 in homozygous mutant mice (**Figure 3A**). In mice from different groups, hair cells were labeled by Myonsin7a (red) while supporting cells expressed Sox2 (white **Figure 3A**). There was no significant change in the height of the OC in any of the three turns of homozygous mutant mice compared with WT mice (**Figure 3B**). The stria vascularis (SV) showed normal three-layered organization and the thickness was not significantly changed in homozygous mutant mice (**Figures 3A,C**). No substantial hair cell loss was observed in heterozygous or homozygous mutant mice at P20 (**Figures 4A–C**).

There Was No Significant Degeneration of Spiral Ganglion Neurons or Auditory Cortical Neurons in Mutant Mice

HE-stained radial sections were used in morphologic studies. A full view of the cochlea of wild type, heterozygous and homozygous mice were showed. The Rosenthal canal (RC) was amplified for further investigation (**Figure 5A**). After quantifying the area of the RC and the number of SGNs, no significant degeneration of the SGNs was observed in homozygous mutant mice, and no significant change in the area of the RC (**Figures 5B,C**). Counting the number of neurons stained by toluidine blue in the auditory cortex (**Figure 5D**) revealed that there was no significant change in the density of auditory cortex neurons in homozygous mutant mice compared with WT mice (**Figure 5E**).

DISCUSSION

The CCDC154 mutant mouse strain exhibits congenital deafness and skeletal abnormalities. This strain displays no tooth root formation but instead shows development of odontoma, a common feature of osteopetrosis, and the skeletal abnormalities are also closely similar to human osteopetrosis (Lu et al., 2009). Moreover, further work demonstrated that there was a ∼5 kb deletion comprising exons 1–6 of the CCDC154 gene in the mutant mice (Liao et al., 2012). However, whether the mutant mice had other osteosclerosis-related phenotypes has not been reported. In the present study, our data demonstrate that the homozygous mutant mice showed severe hearing loss at high frequency and moderate deafness at low frequency, while heterozygous or wild type littermates displayed normal hearing. These data suggest that the CCDC154 fragment deletion can cause syndromic hereditary deafness in mice.

To date, most research into hearing loss has focused on hair cells in the inner ear. Many genes are crucial for the development and survival of hair cells. Zhou et al. (2020) reported that genetic ablation of Atg7 in outer hair cells (OHCs) in mice caused stereocilium damage and electromotility disturbances, which led to the degeneration of OHCs and subsequent early-onset profound hearing loss. Disrupted function of slc4a2b resulted in a decreased number of HCs in zebrafish neuromasts due to increased HC apoptosis (Qian et al., 2020). Knockdown Arhgef6 in mice caused progressive hearing loss due to HC loss and stereocilia deficits (Zhu et al., 2018). Fang et al. (2019) reported that loss of Limk1 and Limk2 did not affect the overall development of the cochlea and the structure of hair bundles.

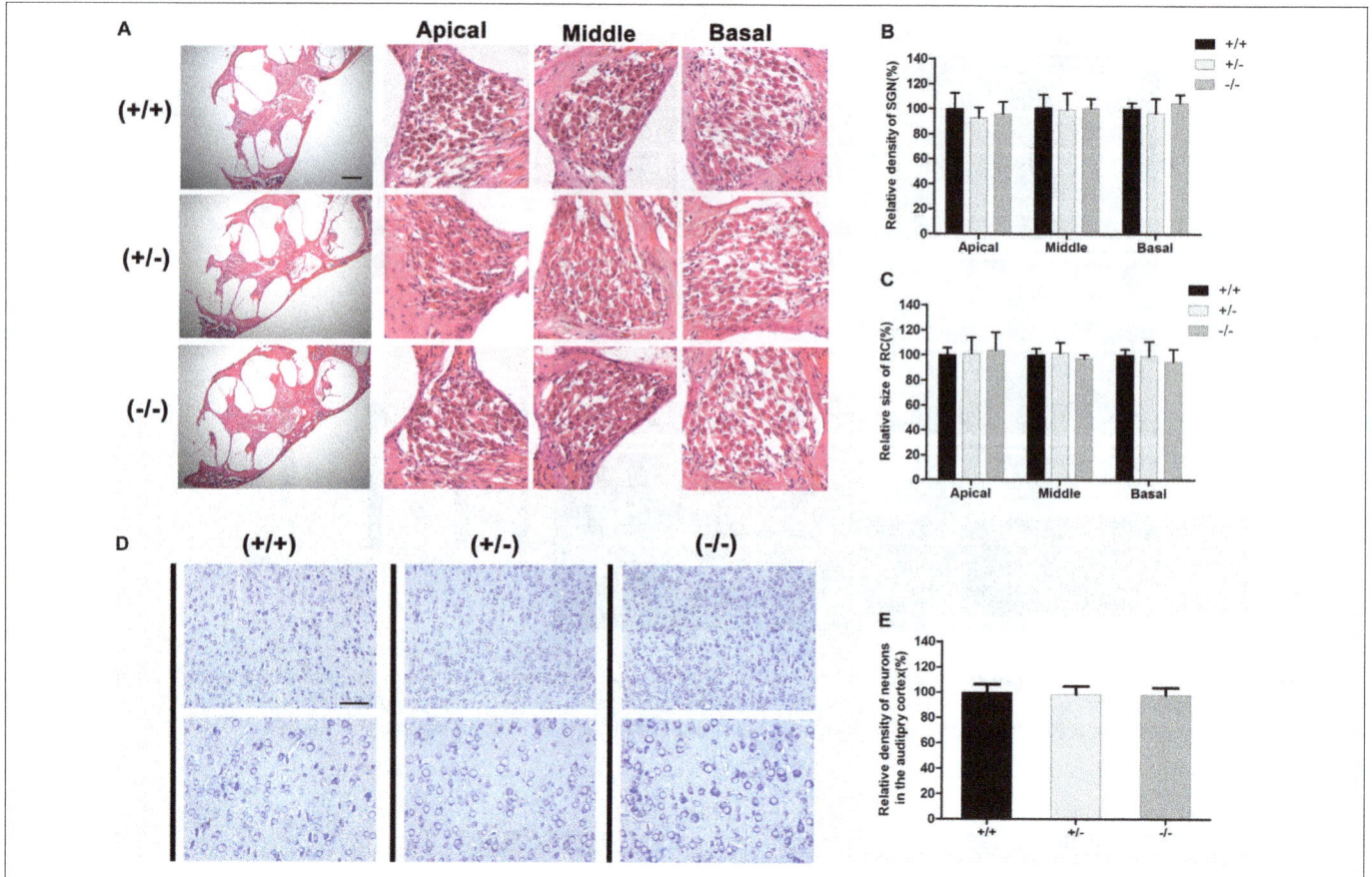

FIGURE 5 | There was no obvious degeneration of spiral ganglion neuron or auditory cortical neurons in mutant mice at P20. **(A)** Full view of the cochlea and representative images of SGN in different turns from the wild type, heterozygous and homozygous mutant mice, respectively. **(B)** Quantifications of SGNs survival at specific cochlear locations in the different groups at P20. **(C)** Quantifications of RC size at specific cochlear locations in the different groups at P20. **(D)** Representative images of neurons in auditory cortical from wild type, heterozygous and homozygous mutant mice, respectively. **(E)** Quantifications of surviving neurons in the auditory cortical from different groups at P20. The scales in panels **(A,D)** represent 200 and 100 μm, respectively.

CCDC154 is not necessary for the survival of hair cells or spiral ganglion cells. The morphology of the OC and the spiral ligament of the cochlea showed normal organization in all turns and there was no substantial hair cell or SGN degeneration in mutant mice. ABRs showed that there was obvious wave I–III at 70–90 dB SPL. These results prove that the inner ear of mutant mice can still transmit acoustic signals to the primary auditory nucleus under high stimulation. In the cuticular plate of hair cells, they are thought to be critical for mammalian hearing (Qi et al., 2019). CCDC154 mutant mice showed normal structure of hair bundles.

Fragment deletion in CDCC154 plays a vital role in bone remodeling of the otic capsule and auditory ossicles. The otic capsule is unique in its composition and pattern of bone remodeling; unlike most bones in the skull that form through intramembranous ossification, the auditory ossicles and otic capsule are formed through endochondral ossification (Tucker et al., 2004). During this process, the hypertrophic chondrocytes and calcified cartilage matrix are absorbed by osteoclasts and the cartilage template is subsequently replaced by bone (Mallo, 2001). The auditory ossicles or otic capsule are almost absent from bone remodeling after development, and the bone remodeling unit has a centrifugal distribution within the inner ear tissues (Frisch et al., 1998). Although osteoclastogenesis is normally suppressed in the ossicles and the auditory otic capsule, osteoclast function is still required to sculpt these bones during development. The reasons for this low level of bone turnover remain unclear. Studies have reported that high levels of OPG in the inner ear may inhibit bone remodeling in the otic capsule (Zehnder et al., 2005). In humans, a disturbed balance of OPG expression in the otic capsule is associated with otosclerosis, a complex bone dystrophy of the human otic capsule leading to conductive and sensorineural hearing loss (Karosi et al., 2011). The typical pathologic feature of otosclerosis is abnormal bony remodeling of the otic capsule, which includes osteoclast-mediated bone resorption and increased vascularization, osteoblast-mediated bone formation and new bone deposition (Quesnel et al., 2018). The active bone remodeling process of the otic capsule in the CCDC154 mutant mice was strikingly similar to that observed in the temporal bone of otosclerosis patients. Typical pathological features of the otic capsule in CDCC154 mutant mice include formation of well-defined hypercellular areas, increased vascularization and new bone or mineralization deposition, which resembles the lesions of active otosclerosis (Parahy and Linthicum, 1984; Quesnel et al., 2018). Zehnder et al. (2006) also observed similar abnormalities of bone remodeling of the otic capsule and hearing loss in OPG knockout mice. Our results suggest that CCDC154 is essential for normal bone remodeling of the otic capsule and auditory ossicles, which is important for maintaining normal auditory function. However, CCDC154 is a novel gene. To date, the function of the CDCC family has been poorly studied. Coiled-coil domain containing (CCDC) family members enhance tumor cell proliferation has been reported. Zhang et al. (2017) reported that CCDC106 promotes non-small cell lung cancer cell proliferation. Overexpression of a novel osteopetrosis-related gene CCDC154 suppresses cell proliferation by inducing G2/M arrest (Liao et al., 2012). Dong et al. (2019) reported that CCDC154 was key proteins involved in the molecular mechanisms of Parkinson's disease (PD), which may be used as novel plasma biomarkers for early diagnosis of PD and the future development of treatments. However, its function in the middle ear or inner ear is unclear. Therefore, more studies are needed to explore the function of CCDC154 in the auditory system.

Otosclerosis is a disease of the bony labyrinth of the inner ear with a prevalence of 0.3–0.4% in the European population but which is rare among Asians and Africans (Declau et al., 2001). The abnormal bone remodeling of the otic capsule results in progressive conductive hearing loss, and up to one-third of patients ultimately develop sensorineural hearing loss in addition to conductive hearing loss (Ishai et al., 2016). However, the etiology of otosclerosis remains poorly understood. Both genetic and environmental factors such as estrogens, fluoride, and viral infection have been implicated in the disease process. To date, several otosclerosis loci named OTSC1–10 have been mapped in families showing segregation of autosomal dominant otosclerosis, although none of the otosclerosis-causing genetic mutations within these locations has been identified so far (Babcock and Liu, 2018). Our results suggest that the CDCC154 mutation may be associated with otosclerosis, even though the mutation has never been found in otosclerosis patients. In future this gene may be worthy of investigation in patients with otosclerosis, and the CDCC154 mutant mouse strain may provide a valuable animal model of human otosclerosis.

ETHICS STATEMENT

The animal study was reviewed and approved by the Committee on Animal Research of Tongji Medical College, Huazhong University of Science and Technology. Written informed consent was obtained from the owners for the participation of their animals in this study.

AUTHOR CONTRIBUTIONS

YS and HL conceived and designed the study. KX, XB, SC, LX, and YQ performed the experiments. KX, XB, and SC wrote the manuscript. YS and HL reviewed and edited the manuscript. All authors read and approved the manuscript.

ACKNOWLEDGMENTS

We are grateful to Xin-Cheng Lu at Wenzhou Medical College for providing osteopetrosis mutant (ntl) mice.

REFERENCES

Aharinejad, S., Grossschmidt, K., Franz, P., Streicher, J., Nourani, F., Mackay, C. A., et al. (1999). Auditory ossicle abnormalities and hearing loss in the toothless (osteopetrotic) mutation in the rat and their improvement after treatment with colony-stimulating factor-1. *J. Bone Miner. Res.* 14, 415–423. doi: 10.1359/jbmr.1999.14.3.415

Babcock, T. A., and Liu, X. Z. (2018). Otosclerosis: from genetics to molecular biology. *Otolaryngol. Clin. North Am.* 51, 305–318. doi: 10.1016/j.otc.2017.11.002

Chen, S., Xu, K., Xie, L., Cao, H. Y., Wu, X., Du, A. N., et al. (2018). The spatial distribution pattern of Connexin26 expression in supporting cells and its role in outer hair cell survival. *Cell Death Dis.* 9:1180. doi: 10.1038/s41419-018-1238-x

Chen, X., Zhao, X., Hu, Y., Lan, F., Sun, H., Fan, G., et al. (2015). The spread of adenoviral vectors to central nervous system through pathway of cochlea in mimetic aging and young rats. *Gene. Ther.* 22, 866–875. doi: 10.1038/gt.2015.63

Declau, F., Van Spaendonck, M., Timmermans, J. P., Michaels, L., Liang, J., Qiu, J. P., et al. (2001). Prevalence of otosclerosis in an unselected series of temporal bones. *Otol. Neurotol.* 22, 596–602. doi: 10.1097/00129492-200109000-00006

Del Fattore, A., Cappariello, A., and Teti, A. (2008). Genetics, pathogenesis and complications of osteopetrosis. *Bone* 42, 19–29. doi: 10.1016/j.bone.2007.08.029

Dong, W., Qiu, C., Gong, D., Jiang, X., Liu, W., Liu, W., et al. (2019). Proteomics and bioinformatics approaches for the identification of plasma biomarkers to detect Parkinson's disease. *Exp. Ther. Med.* 18, 2833–2842. doi: 10.3892/etm.2019.7888

Dozier, T. S., Duncan, L. M., Klein, A. J., Lambert, P. R., and Key, T. L. (2005). Otologic manifestations of malignant osteopetrosis. *Otol. Neurotol.* 26, 762–766. doi: 10.1097/01.mao.0000178139.27472.8d

Fang, Q., Zhang, Y., Da, P., Shao, B., Pan, H., He, Z., et al. (2019). Deletion of limk1 and limk2 in mice does not alter cochlear development or auditory function. *Sci. Rep.* 9:3357. doi: 10.1038/s41598-019-39769-z

Frisch, T., Sørensen, M. S., Overgaard, S., Lind, M., and Bretlau, P. (1998). Volume-referent bone turnover estimated from the interlabel area fraction after sequential labeling. *Bone* 22, 677–682. doi: 10.1016/s8756-3282(98)00050-7

Frolenkov, G. I., Belyantseva, I. A., Friedman, T. B., and Griffith, A. J. (2004). Genetic insights into the morphogenesis of inner ear hair cells. *Nat. Rev. Genet.* 5, 489–498. doi: 10.1038/nrg1377

Ishai, R., Halpin, C. F., Shin, J. J., McKenna, M. J., and Quesnel, A. M. (2016). Long-term incidence and degree of sensorineural hearing loss in otosclerosis. *Otol. Neurotol.* 37, 1489–1496. doi: 10.1097/mao.0000000000001234

Kanzaki, S., Ito, M., Takada, Y., Ogawa, K., and Matsuo, K. (2006). Resorption of auditory ossicles and hearing loss in mice lacking osteoprotegerin. *Bone* 39, 414–419. doi: 10.1016/j.bone.2006.01.155

Kanzaki, S., Takada, Y., Niida, S., Takeda, Y., Udagawa, N., Ogawa, K., et al. (2011). Impaired vibration of auditory ossicles in osteopetrotic mice. *Am. J. Pathol.* 178, 1270–1278. doi: 10.1016/j.ajpath.2010.11.063

Kao, S. Y., Kempfle, J. S., Jensen, J. B., Perez-Fernandez, D., Lysaght, A. C., Edge, A. S., et al. (2013). Loss of osteoprotegerin expression in the inner ear causes degeneration of the cochlear nerve and sensorineural hearing loss. *Neurobiol. Dis.* 56, 25–33. doi: 10.1016/j.nbd.2013.04.008

Karosi, T., Csomor, P., Szalmas, A., Konya, J., Petko, M., and Sziklai, I. (2011). Osteoprotegerin expression and sensitivity in otosclerosis with different histological activity. *Eur. Arch. Otorhinolaryngol.* 268, 357–365. doi: 10.1007/s00405-010-1404-y

Liao, W., Zhao, R., Lu, L., Zhang, R., Zou, J., Xu, T., et al. (2012). Overexpression of a novel osteopetrosis-related gene CCDC154 suppresses cell proliferation by inducing G2/M arrest. *Cell Cycle* 11, 3270–3279. doi: 10.4161/cc.21642

Lu, X., Rios, H. F., Jiang, B., Xing, L., Kadlcek, R., Greenfield, E. M., et al. (2009). A new osteopetrosis mutant mouse strain (ntl) with odontoma-like proliferations and lack of tooth roots. *Eur. J. Oral Sci.* 117, 625–635. doi: 10.1111/j.1600-0722.2009.00690.x

Mallo, M. (2001). Formation of the middle ear: recent progress on the developmental and molecular mechanisms. *Dev. Biol.* 231, 410–419. doi: 10.1006/dbio.2001.0154

Michaelson, M. D., Bieri, P. L., Mehler, M. F., Xu, H., Arezzo, J. C., Pollard, J. W., et al. (1996). CSF-1 deficiency in mice results in abnormal brain development. *Development* 122, 2661–2672.

Parahy, C., and Linthicum, F. H. Jr. (1984). Otosclerosis and otospongiosis: clinical and histological comparisons. *Laryngoscope* 94, 508–512. doi: 10.1288/00005537-198404000-00015

Qi, J., Liu, Y., Chu, C., Chen, X., Zhu, W., Shu, Y., et al. (2019). A cytoskeleton structure revealed by super-resolution fluorescence imaging in inner ear hair cells. *Cell Discov.* 5:12. doi: 10.1038/s41421-018-0076-4

Qian, F., Wang, X., Yin, Z., Xie, G., Yuan, H., Liu, D., et al. (2020). The slc4a2b gene is required for hair cell development in zebrafish. *Aging* 12, 18804–18821. doi: 10.18632/aging.103840

Quesnel, A. M., Ishai, R., and McKenna, M. J. (2018). Otosclerosis: temporal bone pathology. *Otolaryngol. Clin. North Am.* 51, 291–303. doi: 10.1016/j.otc.2017.11.001

Roth, B., and Bruns, V. (1992a). Postnatal development of the rat organ of Corti. I. General morphology, basilar membrane, tectorial membrane and border cells. *Anatomy Embryol.* 185, 559–569. doi: 10.1007/bf00185615

Roth, B., and Bruns, V. (1992b). Postnatal development of the rat organ of Corti. II. Hair cell receptors and their supporting elements. *Anatomy Embryol.* 185, 571–581. doi: 10.1007/bf00185616

Sobacchi, C., Schulz, A., Coxon, F. P., Villa, A., and Helfrich, M. H. (2013). Osteopetrosis: genetics, treatment and new insights into osteoclast function. *Nat. Rev. Endocrinol.* 9, 522–536. doi: 10.1038/nrendo.2013.137

Stocks, R. M. S., Wang, W. C., Thompson, J. W., Stocks, M. C., and Horwitz, E. M. (1998). Malignant infantile osteopetrosis - otolaryngological complications and management. *Arch. Otolaryngol.* 124, 689–694. doi: 10.1001/archotol.124.6.689

Tucker, A. S., Watson, R. P., Lettice, L. A., Yamada, G., and Hill, R. E. (2004). Bapx1 regulates patterning in the middle ear: altered regulatory role in the transition from the proximal jaw during vertebrate evolution. *Development* 131, 1235–1245. doi: 10.1242/dev.01017

Van Wesenbeeck, L., Odgren, P. R., MacKay, C. A., D'Angelo, M., Safadi, F. F., Popoff, S. N., et al. (2002). The osteopetrotic mutation toothless (tl) is a loss-of-function frameshift mutation in the rat Csf1 gene: evidence of a crucial role for CSF-1 in osteoclastogenesis and endochondral ossification. *P. Natl. Acad. Sci. U S A.* 99, 14303–14308. doi: 10.1073/pnas.202332999

Zehnder, A. F., Kristiansen, A. G., Adams, J. C., Kujawa, S. G., Merchant, S. N., McKenna, M. J. et al. (2006). Osteoprotegrin knockout mice demonstrate abnormal remodeling of the otic capsule and progressive hearing loss. *Laryngoscope* 116, 201–206. doi: 10.1097/01.mlg.0000191466.09210.9a

Zehnder, A. F., Kristiansen, A. G., Adams, J. C., Merchant, S. N., and McKenna, M. J. (2005). Osteoprotegerin in the inner ear may inhibit bone remodeling in the otic capsule. *Laryngoscope* 115, 172–177. doi: 10.1097/01.mlg.0000150702.28451.35

Zhang, X., Zheng, Q., Wang, C., Zhou, H., Jiang, G., Miao, Y., et al. (2017). CCDC106 promotes non-small cell lung cancer cell proliferation. *Oncotarget* 8, 26662–26670. doi: 10.18632/oncotarget.15792

Zhou, H., Qian, X., Xu, N., Zhang, S., Zhu, G., Zhang, Y., et al. (2020). Disruption of Atg7-dependent autophagy causes electromotility disturbances, outer hair cell loss, and deafness in mice. *Cell Death Dis.* 11:913. doi: 10.1038/s41419-020-03110-8

Zhou, X. X., Chen, S., Xie, L., Ji, Y. Z., Wu, X., Wang, W. W., et al. (2016). Reduced connexin26 in the mature cochlea increases susceptibility to noise-induced hearing lossin mice. *Int. J. Mol. Sci.* 17:301. doi: 10.3390/ijms17030301

Zhu, C., Cheng, C., Wang, Y., Muhammad, W., Liu, S., Zhu, W., et al. (2018). Loss of ARHGEF6 Causes hair cell stereocilia deficits and hearing loss in mice. *Front. Mol. Neurosci.* 11:362. doi: 10.3389/fnmol.2018.00362

Local Drug Delivery for Prevention of Hearing Loss

Leonard P. Rybak[1,2]*, Asmita Dhukhwa[2], Debashree Mukherjea[1] and Vickram Ramkumar[2]

[1] Department of Otolaryngology, School of Medicine, Southern Illinois University, Springfield, IL, United States,
[2] Department of Pharmacology, School of Medicine, Southern Illinois University, Springfield, IL, United States

*Correspondence:
Leonard P. Rybak
lrybak@siumed.edu

Systemic delivery of therapeutics for targeting the cochlea to prevent or treat hearing loss is challenging. Systemic drugs have to cross the blood-labyrinth barrier (BLB). BLB can significantly prevent effective penetration of drugs in appropriate concentrations to protect against hearing loss caused by inflammation, ototoxic drugs, or acoustic trauma. This obstacle may be obviated by local administration of protective agents. This route can deliver higher concentration of drug compared to systemic application and preclude systemic side effects. Protective agents have been administered by intra-tympanic injection in numerous preclinical studies. Drugs such as steroids, etanercept, D and L-methionine, pifithrin-alpha, adenosine agonists, melatonin, kenpaullone (a cyclin-dependent kinase 2 (CDK2) inhibitor) have been reported to show efficacy against cisplatin ototoxicity in animal models. Several siRNAs have been shown to ameliorate cisplatin ototoxicity when administered by intra-tympanic injection. The application of corticosteroids and a number of other drugs with adjuvants appears to enhance efficacy. Administration of siRNAs to knock down AMPK kinase, liver kinase B1 (LKB1) or G9a in the cochlea have been found to ameliorate noise-induced hearing loss. The local administration of these compounds appears to be effective in protecting the cochlea against damage from cisplatin or noise trauma. Furthermore the intra-tympanic route yields maximum protection in the basal turn of the cochlea which is most vulnerable to cisplatin ototoxicity and noise trauma. There appears to be very little transfer of these agents to the systemic circulation. This would avoid potential side effects including interference with anti-tumor efficacy of cisplatin. Nanotechnology offers strategies to effectively deliver protective agents to the cochlea. This review summarizes the pharmacology of local drug delivery by intra-tympanic injection to prevent hearing loss caused by cisplatin and noise exposure in animals. Future refinements in local protective agents provide exciting prospects for amelioration of hearing loss resulting from cisplatin or noise exposure.

Keywords: intra-tympanic injection, cisplatin, noise, hearing loss, acoustic trauma, ototoxicity

INTRODUCTION

Blood-Labyrinth Barrier

A wide variety of drugs has been used to treat inner ear diseases. However, the efficacy of systemic drug therapy is frequently limited by restricted uptake into the inner ear by a barrier system, the blood labyrinth barrier (BLB). The BLB was a term that was developed from the fact that the inner ear fluids have a composition that is distinct from blood. These features provide a diffusion barrier that excludes many substances from entering the inner ear from the blood. Tracer studies demonstrated that various substances enter the perilymph slowly after systemic injection (Juhn et al., 1981). The rate of penetration into perilymph is generally inversely proportional to the molecular weight of compounds tested. This blood-perilymph barrier appears to be situated in the blood vessels located in the modiolus of the cochlea. Substances traveling in these vessels are transported from blood into perilymph of the scala tympani and scala vestibuli (Zou et al., 2016). The cochlear glomeruli of Schwalbe form vessel loops of capillaries adjacent to both perilymphatic scalae (Franz et al., 1993). This barrier consists of non-fenestrated capillaries with a continuous endothelial lining with tight junctions between endothelial cells.

The perilymph-endolymph barrier consists of tight junctions between cells lining Reissner's membrane (Zou et al., 2016). Substances contained in perilymph may enter endolymph if they are able to penetrate this barrier.

The blood-endolymph barrier consists of endothelial cells of capillaries in the stria vascularis that separate the contents of blood in the capillary lumen from the interstitial fluid of the stria vascularis. These marginal cells have tight junctions between them that can restrict passage of substances from blood to endolymph. Within the stria vascularis, marginal cells and the basal cells comprise the intrastrial compartment which separates fluid in that compartment from endolymph in the scala media. This barrier is called the the intrastrial fluid-blood barrier (Shi, 2016). Additional components of the blood-strial barrier have been recently identified. These include pericytes and perivascular resident macrophage-type melanocytes. These three cell types: endothelial cells, pericytes and perivascular resident macrophages are connected by an extracellular basement membrane. Collectively, these cells together form a "cochlear-vascular unit" in the stria vascularis (Shi, 2016; Nyberg et al., 2019). Substances contained in the blood vessels of the stria vascularis may enter the intra-strial space through the blood-strial barrier and then gain access to the endolymph through the marginal cells lining scala media. The various inner ear barriers are illustrated in **Figure 1**.

Treatments for hearing disorders such as cisplatin ototoxicity and noise-induced hearing loss could be administered systemically. However, this approach poses several difficulties: The potential protective agent may (1) not readily cross the BLB (size of the substance) and thus not reach its intended target cells in the cochlea in effective concentrations, (2) could interfere with the desired therapeutic effect of cisplatin (e.g., sodium thiosulfate), and (3) could cause off-target unwanted side effects, especially if high doses are needed to provide protection against hearing loss. One of these off-target effects could result in exacerbation of hearing loss instead of its amelioration. Local application by intra-tympanic administration is minimally invasive and allows drugs or other therapeutic agents to gain access to the inner ear with few or no systemic side effects and minimal risks of interference with the anti-tumor action of drugs like cisplatin. Intra-tympanic injection involves the instillation of substances through the tympanic membrane (Sheehan et al., 2018), shown schematically as a flowchart in (**Figure 2**) and in detail in (**Figure 3**). Another approach for localized drug delivery is through the bulla into the middle ear cavity or application of drugs directly to the round window membrane (RWM). This paper reviews preclinical strategies for local delivery of drugs by intra-tympanic injection to prevent hearing loss from cisplatin and noise trauma.

Pharmacokinetics of Local Drug Delivery

Salt and Plontke have described the use of a standard pharmacologic acronym to describe the pharmacokinetics of drugs after intra-tympanic delivery to the cochlea (Salt and Plontke, 2009, 2018). This acronym is LADME. This term includes liberation, absorption, distribution, metabolism, and elimination of drugs applied intra-tympanically.

Liberation indicates the release of the agent from the dosage form administered to the tympanic cavity into the inner ear. The use of simple drug solutions may not provide sufficient duration of protection. Therefore, incorporation of the drug into controlled-release vehicles can prolong the presence of the drug in the middle ear cavity for transfer through the round or oval window membrane. A variety of technologies have been developed to allow extended release of drugs injected intra-tympanically. Some examples of these methods to prolong the release of active protective agents to the round or oval window membrane include:

- Implantation of an osmotic or digital mini pump to provide sustained delivery of various antioxidants to the RWM in guinea pigs (Wimmer et al., 2004).
- The development and utilization of OTO-104 which contains micronized dexamethasone 160 in poloxamer gel. Significant levels of dexamethasone were maintained in perilymph for 3 months in guinea pigs and more than 1 month in sheep (Piu et al., 2011).
- The intratympanic injection of a hyaluronic acid liposomal gel for sustained delivery of dexamethasone was tested in the guinea pig. The gel remained for a long time in the middle ear cavity and in the RWM after intra-tympanic injection without any evidence of ototoxicity. This resulted in sustained release of dexamethasone in perilymph for 1 month (El Kechai et al., 2016). This appears to be a promising way to deliver corticosteroids to the inner ear to provide sustained protection against cochlear insults.
- Dormer et al. have developed an innovative system to provide extended release of drugs for intra-tympanic injection (Dormer et al., 2019). It contains a film forming agent (FFA) and microspheres to provide prolonged delivery of betamethasone in a formulation called ORB-202 to the round window and inner ear in mice. This technology has shown that corticosteroids contained in microspheres with FFA were retained on the RWM for up to 5 weeks on necropsy examination. A recent review discusses various approaches to nanotechnology for inner ear applications. Only a few examples will be presented below.
- Li et al. have developed a nanohydrogel delivery system, which combines nanotechnology with a chitosan-glycerophosphate hydrogel delivery system.

Local Drug Delivery for Prevention of Hearing Loss

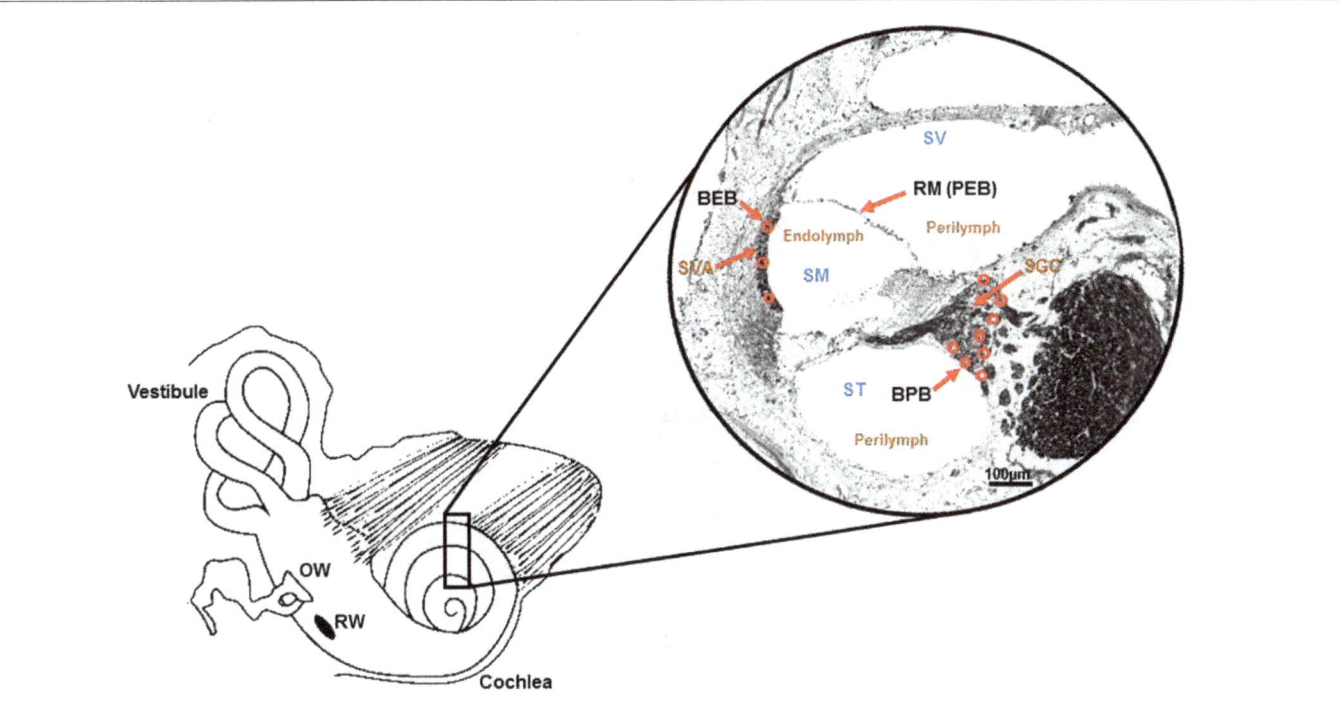

FIGURE 1 | Schematic illustration of barriers within inner ear. Drawing of the cochlea and photomicrograph of a mid-modiolar section of the rat cochlea (stained with Sudan black) demonstrating the various barriers within the inner ear. These include the blood-endolymph barrier (BEB) in the stria vascularis; the blood-perilymph barrier (BPB); and the perilymph-endolymph barrier (PEB) which is formed by Reissner's membrane (RM). Other abbreviations are: SVA (stria vascularis), SGC (spiral ganglion cells), SV (scala vestibuli), ST (scala tympani) and SM (scala media). Perilymph is contained within SV and ST, and endolymph is present in SM. Adapted from Zou et al. (2016).

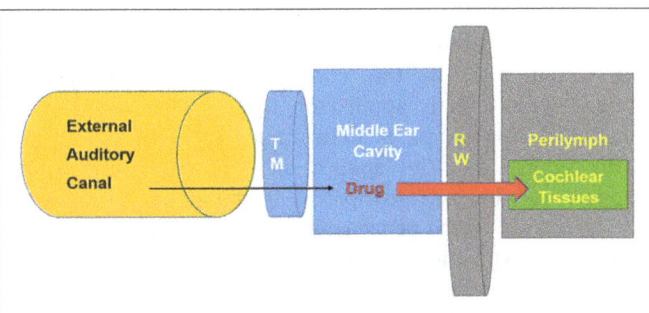

FIGURE 2 | Schematic diagram illustrating method for intra-tympanic injection. The drug is injected through the tympanic membrane (Heinrich et al., 2016) into the middle ear. It then can penetrate the round window membrane (RW) to enter the inner ear fluids (perilymph) and tissues. Modified from the ACS article https://pubs.acs.org/doi/abs/10.1021%2Facs.jmedchem.7b01653 with permission.

These nanoparticles could be delivered across the mouse RWM to reach structures in the scala media (Li et al., 2017).

Liberation can also result from drug generation in the middle ear from gene or cell therapy by which cells are enabled to produce a therapeutic agent (Salt and Plontke, 2018).

A variety of delivery paradigms has been tried to affect liberation. These include rates of injection with pumps, various other devices, and rates of elution among others (Salt and Plontke, 2018).

Absorption describes the passage of the drug from the middle ear cavity to the perilymph through the RWM, oval window or cochlear bone. The RWM in mammals comprises of 3 cellular layers: an epithelial layer that faces the middle ear space; a connective tissue layer in the middle; and a layer that faces the perilymph of the scala tympani (Goycoolea, 1992; Goycoolea and Lundman, 1997). The epithelial layer facing the middle ear cavity has tight junctions between cells (Salt and Plontke, 2009). It appears that the layers of the round window are involved in absorption and secretion of substances to and from the inner ear. Tracer molecules such as cationic ferritin, horseradish peroxidase, and 1 micron latex microspheres instilled into the middle ear pass through RWM, into the inner ear and have been detected in pinocytotic vesicles in the RWM (Goycoolea et al., 1988). Permeability of the RWM depends on molecular weight, solubility in lipids, concentration and charge, as well as the RWM thickness (Goycoolea and Lundman, 1997). Some examples of substances shuttled across RWM are:

- Nanoparticles are translocated across the RWM by endocytosis. This process follows three different mechanisms: macropinocytosis, caveolin-mediated endocytosis, and clathrin-mediated endocytosis (Zhang et al., 2018).

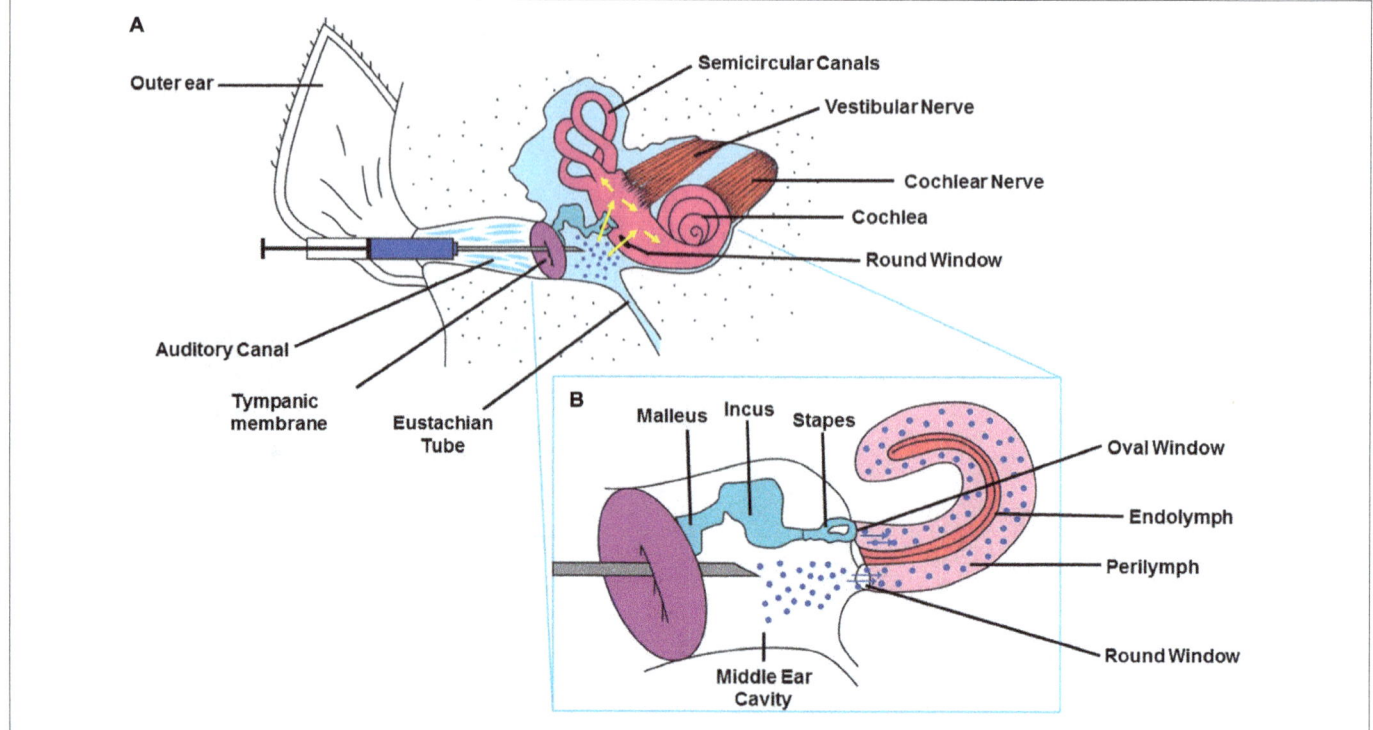

FIGURE 3 | Method for intra-tympanic injection. (A) A syringe with an attached 30 gage needle 1/2 to 5/8th of an inch in length is directed through the external ear canal to the tympanic membrane of anesthetized animal with an operating microscope. A single puncture is made in the anterior inferior region. The desired solution is slowly injected into the middle ear and the rat is left undisturbed for 15 min with injected ear facing upward (Sheehan et al., 2018). (B) Drawing depicting the injected drug traversing the RWM and entering the cochlea. This figure was modified with permission from the image screenshot at 1:59 of the article https://www.jove.com/video/56564/trans-tympanic-drug-delivery-for-the-treatment-of-ototoxicity.

- A study of RW permeation enhancers was carried out using fluorescein tagged dexamethasone applied to the RW niche in guinea pigs. DMSO, N-methylpyrrolidone and benzyl alcohol provided significantly higher entry than that observed in controls (Li et al., 2018).
- Adjuvants were used to enhance the permeation of dexamethasone through the RWM. Application of dexamethasone on a hyaluronic acid sponge with or without histamine or dexamethasone with histamine provided greater penetration into perilymph in guinea pigs than did dexamethasone alone (Creber et al., 2019).
- A novel method to enhance the delivery of siRNA to the cochlea was developed using a recombination protein, double-stranded RNA-binding domains (TAT-DRBDs). The authors showed efficient siRNA transfection to the cochlea of the chinchilla with this delivery system. They were able to demonstrate successful transfection of Cy3-labeled siRNA into cells of the inner ear through the intact RWM, including the IHCs, OHCs, and vestibular cells in the crista ampullaris, macula utriculi, and macula sacculi (Qi et al., 2014).

The oval window and thin bone of the stapes footplate may provide other routes of entry for drugs applied intra-tympanically. Although the oval window has been shown to be permeable to horseradish peroxidase (Tanaka and Motomura, 1981), it is uncertain how much drug would enter by this route (Salt and Plontke, 2009) unless it were directly applied on the stapes footplate (King et al., 2011) or unless it were applied using nanoparticles. In the latter case, the application of fluorescent chitosan nanoparticles by intra-tympanic injection in guinea pigs was associated with penetration of both RWM and oval window, but with much stronger fluorescence in the vestibule than in the cochlea (Ding et al., 2019). On the other hand King et al. showed with MRI that most of the gadolinium applied through tympanic cavity entered perilymph through stapes (King et al., 2011). The bone of the otic capsule may provide a route of transport from the middle ear to the apical regions of the cochlea in guinea pigs (Salt and Plontke, 2009; Salt and Hirose, 2018).

Distribution includes the mechanism by which the drug is spread within and between perilymph and endolymph and how it passes from inner ear fluids into tissues of the cochlea. The distribution of drugs within the cochlear fluids proceeds primarily by passive diffusion but if fluid flow is present, volume flow can occur (Salt and Plontke, 2018). Distribution also includes flow of substances from fluid spaces to extracellular spaces of cochlear tissue compartments, especially in areas where cell layers are not complete or where cells do not possess tight junctions (Salt and Plontke, 2018). Distribution includes all forms of drug movement within the inner ear

(Salt and Plontke, 2018). Distribution may be enhanced by the use of magnetic nanoparticles to cross the RWM and enter the inner ear fluids and tissues. The use of an external magnet can control the delivery of drug packaged in magnetic nanoparticles. After the magnet is taken away, the drug containing nanoparticles can then diffuse through perilymph. Fluorescent magnetic nanoparticles have been shown to traverse the RWM and gain access to the perilymph (Li et al., 2017).

Metabolism is the chemical alteration of drugs administered into the ear. It is also known as biotransformation (Salt and Plontke, 2018). Once a drug enters the inner ear, it can be broken down into substances that are more bioactive or that are inactivated. The intra-tympanic administration of liposomal hyaluronic acid led to the transformation of dexamethasone phosphate, a prodrug, into the active form, dexamethasone (El Kechai et al., 2016). Thus the metabolite may have a greater affinity for its receptors in the inner ear. Changes in physical characteristics of a drug resulting from metabolism can alter its ability to traverse cell membranes and layers in the inner ear. These changes can alter the rate of elimination (Salt and Plontke, 2018).

Elimination includes the processes by which the drug or its metabolites are transferred from the inner ear into other body fluids such as blood or cerebrospinal fluid or transport from the inner ear to the middle ear cavity. From the middle ear cavity a drug administered intra-tympanically can exit be eliminated via the Eustachian tube into the pharynx (Salt and Plontke, 2018). A novel approach to elimination of substances transported into the cochlea is to administer magnetic nanoparticles, then remove them using an external magnet. This has been demonstrated using fluorescently tagged magnetic nanoparticles *in vivo* (Li et al., 2018). Middle ear kinetics of drugs administered intra-tympanically as solutions show rapid decline in concentration within the middle ear cavity, e.g., dexamethasone phosphate, which fell to 10% of the applied concentration at 93 min after injection into the middle ear (Salt and Plontke, 2018). This process could be delayed by the use of slow-release vehicles. The delayed elimination (Hellberg et al., 2013) and prolonged retention of cisplatin for months to years in the cochlea creates challenges for intratympanic protection strategies (Breglio et al., 2017).

Cisplatin Ototoxicity

Cisplatin is frequently used to treat a variety of malignant solid tumors. These include ovarian and testicular cancer, head and neck carcinomas, cervical, bladder, and lung cancer. Although cisplatin is a quite effective antineoplastic drug, dose limiting side effects often occur. Such unintended toxicities include: ototoxicity, neurotoxicity, nephrotoxicity, and bone marrow toxicity. Investigation of potential protective agents to ameliorate cisplatin ototoxicity have not yet yielded an effective drug that has been approved by the United States Food and Drug Administration (FDA). Of great concern is the potential interference of cisplatin efficacy when systemic otoprotective drugs are administered. These otoprotective drugs could neutralize or diminish the anti-tumor effects of cisplatin and may also produce additional side effects, including communication, learning, cognition, and quality of life (Brooks and Knight, 2018). Therefore, numerous preclinical studies have investigated potential protective agents against cisplatin ototoxicity using local therapy, such as intra-tympanic injection. Cisplatin-induced hearing loss is bilateral and permanent. The hearing loss occurs mostly in the high frequencies. It can drastically compromise the quality of life for cancer survivors. Therefore the use of intra-tympanic therapy is attractive since the concentration of putative protective agents will be greater in the basal turn of the cochlea where high frequency hearing is transduced.

Mechanisms Underlying Cisplatin Ototoxicity

Cisplatin ototoxicity and the underlying mechanisms are still being investigated. Several mechanisms have been proposed. These include oxidative stress caused by the production of reactive oxygen species (Kros and Steyger), which can be mediated by activation of a cochlear specific isoform of the enzyme NADPH oxidase (NOX3), and by up regulation of transient receptor potential vanilloid 1 (TRPV1) channels (Mukherjea et al., 2008, 2011; Sheth et al., 2017). Cisplatin mediated damage to mitochondria resulting in cleavage of caspases leading to apoptosis of critical structures in the cochlea (outer hair cells, cells of the stria vascularis and spiral ligament, and spiral ganglion cells); DNA damage with activation of p53 leading to activation of activation of signal transducer and activator of transcription 1 (STAT1) (Zhang et al., 2003; Kaur et al., 2011; Benkafadar et al., 2017; Bhatta et al., 2019), resulting in inflammation and apoptosis (Sheth et al., 2017). Recent reviews of the proposed mechanisms of cisplatin ototoxicity have been published (Karasawa and Steyger, 2015, Sheth et al., 2017, Kros and Steyger, 2018).

Intra-Tympanic Treatments for Cisplatin Ototoxicity

A wide variety of putative protective agents have been reported to ameliorate cisplatin ototoxicity when administered by intra-tympanic injection. A short list of some successful otoprotective agents administered intra-tympanically prior to cisplatin treatment *in vivo* have been categorized as inhibitors, biologicals, siRNA, and dexamethasone and have been listed below:

- Kenpaullone is an inhibitor of multiple kinases, including cyclin-dependent kinase 2 (CDK2). Significant otoprotection was demonstrated in both mice and rats. Mice receiving intra-tympanic kenpaullone demonstrated significant reductions of ABR threshold elevation, at frequencies of 16 and 32 kHz. Morphology of OHCs in the 32 kHz region showed significant protection in kenpaullone treated mice. Even more robust findings were demonstrated in rats. Intra-tympanic kenpaullone provided complete protection against cisplatin ototoxicity in the rat. These findings support the hypothesis that CDK2 inhibition by kenpaullone ameliorates cisplatin ototoxicity by inhibiting mitochondrial ROS production and also preventing cochlear cell death mediated by caspase-3/7 (Teitz et al., 2018).

- Copper sulfate, a copper transporter-1 inhibitor, when administered intra-tympanically 30 min prior to intraperitoneal cisplatin in mice showed significant protection against threshold shifts in ABR using click stimuli and pure tones at 8, 16, and 32 kHz. However, concerns were expressed about the toxicity of copper sulfate. This led to the suggestion that other less toxic inhibitors of CTR1 should be developed and tested (More et al., 2010).
- Thiosulfate, an antioxidant was administered as thiosulphate-hyaluronan gel into the tympanic cavity of guinea pigs 3 h prior to intravenous cisplatin injection. This resulted in high concentrations of thiosulfate in the perilymph of scala tympani and it protected against cochlear hair cell loss from cisplatin. Levels of thiosulfate in blood were kept low, avoiding potential chelation of cisplatin in the blood that could interfere with the anti-tumor efficacy of cisplatin (Berglin et al., 2011).
- KR-22332 (3-amino-3-(4-fluoro-phenyl)-1H-quinoline-2,4-dione) is a novel compound that suppresses ROS. Intra-tympanic administration of KR-22332 in rats protected against cisplatin induced ABR threshold shift to click stimuli. This compound inhibited cisplatin-induced up regulation of NOX3 in the cochlea and reduced the activation of p53, MAP kinases, caspase 3 and tumor necrosis factor-α (TNF-alpha), and TUNEL expression in rat cochlea. KR-22332 may ameliorate cisplatin ototoxicity by reducing the generation of ROS and by preventing mitochondrial dysfunction (Shin et al., 2013).
- Antioxidant vitamins such as vitamin E and vitamin C have been tested for protection against cisplatin ototoxicity. Trolox, a water-soluble form of alpha-tocopherol is an antioxidant. It was applied locally on the round window of guinea pigs treated with cisplatin. Trolox administered in combination with cisplatin prevented ABR threshold elevations and protected against the loss of hair cells (Teranishi and Nakashima, 2003). Another study in rats looked at the effect of intra-tympanic application of vitamin E solution followed by cisplatin administration 30 min later. Significant protection against cisplatin induced ABR threshold shifts was seen in rats (Paksoy et al., 2011). Another strategy employed the intra-tympanic administration of vitamin E polymeric nanoparticles in rats treated with cisplatin. Rats pretreated with vitamin E nanoparticles had significant protection against cisplatin-induced ABR threshold shifts at 12, 20, and 32 (Martin-Saldana et al., 2017). Vitamin C administered by intra-tympanic injection protected against cisplatin-induced decrease in DPOAE amplitudes in rats treated with cisplatin (Celebi et al., 2013).
- Melatonin is a hormone secreted by the pineal gland that has antioxidant properties. It has both indirect antioxidant and direct free radical scavenger activity. Rats treated with intra-tympanic melatonin showed improved ABR thresholds for clicks, 4, 6, and 8 kHz and threshold shifts for DPOAE. Staining for TNF-alpha was diminished in melatonin treated rats receiving cisplatin (Demir et al., 2015).
- Capsaicin is a spicy capsaicinoid, a natural product produced by hot chili peppers, Capsicum fruits. This alkaloid has been used for its analgesic and anti-inflammatory actions (Lavorgna et al., 2019), Capsaicin activates TRPV1 pain receptors, and can produce rapid desensitization of TRPV1. The intra-tympanic administration of capsaicin in rats 24 h prior to cisplatin reduced ABR threshold shifts. Capsaicin appears to prevent cisplatin ototoxicity by increasing the expression of cannabinoid 2 receptors (CB2R) in the cochlea leading to increased activation of pro-survival transcription factor signal transducer and activator of transcription (STAT3) (Bhatta et al., 2019).
- JWH-015 (2-methyl-1-propyl-1H-indol-3-yl)-1-naphthalenylmethanone) is a cannabinoid receptor 2 (CB2) agonist. Pretreatment with intra-tympanic JWH-015, 30 min prior to cisplatin reduced ABR threshold shifts at 8, 16, and 32 kHz and also protected against the loss of OHCs in rats. In addition, this CB2R agonist prevented cisplatin-induced loss of ribbon synapses on inner hair cells (IHCs) and prevented loss of Na^+/K^+-ATPase immunoreactivity in the stria vascularis (Ghosh et al., 2018).
- Pifithrin-alpha is an inhibitor of p53. Pifithrin-alpha was applied on the RWM of the chinchilla prior to the local application of cisplatin. The cochleae that were pretreated with pifithrin were significantly protected from cisplatin-induced increase in ABR threshold shifts at 1,2,4,8, and 16 kHz (Parhizkar and Rybak, 2003).
- R-PIA (R-phenylisopropyladenosine) is an adenosine A1 receptor agonist. Intra-tympanic administration of R-PIA in rats prior to cisplatin reduced cisplatin-induced ABR threshold elevation and OHCs were preserved. This protection was associated with reduced NOX3 expression, STAT1 activation, TNF-α levels, and apoptosis in the cochlea (Kaur et al., 2016).
- D-methionine and L-methionine are amino acids with antioxidant properties and both of these compounds have been shown to protect against cisplatin ototoxicity in preclinical studies. D-methionine applied to the RWM provided complete protection against cisplatin applied to the round window in chinchillas. ABR thresholds and OHCs were completely preserved in animals pretreated with D-methionine (Korver et al., 2002). In a study using guinea pigs, osmotic pumps were implanted to provide continuous administration of D-methionine, sodium thiosulfate, fibroblast growth factor-2, or brain-derived neurotrophic factor in animals treated with cisplatin. Guinea pigs receiving D-methionine demonstrated better OAEs on the 3th and 5th day of a 5 day regimen of cisplatin administration. On 5th and 6th day of the treatment, D-methionine failed to provide protection. It appears that the additional dosing of cisplatin overpowered the effectiveness of D-methionine

on those later 2 days. The other agents provided no significant protection (Wimmer et al., 2004). The efficacy of L-methionine against cisplatin ototoxicity was investigated in rats. Local application of L-methionine prior to cisplatin provided complete protection against cisplatin-induced ABR threshold shifts and preserved the integrity of OHCs against damage by cisplatin (Li et al., 2001).

- L-N-acetylcysteine (L-NAC) is a sulfhydryl compound that can neutralize cisplatin and function as an antioxidant. A 2% solution of L-NAC was administered by intra-tympanic injection in guinea pigs treated with cisplatin. Pretreatment with L-NAC preserved DPOAEs that were otherwise severely affected by cisplatin. This same study successfully utilized lactated Ringer's solution by intra-tympanic injection prior to cisplatin administration. The latter solution was also effective in preserving DPOAEs in cisplatin treated guinea pigs (Choe et al., 2004). A later study showed that intra-tympanic administration of L-NAC was harmful and exacerbated cisplatin ototoxicity in the guinea pig. However, this latter study utilized extremely high concentrations of L-NAC (20%) and this proved to be toxic. Animals receiving this high dose of L-NAC showed severe disruption of OHC stereocilia (Nader et al., 2010). It appears that a more dilute solution of L-NAC is a better preparation to use for intra-tympanic injection to ameliorate cisplatin ototoxicity.
- TNF-alpha antagonist, etanercept, when administered intra-tympanically in rats protected against OHC damage and cisplatin-induced hearing loss. ABR threshold shifts were significantly reduced in rats treated with etanercept 30 min prior to cisplatin. Scanning electron microscopy of etanercept pre-treated animals showed significant protection against cisplatin induced OHC damage (Kaur et al., 2011).
- RNA silencing has been successfully employed using intra-tympanic delivery for protection against cisplatin ototoxicity. In a rat model of cisplatin ototoxicity, it was shown than intra-tympanic administration of siRNA to knock down TRPV1 protected against cisplatin-induced hearing loss and damage to outer hair cells in the cochlea (Mukherjea et al., 2008). It was hypothesized that protection was afforded by reducing down-stream targets, such as the cochlear specific NADPH oxidase -3 (NOX3) enzyme, and STAT-1. Indeed, the intra-tympanic injection of siRNA directed against NOX3 (Mukherjea et al., 2011) or STAT-1 siRNA (Kaur et al., 2011) were each protective against cisplatin induced hearing loss and outer hair cell damage. NOX3 activation results in reactive oxygen species upregulation and STAT-1 can promote inflammation and apoptosis in the cochlea as a result of cisplatin's ototoxic effect. Such deleterious effects can be prevented by the use of these siRNAs.
- Dexamethasone is a glucocorticoid that appears to offer protection against cisplatin ototoxicity by several mechanisms. These include the down-regulation of pro-inflammatory genes that regulate the expression of cytokines; the inhibition of apoptosis; the up-regulation of antioxidant enzymes that could antagonize the effects of ROS (Hazlitt et al., 2018).

  ○ Successful attenuation of cisplatin ototoxicity has been reported in various animal models treated with intra-tympanic dexamethasone. The animals tested include: mouse (Hill et al., 2008), aged mouse (Parham, 2011), rat (Paksoy et al., 2011), and guinea pig (Shafik et al., 2013). Intratympanic dexamethasone delivered 1 day before cisplatin treatment did not protect against cisplatin ototoxicity. However, intra-tympanic dexamethasone administered 1 h before cisplatin provided significant preservation of cochlear structure and function (Shafik et al., 2013). The efficacy of intra-tympanic dexamethasone solution in protecting against cisplatin ototoxicity in various experimental animal models has been rather inconsistent. Results appear to depend on the dose of both dexamethasone and cisplatin and the species of experimental animals (Hazlitt et al., 2018). Therefore, other formulations have been explored for providing sustained release of steroid or increase in penetration into the cochlea, such as the incorporation of dexamethasone into nanoparticles.
  ○ Dexamethasone OTO-104 contains micronized dexamethasone in a poloxamer based hydrogel. This formulation was found to be much more effective than dexamethasone solution alone (Fernandez et al., 2016). A single intra-tympanic injection of 6% OTO-104, provided nearly total protection against cisplatin ototoxicity in guinea pigs receiving acute injection of cisplatin. On the other hand intra-tympanic dexamethasone solution offered no protection. OTO-104 was also very effective in prevention of hearing loss associated with chronic administration of cisplatin (Fernandez et al., 2016).
  ○ Dexamethasone has also been delivered intra-tympanically as nanoparticles. Dexamethasone-PEG-PLA nanoparticles provided significant otoprotection against cisplatin induced ABR threshold shifts at 4 and 8 kHz but not at 16 or 24 kHz in guinea pigs (Sun et al., 2015). Dexamethasone polymeric nanoparticles also protected against cisplatin ototoxicity in rats (Martin-Saldana et al., 2017). Dexamethasone treatment by bullostomy (intra-tympanic administration) successfully reduced hearing loss in all frequencies (from 8 to 32 kHz) tested by auditory steady-state responses (ASSR) (Martin-Saldana et al., 2017).
  ○ Dexamethasone-A666 nanoparticles administered intra-tympanically protected guinea pigs against cisplatin-induced cochlear outer hair cell damage and hearing loss (Wang et al., 2018). This latter study used A666-peptides that were shown to bind to prestin in outer hair cells. This formulation effectively delivered dexamethasone into outer hair cells and was significantly more effective than intra-tympanic injection of free dexamethasone or dexamethasone

incorporated into nanoparticles without A666 (Wang et al., 2018).

- Prednisolone was found to reduce cisplatin induced ABR threshold elevations in mice. Intra-tympanic magnetically delivered prednisolone-loaded nanoparticles resulted in significantly lower elevations of ABR threshold, particularly at the higher frequencies (16 and 32 kHz) compared with intra-tympanic methylprednisolone solution or empty magnetic nanoparticles (Ramaswamy et al., 2017).

We have summarized the studies reporting intra-tympanic drug delivery that protect against cisplatin ototoxicity in **Table 1**.

Noise Induced Hearing Loss and Underlying Mechanisms

Noise induced hearing loss (NIHL) is a global burden with an estimated 16% of the adult population being affected, with significant regional variations (Nelson et al., 2005; Oishi and Schacht, 2011; Basner et al., 2014; Masterson et al., 2018). NIHL is not only characterized by increased thresholds in hearing, speech processing and tinnitus but also associated with sleep disorders, cardiovascular diseases and cognitive decline (Gates et al., 2000; Ohlemiller, 2008; Kumar et al., 2012; Bressler et al., 2017; Cunningham and Tucci, 2017; Le Prell and Clavier, 2017; Munzel et al., 2018).

The sensitivity to noise varies with the intensity and duration of exposure and the mammalian species tested. Auditory threshold shifts after noise exposure can cause either a temporary threshold shift (TTS) or shifts that do not revert back to baseline are known as permanent threshold shifts (PTS) (Kujawa and Liberman, 2009). Permanent hearing loss or PTS occurs when the noise exposure exceeds the capacity of the cochlea to recover. Permanent damage can be inflicted upon various cochlear tissues, including hair cells, spiral ganglion neurons and the lateral wall (stria vascularis and spiral ligament). Intense noise can cause mechanical damage that can result in the mixing of endolymph and perilymph causing high levels of potassium to kill hair cells (Kurabi et al., 2017). NIHL could be caused by a number of molecular events in the cochlea. Acoustic trauma can lead to the production of reactive oxygen species (Kros and Steyger) in the cochlea. ROS can remain in the cochlea for up to 10 days after noise exposure (Yamane et al., 1995). ROS may be generated by enzymes activated by noise exposure, including NADPH oxidases. ROS can oxidize lipids to form vasoactive lipid peroxidation molecules like isoprostanes (Ohinata et al., 2000). These toxic products may reduce cochlear blood flow. ROS can also lead to the formation of inflammatory cytokines that can cause cochlear damage. These include interleukin-6 and tumor necrosis factor-alpha (Kurabi et al., 2017). Reactive nitrogen species (RNS) are also formed in the cochlea of animals subjected to high levels of noise. These products include nitro tyrosine and peroxynitrite (Ohinata et al., 2000). The latter toxic free radical is formed by the reaction of nitric oxide (NO) with superoxide. Toxic noise exposure can produce accumulation of calcium in the inner ear tissues. Excess calcium may cause ROS release from mitochondria and can upregulate mitogen activated kinase (MAPK) including c-Jun-N-terminal kinase (JNK) and other cellular stress molecules. These downstream molecules can lead to OHC apoptosis or necrosis (Kurabi et al., 2017).

Intra-Tympanic Treatments Against Noise Trauma

Protective agents have been reported to ameliorate NIHL when administered by intra-tympanic injection. The following is a short list of some successful otoprotective agents administered intra-tympanically *in vivo*. Interestingly, some of these inhibitors were also protective against cisplatin induced hearing loss. Most otoprotective agents used are either inhibitors of cellular pathways, antioxidants, anti-inflammatory compounds, siRNA trophic factors or dexamethasone and have been listed below:

- A cell-permeable inhibitor of JNK mediated apoptosis, AM-111, was administered on the RWM (in a hyaluronic acid gel formulation or osmotic mini-pump) 1 or 4 h after impulse noise exposure in chinchillas. Three weeks after traumatic noise exposure the PTS were significantly less in animals receiving AM-111 even when it was administered 4 h after noise exposure (Coleman et al., 2007). D-JNKI-1 was found to block the mitogen-activated protein kinase/JNK-mediated activation of a mitochondrial death pathway. D-JNKi-1 administered intra-tympanically to guinea pigs exposed to acoustic trauma also provided excellent protection. The majority of hair cells were preserved in the area of maximum noise damage and resulted in almost no permanent hearing loss. Treatment was effective even when administered up to 12 h after noise exposure. These findings strongly suggest that the mitogen-activated protein kinase/JNK signaling pathway plays a critical role in producing hair cell death from acoustic trauma (Wang et al., 2007).
    - A novel and intriguing refinement of the intra-tympanic delivery of D-JNKi-1 to the cochlea of mice was recently reported. Mice underwent intra-tympanic application of a chitosan glycerophosphate (CGP)-hydrogel system containing targeted and untargeted D-JNKi-1 containing multifunctional nanoparticles (MFNPs) or empty MFNPs. Targeting was directed to the protein prestin in OHCs. Two days after round window application of the hydrogel the mice were exposed to acoustic trauma. ABR threshold shifts at 14 days after noise exposure were significantly lower for 4 and 8 kHz stimuli in mice treated with targeted MFNPs containing D-JNKi-1 compared to untargeted D-JNKi-1 MFNPs but protection was similar at 16, 24 and 32 kHz. At these frequencies, both targeted and untargeted D-JNKi-1-MFNPs provided partial protection that did not significantly differ from each other (Kayyali et al., 2018).

TABLE 1 | This table summarizes pertinent studies demonstrating amelioration of cisplatin-induced ototoxicity using intra-tympanic therapy.

Drug	Animal model	Mechanism	References
Kenpaullone	Mouse, Rat	Cyclin-dependent kinase-2 inhibitor	Teitz et al., 2018
Etanercept	Rat	TNF-alpha inhibitor	Kaur et al., 2011
Copper sulfate	Mouse	CTR1 inhibitor	More et al., 2010
Thiosulfate-hyaluronan gel	Guinea pig	Platinum chelator	Berglin et al., 2011
KR-22332 (3-amino-3-(4-fluoro-phenyl)-1H-quinoline-2,4-dione)	Rat	Suppresses ROS	Shin et al., 2013
Trolox	Guinea pig	Antioxidant	Teranishi and Nakashima, 2003
Vitamin E	Rat	Antioxidant	Paksoy et al., 2011
Vitamin E polymeric nanoparticles	Rat		Martin-Saldana et al., 2017
Vitamin C	Rat	Antioxidant	Celebi et al., 2013
Melatonin	Rat	Antioxidant	Demir et al., 2015
Capsaicin	Rat	CB2R upregulation increase STAT3/STAT1	Bhatta et al., 2019
Dexamethasone	Rat	Anti-inflammatory	Paksoy et al., 2011; Özel et al., 2016
	Mouse		Hill et al., 2008
	Aged mouse		Parham, 2011
	Guinea pig		Murphy and Daniel, 2011; Shafik et al., 2013
Dexamethasone-PEG-PLA nanoparticles	Guinea pig		Sun et al., 2015
Dexamethasone polymeric nanoparticles	Rat		Martin-Saldana et al., 2017
Dexamethasone-A666 nanoparticles	Guinea pig		Wang et al., 2018
Dexamethasone OTO-104	Guinea pig	Antioxidant	Fernandez et al., 2016
Prednisolone magnetic nanoparticles	Mouse	Anti-inflammatory	Ramaswamy et al., 2017
JWH-015	Rat	CB2R upregulation	Ghosh et al., 2018
Pifithrin-alpha	Chinchilla	p53 inhibitor	Parhizkar and Rybak, 2003
R-PIA	Rat	Adenosine A1R	Kaur et al., 2016
D-methionine	Chinchilla	Antioxidant	Korver et al., 2002
	Guinea pig		Wimmer et al., 2004
L-methionine	Rat	Antioxidant	Li et al., 2001
L-N-acetylcysteine	Guinea pig	Antioxidant	Choe et al., 2004
Lactated Ringer's	Guinea pig	–	Choe et al., 2004
TRPV1 siRNA	Rat	Decrease ROS	Mukherjea et al., 2008
NOX3 siRNA	Rat	Decrease ROS	Mukherjea et al., 2011
STAT1 siRNA	Rat	Anti-inflammatory	Kaur et al., 2011

- Rosmarinic acid is a polyphenol that is found in aqueous extracts of spearmint. It has demonstrated antioxidant, anti-inflammatory and neuroprotective properties (Falcone et al., 2019). Rats were exposed to acoustic trauma and underwent ABR measurements before and up to 30 days afterward. One group was treated with systemic rosmarinic acid and a second treatment group was administered intra-tympanic rosmarinic acid. Significant protection against ABR threshold shifts was seen in both treatment groups compared with controls. Less OHC loss and decreased evidence of superoxide production and lipid peroxidation was ascertained using dihydroethidium and 8-isoprostane immunostaining, respectively. These findings strongly suggest that adminstration of rosmarinic acid by both routes of administration protected the hearing and preserved the cochlea of rats exposed to noise trauma (Fetoni et al., 2018).

- Peroxisome proliferator-activated receptors (PPARs) function as lipid sensors and help to regulate redox balance by inhibiting ROS and upregulating antioxidant genes. Pioglitazone is a PPAR-gamma agonist that has been shown to reduce inflammation in patients with type two diabetes and coronary artery disease. This drug seemed to have favorable properties to test as a protective agent against noise trauma. Rats were administered pioglitazone in a temperature sensitive gel intra-tympanically 1 h after acoustic trauma. Pioglitazone significantly protected against threshold shifts in the ABR and significantly reduced the loss of OHCs. These findings were associated with a reduction in superoxide anion expression and lipid peroxidation (8-isoprostane). Anti-inflammatory effects of pioglitazone were demonstrated by its blockade of noise induced upregulation of pNFkB and interleukin 1b (IL-1b). Thus, pioglitazone protection against traumatic noise injury to the cochlea by both anti-oxidant and anti-inflammatory effects (Paciello et al., 2018).

- Caroverine is an antagonist of two glutamate receptors, N-methyl-D-aspartate (NMDA) and alpha-amino-3-hydroxy-5-methyl-4-isoxazolepropionic acid (AMPA). Caroverine was applied onto the RWM with gelfoam in

guinea pigs, followed by noise exposure. ABR threshold shifts were significantly lower in caroverine treated animals (Chen et al., 2004).
- Edaravone is a free radical scavenger and antioxidant. Edaravone solid lipid nanoparticles, were delivered to guinea pigs by intra-tympanic injection. Noise exposure resulted in ABR threshold shifts and induced ROS formation. Edaravone reduced the ABR threshold shift and ROS production in noise-exposed animals compared with controls. Edaravone solid lipid nanoparticles show protective effects against noise-induced hearing loss. However, guinea pigs treated with edaravone had no significant protection of OHCs. More experiments will be needed to see if edaravone could be useful in protecting cochlear tissues from noise injury (Gao et al., 2015).
- Kenpaullone is an inhibitor of CDK2. When kenpaullone was injected intra-tympanically in mice had significantly better ABR thresholds and wave 1 amplitudes than controls. In animals treated with this agent, the presynaptic ribbon density at D14 after the acoustic damage was diminished. These data support the hypothesis that kenpaullone protects against noise-induced hearing loss in mice. It is interesting to note that kenpaullone also protected against cisplatin (see above) (Teitz et al., 2018).
- RNA silencing: Noise exposed mice suffered permanent ABR threshold shifts, loss of OHCs and cochlear synapses. G9a (KMT1C, EHMT2) is an important histone lysine methyltransferase encoded by the human *EHMT2* gene and responsible for histone H3 lysine 9 dimethylation (H3K9me2). The intra-tympanic administration of siRNA against G9a to silence the *EHMT2* gene 72 h prior to noise exposure significantly reduced ABR threshold shifts and resulted in greater survival of OHCs compared to treatment with the control siRNA. These data suggest that pretreatment with siG9a partially ameliorates noise-induced permanent hearing loss via the inhibition of G9a (Xiong et al., 2019).

  o Noise exposure activates two key enzymes in the cochlea of mice: phosphorylated AMP-activated protein kinase-alpha-1 (AMPK-alpha-1) and its upstream kinase, liver kinase B1 (LKB1) in the cochlea. Pretreatment with intra-tympanic siRNA against AMPK-alpha-1 prior to noise exposure inhibited the expression of this enzyme and significantly reduced ABR threshold shifts and loss of OHCs and loss of synaptic ribbons at IHCs. Furthermore, inhibition of LKB1 by intra-tympanic siRNA reduced the noise-induced increase in phosphorylation of AMPK-alpha-1 in OHCs, reduced the loss of IHC synaptic ribbons and OHCs, and protected against ABR threshold shifts. These findings provide interesting new approach to prevent noise-induced hearing loss and cochlear synaptopathy (Hill et al., 2016).

- Neurotrophins have been used successfully for preservation of IHC pre and post-synaptic ribbon synapses: Guinea pigs were exposed for 2 h to 4 to 8 kHz noise at 95 dB. Auditory brainstem responses to pure-tone pips were acquired preoperatively, and at 1 and 2 weeks' post exposure. Immediately after noise exposure neurotrophins (brain-derived neurotrophic factor and neurotrophin-3) were applied to the RWM. ABR amplitude growth recovered in the ears of neurotrophin-treated guinea pigs using 16 kHz tones. Significantly more presynaptic ribbons, post-synaptic glutamate receptors, and co-localized ribbon synapse were seen after neurotrophin treatment. These findings supported the hypothesis that the local application of neurotrophins to the round window immediately after noise exposure will prevent noise-induced "hidden hearing loss" (Sly et al., 2016).

  o Even more exciting is the report that synapses may regenerate with intra-tympanic treatment with NT-3 after noise exposure. Mice exposed to noise ("neuropathic noise") that resulted in loss of up to 50% of synapses in the base of the cochlea within 24 h were treated with intra-tympanic neurotrophic-3 (NT-3 in a poloxamer gel) 24 h after noise exposure. Interestingly, this treatment was associated with regeneration of both pre- and post-synaptic elements at the junction of the IHC and cochlear nerve. Not only did the mice show structural recovery of these synapses, but they also demonstrated functional recovery by restoration of ABR wave 1 suprathreshold amplitudes. These findings have significant potential for healing "hidden hearing loss" in humans (Suzuki et al., 2016).

- Dexamethasone is the most frequently tested glucocorticosteroid by intra-tympanic injection to protect against noise-induced hearing loss. Rats were exposed to noise at 110 dB for 25 min and DPOAE measurements were performed before and after noise exposure. DPOAE measurements were performed before and 7 and 10 days after noise trauma. Rats treated with intra-tympanic dexamethasone had significantly better hearing than controls (Gumrukcu et al., 2018). Guinea pigs receiving intra-tympanic dexamethasone demonstrated significantly smaller ABR threshold shifts and decreased OHC loss compared with controls. They also had significant reduction in malondialdehyde concentration in the cochlea. This suggests that dexamethasone provided antioxidant effects in the treated ears (Chi et al., 2011). Another study showed short-term protection against hearing loss in guinea pigs with intra-tympanic dexamethasone. Animals received dexamethasone by intra-tympanic injection 2 h prior to white noise exposure. ABR thresholds were better and hair cell loss was reduced by this treatment. However, the major flaw of this study is that ABR thresholds and cochlear histology were performed only 2 h after noise exposure (Heinrich et al., 2016). Another study using guinea pigs tested the efficacy of dexamethasone administered intra-tympanically 2 h prior to white noise exposure. One group received dexamethasone solution and

TABLE 2 | This table summarizes pertinent studies of amelioration of noise-induced hearing loss using intra-tympanic therapy.

Drug	Animal model	Mechanism	References
AM-111 (D-JNKi-1)	Chinchilla	Anti-apoptotic	Coleman et al., 2007
d-JNKI-1	Guinea pig	Anti-apoptotic	Wang et al., 2007
D-JNKi-1 multifunctional	Mouse	Anti-apoptotic	Kayyali et al., 2018
Methylprednisolone	Guinea pig, Rat	Anti-inflammatory	Zhou et al., 2009; Ozdogan et al., 2012
Dexamethasone	Guinea pig	Anti-inflammatory	Chi et al., 2011; Heinrich et al., 2016
	Mouse		Han et al., 2015
	Rat		Gumrukcu et al., 2018
Dexamethasone (OTO-104)	Guinea pig		Harrop-Jones et al., 2016
Dexamethasone ultrasonic microbubbles	Guinea pig		Shih et al., 2018
Caroverine	Guinea pig	Glutamate antagonism	Chen et al., 2004
Kenpaullone	Mouse	Cyclin-dependent kinase-2 inhibitor	Teitz et al., 2018
Edavarone solid lipid nanoparticles	guinea pig	Antioxidant	Gao et al., 2015
BDNF + NT3	Guinea pig	Synapse regeneration	Sly et al., 2016
NT3	Mouse	Synapse regeneration	Suzuki et al., 2016
Pioglitazone	Rat	Anti-inflammatory, Antioxidant	Paciello et al., 2018
Rosmarinic acid	Rat	Antioxidant	Fetoni et al., 2018
AMPK-alpha1 siRNA	Mouse	AMPK-alpha 1	Hill et al., 2016
LKB1 siRNA	Mouse	LKB1	Hill et al., 2016
G9a siRNA	Mouse	EHMT2	Xiong et al., 2019

a second group was provided dexamethasone microbubbles with ultrasound irradiation. Compared with controls, dexamethasone in both groups provided protection against hair cell loss and auditory threshold shifts. However, significantly greater protection was afforded to the guinea pigs pretreated with ultrasound delivered microbubbles (Shih et al., 2018).

- Interesting findings were reported in a study of noise exposed mice. Animals were exposed to 110 db white noise for 60 min in a single exposure. One group received intraperitoneal dexamethasone injection (IP) daily for five consecutive days, while another cohort was given intra-tympanic injection of dexamethasone on days one and four after noise exposure. Mice in both treatment groups showed improved ABR thresholds but no apparent improvement in DPOAEs. Interestingly, better preservation of organ of Corti ultrastructure was observed in mice receiving IP drug than in those who were administered dexamethasone by intra-tympanic injection. On the other hand, efferent synapses were damaged in control (noise only), and in both groups treated with dexamethasone. However, there was better preservation of synapses of efferent terminals on OHCs in the group treated with intra-tympanic steroids (Han et al., 2015).
- In efforts to provide sustained release of dexamethasone for prolonged otoprotection against noise the efficacy of OTO-104 was investigated both prior to and following acute acoustic trauma. OTO-104 is a poloxamer-based hydrogel containing micronized dexamethasone. Guinea pigs received a single intra-tympanic injection of OTO-104 and were assessed in a model of acute acoustic trauma. Doses of at least 2.0% OTO-104 offered significant protection against hearing loss induced by noise exposure when administered 1 day prior to trauma and up to 3 days afterward. Otoprotection remained effective even with higher degrees of trauma. In contrast, the administration of a dexamethasone sodium phosphate solution did not protect against noise-induced hearing loss. Activation of the classical nuclear glucocorticoid and mineralocorticoid receptor pathways was required for otoprotection by OTO-104. The sustained release features of OTO-104 provided greater protection than the solution (Harrop-Jones et al., 2016).
- Methylprednisolone was administered intra-tympanically to guinea pigs exposed to impulse noise. Animals receiving this treatment had significantly better ABR thresholds at 4 weeks compared with those treated with saline. Significantly better preservation of hair cells was observed in the cochleae of guinea pigs receiving intra-tympanic methylprednisolone compared to those treated with saline (Zhou et al., 2009). Intra-tympanic methylprednisolone injection in rats administered following acoustic trauma was shown to reduce OHC loss. Although DPOAE measurement within the first week demonstrated significantly better amplitudes in the treated rats compared to controls at 2 weeks, there was no significant difference in DPOAE amplitudes between the treated and control group (Ozdogan et al., 2012).

We have summarized the studies reporting intra-tympanic drug delivery that protect against NIHL in **Table 2**.

CONCLUSION

Studies described in the above review highlight some exciting new research on local drug delivery using intra-tympanic administration of substances to ameliorate ototoxicity of cisplatin and noise-induced hearing loss. These are two very important causes of permanent sensorineural hearing loss for which there are currently no approved treatments on the market. The reports that are discussed include the proposed mechanisms for protection against these two major causes of hearing loss in humans.

The advantages of local delivery include targeted effects on the inner ear while minimizing systemic toxicity or interference with cisplatin antitumor efficacy and the ability to deliver sufficient amount of protective agent within the inner ear while by-passing the blood-labyrinth barrier (BLB), a major obstacle to effective protection delivered by systemic administration. The use of intra-tympanic injection in humans is minimally invasive and can generally be performed in the office under local anesthesia. The exploration of methods to extend the duration of release of protective agents and the investigation of round window permeation enhancers can provide higher concentrations of protectant molecules in the cochlea following intra-tympanic administration. The use of nanoparticles incorporating protective agents to target prestin in outer hair cells is very innovative and exciting. Although the regeneration of hair cells in the cochlea of humans has not been demonstrated, the regeneration of synapses on IHCs in animals after noise-induced synaptopathy using locally applied neurotrophins appears feasible. Future research is likely to reveal new mechanisms and exciting and novel treatments for sensorineural hearing loss.

AUTHOR CONTRIBUTIONS

LR conceived the study. LR and AD wrote the manuscript. DM and VR critiqued and revised the manuscript.

REFERENCES

Basner, M., Babisch, W., Davis, A., Brink, M., Clark, C., Janssen, S., et al. (2014). Auditory and non-auditory effects of noise on health. *Lancet* 383, 1325–1332. doi: 10.1016/s0140-6736(13)61613-x

Benkafadar, N., Menardo, J., Bourien, J., Nouvian, R., François, F., Decaudin, D., et al. (2017). Reversible p53 inhibition prevents cisplatin ototoxicity without blocking chemotherapeutic efficacy. *EMBO Mol. Med.* 9, 7–26. doi: 10.15252/emmm.201606230

Berglin, C. E., Pierre, P. V., Bramer, T., Edsman, K., Ehrsson, H., Eksborg, S., et al. (2011). Prevention of cisplatin-induced hearing loss by administration of a thiosulfate-containing gel to the middle ear in a guinea pig model. *Cancer Chemother. Pharmacol.* 68, 1547–1556. doi: 10.1007/s00280-011-1656-2

Bhatta, P., Dhukhwa, A., Sheehan, K., Al Aameri, R. F. H., Borse, V., Ghosh, S., et al. (2019). Capsaicin protects against cisplatin ototoxicity by changing the STAT3/STAT1 ratio and activating cannabinoid (CB2) receptors in the cochlea. *Sci. Rep.* 9:4131. doi: 10.1038/s41598-019-40425-9

Breglio, A. M., Rusheen, A. E., Shide, E. D., Fernandez, K. A., Spielbauer, K. K., McLachlin, K. M., et al. (2017). Cisplatin is retained in the cochlea indefinitely following chemotherapy. *Nat. Commun.* 8:1654. doi: 10.1038/s41467-017-01837-1

Bressler, S., Goldberg, H., and Shinn-Cunningham, B. (2017). Sensory coding and cognitive processing of sound in Veterans with blast exposure. *Hear. Res.* 349, 98–110. doi: 10.1016/j.heares.2016.10.018

Brooks, B., and Knight, K. (2018). Ototoxicity monitoring in children treated with platinum chemotherapy. *Int. J. Audiol.* 57, S34–S40. doi: 10.1080/14992027.2017.1355570

Celebi, S., Gurdal, M. M., Ozkul, M. H., Yasar, H., and Balikci, H. H. (2013). The effect of intratympanic vitamin C administration on cisplatin-induced ototoxicity. *Eur. Arch. Otorhinolaryngol.* 270, 1293–1297. doi: 10.1007/s00405-012-2140-2

Chen, Z., Ulfendahl, M., Ruan, R., Tan, L., and Duan, M. (2004). Protection of auditory function against noise trauma with local caroverine administration in guinea pigs. *Hear. Res.* 197, 131–136. doi: 10.1016/j.heares.2004.03.021

Chi, F. L., Yang, M. Q., Zhou, Y. D., and Wang, B. (2011). Therapeutic efficacy of topical application of dexamethasone to the round window niche after acoustic trauma caused by intensive impulse noise in guinea pigs. *J. Laryngol. Otol.* 125, 673–685. doi: 10.1017/S0022215111000028

Choe, W. T., Chinosornvatana, N., and Chang, K. W. (2004). Prevention of cisplatin ototoxicity using transtympanic N-acetylcysteine and lactate. *Otol. Neurotol.* 25, 910–915. doi: 10.1097/00129492-200411000-00009

Coleman, J. K., Littlesunday, C., Jackson, R., and Meyer, T. (2007). AM-111 protects against permanent hearing loss from impulse noise trauma. *Hear. Res.* 226, 70–78. doi: 10.1016/j.heares.2006.05.006

Creber, N. J., Eastwood, H. T., Hampson, A. J., Tan, J., and O'Leary, S. J. (2019). Adjuvant agents enhance round window membrane permeability to dexamethasone and modulate basal to apical cochlear gradients. *Eur. J. Pharm. Sci.* 126, 69–81. doi: 10.1016/j.ejps.2018.08.013

Cunningham, L. L., and Tucci, D. L. (2017). Hearing Loss in Adults. *N. Engl. J. Med.* 377, 2465–2473.

Demir, M. G., Altintoprak, N., Aydin, S., Kosemihal, E., and Basak, K. (2015). Effect of transtympanic injection of melatonin on cisplatin-induced ototoxicity. *J. Int. Adv. Otol.* 11, 202–206. doi: 10.5152/iao.2015.1094

Ding, S., Xie, S., Chen, W., Wen, L., Wang, J., Yang, F., et al. (2019). Is oval window transport a royal gate for nanoparticle delivery to vestibule in the inner ear? *Eur. J. Pharm. Sci.* 126, 11–22. doi: 10.1016/j.ejps.2018.02.031

Dormer, N. H., Nelson-Brantley, J., Staecker, H., and Berkland, C. J. (2019). Evaluation of a transtympanic delivery system in Mus musculus for extended release steroids. *Eur. J. Pharm. Sci.* 126, 3–10. doi: 10.1016/j.ejps.2018.01.020

El Kechai, N., Mamelle, E., Nguyen, Y., Huang, N., Nicolas, V., Chaminade, P., et al. (2016). Hyaluronic acid liposomal gel sustains delivery of a corticoid to the inner ear. *J. Control Release* 226, 248–257. doi: 10.1016/j.jconrel.2016.02.013

Falcone, P. H., Nieman, K. M., Tribby, A. C., Vogel, R. M., Joy, J. M., Moon, J. R., et al. (2019). The attention-enhancing effects of spearmint extract supplementation in healthy men and women: a randomized, double-blind, placebo-controlled, parallel trial. *Nutr. Res.* 64, 24–38. doi: 10.1016/j.nutres.2018.11.012

Fernandez, R., Harrop-Jones, A., Wang, X., Dellamary, L., LeBel, C., and Piu, F. (2016). The sustained-exposure dexamethasone formulation OTO-104 offers effective protection against cisplatin-induced hearing loss. *Audiol. Neurootol.* 21, 22–29. doi: 10.1159/000441833

Fetoni, A. R., Eramo, S. L. M., Di Pino, A., Rolesi, R., Paciello, F., Grassi, C., et al. (2018). The antioxidant effect of rosmarinic acid by different delivery routes in the animal model of noise-induced hearing loss. *Otol. Neurotol.* 39, 378–386. doi: 10.1097/MAO.0000000000001700

Franz, P., Aharinejad, S., Bock, P., and Firbas, W. (1993). The cochlear glomeruli in the modiolus of the guinea pig. *Eur. Arch. Otorhinolaryngol.* 250, 44–50.

Gao, G., Liu, Y., Zhou, C. H., Jiang, P., and Sun, J. J. (2015). Solid lipid nanoparticles loaded with edaravone for inner ear protection after noise exposure. *Chin. Med. J.* 128, 203–209. doi: 10.4103/0366-6999.149202

Gates, G. A., Schmid, P., Kujawa, S. G., Nam, B., and D'Agostino, R. (2000). Longitudinal threshold changes in older men with audiometric notches. *Hear. Res.* 141, 220–228. doi: 10.1016/s0378-5955(99)00223-3

Ghosh, S., Sheth, S., Sheehan, K., Mukherjea, D., Dhukhwa, A., Borse, V., et al. (2018). The Endocannabinoid/Cannabinoid Receptor 2 System Protects Against Cisplatin-Induced Hearing Loss. *Front. Cell. Neurosci.* 12:271. doi: 10.3389/fncel.2018.00271

Goycoolea, M. V. (1992). The round window membrane under normal and pathological conditions. *Acta Otolaryngol. Suppl.* 493, 43–55.

Goycoolea, M. V., and Lundman, L. (1997). Round window membrane. Structure function and permeability: a review. *Microsc. Res. Tech.* 36, 201–211.

Goycoolea, M. V., Muchow, D., and Schachern, P. (1988). Experimental studies on round window structure: function and permeability. *Laryngoscope* 98(6 Pt 2 Suppl. 44), 1–20. doi: 10.1288/00005537-198806001-00002

Gumrukcu, S. S., Topaloglu, I., Salturk, Z., Tutar, B., Atar, Y., Berkiten, G., et al. (2018). Effects of intratympanic dexamethasone on noise-induced hearing loss: an experimental study. *Am. J. Otolaryngol.* 39, 71–73. doi: 10.1016/j.amjoto.2017.10.011

Han, M. A., Back, S. A., Kim, H. L., Park, S. Y., Yeo, S. W., and Park, S. N. (2015). Therapeutic effect of dexamethasone for noise-induced hearing loss: systemic versus intratympanic injection in mice. *Otol. Neurotol.* 36, 755–762. doi: 10.1097/MAO.0000000000000759

Harrop-Jones, A., Wang, X., Fernandez, R., Dellamary, L., Ryan, A. F., LeBel, C., et al. (2016). The sustained-exposure dexamethasone formulation OTO-104 offers effective protection against noise-induced hearing loss. *Audiol. Neurootol.* 21, 12–21. doi: 10.1159/000441814

Hazlitt, R. A., Min, J., and Zuo, J. (2018). Progress in the Development of Preventative Drugs for Cisplatin-Induced Hearing Loss. *J. Med. Chem.* 61, 5512–5524. doi: 10.1021/acs.jmedchem.7b01653

Heinrich, U. R., Strieth, S., Schmidtmann, I., Stauber, R., and Helling, K. (2016). Dexamethasone prevents hearing loss by restoring glucocorticoid receptor expression in the guinea pig cochlea. *Laryngoscope* 126, E29–E34. doi: 10.1002/lary.25345

Hellberg, V., Wallin, I., Ehrsson, H., and Laurell, G. (2013). Cochlear pharmacokinetics of cisplatin: an in vivo study in the guinea pig. *Laryngoscope* 123, 3172–3177. doi: 10.1002/lary.24235

Hill, G. W., Morest, D. K., and Parham, K. (2008). Cisplatin-induced ototoxicity: effect of intratympanic dexamethasone injections. *Otol. Neurotol.* 29, 1005–1011. doi: 10.1097/MAO.0b013e31818599d5

Hill, K., Yuan, H., Wang, X., and Sha, S. H. (2016). Noise-induced loss of hair cells and cochlear synaptopathy are mediated by the activation of AMPK. *J. Neurosci.* 36, 7497–7510. doi: 10.1523/JNEUROSCI.0782-16.2016

Juhn, S. K., Meyerhoff, W. L., and Paparella, M. M. (1981). Clinical application of middle ear effusion analyses. *Laryngoscope* 91, 1012–1015.

Karasawa, T., and Steyger, P. S. (2015). An integrated view of cisplatin-induced nephrotoxicity and ototoxicity. *Toxicol. Lett.* 237, 219–227. doi: 10.1016/j.toxlet.2015.06.012

Kaur, T., Borse, V., Sheth, S., Sheehan, K., Ghosh, S., Tupal, S., et al. (2016). Adenosine A1 receptor protects against cisplatin ototoxicity by suppressing the NOX3/STAT1 inflammatory pathway in the cochlea. *J. Neurosci.* 36, 3962–3977. doi: 10.1523/JNEUROSCI.3111-15.2016

Kaur, T., Mukherjea, D., Sheehan, K., Jajoo, S., Rybak, L. P., and Ramkumar, V. (2011). Short interfering RNA against STAT1 attenuates cisplatin-induced ototoxicity in the rat by suppressing inflammation. *Cell Death Dis.* 2:e180. doi: 10.1038/cddis.2011.63

Kayyali, M. N., Wooltorton, J. R. A., Ramsey, A. J., Lin, M., Chao, T. N., Tsourkas, A., et al. (2018). A novel nanoparticle delivery system for targeted therapy of noise-induced hearing loss. *J. Control Release* 279, 243–250. doi: 10.1016/j.jconrel.2018.04.028

King, E. B., Salt, A. N., Eastwood, H. T., and O'Leary, S. J. (2011). Direct entry of gadolinium into the vestibule following intratympanic applications in Guinea pigs and the influence of cochlear implantation. *J. Assoc. Res. Otolaryngol.* 12, 741–751. doi: 10.1007/s10162-011-0280-5

Korver, K. D., Rybak, L. P., Whitworth, C., and Campbell, K. M. (2002). Round window application of D-methionine provides complete cisplatin otoprotection. *Otolaryngol. Head Neck Surg.* 126, 683–689. doi: 10.1067/mhn.2002.125299

Kros, C. J., and Steyger, P. S. (2018). Aminoglycoside- and cisplatin-induced ototoxicity: mechanisms and otoprotective strategies*. *Cold Spring Harb. Perspect. Med.* a033548. doi: 10.1101/cshperspect.a033548

Kujawa, S. G., and Liberman, M. C. (2009). Adding insult to injury: cochlear nerve degeneration after temporary noise-induced hearing loss. *J. Neurosci.* 29, 14077–14085. doi: 10.1523/jneurosci.2845-09.2009

Kumar, U. A., Ameenudin, S., and Sangamanatha, A. V. (2012). Temporal and speech processing skills in normal hearing individuals exposed to occupational noise. *Noise Health* 14, 100–105. doi: 10.4103/1463-1741.97252

Kurabi, A., Keithley, E. M., Housley, G. D., Ryan, A. F., and Wong, A. C. (2017). Cellular mechanisms of noise-induced hearing loss. *Hear. Res.* 349, 129–137. doi: 10.1016/j.heares.2016.11.013

Lavorgna, M., Orlo, E., Nugnes, R., Piscitelli, C., Russo, C., and Isidori, M. (2019). Capsaicin in hot chili peppers: in vitro evaluation of its antiradical, antiproliferative and apoptotic activities. *Plant Foods Hum. Nutr.* 74, 164–170. doi: 10.1007/s11130-019-00722-0

Le Prell, C. G., and Clavier, O. H. (2017). Effects of noise on speech recognition: challenges for communication by service members. *Hear. Res.* 349, 76–89. doi: 10.1016/j.heares.2016.10.004

Li, G., Frenz, D. A., Brahmblatt, S., Feghali, J. G., Ruben, R. J., Berggren, D., et al. (2001). Round window membrane delivery of L-methionine provides protection from cisplatin ototoxicity without compromising chemotherapeutic efficacy. *Neurotoxicology* 22, 163–176. doi: 10.1016/s0161-813x(00)00010-3

Li, L., Chao, T., Brant, J., O'Malley, B. Jr., Tsourkas, A., and Li, D. (2017). Advances in nano-based inner ear delivery systems for the treatment of sensorineural hearing loss. *Adv. Drug Deliv. Rev.* 108, 2–12. doi: 10.1016/j.addr.2016.01.004

Li, W., Hartsock, J. J., Dai, C., and Salt, A. N. (2018). Permeation enhancers for intratympanically-applied drugs studied using fluorescent dexamethasone as a marker. *Otol. Neurotol.* 39, 639–647. doi: 10.1097/MAO.0000000000001786

Martin-Saldana, S., Palao-Suay, R., Aguilar, M. R., Ramirez-Camacho, R., and San Roman, J. (2017). Polymeric nanoparticles loaded with dexamethasone or alpha-tocopheryl succinate to prevent cisplatin-induced ototoxicity. *Acta Biomater.* 53, 199–210. doi: 10.1016/j.actbio.2017.02.019

Masterson, E. A., Themann, C. L., and Calvert, G. M. (2018). prevalence of hearing loss among noise-exposed workers within the health care and social assistance sector, 2003 to 2012. *J. Occup. Environ. Med.* 60, 350–356. doi: 10.1097/JOM.0000000000001214

More, S. S., Akil, O., Ianculescu, A. G., Geier, E. G., Lustig, L. R., and Giacomini, K. M. (2010). Role of the copper transporter, CTR1, in platinum-induced ototoxicity. *J. Neurosci.* 30, 9500–9509. doi: 10.1523/JNEUROSCI.1544-10.2010

Mukherjea, D., Jajoo, S., Sheehan, K., Kaur, T., Sheth, S., Bunch, J., et al. (2011). NOX3 NADPH oxidase couples transient receptor potential vanilloid 1 to signal transducer and activator of transcription 1-mediated inflammation and hearing loss. *Antioxid. Redox Signal.* 14, 999–1010. doi: 10.1089/ars.2010.3497

Mukherjea, D., Jajoo, S., Whitworth, C., Bunch, J. R., Turner, J. G., Rybak, L. P., et al. (2008). Short interfering RNA against transient receptor potential vanilloid 1 attenuates cisplatin-induced hearing loss in the rat. *J. Neurosci.* 28, 13056–13065. doi: 10.1523/JNEUROSCI.1307-08.2008

Munzel, T., Sorensen, M., Schmidt, F., Schmidt, E., Steven, S., Kroller-Schon, S., et al. (2018). The adverse effects of environmental noise exposure on oxidative stress and cardiovascular risk. *Antioxid. Redox. Signal.* 28, 873–908. doi: 10.1089/ars.2017.7118

Murphy, D., and Daniel, S. J. (2011). Intratympanic dexamethasone to prevent cisplatin ototoxicity: a guinea pig model. *Otolaryngol Head Neck Surg.* 145, 452–457. doi: 10.1177/0194599811406673

Nader, M. E., Theoret, Y., and Saliba, I. (2010). The role of intratympanic lactate injection in the prevention of cisplatin-induced ototoxicity. *Laryngoscope* 120, 1208–1213. doi: 10.1002/lary.20892

Nelson, D. I., Nelson, R. Y., Concha-Barrientos, M., and Fingerhut, M. (2005). The global burden of occupational noise-induced hearing loss. *Am. J. Ind. Med.* 48, 446–458. doi: 10.1002/ajim.20223

Nyberg, S., Abbott, N. J., Shi, X., Steyger, P. S., and Dabdoub, A. (2019). Delivery of therapeutics to the inner ear: the challenge of the blood-labyrinth barrier. *Sci. Transl. Med.* 11:eaao0935. doi: 10.1126/scitranslmed.aao0935

Ohinata, Y., Miller, J. M., Altschuler, R. A., and Schacht, J. (2000). Intense noise induces formation of vasoactive lipid peroxidation products in the cochlea. *Brain Res.* 878, 163–173. doi: 10.1016/s0006-8993(00)02733-5

Ohlemiller, K. K. (2008). Recent findings and emerging questions in cochlear noise injury. *Hear. Res.* 245, 5–17. doi: 10.1016/j.heares.2008.08.007

Oishi, N., and Schacht, J. (2011). Emerging treatments for noise-induced hearing loss. *Expert Opin. Emerg. Drugs* 16, 235–245. doi: 10.1517/14728214.2011.552427

Ozdogan, F., Ensari, S., Cakir, O., Ozcan, K. M., Koseoglu, S., Ozdas, T., et al. (2012). Investigation of the cochlear effects of intratympanic steroids administered following acoustic trauma. *Laryngoscope* 122, 877–882. doi: 10.1002/lary.23185

Özel, H. E., Özdoğan, F., Gürgen, S. G., Esen, E., Genç S., and Selçuk, A. (2016). Comparison of the protective effects of intratympanic dexamethasone and methylprednisolone against cisplatin-induced ototoxicity. *J. Laryngol. Otol.* 130, 225–234. doi: 10.1017/S0022215115003473

Paciello, F., Fetoni, A. R., Rolesi, R., Wright, M. B., Grassi, C., Troiani, D., et al. (2018). pioglitazone represents an effective therapeutic target in preventing oxidative/inflammatory cochlear damage induced by noise exposure. *Front. Pharmacol.* 9:1103. doi: 10.3389/fphar.2018.01103

Paksoy, M., Ayduran, E., Sanli, A., Eken, M., Aydin, S., and Oktay, Z. A. (2011). The protective effects of intratympanic dexamethasone and vitamin E on cisplatin-induced ototoxicity are demonstrated in rats. *Med. Oncol.* 28, 615–621. doi: 10.1007/s12032-010-9477-4

Parham, K. (2011). Can intratympanic dexamethasone protect against cisplatin ototoxicity in mice with age-related hearing loss? *Otolaryngol. Head Neck Surg.* 145, 635–640. doi: 10.1177/0194599811409304

Parhizkar, N., and Rybak, L. (2003). "Round Window Application of the P53 Inhibitor Pifithrin-Alpha provides complete protection against Cisplatin Ototoxicity," in *Proceedings of the 26th Annual Midwinter Research Meeting of The Association for Research in Otolaryngology*, Florida, FL.

Piu, F., Wang, X., Fernandez, R., Dellamary, L., Harrop, A., Ye, Q., et al. (2011). OTO-104: a sustained-release dexamethasone hydrogel for the treatment of otic disorders. *Otol. Neurotol.* 32, 171–179. doi: 10.1097/MAO.0b013e3182009d29

Qi, W., Ding, D., Zhu, H., Lu, D., Wang, Y., Ding, J., et al. (2014). Efficient siRNA transfection to the inner ear through the intact round window by a novel proteidic delivery technology in the chinchilla. *Gene. Ther.* 21, 10–18. doi: 10.1038/gt.2013.49

Ramaswamy, B., Roy, S., Apolo, A. B., Shapiro, B., and Depireux, D. A. (2017). Magnetic nanoparticle mediated steroid delivery mitigates cisplatin induced hearing loss. *Front. Cell. Neurosci.* 11:268. doi: 10.3389/fncel.2017.00268

Salt, A. N., and Hirose, K. (2018). Communication pathways to and from the inner ear and their contributions to drug delivery. *Hear. Res.* 362, 25–37. doi: 10.1016/j.heares.2017.12.010

Salt, A. N., and Plontke, S. K. (2009). Principles of local drug delivery to the inner ear. *Audiol. Neurootol.* 14, 350–360. doi: 10.1159/000241892

Salt, A. N., and Plontke, S. K. (2018). Pharmacokinetic principles in the inner ear: influence of drug properties on intratympanic applications. *Hear. Res.* 368, 28–40. doi: 10.1016/j.heares.2018.03.002

Shafik, A. G., Elkabarity, R. H., Thabet, M. T., Soliman, N. B., and Kalleny, N. K. (2013). Effect of intratympanic dexamethasone administration on cisplatin-induced ototoxicity in adult guinea pigs. *Auris Nasus Larynx* 40, 51–60. doi: 10.1016/j.anl.2012.05.010

Sheehan, K., Sheth, S., Mukherjea, D., Rybak, L. P., and Ramkumar, V. (2018). Trans-tympanic drug delivery for the treatment of ototoxicity*. *J. Vis. Exp.* 56564. doi: 10.3791/56564

Sheth, S., Mukherjea, D., Rybak, L. P., and Ramkumar, V. (2017). Mechanisms of cisplatin-induced ototoxicity and otoprotection. *Front. Cell. Neurosci.* 11:338. doi: 10.3389/fncel.2017.00338

Shi, X. (2016). Pathophysiology of the cochlear intrastrial fluid-blood barrier (review). *Hear. Res.* 338, 52–63. doi: 10.1016/j.heares.2016.01.010

Shih, C. P., Chen, H. C., Lin, Y. C., Chen, H. K., Wang, H., Kuo, C. Y., et al. (2018). Middle-ear dexamethasone delivery via ultrasound microbubbles attenuates noise-induced hearing loss. *Laryngoscope* doi: 10.1002/lary.27713 [Epub ahead of print].

Shin, Y. S., Song, S. J., Kang, S. U., Hwang, H. S., Choi, J. W., Lee, B. H., et al. (2013). A novel synthetic compound, 3-amino-3-(4-fluoro-phenyl)-1H-quinoline-2,4-dione, inhibits cisplatin-induced hearing loss by the suppression of reactive oxygen species: in vitro and in vivo study. *Neuroscience* 232, 1–12. doi: 10.1016/j.neuroscience.2012.12.008

Sly, D. J., Campbell, L., Uschakov, A., Saief, S. T., Lam, M., and O'Leary, S. J. (2016). Applying neurotrophins to the round window rescues auditory function and reduces inner hair cell synaptopathy after noise-induced hearing loss. *Otol. Neurotol.* 37, 1223–1230. doi: 10.1097/MAO.0000000000001191

Sun, C., Wang, X., Zheng, Z., Chen, D., Wang, X., Shi, F., et al. (2015). A single dose of dexamethasone encapsulated in polyethylene glycol-coated polylactic acid nanoparticles attenuates cisplatin-induced hearing loss following round window membrane administration. *Int. J. Nanomed.* 10, 3567–3579. doi: 10.2147/IJN.S77912

Suzuki, J., Corfas, G., and Liberman, M. C. (2016). Round-window delivery of neurotrophin 3 regenerates cochlear synapses after acoustic overexposure. *Sci. Rep.* 6:24907. doi: 10.1038/srep24907

Tanaka, K., and Motomura, S. (1981). Permeability of the labyrinthine windows in guinea pigs. *Arch. Otorhinolaryngol.* 233, 67–73.

Teitz, T., Fang, J., Goktug, A. N., Bonga, J. D., Diao, S., Hazlitt, R. A., et al. (2018). CDK2 inhibitors as candidate therapeutics for cisplatin- and noise-induced hearing loss. *J. Exp. Med.* 215, 1187–1203. doi: 10.1084/jem.20172246

Teranishi, M. A., and Nakashima, T. (2003). Effects of trolox, locally applied on round windows, on cisplatin-induced ototoxicity in guinea pigs. *Int. J. Pediatr. Otorhinolaryngol.* 67, 133–139. doi: 10.1016/s0165-5876(02)00353-1

Wang, J., Ruel, J., Ladrech, S., Bonny, C., van de Water, T. R., and Puel, J. L. (2007). Inhibition of the c-Jun N-terminal kinase-mediated mitochondrial cell death pathway restores auditory function in sound-exposed animals. *Mol. Pharmacol.* 71, 654–666. doi: 10.1124/mol.106.028936

Wang, X., Chen, Y., Tao, Y., Gao, Y., Yu, D., and Wu, H. (2018). A666-conjugated nanoparticles target prestin of outer hair cells preventing cisplatin-induced hearing loss. *Int. J. Nanomed.* 13, 7517–7531. doi: 10.2147/IJN.S170130

Wimmer, C., Mees, K., Stumpf, P., Welsch, U., Reichel, O., and Suckfull, M. (2004). Round window application of D-methionine, sodium thiosulfate, brain-derived neurotrophic factor, and fibroblast growth factor-2 in cisplatin-induced ototoxicity. *Otol. Neurotol.* 25, 33–40. doi: 10.1097/00129492-200401000-00007

Xiong, H., Long, H., Pan, S., Lai, R., Wang, X., Zhu, Y., et al. (2019). Inhibition of histone methyltransferase g9a attenuates noise-induced cochlear synaptopathy and hearing loss. *J. Assoc. Res. Otolaryngol.* 20, 217–232. doi: 10.1007/s10162-019-00714-6

Yamane, H., Nakai, Y., Takayama, M., Iguchi, H., Nakagawa, T., and Kojima, A. (1995). Appearance of free radicals in the guinea pig inner ear after noise-induced acoustic trauma. *Eur. Arch. Otorhinolaryngol.* 252, 504–508. doi: 10.1007/bf02114761

Zhang, L., Xu, Y., Cao, W., Xie, S., Wen, L., and Chen, G. (2018). Understanding the translocation mechanism of PLGA nanoparticles across round window membrane into the inner ear: a guideline for inner ear drug delivery based on nanomedicine. *Int. J. Nanomed.* 13, 479–492. doi: 10.2147/IJN.S154968

Zhang, M., Liu, W., Ding, D., and Salvi, R. (2003). Pifithrin-alpha suppresses p53 and protects cochlear and vestibular hair cells from cisplatin-induced apoptosis. *Neuroscience* 120, 191–205. doi: 10.1016/s0306-4522(03)00286-0

Zhou, Y., Zheng, H., Shen, X., Zhang, Q., and Yang, M. (2009). Intratympanic administration of methylprednisolone reduces impact of experimental intensive impulse noise trauma on hearing. *Acta Otolaryngol.* 129, 602–607. doi: 10.1080/00016480802342424

Zou, J., Pyykko, I., and Hyttinen, J. (2016). Inner ear barriers to nanomedicine-augmented drug delivery and imaging. *J. Otol.* 11, 165–177. doi: 10.1016/j.joto.2016.11.002

Permissions

All chapters in this book were first published by Frontiers; hereby published with permission under the Creative Commons Attribution License or equivalent. Every chapter published in this book has been scrutinized by our experts. Their significance has been extensively debated. The topics covered herein carry significant findings which will fuel the growth of the discipline. They may even be implemented as practical applications or may be referred to as a beginning point for another development.

The contributors of this book come from diverse backgrounds, making this book a truly international effort. This book will bring forth new frontiers with its revolutionizing research information and detailed analysis of the nascent developments around the world.

We would like to thank all the contributing authors for lending their expertise to make the book truly unique. They have played a crucial role in the development of this book. Without their invaluable contributions this book wouldn't have been possible. They have made vital efforts to compile up to date information on the varied aspects of this subject to make this book a valuable addition to the collection of many professionals and students.

This book was conceptualized with the vision of imparting up-to-date information and advanced data in this field. To ensure the same, a matchless editorial board was set up. Every individual on the board went through rigorous rounds of assessment to prove their worth. After which they invested a large part of their time researching and compiling the most relevant data for our readers.

The editorial board has been involved in producing this book since its inception. They have spent rigorous hours researching and exploring the diverse topics which have resulted in the successful publishing of this book. They have passed on their knowledge of decades through this book. To expedite this challenging task, the publisher supported the team at every step. A small team of assistant editors was also appointed to further simplify the editing procedure and attain best results for the readers.

Apart from the editorial board, the designing team has also invested a significant amount of their time in understanding the subject and creating the most relevant covers. They scrutinized every image to scout for the most suitable representation of the subject and create an appropriate cover for the book.

The publishing team has been an ardent support to the editorial, designing and production team. Their endless efforts to recruit the best for this project, has resulted in the accomplishment of this book. They are a veteran in the field of academics and their pool of knowledge is as vast as their experience in printing. Their expertise and guidance has proved useful at every step. Their uncompromising quality standards have made this book an exceptional effort. Their encouragement from time to time has been an inspiration for everyone.

The publisher and the editorial board hope that this book will prove to be a valuable piece of knowledge for researchers, students, practitioners and scholars across the globe.

List of Contributors

Xiaomin Tang, Yuxuan Sun, Chenyu Xu, Xiaotao Guo, Jiaqiang Sun, Chunchen Pan and Jingwu Sun
Departments of Otolaryngology-Head and Neck Surgery, The First Affiliated Hospital of University of Science and Technique of China, Hefei, China

Haiying Sun
Department of Otolaryngology-Head and Neck Surgery, Stanford University School of Medicine, Stanford, CA, United States
Department of Otorhinolaryngology, Union Hospital, Tongji Medical College, Huazhong University of Science and Technology, Wuhan, China

Tian Wang, Patrick J. Atkinson, Sara E. Billings, Wuxing Dong and Alan G. Cheng
Department of Otolaryngology-Head and Neck Surgery, Stanford University School of Medicine, Stanford, CA, United States

Zhengqing Hu
John D. Dingell VA Medical Center, Detroit, MI, United States
Department of Otolaryngology-HNS, Wayne State University School of Medicine, Detroit, MI, United States

Fnu Komal, Aditi Singh and Meng Deng
Department of Otolaryngology-HNS, Wayne State University School of Medicine, Detroit, MI, United States

Zhen Chen, Yuhang Huang, Chaorong Yu, Qing Liu and Cui Qiu
MOE Key Laboratory of Model Animal for Disease Study, Department of Otorhinolaryngology Head and Neck Surgery, The Affiliated Drum Tower Hospital of Medical School, Model Animal Research Center of Medical School, Nanjing University, Nanjing, China

Guoqiang Wan
MOE Key Laboratory of Model Animal for Disease Study, Department of Otorhinolaryngology Head and Neck Surgery, The Affiliated Drum Tower Hospital of Medical School, Model Animal Research Center of Medical School, Nanjing University, Nanjing, China
Research Institute of Otolaryngology, Nanjing, China
Jiangsu Key Laboratory of Molecular Medicine, Medical School of Nanjing University, Nanjing, China
Institute for Brain Sciences, Nanjing University, Nanjing, China

Wenqi Liang, Chunli Zhao, Zhongrui Chen, Zijing Yang, Ke Liu and Shusheng Gong
Department of Otolaryngology Head and Neck Surgery, Beijing Friendship Hospital, Capital Medical University, Beijing, China

Jie Wen, Jian Song, Yijiang Bai, Yalan Liu, Xinzhang Cai, Lingyun Mei and Chufeng He
Department of Otorhinolaryngology, Xiangya Hospital Central South University, Changsha, China
Province Key Laboratory of Otolaryngology Critical Diseases, Changsha, China
Department of Geriatrics, National Clinical Research Centre for Geriatric Disorders, Xiangya Hospital, Central South University, Changsha, China

Lu Ma
Department of Otorhinolaryngology, The Affiliated Changsha Central Hospital, Hengyang Medical School, University of South China, Changsha, China

Yong Feng
Department of Otorhinolaryngology, Xiangya Hospital Central South University, Changsha, China
Department of Otorhinolaryngology, The Affiliated Changsha Central Hospital, Hengyang Medical School, University of South China, Changsha, China

Quan Wang, Yilin Shen, Yi Pan, Kaili Chen, Rui Ding, Tianyuan Zou, Andi Zhang, Dongye Guo, Cui Fan, Haixia Hu, Bin Ye, Peilin Ji and Mingliang Xiang
Department of Otolaryngology and Head and Neck Surgery, Ruijin Hospital, Shanghai Jiao Tong University School of Medicine, Shanghai, China
Ear Institute, Shanghai Jiao Tong University School of Medicine, Shanghai, China

Ling Mei
Ear Institute, Shanghai Jiao Tong University School of Medicine, Shanghai, China

Siyu Li, Cheng Cheng, Ling Lu, Xiaoli Zhang, Ao Li, Jie Chen, Xiaoyun Qian and Xia Gao
Department of Otolaryngology Head and Neck Surgery, Affiliated Drum Tower Hospital of Nanjing University Medical School, Jiangsu Provincial Key Medical Discipline (Laboratory), Nanjing, China
Research Institute of Otolaryngology, Nanjing, China

List of Contributors

Xiaofeng Ma
Department of Otolaryngology Head and Neck Surgery, Affiliated Drum Tower Hospital of Nanjing University Medical School, Jiangsu Provincial Key Medical Discipline (Laboratory), Nanjing, China

Zilin Huang, Qiang Xie, Shuang Li, Yuhao Zhou, Zuhong He, Kun Lin, Minlan Yang, Peng Song and Xiong Chen
Department of Otorhinolaryngology, Head and Neck Surgery, Zhongnan Hospital of Wuhan University, Wuhan, China
Sleep Medicine Center, Zhongnan Hospital of Wuhan University, Wuhan, China

Jianyong Chen, Dekun Gao, Junmin Chen, Shule Hou, Baihui He, Yue Li, Shuna Li, Fan Zhang, Xiayu Sun, Lianhua Sun, Jun Yang and Guiliang Zheng
Department of Otorhinolaryngology Head and Neck Surgery, Xinhua Hospital, Shanghai Jiao Tong University School of Medicine, Shanghai, China
Shanghai Jiao Tong University School of Medicine Ear Institute, Shanghai, China
Shanghai Key Laboratory of Translational Medicine on Ear and Nose Diseases, Shanghai, China

Fabio Mammano
Department of Physics and Astronomy "G. Galilei", University of Padova, Padua, Italy
Department of Biomedical Sciences, Institute of Cell Biology and Neurobiology, Italian National Research Council, Monterotondo, Italy

Feng Liang and Xin Fu
Anaesthesia Department, China-Japan Union Hospital, JiLin University, Changchun, China

ShiJian Ding
School of Life Sciences, Shanghai University, Shanghai, China

Lin Li
Department of Otorhinolaryngology Head and Neck Surgery, China-Japan Union Hospital of Jilin University, Changchun, China

Xiaoxiang Xu
Department of Otolaryngology-Head and Neck Surgery, Zhongnan Hospital of Wuhan University, Wuhan, China

Yanyan Ding, Yurong Mu and Weijia Kong
Department of Otorhinolaryngology, Union Hospital, Tongji Medical College, Huazhong University of Science and Technology, Wuhan, China

Renjie Chai
State Key Laboratory of Bioelectronics, Jiangsu Province High-Tech Key Laboratory for Bio-Medical Research, School of Life Sciences and Technology, Southeast University, Nanjing, China
Co-Innovation Center of Neuroregeneration, Nantong University, Nantong, China
Institute for Stem Cell and Regeneration, Chinese Academy of Sciences, Beijing, China
Jiangsu Province High-Tech Key Laboratory for Bio-Medical Research, Southeast University, Nanjing, China
Beijing Key Laboratory of Neural Regeneration and Repair, Capital Medical University, Beijing, China

Ido Badash, Patricia M. Quiñones, Juemei Wang and Frank Macias-Escriva
Caruso Department of Otolaryngology-Head and Neck Surgery, Keck School of Medicine of the University of Southern California, Los Angeles, CA, United States

Kevin J. Oghalai
Viterbi School of Engineering, University of Southern California, Los Angeles, CA, United States

Christopher G. Lui
Department of Otolaryngology-Head and Neck Surgery, Northwestern University Feinberg School of Medicine, Chicago, IL, United States

Brian E. Applegate and John S. Oghalai
Caruso Department of Otolaryngology-Head and Neck Surgery, Keck School of Medicine of the University of Southern California, Los Angeles, CA, United States
Viterbi School of Engineering, University of Southern California, Los Angeles, CA, United States

Zu-Hong He, Song Pan, Hong-Wei Zheng, Qiao-Jun Fang, Kayla Hill and Su-Hua Sha
Department of Pathology and Laboratory Medicine, Medical University of South Carolina, Charleston, SC, United States

Shiwei Qiu
Department of Otolaryngology, Head and Neck Surgery, Institute of Otolaryngology, Genetic Testing Center for Deafness, Chinese PLA General Hospital; National Clinical Research Center for Otolaryngologic Diseases; Key Lab of Hearing Impairment Science of Ministry of Education; Key Lab of Hearing Impairment Prevention and Treatment of Beijing, Beijing, China
The Institute of Audiology and Balance Science, Artificial Auditory Laboratory of Jiangsu Province, Xuzhou Medical University, Xuzhou, China

Weihao Zhao
Department of Otolaryngology, Head and Neck Surgery, Institute of Otolaryngology, Genetic Testing Center for Deafness, Chinese PLA General Hospital; National Clinical Research Center for Otolaryngologic Diseases; Key Lab of Hearing Impairment Science of Ministry of Education; Key Lab of Hearing Impairment Prevention and Treatment of Beijing, Beijing, China
Department of Otolaryngology General Hospital of Tibet Military Region, Lhasa, China

Xue Gao
Department of Otolaryngology, PLA Rocket Force Characteristic Medical Center, Beijing, China

Dapeng Li
Department of Neurobiology, School of Basic Medical Sciences, Beijing Key Laboratory of Neural Regeneration and Repair, Advanced Innovation Center for Human Brain Protection, Capital Medical University, Beijing, China

Weiqian Wang, Bo Gao, Weiju Han, Shiming Yang, Pu Dai and Yongyi Yuan
Department of Otolaryngology, Head and Neck Surgery, Institute of Otolaryngology, Genetic Testing Center for Deafness, Chinese PLA General Hospital; National Clinical Research Center for Otolaryngologic Diseases; Key Lab of Hearing Impairment Science of Ministry of Education; Key Lab of Hearing Impairment Prevention and Treatment of Beijing, Beijing, China

Peng Cao
National Institute of Biological Sciences, Beijing, China

Xue Bai, Sen Chen, Kai Xu, Yuan Jin, Xun Niu, Le Xie, Yue Qiu, Xiao-Zhou Liu and Yu Sun
Department of Otorhinolaryngology, Union Hospital, Tongji Medical College, Huazhong University of Science and Technology, Wuhan, China

He Li
Department of Otolaryngology, The First Affiliated Hospital of Wenzhou Medical University, Wenzhou, China

Leonard P. Rybak
Department of Otolaryngology, School of Medicine, Southern Illinois University, Springfield, IL, United States
Department of Pharmacology, School of Medicine, Southern Illinois University, Springfield, IL, United States

Asmita Dhukhwa and Vickram Ramkumar
Department of Pharmacology, School of Medicine, Southern Illinois University, Springfield, IL, United States

Debashree Mukherjea
Department of Otolaryngology, School of Medicine, Southern Illinois University, Springfield, IL, United States

Index

A
Abnormal Bone Resorption, 213-214
Acoustic Trauma, 2, 66, 78, 97, 102, 158-159, 161-162, 164, 170-171, 173, 186, 203, 209, 219, 226-227, 229-230, 232
Acute Kidney Injury, 64-65
Alzheimer's Disease, 53, 88, 98, 101-102, 112-115, 153, 158-159, 175, 185, 199
Aminoglycoside, 2, 29, 37, 88, 175, 185, 208, 231
Apoptosis, 1-4, 7-15, 19, 37, 53, 55-56, 59-60, 62, 64-65, 78, 81, 84-85, 90-91, 96, 98, 105, 113-114, 120-122, 126, 132, 136, 138-141, 153-154, 175, 183-184, 186-187, 191, 193, 196-200, 208, 215, 223-226, 232
Arachidonic Acid, 90, 94
Auditory Brainstem Response, 1, 3, 29-33, 56, 61, 63, 92, 103, 113, 154, 161, 172, 175-176, 187-188, 199, 211
Auditory Dysfunction, 102, 104-109, 111, 113-114
Auditory Ossicles, 210-211, 213-214, 216-217
Auditory System, 12, 24, 29-30, 35-37, 53-54, 82, 88, 99, 102, 105-108, 111, 115-116, 141, 153, 200, 211, 217
Autophagy, 1-3, 7-15, 53, 55, 65, 84-86, 90, 98-100, 113-114, 122, 124, 126, 136, 139-141, 174-175, 181-186, 188, 191, 193-194, 197-200, 208-209, 218
Autophagy Lysosome, 194

B
Basal Ganglia, 107
Bone Homeostasis, 210-211

C
Cell Division Cycle, 148, 155
Cell Replacement, 37, 153, 158
Central Auditory System, 105
Central Nervous System, 1, 12, 27, 35, 53, 84, 146, 197, 217
Cerebral Cortex, 102
Cochlear Duct, 17-18, 23, 25, 27, 82, 84, 125-129, 156, 162
Cochlear Sensory, 90-91, 97, 140
Columnar Cells, 126, 134, 136
Cortical Neurons, 215-216
Cytoplasm, 59, 92-93, 106, 126, 130, 136, 175, 184, 191, 196

D
Decalcification, 40, 176, 188-189, 211-212
Dementia, 102, 105, 112-115
Diphtheria Toxin, 29-31, 33-35, 37
Dopaminergic Neurons, 107-108, 111

E
Electrical Signal, 126, 156, 194

Endopeptidase Activity, 94
Epithelial Cell, 28

F
Furosemide Injection, 90-92, 97

G
Gastrulation, 17, 20, 24, 76, 80, 82
Gene Therapy, 53-54, 99, 102, 154-155, 158

H
Hair Cell Damage, 13, 15, 29, 34, 55, 62-65, 86, 98, 114, 122-123, 141, 199, 206, 208-209, 225
Homozygous Mutant Mice, 210-216
Huntington's Disease, 101, 105, 112-116, 153, 158

I
Immunofluorescence, 3, 7, 9, 26-27, 30-35, 40-41, 44, 57, 59-60, 70, 73, 76-77, 89, 162, 173, 189, 191
Immunolabeling, 20-21, 163, 165-166, 168, 174-175, 177-182, 214
Interdental Cell, 25

K
Kanamycin, 87-93, 95-98, 140

M
Mechanosensory, 101, 118, 128
Medial Geniculate, 102, 104, 115
Mitochondrial Dysfunction, 2, 13, 55, 107, 196, 224
Mitochondrial Oxidative Stress, 55, 64
Morphology, 23, 32, 36-37, 41, 43, 46, 53, 58, 62, 72, 87, 94, 104, 110, 114, 126, 136, 140, 154, 156-157, 172, 191-192, 194, 211, 214, 216, 218, 223

N
Neural Crest Cell, 82-83
Neurodegenerative Disorder, 102, 107
Neuroinflammation, 88, 98, 104-105
Neurologic Disease, 1, 12
Neuropathology, 103, 105, 108, 111-114, 116
Neurotransmitter, 47, 107, 162
Nicotinamide Riboside, 64-65

O
Osteopetrosis, 210-211, 215, 217-218
Osteosclerosis, 210-211, 215
Otic Capsule, 23, 127, 162, 210-211, 213-214, 216-218, 222
Ototoxic Drugs, 1-2, 29-30, 70, 78, 95, 102, 194, 206, 219

Ototoxicity, 1-2, 12-13, 38, 62, 65, 98, 112, 118, 120-121, 142-143, 150, 175, 183, 186, 208-209, 219-220, 222-227, 229-232

P
Paraformaldehyde, 3-4, 26, 31, 40, 57, 70, 89, 128, 162-163, 176, 188-189, 202, 211-212

Parkinson's Disease, 2, 9, 13-14, 54, 65, 101-102, 107, 112-115, 153, 159, 198, 217

Phosphorylation, 90, 93-94, 113, 228

Pluripotent Stem Cells, 53, 67, 83, 86, 159-160

Postsynaptic Densities, 161-162, 166, 168, 171

Protein-coupled Receptor, 16, 27-28, 80

R
Ribbon Synapse, 62, 161, 173, 198-199

S
Sensory Neuron, 37, 54, 99, 200

Signaling Pathway, 7, 10, 12-14, 28, 52-53, 55, 64-66, 76, 82, 85, 87, 90, 94, 98, 100, 109, 114, 122, 130, 132, 137-141, 149, 155, 158-159, 199, 226

Spiral Ganglion Neurons, 1-2, 5, 7, 16, 18-19, 21, 25, 27, 29, 37-38, 47, 50, 52-53, 55, 77, 84, 87, 89-91, 94-95, 97-100, 102, 104, 112, 122-123, 140, 152-154, 160, 187, 190, 193-196, 200, 209, 211, 215

Spiral Ligament, 115, 127, 214-216, 223, 226

Stem Cell Therapy, 54, 100, 123, 152-154, 158-159, 200

Stereocilia, 13, 83, 85-86, 98-99, 106, 118, 121, 123-124, 159-160, 169, 194, 198-199, 209, 215, 218, 225

Stria Vascularis, 1, 3, 5-7, 19-20, 23-26, 39, 68, 85, 127, 169-170, 220-221, 224, 226

Synaptic Ribbon, 228

T
Toxin Receptor, 29-30, 37

Transcriptome Analysis, 7, 53, 67, 87-88, 95, 99, 140

Transmission Electron Microscopy, 189, 194, 198

U
Ultrasonic Vocalization, 104

W
Waardenburg Syndrome, 67-68, 83-86

Printed in the USA
CPSIA information can be obtained
at www.ICGtesting.com
JSHW060008070923
47937JS00023B/176